MW01108139

Clinical Applications of Antibiotics and Anti-inflammatory Drugs in Ophthalmology

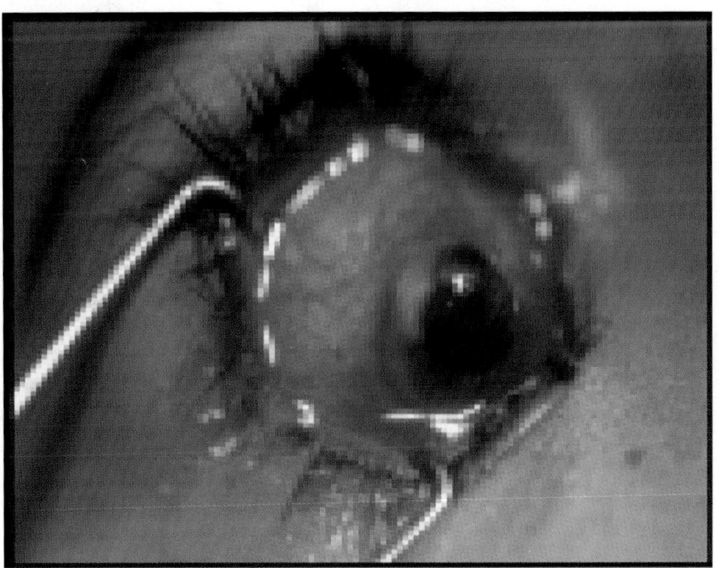

System requirement: 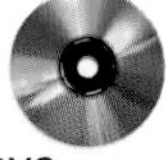

- Windows XP or above
- Power DVD player (Software)
- Windows media player 10.0 version or above (Software)

Accompanying photo CD ROM is playable only in Computer and not in CD player.

Kindly wait for few seconds for CD to autorun. If it does not autorun then please follow the steps:

- Click on my computer
- Click the CD drive labelled **LWW** and after opening the Drive, kindly double click the file **LWW**

CD CONTENTS

Clinical Applications of Antibiotics and Anti-inflammatory Drugs in Ophthalmology

Editors

Ashok Garg MS PhD FIAO (Bel) FRSM ADM FAIMS FICA
International and National Gold Medalist
Chairman and Medical Director
Garg Eye Institute and Research Centre
235-Model Town, Dabra Chowk,
Hisar-125005, India

John D Sheppard MD MMSc
Clinical Director–Thomas R Lee
Center for Ocular Pharmacology
Associate Professor of Ophthalmology
Eastern Virginia Medical School
241 Corporate Boulevard
Norfolk, Virginia 23502, USA

Eric D Donnenfeld MD FCA
Clinical Associate Professor
North Shore University Hospital and
Nassau County Medical Center
Founding Partner, Ophthalmic Consultants of
Long Island Center, New York, USA

Mitchell Friedlaender MD
Head, Division of Ophthalmology,
Director, Laser Vision Center,
Scripps Clinic, 10666, North Torrey
Pines Road, La Jolla, CA 92037,
Rockville, USA

***Foreword*: Christopher J Rapuano**

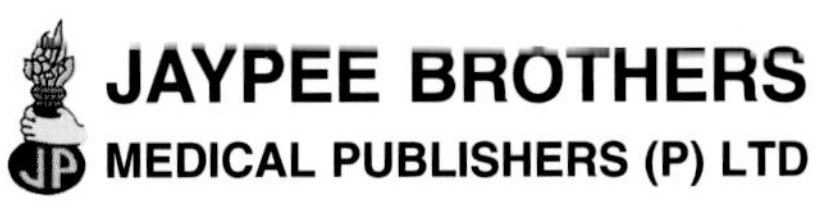

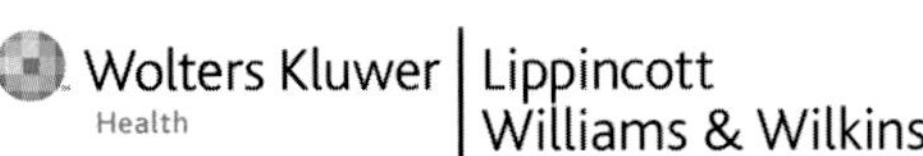

First published in India in 2007 by
Jaypee Brothers Medical Publishers (P) Ltd, New Delhi, India.
EMCA House, 23/23B Ansari Road, Daryaganj, New Delhi 110 002, India
Phones: +91-11-23272143, +91-11-23272703, +91-11-23282021, +91-11-23245672
Fax: +91-11-23276490, +91-11-23245683
e-mail: jaypee@jaypeebrothers.com, Visit our website: www.jaypeebrothers.com

First published in USA by The Lippincott Williams & Wilkins, 530 Walnut Street, Philadelphia, PA 19106, USA. Exclusively worldwide distributor except South East Asia (India, Nepal, Sri Lanka, Bhutan, Pakistan, Bangladesh).

ISBN 978-0-7817-9123-6

DEDICATIONS

To

- *My Respected Param Pujya Guru Sant Gurmeet Ram Rahim Singh Ji for his blessings and motivation.*
- *My Respected Parents, teachers, my wife Dr. Aruna Garg, son Abhishek and daughter Anshul for their constant support and patience during all these days of hard work.*
- *My dear friend Dr. Amar Agarwal, a leading International Ophthalmologist from India for his continued support and guidance.*

Ashok Garg

My wife of 25 years, Clelia, whose understanding and patience have allowed my time to be dedicated to the discovery of new treatments of dry eye and other severe ocular diseases, and whose own experience with dry eye has provided me with marvelous insight into the human side of patient concerns.

John D Sheppard

My wonderful wife and children who make everything possible.

Eric Donnenfeld

My mentors at the Francis I. Proctor Foundation. G. Richard O'Connor, H Bruce Ostler, and Phillips Thygeson.

Mitch Friedlaender

CONTRIBUTORS

Abhiyan Kumar MD
Dr RP Center for Ophthalmic Sciences
AIIMS, Ansari Nagar
New Delhi 110029
India

Alok K Ravi PhD
Department of Ocular Pharmacology
Dr RP Center for Ophthalmic Sciences
AIIMS, Ansari Nagar
New Delhi 110029, India

Anita Panda MD
Professor of Ophthalmology
Dr RP Center for Ophthalmic Sciences
AIIMS, Ansari Nagar
New Delhi 110029, India

Armando Caballero
Louisiana State University Eye Center
2020 Gravier Street, Suite B New
Orleans LA 70112-2234, USA

Arturo Pérez-Arteaga MD
Medical Director
Centro Oftalmologico Tlalnepantla
Dr. Perez - Arteaga Vallarta no. 42
Tlalnepantla, Centro, Estado de
Mexico, 54000, Mexico

Ashim K Mitra MD
University of Missouri-Kansas City
School of Pharmacy, Division of
Pharmaceutical Sciences
Kansas City
MO 64110 2499, USA

Ashok Garg MS PhD FRSM
Medical Director
Garg Eye Institute and
Research Centre
235-Model Town, Dabra Chowk
Hisar 125005, India

Cintia S De Paiva MD
Ocular Surface Centre
Cullen Eye Institute
Baylor College of Medicine
6565 Fannin St, NC 205,
Houston, Texas 77030, USA

Daphne Breshears coa
Division of Ophthalmology
Scripps Clinic
La Jolla, California
USA

De-Quan Li MD PhD
Ocular Surface Centre
Cullen Eye Institute
Baylor College of Medicine
6565 Fannin St, NC 205
Houston, Texas 77030
USA

Douglas W Morck DVM PhD
Department of Ophthalmology
The Eye Care Centre
2550 Willow St., Section G
Vancouver, BC V5Z 3N9
Canada

Emma BH Hume MD
The Co-operative Research Center
for Eye Research and Technology
(CRCERT), Sydney
New South Wales
Australia

Eric Donnenfeld MD FACS
Clinical Associate Professor
North Shore University Hospital and
Nassau County Medical Center
2000 North Village Ave
Rockville Centre, NY 11570
USA

Gagandeep Singh Brar MS
Assistant Professor
Department of Ophthalmology
PGI, Chandigarh, India

Gina Chavez BSc
Department of Ophthalmology
The Eye Care Centre
2550 Willow St., Section G
Vancouver, BC V5Z 3N9
Canada

GK Das MD
Professor of Ophthalmology
UCMS and GTB Hospital
Shahdara, New Delhi
India

Henry D Perry MD FACS
Chief of Cornea Service
Nassau University Medical Center
East Meadow, New York
2000 North Village Ave
Rockville Centre, NY 11570
USA

Hsi-Kung Kuo MD
Department of Ophthalmology
Chang Gung Memorial Hospita-
Kaohsiung Medical Center
123, Ta-PEi Road, Niao-Sung
Hsien, Kaohsiung, Hsien, 883
Taiwan, ROC

Ian Bell MD
Clinical Director
Bell Institute of Ophthalmology
Texas, USA

James M Hill MD
Louisiana State University Eye Center
2020 Gravier Street, Suite B
New Orleans, LA 70112-2234,
USA

Jean Deschénes MD
McGill University
Montreal, Canada

Jerome Bovet MD
Consultant Ophthalmic Surgeon
FMH, Clinique de I'oeil
15, Avenue du Bois-de-la-Chapelle
CH-1213 Onex, Switzerland

John D Sheppard MD MMSc
Associate Professor of
Ophthalmology
Microbiology and Immunology,
Clinical Director, Thomas R. Lee
Centre for Ocular Pharmacology
Eastern Virginia Medical School
Norfolk, Virginia 23501, USA

José L Güell MD
Instituto De Microcirugia Ocular
De Barcelona
Barcelona, Spain

Jorge L Alio MD PhD
Instituto Oftalmologico De Alicante
Avda. Denia 111, 03015
Alicante, Spain

Kirit Mody MS FRCS FRCO
Consulting Eye Surgeon
Salil Eye Clinic and
Contact Lens Centre
506, Om Chambers, Kemps Corner
123, August Kranti Marg
Mumbai 400036, India

Li Gisele MD
McGill University
Montreal, Canada

Madhurjya Gogai MD
Department of Pharmacology
Dr RP Center for Ophthalmic Sciences
AIIMS, Ansari Nagar,
New Delhi 110029, India

Marta Calatayud MD
Instuto De Microcirugia Ocular
De Barcelona, Barcelona
Spain

Mary E Marquart MD
Department of Ophthalmology
Louisiana State University Health
Sciences Center, New Orleans
LA, USA

Mitchell H Friedlaender MD
Head Division of Ophthalmology
Director, Laser Vision Center
Scripps Clinic, 10666, North Torrey
Pines Road, La Jolla, CA 92037
Rockville, USA

Mohammed Ahmed MD
Instituto Oftalmologico De Alicante
Avda. Denia 111, 03015
Alicante, Spain

N Venkatesh Prajna
Aravind Eye Hospital
Madurai, India

Niranjan Nayak MD
Additional Professor of Ocular
Microbiology, Dr RP Center for
Ophthalmic Sciences
AIIMS, Ansari Nagar
New Delhi, India

NR Biswas MD DM
Professor of Ocular Pharmacology
Dr RP Center for Ophthalmic
Sciences
AIIMS, Ansari Nagar,
New Delhi, India

Oscar Gris MD
Instituto De Microcirugia Ocular
De Barcelona, Barcelona,
Spain

Pei-Chang Wu MD
Department of Ophthalmology
Chang Gung Memorial Hospita-
Kaohsiung Medical Center
123, Ta-PEi Road, Niao-Sung
Hsien, Kaohsiung, Hsien, 883
Taiwan, ROC

Rami Pai MS
Senior Research Fellow
Conwest Jain Clinic and Medical
Research Society, Mumbai
India

Rasheena MD
Dr RP Center for Ophthalmic Sciences
AIIMS, Ansari Nagar
New Delhi 110029, India

René Cano-Hidalgo MD
Chairman
Institute of Ophthalmology
Conde de Valenciana
Vitreous and Retina Department
Professor of Ophthalmology
National Institute of Mexico
(UNAM), Mexico

Renee Solomon MD
North Shore University Hospital and
Nassau County Medical Center
2000 North Village Ave
Rockville Centre, NY 11570
USA

Richard J O'Callaghan MD
Louisiana State University Health
Sciences Center
New Orleans, LA, USA

Richard Mathias MD FRCP
Department of Ophthalmology
The Eye Care Centre
2550 Willow St., Section G
Vancouver, BC V5Z 3N9, Canada

Robert Latkany MD
Director and Founder
Dry Eye Clinic NY Eye and Ear Infirmary, Dry Eye Center of New York, Manhattan 212-832-2020
USA

Shalini Mohan MD
Dr RP Center for Ophthalmic Sciences
AIIMS, Ansari Nagar
New Delhi 110029
India

Simon P Holland
MB FRCSC FRCOph
Clinical Professor
Department of Ophthalmology
The Eye Care Centre
2550 Willow St., Section G
Vancouver, BC V5Z 3N9
Canada

SPS Grewal MD
Director, Grewal Eye Institute and Research Center, SCO 168-169
Sector 9-C, Chandigarh, India

Srujana Mohanty MD
Dr RP Center for Ophthalmic Sciences
AIIMS, Ansari Nagar
New Delhi-110029
India

Stephen C Pflugfelder MD
Professor and Director of Ocular Surface Center
Cullen Eye Institute
Baylor College of Medicine
6565 Fannin St, NC 205,
Houston, Texas 77030, USA

Sujith Vengayil MD
Registrar, Dr RP Center for Ophthalmic Sciences
AIIMS, Ansari Nagar
New Delhi 110029, India

Sunita Agarwal MS DO PSVH
Dr Agarwal's Eye Hospital
19, Cathedral Road
Chennai-600086, India
15, Eagle Street, Langford Town
Bangalore, India

Tracy L Lee BSc MPT
Department of Ophthalmology
The Eye Care Centre
2550 Willow St., Section G
Vancouver, BC V5Z 3N9
Canada

Viney Gupta MD
Assistant Professor of Ophthalmology
Dr RP Center for Ophthalmic Sciences
AIIMS, Ansari Nagar
New Delhi 110029
India

Xiadong Zheng MD
Department of Ophthalmology
Ehime University School of Medicine, Ehime, Japan

Yumi G Ohashi BSc
Department of Ophthalmology
The Eye Care Centre
2550 Willow St., Section G
Vancouver, BC V5Z 3N9
Canada

FOREWORD

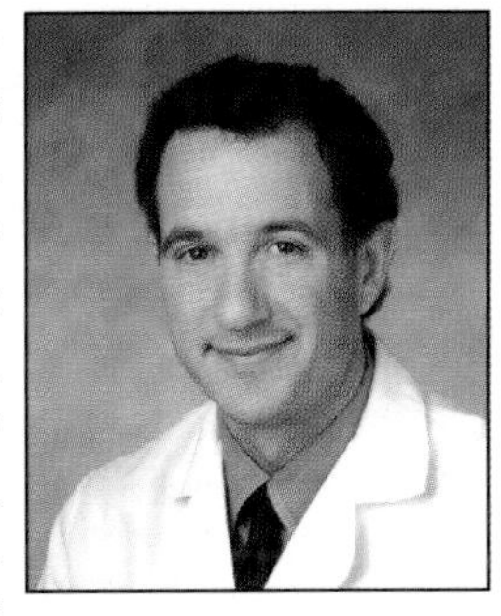

Antibiotic and anti-inflammatory therapy in the treatment of ocular conditions is a critically important area in the field of ophthalmology. For better or worse, it is also rapidly changing. The recent worldwide outbreak of *Fusarium* keratitis related to a specific contact lens disinfection product highlights our need to keep informed not only about new treatments for ocular infections, but also novel methods of infection prevention. Fourth generation topical fluoroquinolones have changed the landscape for treatment of corneal ulcers but also surgical prophylaxis over the last several years. Originally touted as being very difficult medications against which to develop resistance, we are now learning that more and more organisms are becoming resistant to them. New diagnostic technology is better demonstrating some untoward effects of our ocular surgeries. For example, optical coherence tomography has become a widely used, non-invasive tool to diagnose mild cystoid macular edema. We are now better able to identify certain conditions, such as cystoid macular edema, and therefore treat them more effectively. As an added benefit, we are also better able to prevent some side effects from occurring in the first place. As new medications and technologies are developed and new conditions emerge, however, it is increasingly difficult to obtain accurate and up-to-date information in this field.

Dr Ashok Garg has assembled an impressive cast of international authors to accomplish this task. The book begins with Section 1 which covers fundamentals including the ocular defense system, ocular drug delivery systems and drug permeability. Section 2 covers specific antibiotic therapies and clinical applications. New generation fluoroquinolones, new uses of tetracyclines and topical azithromycin are all discussed. Pre- and postoperative cataract surgery regimens, endophthalmitis prophylaxis and management and treatment of corneal ulcers are also covered in detail. Section 3 concentrates on anti-inflammatory conditions and their management. Medical treatment of anterior and posterior uveitis, cystoid macular edema, post refractive surgery inflammation and blepharitis are all covered. The use of nonsteroidal anti-inflammatory therapy to optimize refractive and cataract surgery outcomes is expertly reviewed. The 4 and final section discusses recent advances in antibiotic and anti-inflammatory therapies including toxic anterior segment syndrome, topical immune therapy and nanotechnology in ophthalmology. **Dr Garg and his co-editors conclude the book with a look into future drugs in ophthalmology. They have splendidly completed their mission of putting together a world-class text that should be beneficial to all practicing ophthalmologists.**

Dr Christopher J Rapuano MD
Co-Director, Cornea Service, Wills Eye Institute
Co-Director, Refractive Surgery Department, Wills Eye Institute,
Professor of Ophthalmology, Jefferson Medical College,
Thomas Jefferson University, Philadelphia, Pennsylvania
Cornea Service, Wills Eye Institute, 840 Walnut Street, Suite 920,
Philadelphia, PA 19107, USA
Phone: 215-928-3180 Fax: 215-928-3854
E-mail: cjrapuano@willseye.org

PREFACE

Pre- and postoperative prophylaxis is an essential component of both cataract and refractive surgeries. Corneal refractive surgeons are specially concerned with two classes of microorganisms those that likely exist on patient ocular surface and those that are introduced during surgery. In last few years tremendous research work has been done specially in the field of Topical Antibiotics and Anti-inflammatory drugs. Fourth generation Fluoroquinolones specially Moxifloxacin and Gatifloxacin best achieve the two main goals of antibiotic prophylaxis sterilizing the ocular surface and preventing infections. Excellent potency, therapeutic penetration, broad coverage and low toxicity also make these antibiotics ideal for clinical use against ocular external infections. Recently introduced NSAID topical Nepafenac holds great promise for Refractive lens procedures and CME management. Proper NSAID and Anti-infective regimen is critical for cataract prophylaxis.

Present book has been written with the aim of providing complete up to date pharmacotherapeutic information about commercially available Antibiotics and Anti-inflammatory drugs in ophthalmology. Clinical and surgical applications of these in various ocular conditions is special attraction of this book. A number of known international ophthalmologists who are masters in ocular therapeutics field have shared their experiences in form of 45 chapters of this book. A Photo CD ROM provided with this book shall provide insight into Atlas of typical ocular infective and inflammatory conditions which are faced by ophthalmologists in their day-to-day practice.

Our special gratitude to Shri Jitendar P Vij (CEO), Mr Tarun Duneja (General Manager, publishing) and all staff members of M/s Jaypee Brothers Medical Publisher who took keen interest in this project and completed it expeditiously.

Last but not the least we are hopeful this practical handbook shall be useful companion of every ophthalmologist OPD Desk as a primary reference book to reduce visual threatening infections and blindness.

Editors

CONTENTS

Section One: Fundamentals and Preliminary Considerations in Ocular Therapeutics

Section Two: Classification of Antibiotics and their Clinical and Surgical Applications in Ophthalmology

Section Three: Classification of Anti-inflammatory Drugs and their Clinical and Surgical Applications in Ophthalmology

Section Four: Recent Advances in Antibiotics and Anti-inflammatory Drugs in Ophthalmology

SECTION ONE

Fundamentals and Preliminary Considerations in Ocular Therapeutics

Chapter 1

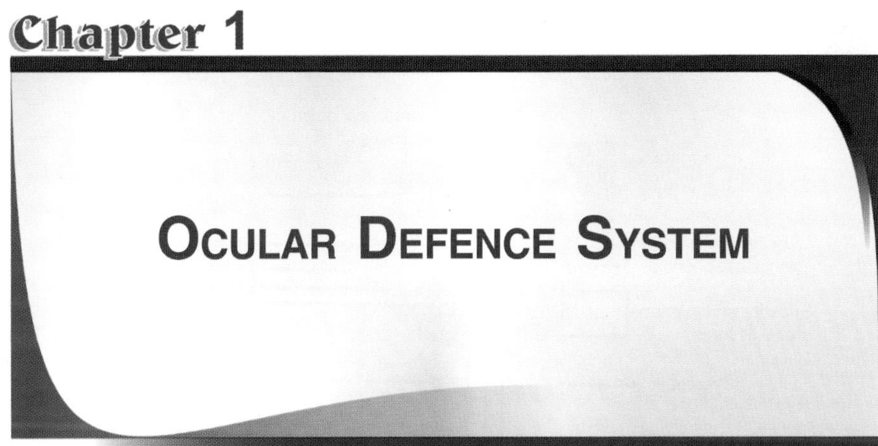

OCULAR DEFENCE SYSTEM

Ashok Garg (India)

Eye like the other parts of the body has natural defence mechanism.

Eye is one of the highly specialized sensory organ of the body. Nature has provided eye with bony and anatomical protection and physiological reflexes. Eyes are protected from radiational hazards. Immunological process, Biochemical and enzymatic systems protect the eyes from ocular inflammation. Ocular defence system is broadly classified in two categories:

a. Physical protection
b. Physiological protection

Physical Protection

Eye balls are well protected in the bony orbit. The eye lies in the front half of the orbit surrounded by Fat and connective tissue and is supported by a Fascial hammock. The eyeball lies in a quadrilateral pyramid or pear shaped bony cavity situated on the either side of the root of the nose called orbit. Orbit stalk is the optic canal. The orbit lies behind the orbital septum and has a roof, a floor; a medial wall and a lateral wall. The protective orbit is made up of seven bones namely Maxilla, frontal, zygomatic, lacrimal, ethmoid, sphenoid and palatine. The bones of the anterior margin of the orbit are thick and strong but most of the walls are thin. Its two medial walls are parallel and two lateral walls from a 90° angle with each other. Each eyeball is suspended by extraocular muscles and their facial sheath. The anterior part of eyeball and center of cornea are just at the level of line joining the upper and lower bony orbital margins so that eyeball is protected from any kind of damage as a result of fall on the face side or when a large object hits the orbits. The eyeball is also protected by orbital fat to absorb any shock or vibrations specially in condition of concussion and free fall injury and provides a protective cushion. However, in counter coup injury the medial wall of the bony orbit give way as these are the weakest part of the orbits (Figs 1.1 and 1.2).

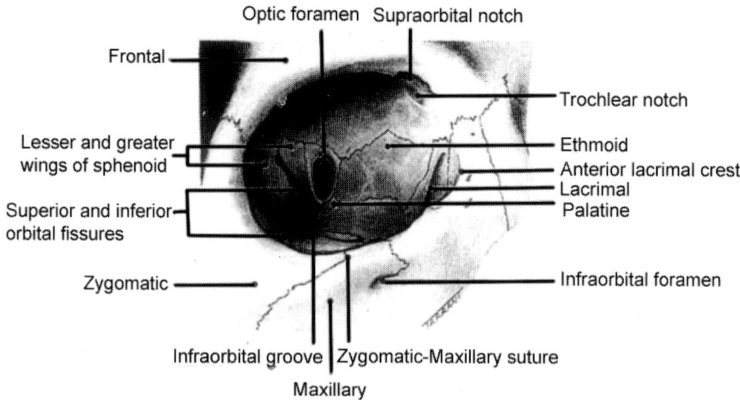

Fig. 1.1: Anatomy of the orbital cavity (Physical defense system of the eye). *Courtesy*: Kanski Clinical Ophthalmology, Butterworths International Edition

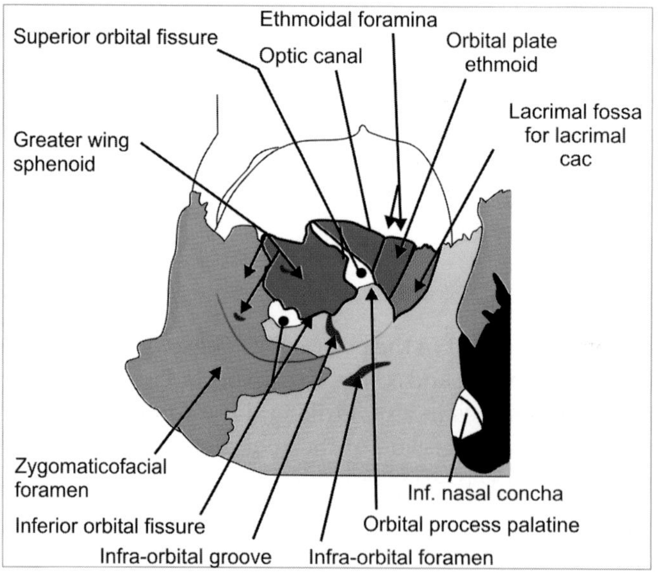

Fig. 1.2: Walls of the orbit

Lattice arrangement of collagan fibers adds to the strength of the cornea. Descemet membrane elasticity reduces the risk of corneal perforation. Criss-Cross pattern of zonular fibers hold the lens in place.

Condensed part of the peripheral vitreous supports the retina.

The special physical protection in term of anatomical safeguards is provided by extra length of the optic nerve between scleral entry and optic canal so that even if the eye is temporarily explused, the optic nerve cannot detach itself away from the eye ball. The firm attachment of optic nerve to the bony optic canal through its dural covering also ensures that optic nerve cannot be pulled out of intra cranial cavity. The intra-orbital portion of optic nerve is much longer (25 mm) than the distance between the back of globe to the optic formen (18 mm). This allows for significant forward displacement of globe without causing exessive stretching of the optic nerve.

Physiological Protection

A number of physiological factors provide protection to the eye.

The blinking reflex of the eye protects and helps to moisten and lubricate the exposed part of the eyeball. The eye lashes acts as antenae to warn against any foreign body coming near to eyeball and reflexly stimulate the closure of eye-lids. Eye lashes also produce physical obstruction against flying particles, dust and dirt etc. The Bells phenomenon protects the cornea from exposure and injury. The pupil regulates the entry of light into the eyes. Iris diaphragm makes the posterior segment a dark room.

The pigment epithelium of the retina adsorbs the light after it passes through the anterior layers of retina. Cilioretinal arteries also acts as nutrition of the the macula in CRA occlusion cases.

The cornea absorbs most of the infrared rays of the sunlight. The lens by its biochemical mechanism absorbs most of the UV rays of the sunlight so that retina is protected from the harmful effects of the sunrays.

Intact corneal epithelium acts as a strong barrier against invasion by most of the micro-organisms and also acts as selective permeable membrane. Micro polysaccharides in the corneal stroma prevents swelling of the cornea.

Descement membrane acts as a strong barrier against invading organisms. Due to absence of blood vessels in the cornea and lens, these two structures do not suffer from primary inflammation and also from neoplastic pathology.

The optical integrity and normal function of the eye depend on an adequate supply of fluid covering its surface. The exposed part of the globe-the cornea and the bulbar conjunctiva is covered by a thin fluid film known as pre-ocular tear film. Tears refer to fluid film known as pre-ocular tear film, and the conjunctival sac.

The volume of the tear fluid is about 5-10 microliter and about 95% of it is produced by the goblet cells and the accessory lacrimal glands of the conjunctiva, in healthy invidual s.

Tear film is a complete trilaminar structure which is directly in contact with the environment and is critically important for protecting the eye from external influences.

The pre-corneal tear film consists of three layers each of which has separate functions (Figs 1.3 and 1.4).

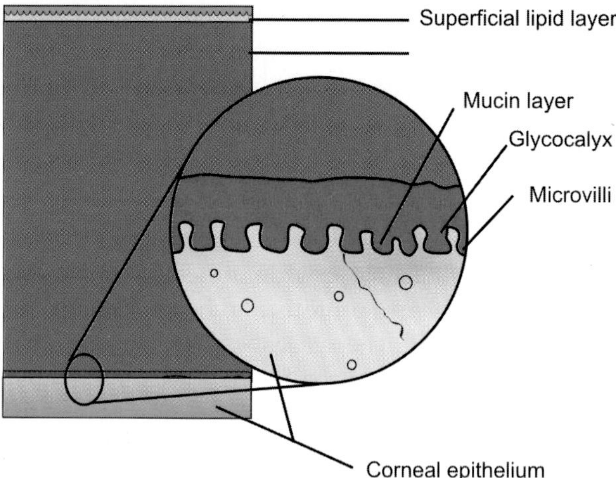

Fig. 1.3: Tear film layers (Physiological protection of the eye). *Courtesy*: Allergan India Limited

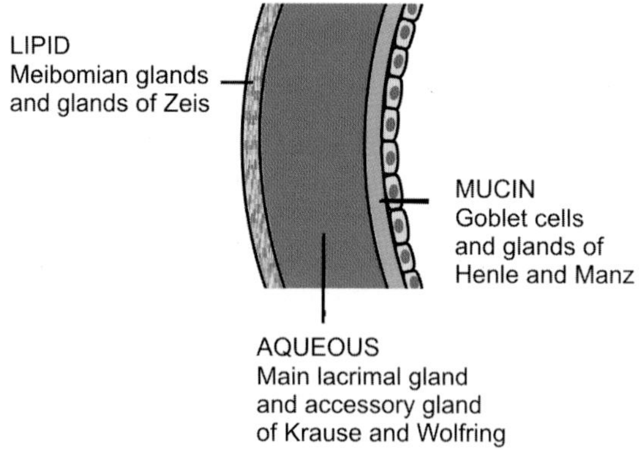

Fig. 1.4: Three layers of precorneal tear film. *Courtesy*: Kanski Clinical Ophthalmology, Butterworths International Edition

Outer Lipid Layer

It is secreted by meibomian glands and has three main functions.

i. To retard the evaporation of the aqueous layer of the tear film.
ii. To increase surface tension and assist in the vertical stability of the tear film so that tears do not overflow the lower lid margin.
iii. To lubricate the eyelids as they pass over the surface of the globe.

The Middle Aqueous Layer

This is secreted by main lacrimal gland and the accessory lacrimal glands and has four main functions -

i. It supplies atmospheric oxygen to the corneal epithelium.
ii. It has antibacterial substances like Lactoferrin and Lysozyme.
iii. It provides a smooth optical surface by abolishing any minute irregularities of the cornea.
iv. It washes away debris from the conjunctiva and cornea.

The Inner Mucin Layer

This is very thin and is secreted by the goblet cells in the conjunctiva and also by the Crypts of Henle and glands of Manz. The main function of this layer is to convert the corneal epithelium from a hydrophobic to the hydrophilic surface. An aqueous solution form a smooth and even layer when dropped on to a hydrophilic surface. This layer enables the corneal epithelium to be adequately wetted.

In addition to adequate amounts of aqueous tears and mucin, three other factors are necessary for effective resurfacing of the cornea by the pre-corneal tear film.

1. A normal blink reflex which ensure that the mucin is brought from the inferior conjunctiva and rubbed into the corneal epithelium.
2. Congruity between the external ocular surface and the eyelids ensures that the precorneal tear film spread evenly over the entire cornea.
3. Normal epithelium is necessary for the adsorption of mucin is necessary for the adsorption of mucin on to its surface cells.

The chemical composition of human tear is quite complex containing proteins, lipids, metabolites, enzymes, electrolytes and other elements which play an important role in the defence of the outer eye.

The tear protein fraction forms the first line of defence against external influences.

In normal human tears three types of immunoglobulins namely IgA, IgG and IgM are present.

In normal tears secretary IgA and IgG forms the first line of ocular defence and may act to modulate the normal flora of Ocular adnexa allowing saprophytic growth which prevents pathological flora colonizing the ocular surface.

These Globulins also prevents adherance of bacteria to the muscosal surface and neutralize viruses and toxins.

Tears transport metabolic products and provide a pathway for WBC in cases of injury.

Avascularity of the cornea is an important factor for antigenicity.

HDA in the peripheral cornea allows tissue immune reaction only when the blood vessels invade the corneal tissue.

In short the eye is physically well protected and the physiological mechanisms retain the transparency of media and Visuosensory Character of the retina. Cornea and lens are immunologically well protected.

The ocular defence system during physical or pathological attacks is too strong to break the defence barrier.

BIBLIOGRAPHY

1. Adler. Physiology of the Eye. CV Mosby, 1992.
2. Agarwal Amar. Text book of ophthalmology, ed.1, New Delhi: Jaypee Medical Publishers, 2002.
3. Bartlett JD. Clinical Ocular Pharmacology, ed. 4, Boston: Butterworth-Heinemann, 2001.
4. Bartlett JD. Ophthalmic Drug facts : Lippincott – William and Wilkins, 2001.
5. Crick RP, Trimble RB. Textbook of clinical ophthalmology : Hodder and Stoughton, 1986.
6. Chong. Clinical Ocular Physiology: Lippincott – William – Wilkins, 1997.
7. Duane TD. Clinical ophthalmology, ed. 4: Butterworth – Heinemann, 1999.
8. Duvall. Ophthalmic Medications and Pharmacology : Slack Inc, 1998.
9. Ellis PP. Ocular Therapeutics and Pharmacology, ed. 7 : CV Mosby, 1985.
10. Fechner. Ocular Therapeutics : Slack Inc., 1998.
11. Fraunfelder. Current Ocular Therapy, ed. 5: WB Saunders, 2000.
12. Garg Ashok. Current Trends in ophthalmology, ed. 1, New Delhi : Jaypee Medical Publishers, 1997.
13. Garg Ashok. Manual of Ocular Therapeutics, ed. 1, New Delhi : Jaypee Medical Publishers, 1996.
14. Garg Ashok, Ready Reckoner of Ocular Therapeutics, ed.1, New Delhi : 2002.
15. Goodman LS, Gilman A. Pharmacological basis of Therapeutics, ed.7, New York: Macmillan, 1985.
16. Havener's. Ocular Pharmacology, ed. 6: CV Mosby, 1994.
17. Kanski. Clinical ophthalmology, ed. 4: Butterworth – Heineman, 1999.
18. Kershner. Ophthalmic Medications and Pharmacology: Slack. Inc., 1994.
19. Korb. The Tear Film: Butterworth – Heinemann, 2001.
20. Lens. Ocular Anatomy and Physiology, Lippincott – William and Wilkins, 1999.
21. Olin BR et al. Drugs Facts and Comparisons : Facts and Comparisons, St. Louis, 1997.
22. Onofrey. The Ocular Therapeutics; Lippincott-William and Wilkins, 1997.
23. Rhee. The Wills Eye drug Guide : Lippincott – William and Wilkins, 1998.
24. Saude. Ocular Anatomy and Physiology : Blackwell Science, 1993.
25. Snell. Clinical Anatomy of the Eye : Blackwell Science, 1998.
26. Steven Podos. Textbook of ophthalmology, New Delhi: Jaypee Medical Publishers, 2001.
27. Zide. Surgical Anatomy of the Orbit: Lippincott – William and Wilkins, 1985.
28. Zimmerman. Textbook of Ocular Pharmacology : Lippincott and William and Wilkins, 1997.

Chapter 2

Routes of Administration and Drug Delivery Systems in Ophthalmology

Ashok Garg (India)

For ocular drugs to be effective an ideal drug delivery system (DDS) should deliver the drug at the receptor site in ocular tissues in relatively high concentration to elicit the desired pharmacological response. Most of the ophthalmic drugs are applied topically in the form of eye drops. The time course of drug deliver from an eye drop follows a first order kinetics. It is well known that about 1% or less of an applied dose is absorbed across the cornea topically to reach the anterior segment of eye.

The major problem in the drug treatment (topical) of ocular diseases is the difficulty of achieving a sufficient quantity of drug at the desired site of action. The tight junctions of iris capillaries and retina act as a barrier to the diffusion of drugs from the blood into the aqueous and vitreous and the cornea acts as a barrier to drugs applied locally. Another factor quite important is the rate of removal from the eye of any drug that does actually penetrate into the aqueous or vitreous because although inflammation may reduce the barrier to penetration of the drug into the eye, the associated hyperemia will also speed the removal of the drug from the eye.

During the last decade research is going on in ophthalmic field for a suitable mode of ocular therapy to provide higher and sustained penetration of the drugs into the ocular tissues and anterior chamber promptly and effectively.

Most important factor which modify drug penetration is slow release of the drug thereby increasing the contact time of the drug to the ocular structures. The duration of drug action in the eye can be extended by:

a. Reducing drainage through the use of viscosity enhancing agents.
b. Improving corneal drug penetration. An ideal drug delivery system should have (i) Spatial placement, (2) Controlled drug delivery.

The route of administration are local and systemic for ocular diseases.

Local Application

Local application of drugs for the treatment of superficial eye diseases is a very satisfactory route. When the desired site of action of the drug is inside the eye then the problems of ocular barrier arises.

Corneal Barrier

For practical purposes cornea can be considered to consist of three layers. The outer and inner layers). The epithelium and the endothelium) prevent water soluble agents, e.g. ionized molecules passing into the eye, but permit the passage of lipid soluble agents where as the corneal stroma resists the passage of lipid soluble agents but freely allows the passage of water soluble agents. Drugs with dual capability are usually capable of changing from lipid solubility to water solubility of ionization. The effectiveness of corneal barrier may be considerably reduced by damage to the corneal epithelium.

Scleral Barrier

The sclera unlike cornea does not act as a differential solubility barrier and is relatively porous. However, there is unidirectional flow across the sclera from the inside to the outside of the eye. The intraocular pressure may be partially responsible for this.

Methods of Local Application of Drugs

a. Application to corneal surface
b. Subconjunctival route
c. Retrobulbar route
d. Direct injection into the aqueous or vitreous.

Application to the Corneal Surface

The drug through this route must fulfil the necessary criteria for passing the corneal barrier to penetrate into the eye.

Formally, the drug delivery kinetics passing through this route can be divided in two parts.

First order kinetics: In this concentration of drug available for penetration falls off exponentially as the medication is diluted and washed away by the tear film and drug concentration achieved in posterior segment of the eye is very less. This type of drug delivery is provided by aqueous or high viscosity solutions, ointments or hydrogel drug delivery system.

Zero order kinetics: In this system drug is held in reserviour and is released into the tear film at the constant rate to provide constant drug concentration in the cornea or aqueous.

This drug delivery system is provided by ocuserts, soluble ophthalmic drug inserts (SODI) and the osmotic pumps, and liposomal drug delivery system, Cotton pledgets and filter paper strips.

Application to the corneal surface may be in form of topical drops, ointments, gels viscous preparations, constant release membranes and soft lenses. Topical drops route is commonly used to treat various ocular infections, inflammation and as topical anesthesia in modern cataract surgery phacoemulsification and LASIK surgery.

The passage of the drug is aided by damage to the corneal epithelium and on the amount of drug in contact with cornea and duration of contact.

When topical drops are used, much is lost because it is washed away by the tears.

Viscous and ointment preparations of drugs including oil suspensions and methyl cellulose solutions prolong contact time. This reduces the total quantity of drug given to the patients as well as reducing the unwanted frequency of medication giving better patient compliance.

Membrane Bound Devices

Ocusert System

This system was the first ophthalmic drug delivery system approved by US FDA for use in human beings.

Ocuserts provide zero order kinetics drug release.

The ocuserts is a device with a two membrane sandwich with a pilocarpine reservior in the center. The copolymeric membrane is ethyline Vinylacetate also encased between the membranes is a white titanium dioxide ring that aids in visualizing and handling the inserts.

Ocuserts not only provides zero order delivery of the drug but the total amount of drug needed for therapeutic effect is much less than what used as drops or suspension.

Ocuserts are soft and extremly flexible and can be placed either under the upper or lower lid.

The problems with ocuserts can be cost factor, foreign body sensation or incidental loss of ocusert from the cul-de-sac. Other type of ocuserts are diffusible units osmotic units and erodible units. Drugs that can be delivered through ocuserts are pilocarpine, antibiotics, steroids carbachol or a combination.

Drug Impregnated Inserts

Soluble ophthalmic drug inserts (SODI) were first introduced in seventies and are made of polymers of acrylamide, ethylacrylate and Vinyl pyrolidone. SODI dissolve in the cul-de-sac and is capable to provide detectable drugs levels in the cornea upto 48 hours.

Wafers were introduced into Eighties. Wafers are soluble ophthalmic inserts made of succinylated collagen. These wafers are 6 × 12 mm in size and are inserted into the inferior cul-de-sac. Antibiotics can be delivered through this route.

Hydrogel Contact Lens Delivery

The hydrogel contact lenses (soft lenses) by virtue of their high water content and large intermolecular pore size, absorb water soluble drugs and release them initially in a high pulse and then release gradually. Hydrogel lenses can be used to deliver water soluble drugs like dexamethasone, antibiotics and pilocarpine. These lenses can be an excellant route of administration. The lens is inserted into the eye after being presoaked in the drug solution. This device is often used in the management of dry eye disorders.

Osmotic Pumps

Osmotic pump recently introduced is the drug delivery system of future to treat various ocular diseases commonly. Osmotic pumps, contain salt enclosed in one compartment and drug enclosed in an adjacent compartment. Both compartments have flexible walls.

This type of device can deliver any type of medication into the eye regardless of its solubility or molecular weight. The development of new polymeric membranes for use as drug inserts envelops, has recently begun.

Research work is going on suitable new site specific drugs delivery system, one side coated hydroly propyl cellulose inserts, sub-Tenon administration of drug through collagen sponges connected with silicon tube work is going on Margan therapeutic lens as continuous corneal perfusion system and on colloidal suspension capsules with an oily core in which drugs is dissolved (nano capsules).

Periocular Administration

When higher concentrations of drugs are required they can be injected locally into the periocular tissues. Periocular drug administration include injection under bulbar conjunctiva, under Tenon capsule (Sub-Tenon's) and behind globe itself and peribulbar route (Fig. 2.1). Drugs most often delivered in this manner include steroids and antibiotics. Local anesthetics are commonly injected through peribulbar route prior to cataract extraction and other intra-ocular surgical procedures.

Subconjunctival Route

This route including injection under the bulbar conjunctiva used to achieve high concentrations of drug in the anterior chamber. Antibiotics, steroids, mydriatics can be given by this route.

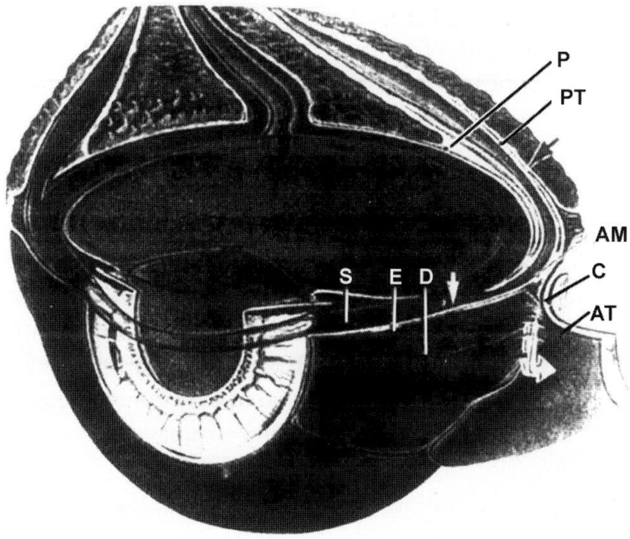

Fig. 2.1: Sub-Tenon's plane relationship (cross-section view)

Subconjunctival injections are painful so this route is used only in severe cases of ocular inflammation or infection of the anterior segment.

Retrobulbar Route

Drugs can be delivered to the back of the orbit by retrobulbar injections. This is the route for local anesthesia in ocular surgery. Steroids may also be injected by this route to reduce optic nerve or posterior segment inflammation (Fig. 2.2).

Intracameral Administration

Intracameral administration involves placing drug directly into the anterior chamber of the eye. This is most commonly associated with cataract extraction,

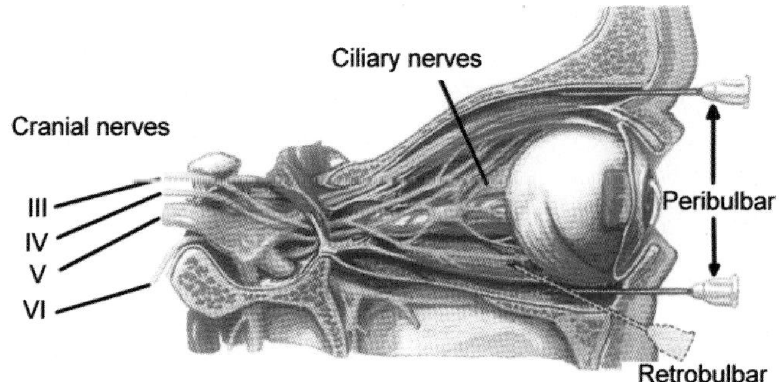

Fig. 2.2: Retrobulbar and peribulbar anesthesia (needle positions)

IOL implantation and phacoemulsification during which a viscoelastic substance is injected into the anterior chamber to protect the corneal endothelium. Antibiotics are not routinely injected into the anterior chamber as there is significant risk of complications as well as drug toxicity.

Intravitreal Administration

The intravitreal injection is primarily reserved as a last effort to save eye with severe acute infection or intraocular inflammation. Intravitreal antibiotics is the treatment of choice for endophthalmitis. Intravitreal liquid silicone is used for the treatment of complicated retinal detachment. Recently intravitreal ganciclovir has been used with success in treating cytomegaloretinitis in patient with AIDS.

Parabulbar (Flush) Administration

This is new administration route for local anesthesia which is highly useful, safe, effective and technically easier. In this method consisting of a limbal sub-Tenon administration of retrobulbar anesthesia using a blunt irrigating cannula. This technique can be used involving anterior and posterior segment surgery (Figs 2.3 and 2.4).

Peribulbar Administration

Peribulbar administration is mainly used for giving local anesthesia for modern intraocular surgery. Since the exit of retrobulbar route peribulbar is safe and

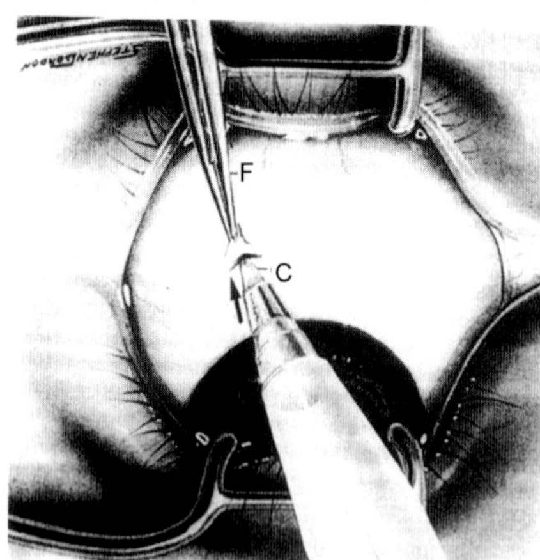

Fig. 2.3: Parabulbar (flush) local anesthesia (Surgeon's view)

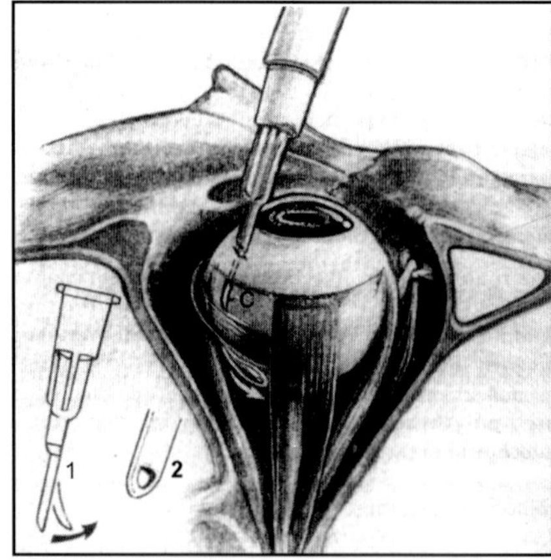

Fig. 2.4: Parabulbar (flush) local anesthesia (cross-section view)

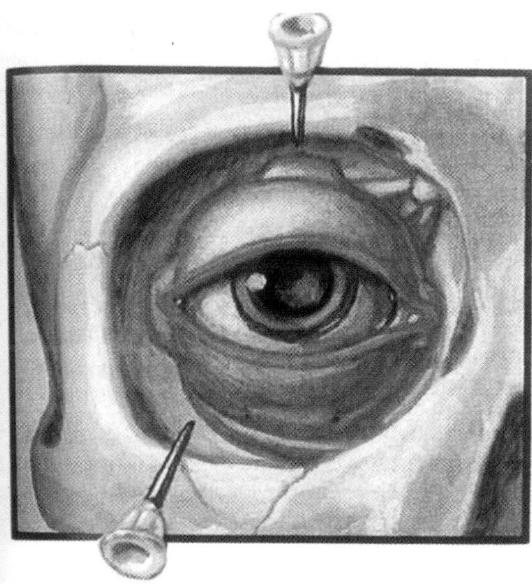

Fig. 2.5: Needle positions for retrobulbar or peribulbar anesthesia (frontal view)

effective route of administrating local anesthesia. Peribulbar route is safe because here local injection is given out of muscle cone and complications like intraconal hemorrhage or damage to optic nerve are ruled out.

In this method a cocktail of lignocaine and bupivacaine is injected at the junction of lateral 1/3rd and medial 2/3rd of inferior orbital rim by 26 gauge 1″ long needle which is directed backward and medially to its whole length. At present after topical anesthesia, Peribulbar anesthesia is most commonly used method of giving local anesthesia world wide (Fig. 2.5).

Direct Injection into the Globe

Drugs are often introduced into the eye during ocular surgery. Care is taken that the concentration of drug the vehicle and the type of preservative is suitable. Antibiotics may be injected directly into the aqueous and vitreous in cases of endophthalmits.

Systemic Administration

General rules for system drug administration apply but there is an effective blood aqueous and blood vitreous barrier so that intraocular levels of systemically administered drugs are usually lower than the serum.

Most drugs will cross the aqueous and vitreous in cases of ocular inflammatory diseases which increases permeability. In systemic administration drugs can be given orally or by intramuscular intravenous injections.

Although most ocular diseases respond to topical therapy but certain ocular disorders require systemic drug administration. Oral administration of certain drugs may be most effective route of drug delivery. Carbonic anhydrase inhibitors for treatment of glaucoma, steroids for optic neuritis, uveitis, analgesics for the management of pain associated with ocular trauma, antibiotic therapy for ocular infections and antihistaminic therapy for acute ocular allergy are few examples of oral administration.

Parental administration include intramuscular (IM) and intravenous (IV) injections. Hydroxy cobalamin (Vitamin B_{12}) and certain antibiotics are given through IM route. Continuous IV infusion of various antibiotics may be required for treatment of endophthalmitis and other severe ocular infections.

The futuristic considerations in ocular drug delivery system is to make drug delivery in therapeutic concentration in the posterior segment of the globe. The new modifications in ocular DDS design must not only work on the corneal route for drug absorption but also of other routes like scleral route. There is also need of sophisticated technology to monitor the pharmacokinetics.

Medications forms used in Ophthalmology

Solutions and Suspensions

This is one of the most common form of drug delivery system being used in ophthalmology today. Most of the topical ocular preparations are commercially available as solutions or suspensions which are applied directly to the eye from the bottle via sterile eye dropper provided alongwith.

Patient should be cautioned about touching the dropper tip to the eye as it can lead to contamination of the medication beside causing ocular injury. Patient should not also touch tip of the dropper with hand to avoid contamination of preparation. Suspension forms should be shaken before use to provide an accurate dosage of drug.

Ointments

This is second most common form of drug delivery system used in ophthalmology. The main purpose for an ophthalmic ointment vehicle is to prolong drug contact time with the eye. Ointments are specially useful for treating children who may not cooperate for topically applied solutions ointments are especially useful for medicating ocular injuries such as corneal abrasions where the eye needs to be patched. Always administer solutions before ointments as ointments preclude entry of subsequent drops. In general put 0.25-0.50 inch ribbon of ointment with a sweeping motion inside the lower lid by squeezing the tube gently and slowly release the eyelid. Ask the patient to close the eye for 1-2 minutes and remove excessive ointment around the eye. Patients should be cautioned about temporary blurring of vision due to ointment. Patients should avoid activities requiring visual acuity until blurring clears.

Gels

In modern ophthalmic drug delivery systems gels are fast gaining importance. Ophthalmic gels are similar in viscosity and clinical usage to ophthalmic ointments. Gels provide prolonged contact time for medication with in the precorneal tear film.

Sprays

Some ophthalmic medications like mydriatics and cycloplegics alone or in combination can be administered as spray to the eye to dilate pupil or cycloplegic examination. This form is especially used for pediatric patients and solution is administered using a sterile perfume atomizer or plastic spray bottle.

Lid Scrubs

Certain commercial ophthalmic preparations (eye lid cleansers, antibiotic solutions or ointments) can be applied directly to eyelid margin for the treatment of non-infectious blepharitis. This is ideally achieved by applying the medication to the end of the special cotton tipped applicator and then scrubbing the eyelid margins several times daily. Gauze pads supplied with commercially available eyelid cleansers are also suitable.

Drug delivery implants:
- Vitrasert implant
- Retisert
- Posurdex
- Encapsulated cell therapy.

Vitrasert implant: One of the initial drug delivery devices for vitreoretinal disease is the Vitrasert implant for AIDS-related cytomegalovirus retinitis. The product was developed by control delivery systems (Watertown mass) using its Aeon technology, a controlled rate and duration of release delivery system. The device is surgically implanted into the vitreous where it releases the antiviral drug ganciclovir. The device is replaced when the drug is depleted, usually after six to eight months.

Retisert: Using a technology similar to Vitrasert called Envision TD. Bausch and Lomb and control delivery systems are developing Retisert, an intravitreal device containing the steroid fluocinolone acetonide, which is currently in clinical studies for posterior uveitis, diabetic macular edema and AMD.

Posurdex: Another steroid-releasing device being developed by Oculex is Posurdex, a slow-released dexamethasone intravitreal implant currently in human trials for persistent macular edema associated with diabetic retinopathy, uveitis, vein occlusion and Irvine-Gass syndrome. Posurdex uses a completely biodegradable polymer that dissolves over time.

Encapsulated cell therapy: An interesting technology being developed by Paris' Neurotech SA is encapsulated cell therapy. Their lead product, NT-501, consists of encapsulated retinal pigment epithelial cells, which are genetically modified to secrete ciliary neurotrophic factor for the treatment of retinitis pigmentosa. CNTF is a protein that may prevent generation of photoreceptors in RP. The cells are inside a membrane designated to permit the intake of oxygen and nutrients and the release of CNTF. The cells are maintained in a biological matrix that supports their long-term survival *in vivo*. The current prototype is about 10 mm long and may be able to be implanted into the vitreous and anchored to the sclera in 15 minutes.

Iontophoresis: As an alternative to parenteral or systemic delivery, iontophoresis is being investigated for ocular uses. By applying an electrical current to a topically applied drug, iontophoresis is capable of pushing it through specific tissues to a target treatment area. Depending on the charge of the drug, a positive or negative charge can propel it. Iontophoresis has been used for transdermal delivery of anti-inflammatory drug.

Eyegate and Ocuphor are two ophthalmic iontophoresis systems being investigated. Similar to transdermal delivery, iontophoresis may offer a less invasive alternative to injections or delivery implants.

Medication devices used in Ophthalmology

Contact Lenses

Therapeutic soft contact lenses with high water content are of great benefit in treating several ophthalmic diseases. Soft contact lenses can absorb water soluble drugs and release them into the eye over a prolonged duration. These lenses are especially useful in promoting substained release of solutions or suspensions that normally would be removed quickly from the external ocular tissues. Therapeutic soft contact lenses are used commonly as drug delivery devices in the management of dry eye disorders. Sometimes these lenses are also used for the treatment of ocular infections especially bacterial corneal ulcers.

Corneal Shields

Porcine or bovine scleral collagen shields are commercially available which are usually non-cross linked and homogenized. Corneal shields are generally placed as a bandage on the cornea following surgery or injury to protect and lubricate the cornea. For treating bacterial corneal ulcers corneal shields are used in conjunction with topical antibiotics with good results.

Cotton Pledgets

Small cotton pieces can be soaked with topical ophthalmic solutions and placed in conjunctival sac. Such devices certainly allow a prolonged ocular contact time with solutions that are normally instilled topically into the eye. Generally cotton pledgets are used for the administration of mydriatic solutions. This drug delivery device promotes maximum mydriasis in an effort to break posterior synechiae or to dilate sluggish pupils.

Filter Paper Strips

Fluorescein strips are commercially available as drug impregnated filter paper strips (Sodium Fluorescein, Rose Bengal or Flurexon). These filter strips help to ensure sterility of sodium Fluorescein which can be easily contaminated with *Pseudomonas aeruginosa* when prepared in solution. These tests strips are used diagnostically to identify corneal injuries and infections. Schirmer tear test strips are also available commercially for diagnosing dry eye disorders.

Artificial Tear Inserts

An especially designed rod shaped pellet of hydroxy propyl cellulose without preservative is commercially available to be inserted into the inferior conjunctival sac with a special applicator. Following insertion, these devices absorbs fluid, swells and then releases the non-medicated polymer to the eye for a duration of 24 hours. Ocuserts are especially used in the treatment of dry eye disorders.

Membrane Bound Inserts

Ocuserts are membrane controlled drug delivery system which deliver a constant quantity of medication to the eye for a week continuously, Pilocarpine Ocuserts are commonly used in the treatment of glaucoma. These Ocuserts are placed on to bulbar conjunctiva under the upper or lower eyelid. pilocarpine Ocusert is a useful substitute for Pilocarpine drops or gel in glaucoma patients who have poor compliance with more frequent drug instillation.

Practical Tips for Use of Various Ophthalmic Medications

Proper administration of ophthalmic drugs is absolutely essential to achieve optimal therapeutic results. Here I shall describe several common practical points which should be informed to the patients before starting any ophthalmic formulation.

a. Never instill more than one properly placed drop of ophthalmic solution or suspension into the affected eye. Normal eye retans 10 mcl of fluid on an average. Generally eye dropper delivers 25-50 mcl/drop of fluid.

For proper placement of drop into the eye ask the patient to tilt head backward or lie down in supine position with gaze upward. Gently grasp lower eyelid below eyelashes and pull the eyelid away from the eye to form a pouch. Put dropper directly over eye. Avoid contact of dropper with the eye. Keep the dropper tip about one inch away from the eye. Look upward before instilling the drop. Release the lid slowly and close eye gently for 2-3 minutes.

b. Systemic absorption of ophthalmic solution or suspension can be minimized by compressing the canaliculus and lacrimal sac for 3-5 minutes after instillation. This compressing certainly retards the passage of drops via nasolacrimal duct into the areas of potential absorption like nasal and pharyngeal mucosa.
c. When multi solution therapy is indicated ideally instill the drops separately at 5 minutes interval. This ensures that first solution drop is not flushed away by the second or second is not diluted by first one.
d. Certain ophthalmic factors may increase absorption from ophthalmic dose forms like lax eye lids especially in elderly patients and diseased eyes which forms a great pool for retention of topical solution or suspension.
e. Discourage the use of eye cup in cases of eye lotions due to risk of contamination and spreading disease.
f. Ophthalmic suspensions generally mix with tears poorly and remain in the lower cul-de-sac longer than solutions.
g. Ophthalmic ointments are helpful in maintaining contact between ocular tissues and drug by decreasing the rate as slow as 0.5% per minute. Ophthalmic ointments provide maximum contact between drug and ocular tissues.
h. Ophthalmic ointments should be instilled preferably at bed time as it may impede delivery of other ophthalmic drugs to the affected eye by acting as a barrier to contact.
i. Ointments may blur vision during waking hours so bed time use is generally recommended.
j. Monitor expiration dates of ophthalmic medications. Do not use outdated drugs.
k. Ophthalmic solutions and ointments are generally misused. Patient use these medications on their own without conselling ophthalmologists. Appropriate patient education and counseling with prescribing and dispensing of ophthalmic medicines is essential.

BIBLIOGRAPHY

1. Agarwal Amar. Textbook of Ophthalmology, ed.1, New Delhi : Jaypee Medical Publishers, 2002.
2. Bartlett JD. Clinical Ocular Pharmacology, ed.4, Boston : Butterworth-Heinemann, 2001.

3. Bartlett JD. Ophthalmic Drug Facts : Lippincott – William and Wilkins, 2001.
4. Crick RP, Trimble RB. Textbook of Clinical Ophthalmology: Hodder and Stoughton, 1986.
5. Duane TD. Clinical Ophthalmology, ed. 4 : Butterworth – Heinemann, 1999.
6. Duvall. Ophthalmic Medications and Pharmacology : Slack Inc, 1998.
7. Ellis PP. Ocular Therapeutics and Pharmacology, ed. 7: CV Mosby, 1985.
8. Fechner. Ocular Therapeutics : Slack Inc., 1998.
9. Feibel RM. Current Concepts in Retrobulbar Anaesthesia: Surv Ophthalmol, 1985;30:102.
10. Fraunfelder. Current Ocular Therapy, ed. 5 : WB Saunders, 2000.
11. Fraunfelder FT, Ophthalmic Drug Delivery Systems : Surv Ophthalmol 1974; 18:292.
12. Garg Ashok. Current Trends in Ophthalmology, ed. 1, New Delhi : Jaypee Medical Publishers, 1997.
13. Garg Ashok. Manual of Ocular Therapeutics, ed. 1, New Delhi : Jaypee Medical Publishers, 1996.
14. Garg Ashok. Ready Reckoner of Ocular Therapeutics, ed.1, New Delhi : 2002.
15. Goodman LS, Gilman A. Pharmacological Basis of Therapeutics, ed.7, New York: Macmillan, 1985.
16. Halberg GP. Drug Delivery Systems for Topical Ophthalmic Medication, Ann. Ophthalmol, 1975;7:1199.
17. Havener's Ocular Pharmacology, ed. 6 : CV Mosby, 1994.
18. Kanski. Clinical ophthalmology, ed. 4 : Butterworth – Heineman, 1999.
19. Kershner. Ophthalmic Medications and Pharmacology : Slack. Inc., 1994.
20. Olin BR, et al. Drugs Facts and Comparisons : Facts and Comparisons, St. Louis, 1997.
21. Onofrey, The Ocular Therapeutics; Lippincott-William and Wilkins, 1997.
22. Rhee, The Wills Eye Drug Guide : Lippincott – William and Wilkins, 1998.
23. Robin JS. Ophthalmic ointments; Surv Ophthalmol 1978;22:335.
24. Steven Podos. Textbook of Ophthalmology, New Delhi:Jaypee Medical Publishers, 2001.
25. Zimmerman TJ. Therapeutic index of topically applied ocular drugs, Arch. Ophthalmol 1984;102:551.
26. Zimmerman. Textbook of Ocular Pharmacology : Lippincott—William and Wilkins, 1997.

Chapter 3

Microorganisms and Ocular Diseases

Ashok Garg (India)

About every known pathogenic micro-organism can cause ocular infection, some pathogens have specific affinity for special ocular structures.

For Ex. Gonococcus causes conjunctivitis but does not involve lacrimal apparatus. For the purpose of discussion, organisms affecting the eye may be classified as follows :

Bacteria

On the basis of gram reaction and shape they are divided into

Gram-positive rods
Gram-negative rods
Gram-positive cocci
Gram-negative cocci
} Aerobic and anaerobic

1. Most pathogenic cocci are gram-positive these are:
   1. *Staphylococcus aureus*
   2. *Staphylococcus epidermidis*
   3. *Staphylococcus saprophyticus*
   4. *Streptococcus pyogenes*
   5. *Streptococcus pneumoniae*
   6. *Pneumococcus* (*Diplococcus pneumoniae* and *Streptococcus pneumoniae*
   7. Anaerobic *Strepstococcus* (*Peptostreptococcus*)
   8. α and β Hemolytic *Streptococcus*.
2. Gram-negative cocci are:
   1. *Meningococcus*
   2. *Gonococcus*
   3. *Neisseria*
   4. *Branhamella*

   } *Pharyngis flavescens mucosa sicca*

3. Most pathogenic rods are gram-negative. These are:
   - *Pseudomonas aeruginosa*
   - *Pseudomonas cepacia*
   - *Haemophillus influenzae* and *aegyptius*
   - *Moraxella* } *M. lacunata*, *M. non liquefaciens*, *M.bovis*
   - *Acinetobacter*
   - *Klebsiella* } *K.pneumoniae*, *K.oxytoca*
   - *E. coli*
   - *Shigella* } *S.sonnei*, *S.flexneri*
   - *Brucella* } *B. abortus*, *B.suis*, *B.melitenesis*
   - *Serratia* } *S. marcescens*, *S. flexneri*
   - *Proteus* } *P. merabilis*, *P. vulgaris*
4. Gram-positive rods are:
   - *Bacillus subtilis*
   - *Bacillus anthracis*
   - *Bacillus cereus*
   - *Clostridia* (*Welchi*, Diphtherial)
   - *Cl. tetani*
   - *Corynebacteria* } *C. diphtheria*, *C. xerosis*, *C.pseudodiphtheriticum*, *C. haemolyticus*
   - *Listeria monocytogenes*
5. Mycobacteria (acid-fast bacilli)
   - *Mycobacterium tuberculosis*
   - Atypical mycobacteria
   - *Mycobacterium leprae*

6. Higher bacteria (*Actino mycetales*)
   - *Actinomyces israelii*
   - *Nocardia* species — *N. asteroides*, *N. caviae*, *N. basilienscs*
   - *Streptothrix*
7. Spirochaetes
   - *Treponema pallidum*
8. *Chlamydia* (Between bacteria and virus)
   - *Chlamydia trachomatis*
   - *Chlamydia psittaci*

Fungi

1. Yeast and yeast like fungi:
   - *Cryptococcus*
   - *Candida* (*albicans*, *parapsilosis* and *tropicalis* species)
2. Filamentous fungi:
   i. Aseptate fungi
      - Mucor
      - Rhizopus

   ii. Septate fungi:
      - *Aspergillus* — *A. fumigatus*, *A.flavus*, *A.niger*, *A.terreus*
      - *Fusarium* (*F.solani*, *oxysporum*, *episphaeria* and *monilformae* species)
      - *Dematiaceous fungi* – *Drechslera* species
      - *Curvularia lunare*
      - *Cladosporium species*
      - Alternaria
      - *Penicillium sp.*
      - *Cephalosporium* (*Acremonium* sp.)

   iii. Dimorphic (*Histoplasma capsulatum*)

   iv. *Rhinosporidium seeberi*

Viruses

i. DNA Viruses
   - Herpes Group :
   - Herpes Simplex (HSV_1 type and HSV_2 type)
   - Varicella Zoster
   - Cytomegalovirus

- Adenoviruses (8 and 19, 3 and 7 type)
- Variola and vaccinia
- *Molluscum contagiosum*
- Human Papova virus

ii. RNA Viruses
- Picorna viruses - Enterovirus type 70
- Coxsackie A 24
- Measles
- Mumps
- Rubella

Parasites:

i. *Taenia solium*
ii. *Cysticerus cellulosae*
iii. *Echinococcus granuloses*
iv. *Toxoplasma gondii*
v. *Toxocara canis*
vi. *Loa loa*
vii. *Wuchereria bancrofti*
viii. *Onchocerca volvulus*
ix. *Acanthamoeba* (*Castellanii, Culberisono* and *polyphaga* species)
x. *Demodex organisms* (*Folliculorum* and *brevis*)
xi. *Phthirus pubis*

Common Microbiological Stains used in Ophthalmology

Diff Quick Stain

Used to differentiate white blood cell types in eye disease like:
- Bacterial—neutrophils
- Viral— lymphocytes
- Allergic—Eosinophils and Basophils
- Vernal—mast cells/lymphocytes

Gram Stain

To differentiate gram-positive (blue) and gram-negative (red) organisms.

Giemsa Stain

To identify cellular inclusion bodies in chlamydial infection.

Wright Stain

To reveal the condition and character of epithelial cells and inflammatory cells.

Calcofluor Stain

For identification of *Acanthamoeba*

Ziehl-Neelsen's Stain

For differential staining of acid-fast bacilli

Kinyoun's Method

For identifying *Nocardia* species

Lactophenol Cotton Blue Mount

For filamentous fungal culture

Hansel Stain

For rapid identification of any eosinophilic response.

COMMON OPHTHALMIC CULTURE MEDIA AND USAGE (TABLE 3.1)

Table 3.1: Different culture media and their usage

Media	*Composition*	*Usage*
1. Blood agar	Defibrinated sheep's blood	To detect hemolytic activity
2. Chocolate agar	Heat denaturalized Sheep's blood and nutrients	Best medium for Haemophilus and Neisseria
3. Sabaroud's medium	Glucose/peptone and antibiotics	Fungal culture media
4. Thioglycolate broth	Sodium thioglycolate	General culture media
5. Brain-heart infusion broth	Beef brain and Heart/ protease/Dextrose/ neopeptone/antibiotic	Fungal growth media
6. Page's medium	*E.coli* plates	for *Acanthamoeba*
7. Thayer-Martin medium	Modified Chocolate agar with nutrients and selected antibiotics	Best for *Neisseria*
8. Lowenstein-Jensen	Media for Mycobacteria	
9. Viral carrier medium	Contain Hank's BSS to human cell tissue culture	for Herpes Simplex, Zoster and adenovirus

NORMAL MICROBIAL FLORA OF THE EYE

The conjunctival sac and eye lid margins harbour a variety of microorganisms. The inner structures are sterile. The normally present flora can be divided in two groups—the resident flora and transient flora.

Resident Flora

It consists of fixed type of microorganisms regularly found in the eye. The predominant of these microorganisms are *Staphylococcus epidermidis* and *Corynebacterium Xerosis*.

Transient Flora

It consists of nonpathogenic or potentially pathogenic microorganisms that inhabit the eye for short duration. They may be derived from the environment (Exogenous) or from other parts of the body (Endogenous). Members of transient flora are generally of little clinical significance as long as the normal resident flora and host resistance remain intact. However, under favourable pathological conditions, these transient microorganisms may colonize, proliferate and produce clinical ocular diseases. The various organisms that may be encountered as transient flora are:

Gram-positive bacteria
- Diphtheroids (*Corynebacterium* species)
- *Staphylococcus aureus* and other species
- Hemolytic and non-hemolytic stereptococci
- Aerobic spore beares (*Bacillus* species)

Gram-negative bacteria
- *Haemophillus* species
- *Moraxella* species
- *Neisseria* species

Enteric bacilli
- *E. coli*
- *K. pneumoniae*
- *Enterobacter* species

Fungi
Due to Omni presence of fungal spores in air, they are some times present in the conjunctival sac. The common fungi are *Aspergillus fumigatus, Aspergillus flavus, Mucor* species, *Dematiaceous* fungi (*Alternaria, Curvularia, Helmintho sporium* etc.), *Penicillium* species etc.

The microbial flora of the conjunctiva is normally held in check by the following factors.
- Flushing mechanism provided by tears.
- Bactericidal action of lysozyme present in tears.
- Phagocytosis by epithelial cells and inflammatory cells.
- Mechanical barrier of intact mucous membrane.
- Blinking action of lids.

BIBLIOGRAPHY

1. Apple. Ocular Pathology, ed. 5; CV Mosby, 1998.
2. Agarwal Amar. Text book of ophthalmology, ed.1, New Delhi: Jaypee Medical Publishers, 2002.
3. Bartlett JD. Clinical Ocular Pharmacology, ed. 4, Boston: Butterworth-Heinemann, 2001.
4. Bartlett JD. Ophthalmic Drug facts : Lippincott – William and Wilkins, 2001.
5. Crick RP, Trimble RB. Text book of clinical ophthalmology:Hodder and Stoughton, 1986.
6. Duane TD. Clinical ophthalmology, ed. 4 : Butterworth – Heinemann, 1999.
7. Duvall. Ophthalmic Medications and Pharmacology : Slack Inc, 1998.
8. Ellis PP. Ocular Therapeutics and Pharmacology, ed. 7 : CV Mosby, 1985.
9. Fechner, Ocular Therapeutics : Slack Inc., 1998.
10. Fraunfelder. Current Ocular Therapy, ed. 5 : WB Saunders, 2000.
11. Garg Ashok. Current Trends in ophthalmology, ed. 1, New Delhi: Jaypee Medical Publishers, 1997.
12. Garg Ashok. Manual of Ocular Therapeutics, ed. 1, New Delhi : Jaypee Medical Publishers, 1996.
13. Garg Ashok. Ready Reckoner of Ocular Therapeutics, ed.1, New Delhi, 2002.
14. Goodman. LS, Gilman A. Pharmacological basis of Therapeutics, ed.7, New York: Macmillan, 1985.
15. Harry, Clinical Ocular Pathology : Butterworth–Heinemann, 1993.
16. Havener's. Ocular Pharmacology, ed. 6: CV Mosby, 1994.
17. Kanski. Clinical ophthalmology, ed. 4 : Butterworth–Heineman, 1999.
18. Kershner. Ophthalmic Medications and Pharmacology : Slack. Inc., 1994.
19. Olin BR, et al. Drugs Facts and Comparisons: Facts and Comparisons. St. Louis, 1997.
20. Onofrey. The Ocular Therapeutics. Lippincott-William and Wilkins, 1997.
21. Rhee. The Wills Eye drug Guide : Lippincott – William and Wilkins, 1998.
22. Steven Podos. Textbook of ophthalmology. New Delhi: Jaypee Medical Publishers, 2001.
23. Zimmerman. Textbook of Ocular Pharmacology: Lippincott and William and Wilkins, 1997.

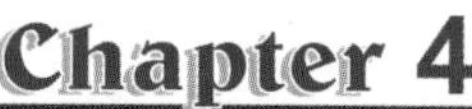

Chapter 4

TEAR FILM PHYSIOLOGY

Ashok Garg (India)

INTRODUCTION

The exposed part of the ocular globe—the cornea and the bulbar conjunctiva is covered by a thin fluid film known as preocular tear film. **Tear film is that surface of the eye, which remains most directly in contact with the environment.** It is critically important for protecting the eye from external influences and for maintaining the health of the underlying cornea and conjunctiva. The optical stability and normal function of the eye depend on an adequate supply of fluid covering its surface.

The tear film is a highly specialized and well-organized moist film which covers the bulbar and palpebral conjunctiva and cornea. It is formed and maintained by an elaborate system—the lacrimal apparatus consisting of secretory, distributive and excretory parts. The secretory part includes the lacrimal gland, accessory lacrimal gland tissue, sebaceous glands of the eyelids, goblet cells and other mucin-secreting elements of the conjunctiva (Fig. 4.1). The elimination of the lacrimal secretions is based on the movement of tears across the eye aided by the act of blinking and a drainage system consisting of lacrimal puncta, canaliculi, sac and nasolacrimal duct (Fig. 4.2).

By definition, a film is a thin layer that can stand vertically without appreciable gravitational flow and the tear film meets this criteria very well. The presence of continuous tear film over the exposed ocular surface is imperative for good visual acuity and wellbeing of the epithelium and facilitates blinking. Tear film serves:

- An optical function by maintaining an optically uniform corneal surface
- A mechanical function by flushing cellular debris, foreign matter from the cornea and conjunctival sac and by lubricating the surface
- A corneal nutritional function
- An antibacterial function.

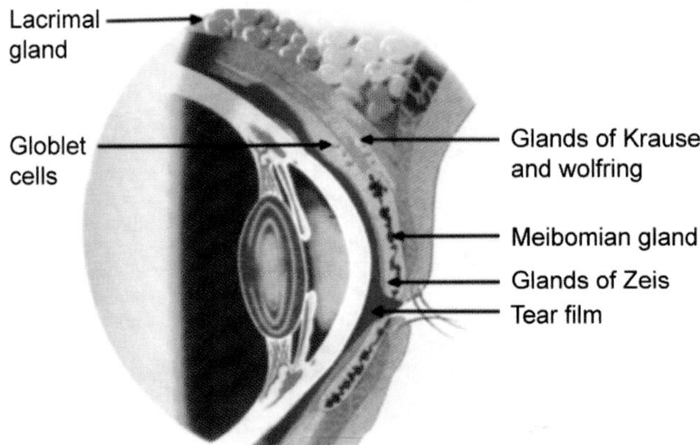

Fig. 4.1: Cross-section of eye showing tear film (blue) in its natural distribution along with tear producing glands (*Courtesy* Allergan India Limited)

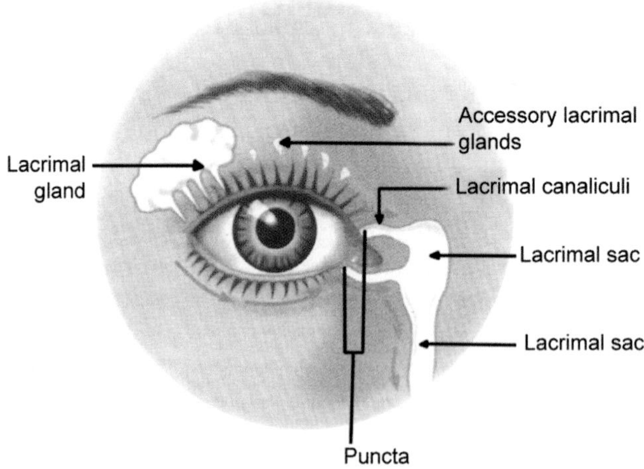

Fig. 4.2: Tear drainage system (*Courtesy* Allergan India Limited)

The composition of the tear film must be kept within rather narrow quantitative and qualitative limits in order to maintain the wellbeing and proper functioning of the visual system. Abnormalities of the tear film affecting its constituents or volume lead to serious dysfunction of the eyelids and the conjunctiva with the concomitant loss of corneal transparency. A thin tear film is uniformally spread over the cornea by blinking and ocular movements. The tear film can be arbitrarily divided into four main parts:

- The marginal tear film along the moist portions of the eyelid which lie posterior to the lipid strip secreted by the tarsal glands

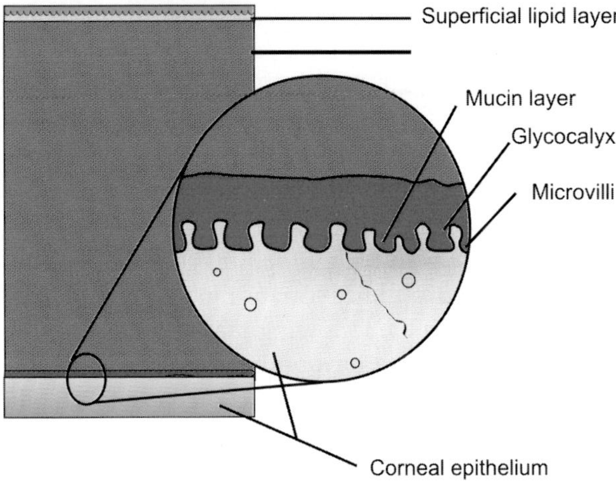

Fig. 4.3: Tear film layers (*Courtesy* Allergan India Limited)

- Portion covering the palpebral conjunctiva
- Portion covering the bulbar conjunctiva
- Precorneal tear film which covers the cornea.

The marginal, palpebral and conjunctival portions are regarded as making the preocular tear film.

Tears refers to the fluid present as the precorneal film and in the conjunctival sac. The volume of tear fluid is about 5 to 10 ml with normal rate of secretion about 1 to 2 ml/minute. About 95 percent of it is produced by the lacrimal gland and lesser amounts are produced by goblet cells and the accessory lacrimal glands of the conjunctiva. The total mass of the latter is about one-tenth of the mass of the main lacrimal gland.

The secretory part of the lacrimal apparatus provides the aqueous tear, lipids and mucus all the important components of the tear film and its boundary.

The tear film is composed of three layers (Fig. 4.3).

1. Superficial Lipid Layer

The superficial layer at the air-tear interface is formed over the aqueous part of the tear film from the oily secretions of meibomian glands and the accessory sebaceous glands of Zeis and Moll. The meibomian gland openings are distributed along the eyelid margin immediately behind the lash follicles.

The chemical nature of the lipid layer is essentially waxy and consists of cholesterol esters and some polar lipids. The thickness of this layer varies with the width of the palpebral fissure and is between 0.1 and 0.2 mm. Being oily in nature it forms a barrier along the lid margins that retains the lid margin tear strip and prevents its overflow on to skin. This layer is so thin that there are no interference color patterns such as one normally sees on an oily surface.

However, if one squints, the oily layer thickness and distinct interference colors may be seen.

While the bulk of tarsal gland secretions are nonpolar lipid compounds which do not spread over an aqueous surface alone, many surface active components are also present. It appears that the tarsal gland secretions which are transported to the cornea in the tear film are massaged into the outermost layer of corneal epithelial cells by eyelid action and then possibly are changed by local metabolic processes in the epithelium combining with conjunctival mucus to form a stable hydrophilic base for the precorneal tear film.

This outer lipid layer has the following main functions:

- It reduces the rate of evaporations of the underlying aqueous tear layer.
- It increases surface tension and assists in the vertical stability of the tear film so that tears do not overflow the lower lid margin.
- It lubricates the eyelids as they pass over the surface of the globe.

2. Middle Aqueous Layer

The intermediate layer of tear film is the aqueous phase which is secreted by the main lacrimal gland and the accessory glands of Krause and Wolfring.

This layer constitutes almost the total thickness of the tear film 6.5 to 10 μm, many times thicker than the fine superficial oily layer. This layer contains two phases—a more concentrated and a highly dilute one. The interfacial tension at the adsorbed mucin-aqueous layer is apt to be rather small due to the intensive hydrogen bond formation across the interface. This layer contains inorganic salts, water proteins, enzymes, glucose, urea, metabolites, electrolytes, glycoproteins and surface active biopolymers. Uptake of oxygen through the tear film is essential to normal corneal metabolism. This layer has four main functions:

- Most importantly it supplies atmospheric oxygen to the corneal epithelium.
- It has antibacterial substances like lactoferrin and lysozyme. Therefore, dry eye patients are more susceptible to infection than a normal eye.
- It provides smooth optical surface by removing any minute irregularities of the cornea.
- It washes away debris from the cornea and conjunctiva.

3. Posterior Mucin Layer

The innermost layer of tear film is a thin mucoid layer elaborated by goblet cells of the conjunctiva and also by the crypts of Henle and glands of Manz. It is the deepest stratum of the precorneal tear film. This layer is even thinner than the lipid layer and is 0.02 to 0.04 μm thick. This adsorbs on the epithelial surface of the cornea and conjunctiva rendering them hydrophilic. It assumes the ridged appearance of the microvilli of superficial epithelial cells which it covers. The preocular tear film is dependent upon a constant supply of mucus which must be of proper chemical and physical nature to maintain corneal and conjunctival surfaces in the proper state of hydration. The mucous threads present in the tear film provides lubrication allowing the eyelid margin and palpebral conjunctiva to slide smoothly over one another with minimal energy lost as friction during blinking and ocular rotation movements. They also cover foreign bodies with a slippery coating thereby protecting the cornea and conjunctiva against the abrasive effects of such particles as they are moved about by the constant blinking movements of eyelids. The mucus contributes stability to the preocular tear film as well as furnishing an attachment for the tear film to the conjunctiva but not to the corneal surface. The corneal surface is covered with a myriad of fine microvilli which provides some support for the tear film. The mucus dissolved in the aqueous phase facilitates spreading of the tear film by smoothening the film over the corneal surface to form a perfect, regular refracting surface.

So the mucin layer which is a glycoprotein converts a hydrophobic surface into a hydrophilic surface and enables the corneal epithelium to be adequately wetted.

In addition to sufficient amounts of aqueous tears and mucin three other important factors are necessary for effective resurfacing of the cornea by the precorneal tear film.

- A normal blink reflex is essential to ensure that the mucin is brought from the inferior conjunctiva and rubbed into the corneal epithelium. Patients suffering from facial palsy and lagophthalmos therefore develop corneal drying.
- Congruity between external ocular surface and the eyelids ensures that the precorneal tear film shall spread evenly over the entire cornea. Patients suffering from limbal lesions like dermoids face the problem of apposition of the eyelids to the globe leading to local selective areas of drying.
- Normal epithelium is necessary for the adsorption of mucin on to its surface cells. Patients suffering from corneal scars and keratinizations have problem of interference with the corneal wetting.

The tear film is not visible apparently on the surface of the eye but at the upper and lower lid margins a 1 mm strip of tear fluid with concave outer surface can be seen. It is here that the oily surface prevents spillage of the tear fluid over the lid margin. Tears forming the upper tear strip are conducted nasally from the upper temporal fornix. At the lateral canthus the tears fall by gravity to form the lower strip, spreading medially the upper and lower strips reach the plica and caruncle where they join together. The tear fluid does not flow over the eye by gravity but a thin film is spread over the cornea by blinking and eye movements.

TEAR FILM FORMATION DYNAMICS

It is interesting to know the tear film formation. Generally during the closure of the eyelids the superficial lipid layer of the tear film is compressed by the eyelid edges because it is energetically unfavorable for the lipid to penetrate under the lids into the fornix. The thickness of lipid layer therefore increases by a factor of 1000 resulting in thickness of 0.1 mm which is easily contained between the adjacent eyelid edges. The aqueous tear layer remains uniform under the lids and acts as a lubricant between the eyelids and the globe. In a complete blink phenomenon, the two tear minisci join and most of their bulk is held at their junction to fill the slight bridge formed by the meeting eyelids and at the canthus.

When the eyelids open, first they form an aqueous tear surface on which the compressed lipid rapidly spread. Monomolecular lipid layer is the first to spread at speeds limited only by the moving eyelid. Following the spread of lipid monolayer, the excess lipid and associated macromolecules shall distribute themselves over the tear film surface at a lower speed, usually the lipid layer ceases within 1 second after the opening of the eye.

Under normal conditions a person blinks on an average 15 times per minute. Some of these blinks may not be complete (the upper eyelid descends only half way towards the lower eyelid). Normally the tear film break up time (BUT) is longer than the interval between blinks and no corneal drying occurs.

A deficiency in the conjunctival secretions can lead to dry eye symptoms even in the presence of an adequate aqueous tear component (Fig. 4.4).

BUT (Break up Time) is generally determined after the instillation of a drop of fluorescein solution in the eye or after staining the tear miniscus and the tear film by a wetted paper strip containing fluorescein. Normal BUT value ranges from 10 to 40 seconds for normal eyes (Fig. 4.5) when the BUT is

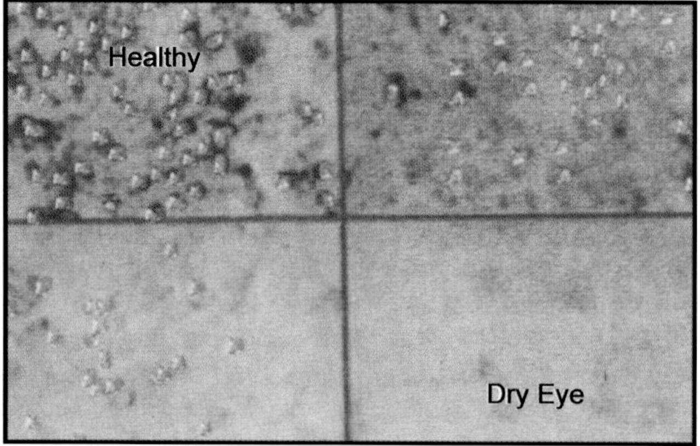

Fig. 4.4: Impression cytology mapping (*Courtesy* Allergan India Limited)

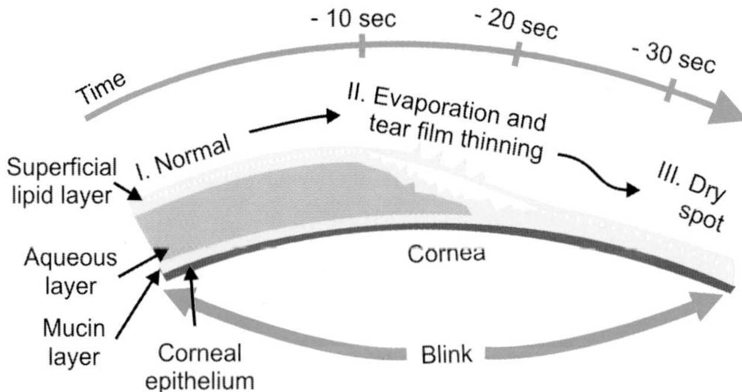

Fig. 4.5: Mechanism of tear film break up (*Courtesy* Allergan India Limited)

determined by a non-invasive method (e.g. by the toposcope). BUT values of as long as 3 to 5 minutes can be recorded.

If the BUT is shorter than the average time interval between two consecutive blinks, tear film rupture can cause pathological changes in the underlying epithelium. The tear film breaks up prematurely over the damaged epithelial surface thereby exacerbating the injury.

Generally there is balance between the secretion and excretion of tears and the rate of tear drainage increases with increased tear volume.

NORMAL TEAR DRAINAGE

In the normal tear film between 10 and 25% of the total tears secreted are lost by evaporation. Evaporation rate is low because of the protective oily surface.

In the absence of the protective oily layer the rate of evaporation is increased 10 to 20 times. Normally tear flows along the upper and lower marginal strips and enters the upper and lower canaliculi by capillarity and possibly by suction also. About 70% of tear drainage is via the lower canaliculus and the remaining through the upper canaliculus. With each blink the superficial and deep heads of pretarsal orbicularis muscle compress the ampullae, shorten the horizontal canaliculi and move the puncta medially. Simultaneously the deep heads of preseptal orbicularis muscle which are attached to the fascia of the lacrimal sac contract and expand the sac. This creates a negative pressure which sucks the tears from the canaliculi into the sac. When the eyes are opened the muscles relax, the sac collapses and a positive pressure is created which forces the tear down the duct into the nose. Gravity also plays an important role in the sac emptying. The puncta move laterally, the canaliculi lengthen and become filled with tears.

TEAR COMPOSITION

Tears contain 98.2% water and 1.8% solids. The high percentage of water in tears is a natural consequence of the need for lubrication of the conjunctiva and corneal surface (Tables 4.1 and 4.2). The evaporation of water between blinks may influence the concentration of the tear film. The evaporation rate of water from the intact precorneal tear film through the superficial lipid layer has been shown to be 8×10^{-7} $cm^{-2}.sec^{-1}$. In a time interval of 10 seconds (between two consecutive blinks) the thickness of the tear film decreases about 0.1 mm resulting in nearly 1 to 2% decrease in water concentration. The solute concentration, however, increases about 20%.

Table 4.1: Relative water contents of tears and other body fluids

Fluid	*Percentage of water*
Tear	98.2
Aqueous humor	98.9
Vitreous humor	99.0
Blood	79.5
Serum	91.0
Urine	96.5

PHYSICAL PROPERTIES OF TEARS

Tear pH

The pH of unstimulated tears is about 7.4 and it approximates that of blood plasma. Although wide variations are found in normal individuals (between 5.0 and 8.35) the usual range is from 7.3 to 7.7. **A more acidic pH of about 7.25 is found following prolonged lid closure possibly due to carbon dioxide produced by the cornea and trapped in the tear pool under the eyelids.** Tear pH is characteristic for each individual and the normal buffering mechanism maintain the pH at a relatively constant level during waking hours. The permeability of the corneal epithelium does not seem to be affected by wide variations in the pH of tear fluid.

Osmotic Pressure

The osmotic pressure in tears mainly caused by the presence of electrolytes is about 305 mOsm/kg equivalent to 0.95% sodium chloride. Individual values over the waking day may range from 0.90 to 1.02% NaCl equivalents. A decrease to an average of 285 mOsm/kg equivalent to 0.89% NaCl has been reported following prolonged lid closure which accounts for the reduced evaporation. When the aqueous component of tears decreases, the tears become markedly hypertonic (0.97% NaCl solution or more) and corneal dehydration results. When the eyes are closed, there is no evaporation of tears and the precorneal tear film is in osmotic equilibrium with the cornea. When the eyes are open evaporation takes place, increasing the tonicity of the tear film and

Table 4.2: Composition of human tears and plasma

Tears		*Plasma*
Physical properties		
pH	7.4 (7.2-7.7)	7.39
Osmotic pressure	305 mOsm/kg Equiv. 0.95% NaCl	6.64 atm
Refractive index	1.357	1.35
Volume	0.50-0.67 g/16 hour (waking)	
Chemical properties		
1. General tear composition		
Water	98.2 g/100 ml	98 g/100 ml
Solids (total)	1.8 g/100 ml	8.6 g/100 ml
Ash	1.05 g/100 ml	0.6-1.0 g/100 ml
2. Electrolytes		
Sodium	120-170 mmol/l	140 mmol/l
Potassium	26-42 mmol/l	4.5 mmol/l
Calcium	0.3-2.0 mmol/l	2.5 mmol/l
Magnesium	0.5-1.1 mmol/l	0.9 mmol/l
Chloride	120-135 mmol/l	100 mmol/l
Bicarbonate	26 mmol/l	30 mmol/l
3. Antiproteinasis		
α_1-Anti trypsin(a_1-at)	0.1-3.0 mg%	280 mg%
α_1-Anti Chymotrypsin	1.4 mg%	24 mg%
Inter-α trypsin inhibitor	0.5 mg%	20 mg%
α_2 Macroglobulin	3-6 mg%	—
4. Nitrogenous substances		
Total protein	0.668-0.800 g/100 ml	6.7 g/100 ml
Albumin	0.392 g/100 ml	4.0-4.8 g/100 ml
Globulin	0.2758 g/100 ml	2.3 g/100 ml
Ammonia	0.005 g/100 ml	0.047 g/100 ml
Uric acid		
Urea	0.04 mg/100 ml	26.8 mg/100 ml
Total nitrogen	158 mg/100 ml	1140 mg/100 ml
Nonprotein nitrogen	51 mg/100 ml	15-42 mg/100 ml
5. Carbohydrates		
Glucose	2.5 (0-5.0) mg/100 ml	80-90 mg/100 ml
6. Sterols		
Cholesterol and cholesterol esters	8-32 mg/100 ml	200-300 mg/100 ml
7. Miscellaneous		
Citric acid	0.6 mg/100 ml	2.2-2.8 mg/100 ml
Ascorbic acid	0.14 mg/100 ml	0.1-0.7 mg/100 ml
Lysozyme	1-2 mg/ml	—
Amino acid	7.58 mg/100 ml	—
Lactate	1-5 mmol/l	0.5-0.8 mmol/l
Prostaglandin	75 pg PF/ml 300 pg PF/ml	80-90 pg PF/ml
Catecholamine	0.5-1.5 µg/ml	
Complement	1:4 dilution (Hemolytic assay)	1.32 dilution (Hemolytic assay)

producing an osmotic gradient from the aqueous through the cornea to the tear film. This direction of flow will continue as long as evaporation maintains the hypertonicity of the tear film. Osmotic pressure is sensitive to changes in tear flow. Reflex stimulation of tears in early adaptation to contact lenses results in a decrease in electrolytes and in total protein leading to hypotonicity. This relative hypotonicity may account for the corneal edema often seen in early stages of contact lens wearing.

Other Physical Properties of Tear (Table 4.2)

- Refractive index—1.357
- Tear volume—0.50-0.67 g/16 hr (waking).

CHEMICAL COMPOSITION OF TEAR FLUID

The chemical composition Table 4.2 of tear fluid is quite complex. The first chemical analysis of tears was studied in 1791 by Fourcroy and Van Que Lin Fleming (1922) and Ridley (1934) demonstrated the detailed chemical composition of normal tears.

Immunoelectrophoretic studies have shown that tears contain lipids, proteins, enzymes, metabolites, electrolytes and hydrogen ions, etc.

Lipids

Lipids are present in small amount in tears as they are contained only in the very thin superficial lipid layer of the tear film. Chromatographic studies of meibomian lipids reveal the presence of all possible lipid classes mainly waxy esters, hydrocarbons, triglycerides, cholesterol esters and in lesser amount diglycerides, monoglycerides, free fatty acids, free cholesterol and phospholipid. However, great individual variations occur in lipid composition.

Cholesterol

Cholesterol has been reported to be present in tear fluid in concentrations of about 200 mg% which is same as in the blood. Like all lipids in biological fluids cholesterol has to be transported by α and β lipoproteins. In normal tears the very low protein content and the absence of lipoproteins is incompatible with a cholesterol concentration of 20 mg%.

Proteins

About 60 components to tear protein fraction have been reported which form the first line of defense against an external infection and seen to be more effective than systemically produced antibodies. The protein content of tears differ from that of blood plasma in several respects. Proteins can be divided in two groups.

Group A: Proteins which are similar to serum proteins with a low concentration representing less than 15% of all tear proteins. Some of them are always present in tears. Table 4.3 namely albumin, IgG, α-L antitrypsin, transferrin, α-L anti-chymotrypsin and β-2 microglobulin others which appears sporadically are ceruloplasmin, haptoglobin and Zinc α-2 glycoprotein.

Group B: Specific proteins synthesized by tear gland are RMP (rapid migration protein) and some other proteins (Tables 4.4 and 4.5) which are also present in other external secretions (lysozyme, lactoferrin and IgA).

Tear Albumin

Albumin represents about 60% of the total protein in tears as it does in plasma. Tear albumin is a unique protein fraction. It is electrophoretically a prealbumin

Table 4.3: Amino acid composition of human tear lysozyme

Amino acids	*Residues (gm/100 g protein)*
Aspartic acid	13.23
Arginine	13.05
Glutamic acid	8.55
Tryptophane	6.89
Alanine	6.36
Leucine	6.11
Trypsin	5.65
Glycine	4.94
Lysine	4.92
Valine	4.62
Serine	4.02
Half-cysteine	4.01
Threonine	3.67
Isoleucine	3.59
Phenylalanine	1.97
Proline	1.72
Methionine	1.50
Histidine	1.01

Table 4.4: Relative quantity of various protein fractions in tears

Fractions	*Normal tears (Percentage)*	*Stimulated flow (Tears) Percentage*
Albumin	58.2	20.2
Globulin	23.9	56.9
Lysozyme	17.9	22.9

Table 4.5: Origin of various tear protein fractions

Protein fraction	*Lacrimal gland proper*	*Accessory lacrimal gland*	*Goblet cells*
Lysozyme	+	—	—
Component-I	—	+	±
Component-II	+	±	±
Component-III	+	±	±
Serum albumin	—	—	+
Tear albumin	+	—	—
Mucin	—	—	+

\+ means fraction is present
— means fraction is absent
± Means fraction is indifferently present

and migrates to a position similar to serum prealbumin. Genetic polymorphism has been reported of the tear albumin.

Electrophoresis of tears shows several peaks of migration. These peaks are main which correspond to proteins synthesized by the lacrimal gland—rapid migrant proteins and lactoferrin migrating to the anode and lysozyme migrating to the cathode.

The total tear proteins content strongly depends upon the method of collection of tears. Small unstimulated tears show levels of about 20 mg/ml while stimulated tears show much lower values in the range of 3 to 7 mg/ml reflecting the level of lacrimal gland fluid.

Lysozyme

Fleming first discovered an antibacterial substance and showed that this substance is an enzyme which he named lysozyme because of its capacity to lyze bacteria. In normal tears concentration of lysozyme is much higher than in any other body fluid. The normal level for human tear lysozyme (HTL) is 1 to 2 mg/ml. The enzymic activity of lysozyme is optimal at pH 5.2 and decreases above and below this pH value.

Lysozyme is a long chain, high molecular weight proteolytic enzyme produced by lysosomes—a known cellular ultra structure. Lysozyme acts upon certain bacteria and dissolves them by cleaning the polysaccharide component of their cell walls. As the function of cell wall in bacteria is to confer mechanical support a bacterium devoid of its cell wall usually bursts because of the high osmotic pressure inside the cell.

Lysozyme level in tears can be measured with a diffusion method or with a spectrophotometric assay.

In addition to lysozyme, presence of other antibacterial factors in human tears have been shown. The nonlysozymal bactericidal protein beta lysin has been reported to be derived chiefly from platelets but it exists in higher concentration in tears than in blood plasma. The lysozyme and beta lysin protein fractions can be separated by filtering the tears. The antibacterial activity of the filtrate results from lysozyme but in whole tears beta lysin is responsible for three-fourth of the bactericidal effect. Beta lysin acts primarily on cellular membrane while lysozyme dissolves bacterial cell walls.

The action of lysozyme depends on the pH. The optimum pH for lysis varies with the solubility of the bacterial proteins but in general it ranges between 6.0 and 7.4. Low salt concentrations favor lysis by increasing solubility.

Human tear lysozyme (HTL) levels have been shown to be greatly decreased in tears of patients suffering from Sjögren's syndrome and ocular toxicity from long-term use of practolol therapy thus making it a useful diagnostic aid. Other disease states where HTL level is lowered include herpes simplex virus infection and malnutrition in children.

Lactoferrin

It is an iron carrying protein and appears to be a major tear protein in the intermediate fraction. Its property of iron binding (Fe III) is 300 times stronger than the other iron binding protein (transferrin). This is probably significant for its bacteriostatic activity in tears making essential metal ions unavailable for microbial metabolism.

Transferrin

Transferrin has been shown to be present in tears. Transferrin along with serum albumin and IgG can be detected only after mild trauma to the mucosal surface of the conjunctiva or in tears.

Ceruloplasmin

Ceruloplasmin, a copper carrying protein is regularly found in tears. In electrophoresis the migration rate of tear ceruloplasmin varies from its serum counter part.

Immunoglobulins

Tiselius (1939) for the first time separated the plasma proteins by electrophoresis and isolated three types of globulins—alpha, beta and gamma. Antibody property of the immune serum resides in the gamma globulin fraction. Immunoglobulins are elaborated by plasma cells following transformation of antigen stimulated B-lymphocytes. This elaboration constitutes the humoral immune system.

Five major classes of immunoglobulins have been recognized (Table 4.6). These are:

Immunoglobulin A (IgA)
Immunoglobulin G (IgG)
Immunoglobulin M (IgM)
Immunoglobulin E (IgE)
Immunoglobulin D (IgD)

Immunoglobulin A (IgA): It is the major immunoglobulin present in tears, saliva and colostrum. Almost all of the IgA have a secretory component attached to them when they occur in external secretions. It participates in the functioning of IgA as antibody in the external environment. The possible functions of secretory IgA include prevention of viral and bacterial infections that may have an access to the external secretions, e.g. tears and participate as opsonins in the phagocytosis process.

The average levels of IgA—the predominant immunoglobulin in normal human tear is 14 mg/dl.

In the human lacrimal gland, IgA appears to be synthesized by interstitial plasma cells and after entry into the intercellular spaces it is coupled to SC and secreted as secretory IgA (IgA-SC) through the blood-tear barrier involving intracellular transport by acinar epithelial cells into the lumens. In the conjunctiva IgA and plasma cells are located in the substantia propria. Only in the acinar epithelium of the accessory lacrimal glands can SC material be present indicating that these are the sites of synthesis of secretory IgA of the conjunctival secretions. Depending upon the method of tear collection IgA values can vary from 10 to 100 mg%.

Immunoglobulin G (IgG): It is present in very low concentrations in normal tears. However, after mild trauma to the mucosal surface of the conjunctiva it can be easily detected.

IgG is the most prominent circulating (serum) immunoglobulin present in concentrations five times that of IgA. The average level of IgG in normal human tears range from 17 to 20 mg/100 ml.

Table 4.6: Immunoglobulin levels in tear and serum

Ig class	*Tears*	*Serum*
Total proteins	800 mg/100 ml	6500 mg/100 ml
IgA	14-24 mg/100 ml	170-200 mg/100 ml
IgG	17 mg/100 ml	1000 mg/100 ml
IgM	5-7 mg/100 ml	100 mg/100 ml
IgE	26-250 mg/ml	2000 mg/ml

The serum level of IgG is about 1000 mg/dl. IgG molecule has a molecular weight of about 150,000. Each molecule of IgG consists of 2 L chains and 2 H chains linked by 20-25-S-S bonds. The antigenic analysis of IgG myelomas show four subclasses now termed as IgG_1, IgG_2, IgG_3, and IgG_4,. IgG_1 is the predominant variant and together with IgG_3 possesses the ability to combine with complement to bind to macrophages and to cross the placenta. IgG synthesis in humans is about 35 mg/kg/d and its half-life is about 23 days. IgG molecules are Y-shaped with a hinge region near the middle of the heavy chain connecting the 2 Fab segments to the Fc segment.

During the secondary response, IgG is the major immunoglobulin to be synthesized probably because of its small size, IgG diffuses more readily than other immunoglobulins into the tears, therefore as the predominating immunoglobulin it carries the major burden of neutralizing bacterial toxins and of binding to microorganisms (specially streptococci, pneumococci and staphylococci) to enhance their phagocytosis. IgG is most efficient in killing and stopping the progress of microorganism's invasion.

Immunoglobulin M (IgM): It is present in very low concentrations in normal tears. The average level of IgM in normal tears range from 5 to 7 mg%. Barnett (1968) reported first the presence of IgM in normal tears.

The serum level of IgM is about 100 mg/dl. The IgM molecule with a molecular weight 900,000 is the largest of the immunoglobulins. Often referred to as macroglobulin because of its size, the IgM molecule are pentamers with a high valency or anticombining capacity. Due to its high valency IgM is extremely efficient agglutinating and cytolytic agent and is the first type of antibody which is formed after the initial encounter with antigen. It appears early in response to infection and is confined mainly to the bloodstream.

Even minimum trauma to conjunctiva would cause serum proteins to leak into the tears. There is increased concentrations of IgA, IgG and IgE in tears. Either these immunoglobulins are selectively excreted into the tears or they are locally synthesized. Increased concentrations of IgA, IgG and IgM are reported in cases of blepharoconjunctivitis, herpes keratitis, vernal conjunctivitis, acute follicular conjunctivitis, phlyctenular conjunctivitis, keratomalacia, corneal ulcer and acute endogenous uveitis.

Immunoglobulin E (IgE): It is mostly extravascular in distribution. IgE values ranges from 26 to 144 mg/ml in normal tears. Normal serum contains only traces of IgE but greatly elevated levels are seen in atopic conditions.

Immunoglobulin D (IgD): IgD levels are quite low in tears as well as in serum. It is mostly intravascular.

Complement

Complement in tears has been shown in hemolytic assays up to dilution of 1.4 whereas serum is active in this system up to 1:32.

Glycoproteins

Glycoproteins are present in the mucoid layer as well as in the tear fluid since they are highly soluble in water. Glycoproteins contribute significantly to the stickiness of the material forming the mucoid layer. N-acetyeneuraminic acid (a sialic acid) has been indentified in normal tears. Glycoproteins may play a critical role in the lubrication of the corneal surface by rendering its hydrophobic surface more hydrophilic permitting spreading and stabilization of the tear film. The mucus is secreted by the conjunctival goblet cells as a solution of glycoproteins (mucoids) and this sticky mixture adheres to the surface of the epithelium even though the glycoproteins are water soluble.

The glycoproteins are carbohydrate-protein complexes characterized by the presence of hexosamines, hexoses and sialic acid. In normal tears relative hexosamine content of the protein which is used as indicator for glycoproteins varies from 0.5 to 17%, the hexosamine concentration from 0.05 to 3 g/l. Sialic acid concentration of human tears has been reported to be 114 mmol/100 ml.

Antiproteinases

Antiproteinases, inhibitors of proteinases are present in tears at levels much lower than in plasma (Table 4.7).

Table 4.7: Antiproteinasis concentration in tears and plasma

Antiproteinasis	*Plasma*	*mg percentage Tears*
α_1-antitrypsin ($\alpha_1$at)	280	0.1-0.4
α_1-antichymotrypsin		1.5
		3.0
α_1-antichymotrypsin	24	1.4
Inter-α-trypsin inhibitor	20	0.5
α_2-macroglobulin		3
		6

These includes α_1-antitrypsin, α_1-antichymotrypsin, inter-α-trypsin inhibitor and α_2-macroglobulin. The source of-α_1 antitrypsin is the lacrimal gland while other antiproteinases originate from corneal and conjunctival surfaces. In various inflammatory conditions of the eye the levels of α_1-at and α_2-m in tear fluid are increased.

In bacterial and viral infections of the eye (Table 4.8) and in corneal ulceration the levels of α_1-at and α_2-m in tear fluids are increased. Using albumin as a marker protein there is evidence suggesting that these two collagenase inhibitors are derived either from plasma by a general increase in vascular permeability to proteins or they are produced locally.

Table 4.8: Antimicrobial factors in tears

Compound	*Evidence*
Lysozyme	+
IgA	+
IgG	±
IgE	+
IgM	±
Complement	+
Lactoferrin	+
Transferrin	±
Betalysin	+
Antibiotic producing Commensal organism	+

+Present in normal tears.
± Present in tears after stimulation (mild trauma to the conjunctiva).

Metabolites

A number of metabolites have been reported to be present in normal human tears. These include organic constituents of low molecular weight like glucose, urea, amino acids and other metabolites like lactate, histamine, prostaglandins and catecholamines.

Glucose

Glucose is present in minimal amounts of about 0.2 mmol/liter in tear fluids of normal glycemic persons. This low concentration of glucose appear to be insufficient for corneal nutrition. There is no definitive evidence that cornea metabolizes glucose emanating from the tears.

It has been shown that some glucose in tears originates from the goblet cells of the conjunctiva. There is corresponding rise in tear glucose level with elevation of plasma glucose level above 100 mg%. However, there is no significant rise in tear glucose levels in diabetics with blood glucose level of more than 20 mmol/liter which demonstrates the barrier function of the corneal and conjunctival epithelium against loss of glucose from the tissues into the tear fluid. It is the tissue fluid which contributes to the tear glucose after mechanically stimulated methods of tear collection.

Urea

Urea concentration in tear fluid and plasma have been found to be equivalent suggesting an unrestricted passage through the blood-tear barrier in the lacrimal gland. Urea concentration in tears decreases with increasing secretion rate.

Amino Acids

Free amino acid concentration in tears is reported to be 7.58 mg/100 ml. This value is 3 to 4 times higher than the free amino acid concentration in serum.

Lactate

Lactate levels of 1 to 5 mmol/l in tears are far higher than the normal blood levels of 0.5 to 0.8 mmol/l. Pyruvate from 0.05 to 0.35 mmol/l is about the same as is normal for blood (0.1-0.2 mmol/l). These levels do not show significant alterations after mechanical irritation. The epithelium does not possess a barrier function for lactate and pyruvate.

Histamine

Histamine is present in normal tears collected from the conjunctival sac at a level of about 10 mg/ml. In vernal conjunctivitis specifically a variable increase up to 125 mg/ml has been observed.

Prostaglandins

Prostaglandins are present in normal tears at the level of 75 pg prostaglandin F/ml and it is little lower than in serum. In inflammatory conditions of the eye significant higher values are found up to 300 pg/ml of tears.

Catecholamines, Dopamine, Noradrenaline and Dopa

Catecholamines, dopamine, noradrenaline and dopa have been found in the tear fluid. The levels vary from 0.5 to 1.5 mg/ml. Dopamine has values as high as 280 mg/ml.

In glaucoma patients lower values have been reported for these compounds which reflect the diminished activity of the sympathetic innervation of the eye. The determination of catecholamines in tears has been advocated as a test in glaucoma diagnosis.

Electrolytes and Hydrogen Ions

The predominant positively charged electrolytes (cation) in tears are mainly sodium and potassium while the negative ions (anions) are chloride and bicarbonate (Table 4.9).

Sodium

Sodium concentration in tears 120 to 170 mmol/liter is about equal to that in plasma suggesting a passive secretion into the tears. While potassium with an average value of about 20 mmol/l is much higher than the corresponding plasma concentration of about 5 mmol/l. This indicates an active secretion of

Table 4.9: Human tear electrolytes

	Concentration in mmol/l					
	Na^+	K^+	Ca^{++}	Mg^{++}	Cl^-	HCO_3^-
Tears	120-170	6-26	0.5-1.1	0.3-0.6	118-138	26
	145	24	0.4-1.1	0.5-1.1	106-130	
	134-170	26-42	0.3-2.0		120-135	
Serum	140	4.5	2.5	0.9	100	30

potassium into the tears. It is interesting to observe that while the main cationic constituent of the aqueous and vitreous humor is sodium while cornea (mainly corneal epithelium) contains a much higher concentration of potassium than sodium. These two cations play an essential role in the osmotic regulation of the extracellular and intracellular spaces and in general changes in sodium level are the reverse of changes in potassium level.

Calcium

Calcium is independent of the tear production and is lower than the free fraction of plasma. In cystic fibrosis patients have much higher calcium values. An average of 2.5 mmol/l have been shown only at slow rates concomitant with lower tear sodium values.

Magnesium

Magnesium in tears is little lower than corresponding serum value possibly reflecting the free fraction of magnesium. Both calcium and magnesium play a role in controlling membrane permeability.

Chloride

Chloride, an anion essential to all tissues also plays an important role in osmotic regulation much like sodium and potassium. The chloride concentration is slightly higher in tears than in serum.

Bicarbonate

The bicarbonate together with the carbonate ions in tears may be involved in the regulation of pH. This buffer system maintains the near neutral pH of the tear film, the surface of which is exposed to atmospheric changes.

Enzymes

Enzymes of Energy Producing Metabolisms

Glycolytic enzymes and enzymes of tricarboxylic acid cycle can be detected in high values only in human tear samples. These enzymes form a blood-tear barrier against penetration from the blood. The source of these enzymes is in the conjunctiva where they are secreted in small amounts. The lacrimal gland apparently does not secrete these enzymes. These enzymes can be obtained during mechanical irritation.

Lactate Dehydrogenase

Lactate dehydrogenase (LDH) is the enzyme in the highest concentration in tears. It can be separated electrophoretically into its five isoenzymes showing a pattern with more of the slower migrating muscle type isoenzymes. This is closely related to the distribution pattern of corneal tissue in contrast to serum LDH where the faster migrating heart type isoenzymes prevail.

These findings indicate that tear LDH originates from the corneal epithelium. Therefore, in patients suffering from corneal disease, the distribution of LDH isoenzymes in tears differs from those found in healthy individuals. LDH isoenzymes bound to immunoglobulin have been found in blood and it is probable that here an analogous binding takes place in tears.

Lysosomal Enzymes

Lysosomal enzymes include a number of lysosomal acid hydrolases which are present in tears in concentration of 2 to 10 times than those in serum. **The lacrimal gland is the main source of the lysosomal enzymes but conjunctiva may act as a second source for lysosomal enzymes after mild trauma.** The relative high values are found in tear fluid collection where the epithelial cells of conjunctiva remain intact and contain very low levels of lactate dehydrogenase or other cytoplasmic enzymes. Lysosomal enzyme activities in tears are used for diagnosis and identification of carriers of several inborn errors of metabolism.

The concentration of β-hexosaminidase in tears collected on filter paper strips is an index for the development and prognosis of diabetic retinopathy. The tears would reflect the decreased enzyme activity of β-hexosaminidase and of other lysosomal glycosidases in the retina showing a negative correlation with the increased plasma levels of these enzymes.

Amylase

Amylase is the enzyme present in tear fluid in relatively moderate levels. The origin of this enzyme is in lacrimal gland. The reported presence of amylase in the cornea might be due to contamination by tear fluid.

Peroxidase

Peroxidase (POD) is present in human tears originating from the lacrimal gland and not from the conjunctiva. The level of tear POD in human tears is 10^3 μ/l. POD activity found in the conjunctiva is probably derived from the tears.

Plasminogen Activator

Plasminogen activator has been demonstrated in tear fluid and corneal epithelium is suggested to be the source of this urokinase-like fibrinolytic activity.

Collagenase

Collagenase has been shown to be present in tear fluid in the presence of corneal ulceration, due to infection, chemical burn, trauma and desiccation. Corneal collagenase is present as an inactive precursor "latent collagenase" which can be activated with trypsin and *in vivo* possibly by plasmin resulting from plasminogen activator activity in tears.

Drugs Excreted in Tears

Tears represent a potentially more stable body fluid of low protein content and with modest variations of pH. Passage of drugs from the plasma to the tears apparently takes place by diffusion of the non-protein bound fraction. However, presence of tight junctions between the acinar epithelial cells in the lacrimal gland forming a blood-tear barrier, the lipid solubility is expected to play a major role. The blood-tear barrier shows the same characteristics as that of cell membrane. Phenobarbital and carbamazepine are excreted in tears in about 0.5% of corresponding plasma concentration.

Methotrexate, an antimetabolite reaches tear levels of 5% of the corresponding plasma concentrations and is in equilibrium with the unbound fraction in plasma. Ampicillin is present in tears in concentration of about 0.02 of the corresponding serum level.

APPLIED PHYSIOLOGY

Basic secretion of tear fluid is made up of the secretions of the lacrimal gland and accessory lacrimal gland tissue together with the secretions of meibomian glands and the mucous glands of the conjunctiva. Reflex secretions of tears is hundreds time greater than basal or resting secretion. The stimulus to reflex secretions appears to be derived from the superficial corneal and conjunctival sensory stimulation as a result of tear break up and dry spot formation. The secretory stimulus to the lacrimal glands is parasympathetic with reflex secretions occurring in both eyes following superficial stimulation of one eye. The whole mass of lacrimal tissue responds as one unit to reflex tearing. Reflex secretion is reduced by topical corneal and conjunctival anesthesia.

HYPOSECRETION OF TEARS

Hyposecretion means decreased formation of tears.

Lacrimal hyposecretion may be congenital although not very common. Acquired lacrimal hyposecretion may be due to:

- Atrophy and fibrosis of lacrimal tissue due to a destructive infiltration by mononuclear cells as in keratoconjunctivitis sicca and Sjögren's syndrome.
- Local inflammatory diseases of the conjunctiva commonly conjunctival scarring secondary to bacterial or viral infection.
- Chronic inflammatory disease of the salivary and lacrimal glands (Mikulicz's syndrome).
- Damage or destruction of lacrimal tissue by granulomatous (sarcoidosis), pseudotumor or neoplastic lesions.
- Absence of lacrimal gland.
- Blockage of excretory ducts of the lacrimal gland.
- Neurogenic lesions.
- Meibomian gland dysfunction.

Diagnostic Tests for Tear Hyposecretions (Table 4.10)

Tear Film Break-up Time (BUT)

The tear film break-up time is a simple physiological test to assess the stability of the precorneal tear film. This test is performed by instilling fluorescein into the lower fornix, taking precaution not to touch cornea. The patient is asked to blink several times and then to refrain from blinking. The tear film is scanned with a broad beam and cobalt blue filter. After an interval of time black spots or line indicating dry spots appear in the tear film. **BUT is the interval between the last blink and appearance of the first randomly distributed dry spot.** Ideally average of three measurements is taken. A normal BUT is more than 10 seconds and a BUT of less than 10 seconds is considered abnormal. This test may also be abnormal in eyes with mucin or lipid deficiency.

Table 4.10: Diagnostic tests and drug assays in tears

Compound	*Diagnosis*	*Usefulness*
Lysozyme	Sjögren's disease	+
	Practolol induced toxicity	+
	Traumatic inflammation of eye	+
Lysosomal enzymes	Lysosomal storage disease	+
Collagenase	Corneal ulceration	+
α_1-Antitrypsin	Bacterial infections	±
Glucose	Diabetes mellitus	±
Tear albumin	Genetic marker	+
Immunoglobulins (IgA, IgG and IgM)	Iatrogenic inflammation of anterior-segment	+

+ Useful
± Comparatively useful

Schirmer's Test

The rate of tear formation is estimated by measuring the amount of wetting on a special filter paper which is 5 mm wide and 35 mm long (Fig. 4.6).

Previously Schirmer's test 1 and 2 were used in diagnostic practice but nowadays modified Schirmer-I test is employed. This test is performed as follows.

Schirmer strips are prepared by cutting out Whatman filter paper No. 41 into the strips of 5 × 35 mm dimensions. A 5 mm tab is folded over at one end. Before use, these strips are autoclaved.

The bent end is placed into lower conjunctival sac at the junction of lateral one-third and medial two-third of the lower eyelid so that a 5 mm bent end rests on the palpebral conjunctiva and the folding crease lies over the eyelid margin. This test is usually performed in sitting posture in dim light.

The patient is asked to keep the eyelid open and look slightly upwards at a fixation point. Blinking is allowed while the patient gazes at the fixation point.

After one minute, the strips are carefully removed and moistening of the exposed portion of the strip is measured in millimeters with the help of a millimeter ruler.

The measurements are made from the notch at the bend of the Schirmer strip to the distal end of the wetting on the strip (excluding the folded over tab). The amount of wetting of the Schirmer strip in one minute is multiplied by three to correspond roughly to the amount of wetting that would have occurred in five minutes (Jones, 1972). It is a measure of the rate of tear secretion in a five-minute period.

A normal eye will wet between 10 and 25 mm during that period. Measurements between 5 and 10 mm are considered borderline and values less than 5 mm is indicative of impaired secretion.

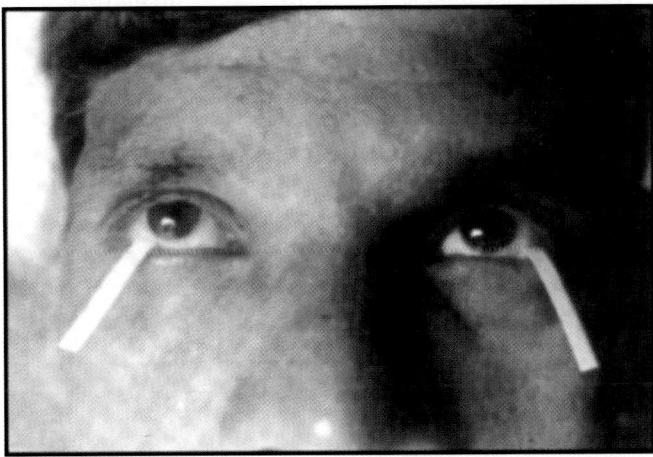

Fig. 4.6: Modified Schirmer's test

Vital Dye Staining

- Rose Bengal 1% has an affinity for devitalized epithelial cells and mucus in contrast to fluorescein which remains extracellular and is more useful in showing up epithelial defects. Rose Bengal is very useful in detecting even mild cases of keratoconjunctivitis sicca (KCS) by staining the interpalpebral conjunctiva in the form of two triangles with their base at the limbus.

  The only disadvantage with Rose Bengal staining is that it may cause ocular irritation specially in eyes with severe KCS. In order to reduce that amount of irritation only a small drop should be instilled into the eye. A topical anesthetic should not be used prior to the instillation of Rose Bengal as it may produce a false-positive result.
- Alcian blue has similar properties as Rose Bengal and is less irritant but it is not generally available.

Lysozyme Assay

Lysozyme assay is based on the fact that in hyposecretion of tears, there may be reduction in the concentration of lysozyme. This test is performed by placing the wetted filter strip into an agar plate containing specific bacteria. The plate is then incubated for 24 hours and the zone of the lysis is measured. The zone will be reduced if the concentration of lysozyme in the tears is decreased.

Tear Globulin Assay

Tear IgA levels are measured in this test. This test is also based on the principle that decreased tear formation will lead to decreased IgA (immunoglobulin A) levels in tears. This test is performed on a specific tripartigan immunodiffusion plates containing specific agar gel in wells (Figs 4.7 and 4.8). 20 ml of tear samples is put into these wells and plates are incubated for 48 hours. The diffusion of rings around wells are measured to the nearest 0.1 mm with a partigen ruler. The ring will be reduced if the concentration of IgA in tears is decreased. This is a reliable test for measuring tear globulins.

Tear Osmolarity

Tear osmolarity is increased in cases of hyposecretion.

Biopsy of the Conjunctiva

Biopsy of the conjunctiva and an estimation of the number of goblet cells are other tests which can be done. In mucin deficiency states the number of goblet cells shall be decreased.

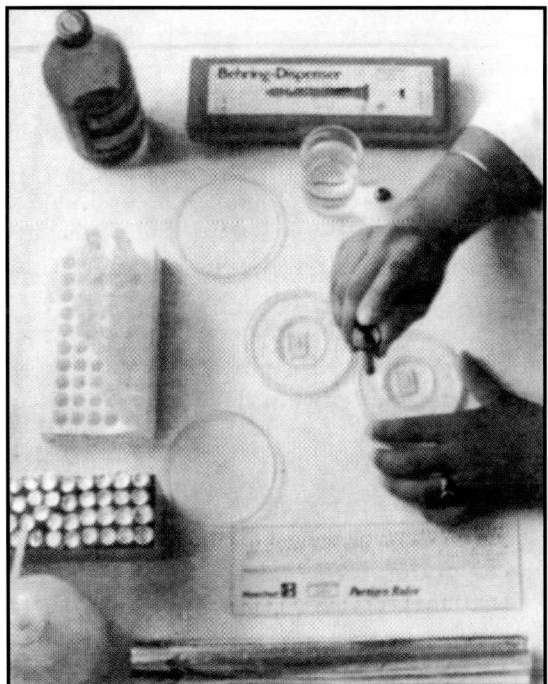

Fig. 4.7: Tear globulin assay (diagnostic test)

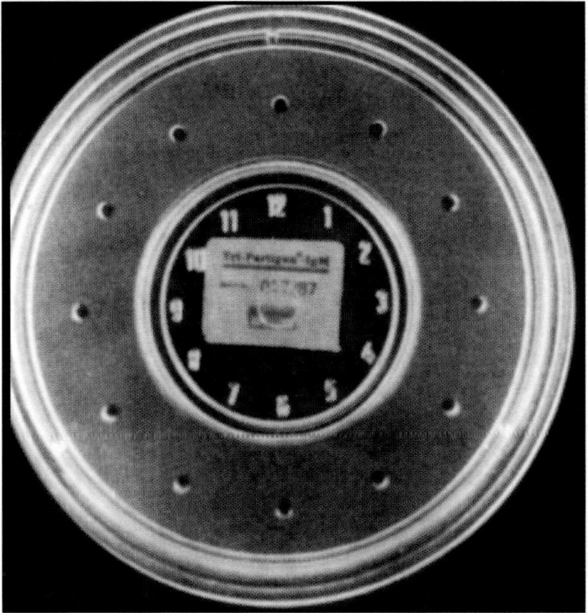

Fig. 4.8: Tripartigen immunodiffusion plates (diffusion of rings around agar wells is measured up to 0.1 mm)

HYPERSECRETION OF TEARS

In practice when patient complains of a wet eye there are two possibilities of excessive watering of the eye.

- Lacrimation from reflex hypersecretion due to irritation of cornea and conjunctiva.
- Obstructive epiphora as a result of failure of tear drainage or evacuation system. The main causes are lacrimal pump failure due to lower lid laxity or weakness of the orbicularis muscle and more commonly due to mechanical obstructions of the drainage system.

If the wet eye is caused by hypersecretion the Schirmer's test values (technique already mentioned) will be increased and the Jones Fluorescein dye test will reveal normal outflow function.

Physiological Diagnostic Test for Hypersecretions

Jones I (Primary) Test

This is a physiological test which differentiates an excessive watering due to a partial obstruction of the lacrimal passages from primary hypersecretion of tears (Fig. 4.9).

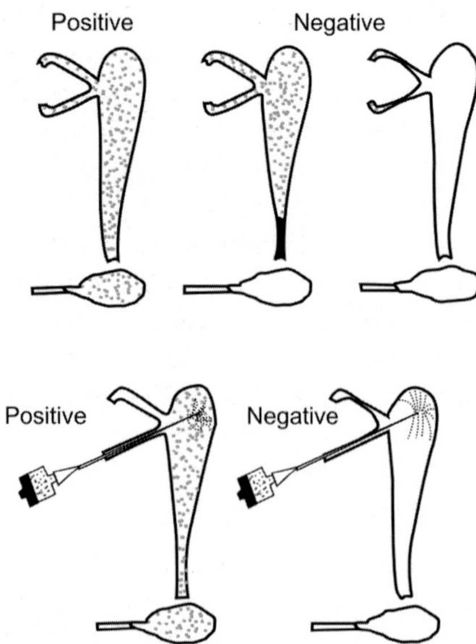

Fig. 4.9: Dye testing: Jones primary test (top) and Jones secondary test (bottom) (*Courtesy* Kanski Clinical Ophthalmology Butterworth International)

In this test 1 drop of 2% fluorescein solution is instilled into the conjunctival sac. After about 5 minutes a cotton-tipped bud or applicator (moistened in coccaine 4% or proparacaine 0.75%) is inserted under the inferior turbinate at the nasolacrimal duct opening. This is situated about 3 cm from the external nares.

The results are interpreted as follows:

- If the fluorescein is recovered from the nose on the applicator and aqueous solution passes from the conjunctival sac to the nose in 1 minute then the excretory system is patent and cause of watering is primary hypersecretion. No further tests are required then and the test is inferred as positive.
- If no dye is recovered from the nose a partial obstruction is present or there is failure of the lacrimal pump mechanism. In this situation secondary dye test or Jones II test is required.

Jones II (Secondary Irrigation) Test

This test helps to identify the probable site of partial obstruction.

In this procedure topical anesthesia (4% Xylocaine or 0.5% proparacaine) is instilled into the conjunctival sac and any residual fluorescein is washed out. The nasolacrimal system is then irrigated with normal saline. The patient is positioned with his or her head down by about 45° so that the saline runs out of the nose into white paper tissues and not into the pharynx.

This test is interpreted as follows.

- Positive—if fluorescein-stained saline is recovered from the nose, the dye must have reached the lacrimal sac during the primary dye test but was stopped from entering the nose by a partial obstruction in the nasolacrimal duct. However, syringing of the lacrimal system had pushed the dye past the obstruction into the nose. A positive secondary dye test indicates a partial obstruction to the nasolacrimal duct which can be treated by a dacryocystorhinostomy (DCR) procedure.
- Negative—if unstained saline is recovered from the nose it means that no dye has entered the lacrimal sac during the primary dye test. This means a partial obstruction in the upper drainage system (punctum, canaliculi or common canaliculus) or a defective lacrimal pump mechanism. In such a situation DCR would fail and some other operative procedure will be required.

Fluorescein Dye Disappearance Test

An accurate status of the excretory capability of the lacrimal system can be obtained by observing the behavior of a single drop of 2% fluorescein solution instilled into the inferior conjunctival cul-de-sac. The color intensity after 5 minutes is measured and graded on a scale of 0 to 4+. The normal excretion of the retained fluorescein shall be 0-1+. Any greater residual then is indicative of impaired outflow. However, by this test one cannot distinguish between impairment of the upper and lower segments of the system, but it may complement the Jones tests.

- Nasal examination should be performed in order to determine the position of normal nasal structures specially the position of the anterior end of the middle turbinate when surgery is contemplated. It will also detect the presence of polyps or tumors, etc.

Special Tests

Intubation Dacryocystography

The conventional method of dacryocystography consists of injecting contrast medium into one of the canaliculi followed by the taking of posteroanterior (PA) and lateral views, radiographs. However, far superior status of the canalicular system can be obtained by using a technique that combines injection of lipoidol ultra fluid through a catheter with macrography. In common canalicular lesions, subtraction macrodacryocystography may provide more sophisticated details.

These specific investigations are not only extremely valuable in depicting the exact location of the obstruction but they are also of help in the diagnosis of diverticula, fistulae, filling defects due to tumors, stones and infections by streptothrix species.

Scintillography (Radionuclide Testing)

This test involves the labeling of tears with gamma-emitting substances such as technetium-99m and monitoring their progress through the drainage system. This is a sophisticated and reliable test for better understanding of excretory physiology.

Color Doppler Scanography

Color Doppler scanography is the latest technique for evaluating the status of the drainage system. It is a recently introduced test with accurate results.

Chapter 5

Unique Ocular Drug Delivery Systems

Xiadong Zheng (Japan), Mary E Marquart (USA), Ashim K Mitra (USA), James M Hill* (USA)

INTRODUCTION

Drug delivery, as it pertains to ocular tissues, is defined as an approach to controlling and ultimately optimizing delivery of the drug to its target tissue in the eye or its adnexal tissues.[1] Ocular drug delivery is one of the most interesting and challenging endeavors facing ophthalmologists and pharmaceutical scientists. The anatomy, physiology, and biochemistry of the eye render this organ exquisitely impervious to foreign substances. However, the eye is vulnerable to endogenous inflammation and exogenous infectious agents, such as bacteria and viruses. Effective ocular drug delivery depends on numerous factors, such as concentration of the drug, the contact time at the corneal surface, the route of drug delivery, and the physical chemical properties of the compound. An optimal topical drug delivery system would be one that can be administered in eyedrop form with no blurred vision or irritation and that would need no more than one instillation each day to maintain therapeutic effect. The benefits to patients are simplicity, higher efficacy, lower toxicity, and minimal side effects.

Conventional ocular drug delivery systems, such as topical administration of ophthalmic suspensions, solutions, or ointment, account for 90 percent of the currently accessible marketed formulations. One of the major problems encountered with the conventional topical delivery of ophthalmic drugs is the rapid and extensive precorneal loss caused by drainage and high tear fluid turnover. After instillation of an eyedrop, in most cases only 10 percent of applied dose is absorbed.[2] Most of the applied drug is immediately diluted in the tear film and rapidly drained from the conjunctival sac to the nasolacrimal duct (tear turnover). The drainage rate becomes even higher when the formulation is irritating. Also, overflow of eyedrops onto lids and evaporation of tear film contribute to loss and waste of the drug. The ocular disposition of ophthalmic formulations is diagrammed in Figure 5.1.

*Recipient of award for the Research to prevent Blindness Senior Scientific Award

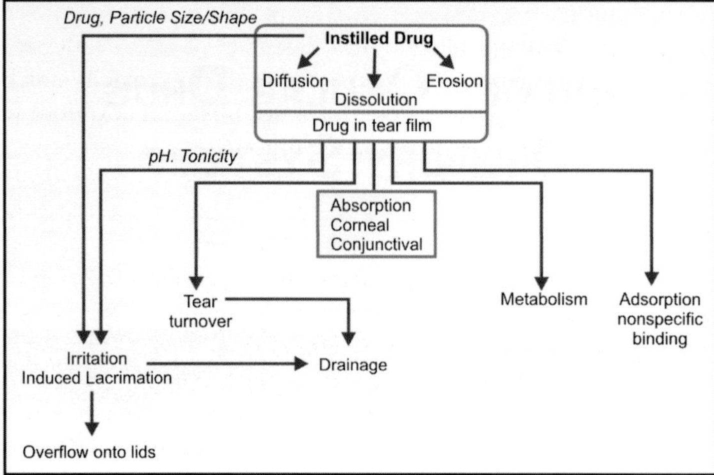

Fig. 5.1: The ocular disposition of ophthalmic formulations. About 10% of the applied drug is actually absorbed by the cornea. The majority of the drug is lost by drainage (Reprinted with permission from Mitra AK (Ed): *Ophthalmic Drug Delivery Systems*, Marcel Dekker: New York, 178, 1993)

Behind the tear film, the corneal epithelial layer is the second barrier for drug penetration. The epithelium facing the tear film is a lipophilic layer. This layer retards the diffusion of water-soluble (hydrophilic) substances through both the apical superficial cell membranes and the paracellular pathways between cells, which are filled with a continuous band of tight junctions. The stromal layer allows for relatively free diffusion of drugs because of its aqueous environment. Although lipid-soluble (hydrophobic) substances permeate cell membranes with ease, they are immiscible in the aqueous phase of the tear film. Therefore, biphasic compounds that possess both lipid and water solubility are necessary components of topical drugs for adequate penetration of the corneal barrier.[3]

All factors considered, the challenge to the formulator is to circumvent the protective barriers of the eye without causing permanent tissue damage. The specific aim of designing a drug delivery system is to achieve a sustained therapeutic concentration of medication to the targeted site(s) while bypassing healthy tissue and lowering nonproductive loss for the appropriate duration, thereby improving the ratio of effectiveness to toxicity. To date, scientists have attempted to improve the bioavailability of topical ocular drugs by extending the drug contact time, using techniques such as subconjunctival injection, application of nanoparticles, liposomes, gels, inserts, latex systems, and muco-adhesives. Others have attempted to increase specific drug penetration by using prodrugs generated by modification of the drug's chemical structure. Attempts have also been made to improve the corneal permeability of drugs by iontophoresis or transiently modifying the integrity of the corneal epithelium through chelating agents and surfactants. However, effective ocular drug delivery has never been fully achieved and drug toxicity has been an obstacle for physicians and pharmaceutical scientists. In addition, with the emergence of virulent uveitis and retinopathies that patients develop after potent immunosuppressant therapy or with acquired immunodeficiency syndrome, the traditional ophthalmic solutions, suspensions, and ointment dosage forms are clearly no longer sufficient to combat these diseases. Poor penetration, lack of specificity, and toxicity when administered in high concentrations render conventional drug delivery systems of limited use in the treatment of posterior global diseases. Therefore, the need to develop even more efficient ocular drug delivery systems is becoming urgent.

Current research in ophthalmology has greatly increased our understanding of the physiological and biochemical constraints that determine the relatively low ocular bioavailability of many drugs. Progress in the chemical and pharmaceutical industry has explored a great number of new chemical entities and novel devices for ocular delivery in experimental eye research and clinical trials. In this chapter, we introduce some representative achievements in the development of unique ocular drug delivery systems, specifically, corneal collagen shields, iontophoresis, liposomes, and dendrimers. We will also review some of the alternative ophthalmologic drug delivery systems including those that have been tested, are being refined, or are still in the developmental stages.

UNIQUE OCULAR DRUG DELIVERY SYSTEMS

Corneal Collagen Shield

Development of Collagen Shield

The development of the corneal collagen shield as an ocular drug delivery system stems from two innovative approaches in ophthalmology. The first is to use bandage shields to protect eyes from ocular insults, such as postoperative recovery from corneal transplantation, refractive surgery, and recovery from recurrent epithelial erosions after ocular infection. The second approach is to use the soft contact lens to deliver drugs across the cornea. In this procedure, the hydrophilic lens is placed on the cornea and the drug is administered topically onto the surface of the lens. The contact lens is thought to act as a drug depot, binding the drug and releasing it slowly, thereby increasing retention of the therapeutic agent in the tear film. Although these soft lenses can enhance healing and deliver drugs for an extended period while allowing the eye to remain open, their cost is relatively high. Also, the contact lens must be fitted accurately and usually needs to be inserted and removed only in the ophthalmologist's office. Furthermore, soft contact lenses could harbor ocular pathogens, which can cause secondary infection of the treated eye. In addition, the drug releasing time has been found to be relatively shorter than expected. Ocular drug delivery by soft contact lenses, therefore, is not an ideal approach to effective, safe ocular disease treatment.

Over nearly two decades, interest in the use of the collagen shield as a unique ocular drug delivery system has been intensively pursued in numerous animal experiments and clinical trials.[4-33] Of the drug delivery systems described in this chapter, only collagen shields have been used in routine clinical practice.

Principle and Properties

The corneal collagen shield is fabricated from porcine or bovine scleral tissue, which bears a collagen composition similar to that of the human cornea. Therefore, the collagen shield displays characteristics of high biocompatibility and low immunogenicity. The collagen shield is shaped like a contact lens. Multiple base curves are not necessary because the shield can easily conform to the shape of the cornea. The mechanical properties of the shield are to protect the corneal epithelium from the action of the eyelids and the collagen acts as a drug reservoir for long-term release.

The collagen shield is packaged in a dehydrated form to be rehydrated before application. Typically, the drug is loaded into the collagen shield simply by soaking the shield in the intended drug solution prior to application. The hydrated shield forms a clear, pliable, thin film approximately 0.1 mm in thickness, with a diameter of 14.5 mm and base curve of 9 mm that conforms to the corneal surface. Drug delivery by collagen shields is dependent on absorption and subsequent release of the medication by the shield. When a water-soluble drug is used for rehydration, the drug becomes trapped in the interstices of the collagen matrix. Some drugs undergo reversible binding to collagen. The shield is designed to dissolve slowly within 12, 24, or 72 hours, thereby releasing the drug. For water-insoluble drugs such as cyclosporine, the drugs need to be incorporated into the shield at the time of manufacturing.

In the manufacture of collagen shields, the ability to control the amount of crosslinking in the collagen subunits by exposure to ultraviolet (UV) light is an important physiochemical property, because the amount of crosslinking is related to the dissolution time of the shield on the corneal surface. Some of the properties of commercially available corneal collagen shields, such as Medilens and Bio-Cor 24 have been described elsewhere.[34]

The collagen shield offers the advantage of being entirely soluble so that it does not need to be removed from its site of application. Other advantages of collagen shields include prevention of delay in treatment and maintenance of high concentrations of a variety of drugs in the eye. Collagen shields avoid some of the disadvantages of bandage soft contact lenses, such as the "suck-on syndrome" and the risk of infection; neovascularization can also be prevented, as the shield seems to increase oxygen absorption as it dissolves. In addition, collagen shields have shown to cause no systemic side effects and minimal corneal surface irritation in comparison to common preservatives in conventional ophthalmic antibiotics.[35]

Therapeutic Approach in Ophthalmology

A number of studies have described the ocular pharmacokinetics of dyes such as fluorescein[4] and other drugs by collagen shields, as well as the use of collagen shields in the chemotherapy of various disorders. The drugs that have been investigated include antibiotics, such as tobramycin,[5-13] gentamicin,[6,14-19] vancomycin,[19] and ofloxacin,[20,21] antifungal agents, such as amphotericin B,[22,23] antiviral agents, such as trifluorothymidine,[24,25] anti-inflammatory agents, such as dexamethasone,[5,6,14,15,26] prednisolone,[27] anticoagulants, such as heparin,[28] and immunosuppressive agents, such as cyclosporin A.[29-32] In the majority of instances in experimental studies, there is moderate to marked improvement in ocular drug absorption. The ability of the shield to deliver a drug to the cornea adds benefit to its usual purpose of promoting wound healing.

However, some recent clinical studies have shown that the use of corneal collagen shields to prevent ocular infection is not warranted. Taravella et al,[5] for example, conducted a prospective, randomized study of 32 patients undergoing cataract surgery. Compared with the conventional eyedrop group, eyes preoperatively treated with collagen shields did not show any difference in the delivery of tobramycin-dexamethasone combination into aqueous humor. Studies by the same group also showed that collagen shields did not enhance delivery of trifluorothymidine to the corneas with intact epithelium before penetrating keratoplasty.[24] Callizo et al found that there were no differences in the time course of the healing process between control and collagen shield treated eyes after keratectomy. There was an important polymorphonuclear infiltration in shield treated eyes, indicating a subacute inflammatory immunological reaction.[33]

In addition, there are a number of difficulties related to the design and use of collagen shields. Hydrated shields are difficult to handle and need to be inserted by ophthalmologists, often producing some discomfort, and interfering with vision. Shields are not individually tailor-made to fit each patient, and therefore, expulsion of the shield may occur.[34,36]

Conclusion

The collagen shield has provided a means of delivery of a variety of medications to ocular tissues. There are many indications that the shields deliver drugs as well as, if not better, than topical drops. Because of their biological inertness, structural stability, good biocompatibility and low cost of production, collagen shields could become promising carriers for ocular drugs. However, some problems exist and the collagen shield, in its present form, is not the most ideal sustained ocular drug delivery system. Collagen shields are not indicated for most patients with conditions requiring chronic rather than acute therapy. For it to be useful in sustained drug delivery, the existing biomaterials in the collagen shield must be modified or new biomaterials must be used. Also more clinical trials are needed to further determine its clinical efficacy and safety.

Iontophoresis

Principle and Properties

Ion transfer (Greek: iontophoresis) is a procedure whereby ions are driven across a barrier by an electric current. The mechanism of iontophoresis is based on the following physical principle *like charged ions repel and oppositely charged ions attract.*

In ocular drug delivery, iontophoresis transiently modifies the integrity of the corneal epithelium or sclera, by physical means, hence facilitating the penetration of ionized drugs across or into the targeted tissues. For best delivery, the solution of medication to be iontophoresed should have a minimum of extraneous ions. The molecule to be delivered by iontophoresis should have a strong net charge: anions (negative ions) or cations (positive ions). In general, the concentration of the ionized drug in solution can range from 0.01 to 5.0 percent. Other physicochemical characteristics, such as pH, conductivity, and ionic strength of the solution, often need to be taken into consideration for the specific drug to be iontophoresed.

One major advantage of iontophoresis for drug delivery is the elimination of systemic toxicity. This procedure can deliver a high concentration of drug to the targeted tissue where it can achieve the maximum benefit with little waste or systemic absorption. This physical approach can be precisely controlled by using the directly applied current. Another advantage is the very rapid delivery with improved consistency in the drug penetration to a specific ocular site.

Device and Procedure

The iontophoretic equipment consists of a device to deliver direct current with a current meter, a rheostat to control the amount of current flowing through the system, and two electrodes. Platinum is the best material for the electrode, since it releases almost no ions, undergoes degradation at a very slow rate, and is nontoxic.

Iontophoresis can be used in ophthalmology to deliver drugs by two approaches. *Corneal iontophoresis* delivers high concentrations of a drug to the anterior segment of the eye (cornea, aqueous humor, ciliary body and lens).

In phakic eyes, the lens-iris-diaphragm limits penetration of a drug into the posterior tissues of the eye such as the posterior vitreous and retina. This barrier can be overcome by applying the current through the *pars plana (transscleral iontophoresis),* which can produce significantly high and sustained drug concentration in vitreous and retina.

Transcorneal iontophoresis: In this procedure, an eyecup, which is filled with medication, is placed over the cornea. A platinum electrode is positioned in contact with the top of the solution. To drive electropositive drugs (cations) from the eyecup solution into the cornea, the positive pole of the circuit (anode) is connected to the eyecup electrode. The negative pole (cathode) is attached to the neck, hand or ear of the subject. Figure 5.2 shows a diagram of transcorneal iontophoresis of a positively charged drug (e.g. gentamicin, epinephrine) in a rabbit eye model.

Transscleral iontophoresis: For transscleral iontophoresis, the drug solution is contained in a narrow tube within an eyecup held to the conjunctiva by suction. The tube is placed over the *pars plana* to avoid current damage to the retina. This technique circumvents the lens-iris barrier and delivers drugs into the vitreous or retina. Figure 5.3 shows a diagram of transscleral iontophoresis.

Therapeutic Approaches in Ophthalmology

Iontophoresis was employed in ophthalmology as early as 1908 by Wirtz who passed an electric current through electrolyte-saturated cotton sponges placed over the eye for the treatment of conditions such as corneal ulcers, keratitis,

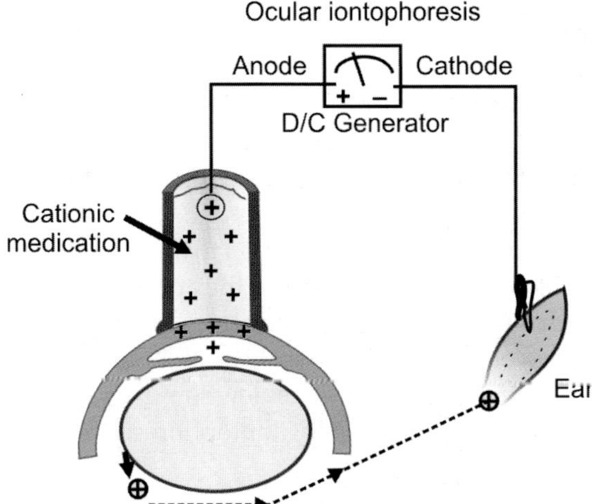

Fig. 5.2: Transcorneal iontophoresis in the rabbit. A positively-charged drug is passed through the cornea by means of a direct electric current (Reprinted with permission from AK Mitra, (Ed): *Ophthalmic Drug Delivery Systems*, Marcel Dekker: New York, 332, 1993)

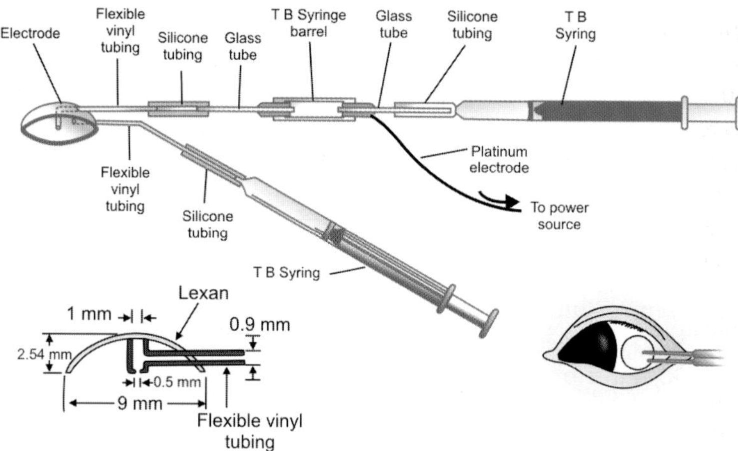

Fig. 5.3: Diagram of apparatus used for transscleral iontophoresis. Drug is delivered to the vitreous or retina by passing the drug through the conjunctiva. A syringe delivers the drug to a small eyecup that is suctioned to the conjunctiva (Reprinted with permission from AK Mitra, (Ed): *Ophthalmic Drug Delivery Systems*, Marcel Dekker: New York, 341, 1993)

and episcleritis.[37] During the first half of the twentieth century iontophoresis was used all over the world and studied extensively in the field of ophthalmology. Hill et al in the 1993 edition of the book of *Ophthalmic Drug Delivery Systems*, reviewed the use of iontophoresis in ophthalmology.[38] In general, iontophoresis has been used as a noninvasive, effective drug delivery system to deliver high concentrations of dyes, antibiotics, antifungal agents, anesthetic agents, and adrenergic agonists and antagonists. Ocular iontophoresis offers a fast, painless, safe, reliable and sustained concentration of drug delivery. Experimentally, iontophoresis has proven extremely useful as a reliable system for inducing reactivation of herpes virus in various models of this ocular disease.[39-44] Clinically, studies have found that this unique drug delivery system is promising in the delivery of dyes and drugs for a variety of ocular diseases. Within the past 10 years, in addition to the review chapter mentioned above, a number of authors have reviewed the application of iontophoresis in therapeutic approaches in ophthalmology with its advantages and disadvantages, such as Pillai et al,[45] Sasaki et al,[46] Sarraf and Lee,[47] Callegan et al.[48] In the following paragraphs, we review some of recent studies in animal models and human approaches utilizing iontophoresis as a unique ocular drug delivery system.

Studies by Frucht-Pery et al[49] showed that although higher current intensity did not significantly enhance drug concentration in the cornea, adequate bactericidal concentrations of gentamicin could be obtained in iontophoresis-treated corneas. In an animal study, Yoshizumi et al[50] found that transscleral iontophoresis of foscarnet represents a noninvasive drug delivery system for the local treatment of cytomegalovirus (CMV) retinopathy.

Frucht-Pery et al[51] also studied the distribution of gentamicin in the rabbit cornea following transcorneal iontophoresis. The highest concentration of the drug remained in the central cornea while the midperipheral cornea had higher levels than the peripheral cornea. Rieger et al[52] investigated iodine distribution in a porcine eye model following iontophoresis and found that the rank of iodine content in the ocular tissues in descending order was cornea> retina> vitreous> anterior chamber fluid> lens. This result provided evidence for the possible approach to protective, antioxidative treatment of ocular tissues by iontophoresis.

Behar-Cohen et al investigated the efficacy of the iontophoretic system in the delivery of dexamethasone for the treatment of rat endotoxin-induced uveitis. They found that iontophoretic administration of dexamethasone exerted a therapeutic effect on the posterior as well as anterior segment of the eye, and there was no clinical and histological damage caused by this technique, indicating that this system presents a safe, viable alternative to systemic administration of glucocorticoids in severe ocular inflammations.[53]

Yoshizumi et al are the first to study the ocular toxicity in multiple applications of foscarnet iontophoresis. They applied foscarnet to rabbit eyes by transscleral iontophoresis for a total of 7 regimens over a period of 21 days. Therapeutic concentrations of foscarnet in the vitreous capable of treating CMV retinitis was achieved. Electroretinography (ERG) and slit-lamp biomicroscopy revealed no evidence of ocular toxicity, indicating multiple applications of transscleral iontophoresis can safely deliver high concentrations of the drug into vitreous.[54]

Another potential application of iontophoresis worth mentioning is the delivery of dyes for gonioscopic pulsed dye laser sclerostomy. Studies have been reported in which dyes were delivered to the sclera by transscleral iontophoresis. Grossman et al[55] delivered methylene blue into rabbit eyes, Melamed et al[56] delivered methylene blue into the sclera of glaucoma patients, and Sarraf et al[57] delivered reactive black 5 dye into rabbit eyes. These three studies reported the delivery of a pulsed dye laser beam to the stained area through a goniolens to treat glaucoma. Iontophoresis was used to effectively deliver dyes into sclera. This system is technically feasible and could be a viable adjunct to pulsed dye laser sclerostomy procedures in ophthalmology.

Conclusion

Iontophoresis offers a unique ocular drug delivery system that is fast, painless, safe, and, in most cases, results in the delivery of a high concentration of the drug to a specific target tissue. In glaucoma studies, iontophoresis applications include fluorescein to study aqueous humor dynamics,[58-60] adrenergic agents for treatment of glaucoma,[61,64] and 5-fluorouracil for control of cellular proliferation after glaucoma surgery.[65] In ocular anesthesia, iontophoresis can be used before ocular surgery.[66,67] In the treatment of ocular infections, antibiotics and antifungal agents can be delivered transcorneally or transsclerally according to the site of infection.[68-72] In the treatment of ocular inflammation, steroids can be delivered efficiently to animal or human eyes.[53,73,74] In the treatment and study of ocular herpes simplex virus infection, antivirals and adrenergic agents have been tested in various animal models.[39-44] In addition, alternative substrates have been tested for the diagnosis and/or treatment of ocular disorders.[75,76] However, this procedure is not a panacea for all eye disorders, but has importance for those substances that are not amenable to topical delivery and require repeated administration over an extended period of time. The role of iontophoresis in the field of clinical ophthalmology is currently being redefined. With this renewed interest, more and more clinical approaches utilizing this unique ocular drug delivery system need to be tested before it becomes a routine clinical procedure to treat patients.

Liposomes

Principle and Property

Liposomes are microscopic vesicles formed when certain phospholipid molecules interact to form a lipid bilayer in an aqueous environment. According to their size, liposomes are known as either small unilamellar vesicles (SUV; 10-100 nm) or large unilamellar vesicles (LUV; >100-3000 nm). If more bilayers are present, they are referred to as multilamellar vesicles (MLV). All the vesicles share the property of a liquid crystalline bilayer, similar to an outer cell membrane. Depending on the composition, liposomes can have a positive, negative, or neutral surface charge.[77]

Figure 5.4 depicts two commonly used methods for liposome preparation, sonication and reverse phase evaporation. Since liposomes are composed of lipids similar to those present in biological membranes, they are expected to be biocompatible and biodegradable. If the liposomes are formed in the presence of a drug, the drug will be incorporated into either the aqueous compartment or the lipid layer depending on its solubility. Thus, liposomes can accommodate both hydrophilic and lipophilic compounds.

A drug can be incorporated into a liposome in several ways depending on its chemical properties. In general, a water-soluble drug is dissolved in the aqueous phase in the interior compartment, whereas a more hydrophobic drug may be incorporated into the lipid bilayer itself, forming part of the vesicle membrane. The oil/water partition coefficient of the drug determines the stability of the drug in the liposome.

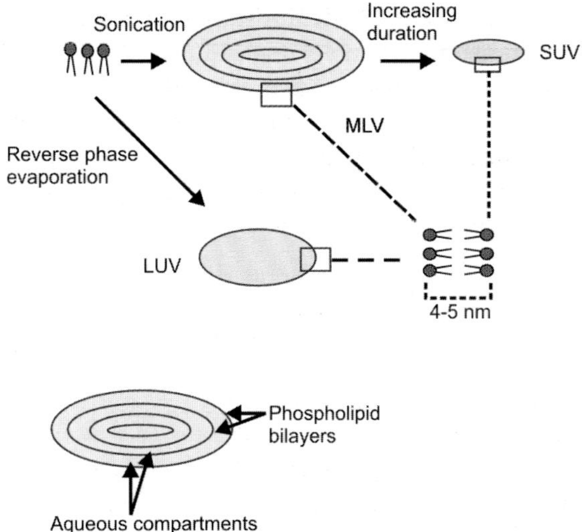

Fig. 5.4: Liposome preparation. Liposomes are made by constructing phospholipid bilayers into spherical structures containing hydrophilic molecules in an inner aqueous compartment, or hydrophobic molecules within the lipid bilayer. Sonication produces multilamellar vesicles (MLV) or small unilamellar vesicles (SUV). Reverse phase evaporation produces large unilamellar vesicles (LUV) (Reprinted with permission from AK Mitra, (Ed): *Ophthalmic Drug Delivery Systems*, Marcel Dekker: New York, 290, 1993)

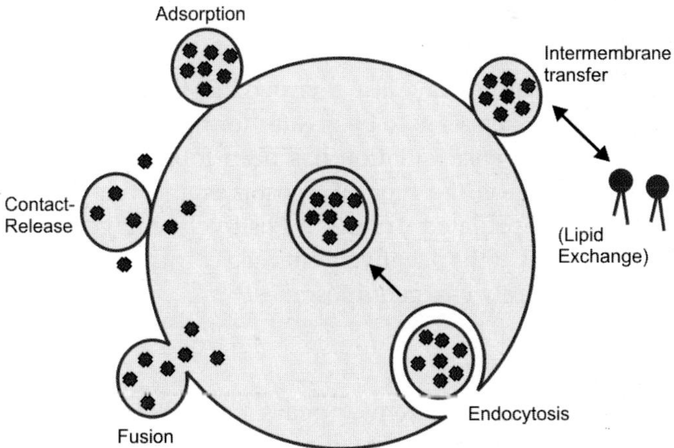

Fig. 5.5: Possible liposome-cell interactions (Reprinted with permission from AK Mitra, (Ed): *Ophthalmic Drug Delivery Systems*, Marcel Dekker: New York, 293, 1993)

Probable mechanisms by which liposomes interact with cells include: (i) intermembrane transfer; (ii) contact release; (iii) adsorption of the liposome to the cell surface via nonspecific means or specific ligands such as antibodies, hormones, and lectins; (iv) fusion of the liposomes with the cell membranes and (v) endocytosis of the liposomes by the cell (Fig. 5.5).

Therapeutic Approaches in Ophthalmology

Liposomes have been widely studied for nearly two decades with the objective of increasing the specificity of action of drugs towards specific targets, to facilitate the bioavailability of drugs through biological membranes, or to protect a drug against enzyme inactivation. Their use in topical administration and especially in ocular administration has not received as much attention as other routes of administration.[77]

Although there is no commercially available product for repeated application in the eye, this colloidal system has been intensively studied as a means to improve and facilitate corneal drug transport. A great number of drugs and even some types of genes have been tested in this unique drug delivery system by experimental research or clinical trials.[35,77-81]

Three approaches have attempted utilizing liposomes as drug delivery systems: (i) topical application;[82-85] (ii) subconjunctival and intravitreal injection,[86-91] and (iii) targeting liposomal drug release with antibody,[92,93] laser,[94-96] and microwave radiation.[97,98] Most of the results have indicated that liposomes as drug carriers provide the possibility of controlled selective drug delivery and improved bioavailability. However, their usefulness is hindered by short shelf-life, limited drug loading capacity, and difficulty in sterilizing the drug preparations[35,77,81]

In addition, these studies have also revealed that the potential of liposomes in ocular drug delivery appears to be greater for lipophilic than hydrophilic compounds. Liposome encapsulation has been found to alter ocular drug disposition depending on the type of liposomes and the physicochemical properties of the encapsulated drug.[99,100] Positively charged liposomes are preferentially captured at the negatively charged corneal surface as compared with neutral or negatively charged liposomes.[101]

Conclusion

Liposomal drug delivery system appears to have potential for ocular applications on the basis of studies in animal models. Liposomes can be easily prepared from nontoxic lipid materials, which are nonirritant and do not obscure vision. Although the potential of liposomes in ocular drug delivery appears greater for lipophilic than hydrophilic compounds, liposomes as drug carriers provide the possibility of controlled and selective drug delivery and improved bioavailability. Further research is needed to refine the procedures for use in humans and to elucidate the various parameters, which may influence the liposome as a means of ocular drug delivery.

Dendrimers

Property and Principle

In the past decade, a new macromolecular architecture has been developed. This new architecture mimics the dendritic branching of trees and is referred to as dendrimers, dendrons or dendrigrafts.[102-105] Dendrimers are different from all other classical synthetic polymers both by their unprecedented structure control, as well as by the fact that they are solvent-soluble, covalently fixed, three-dimensional megamolecules.[102] This unique macromolecular structure has been referred to as the fourth inventive architectural class of polymer that chemists have developed this century.

Dendrimers can be designed to mimic proteins and also be made in very robust forms to withstand both severe thermal and hydrolytic conditions. They are indeed reminiscent of biological cells, displaying three major architectural components: a core, an interior and a surface (Fig. 5.6).

One of the most remarkable features of dendrimers is that these molecules are nanoscale in size and shape. The compounds closely match the sizes and contours of many important proteins and bioassemblies. For example, insulin (≅30A), cytochrome C (≅40A) and hemoglobin (≅55A) are roughly the same

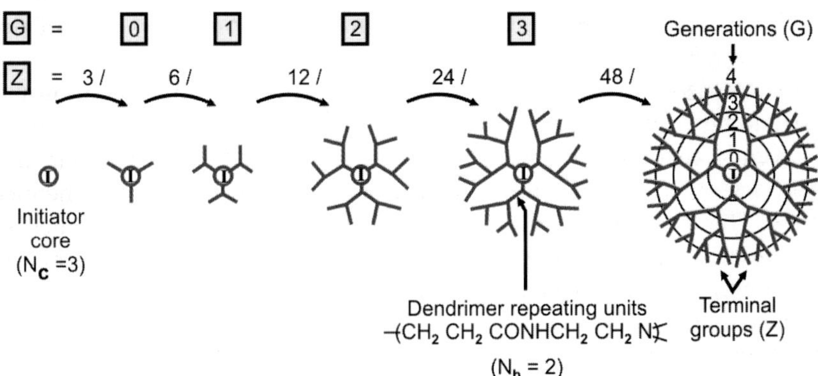

Fig. 5.6: Dendrimer formation. Through successive generations (G), terminal chemical groups (Z) are added to a starting structure, the initiator core. The initiator core depicted is one that allows three terminal groups to be added onto it in the first generation, G_0. Each generation allows two more terminal groups to be added to each terminal group from the preceding generation. By the fourth generation (G_3), there are 48 terminal groups. (Kindly provided by Donald A Tomalia, Michigan Molecular Institute, Ann Arbor, Michigan)

size and shape, respectively, as generations 3, 4 and 5 of ammonia core, PAMAM (polyamidoamines) dendrimers.[102-105]

Another important asset of dendrimers is their ability to present functional groups or be transformed into a wide variety of nanoscaled chemical surfaces. Nanoscopic reagents such as DNA, antibodies or proteins have been combined with dendrimers to produce new gene delivery vectors.[106-110] This architectural function of the dendrimer is related to its guest-host, containment property, known as the "dendrimer box". There are now numerous examples demonstrating the cargo space that can be found in various dendrimer families. For example, the PAMAM dendrimers can host as much as three times the weight of aspirin or agricultural chemicals compared with dendrimer weight. Very recent research has shown that this space has unique shape-specific recognition properties for guest molecules that will undoubtedly offer exciting options for "smart drug delivery" systems.[102,105]

Potential Application of a Unique Drug Delivery System

One practical use of dendrimers in medicine is in gene therapy. Dendrimers can be made into the size and shape of histones, the proteins that carry DNA in cells. In an *in vitro* experiment, Tomalia et al has combined histone-like dendrimers and the luciferase gene with close to 30 different types of cells from various species, including humans. In nearly all cases, the dendrimers successfully transported genetic material into the cells and luciferase protein was expressed as a reporter. Although the exact mechanisms of how this dendrimer-DNA unit delivers the DNA of interest into cells has not been completely determined, this research shows the promising avenue of new gene therapy.[105] The profound advantages of this unique system include great capacity of delivery, nontoxicity, and non-immunogenicity, unlike conventional modified viral vectors.

Recently, many research teams are developing techniques for transporting other classes of drug molecules to selected targets in the body including ocular tissues. The dissolution of water insoluble ibuprofen in dendrimer host molecules clearly demonstrates the exciting potential in this area. Esfand *et al* have shown that the aqueous solubility of ibuprofen increases significantly in the presence of dendrimers.[111] Other related researches include the study of biodistribution of lipidic peptide dendrimer carrier after oral administration in rats,[112] an *in vitro* study of the interaction of synthetic oligonucleotide with mycobacteria after treatment of fourth generation dendrimers,[113] and a study of antisense pharmacology in the potential treatment of cancer.[106] For the practicing ophthalmologist, drug-releasing dendrimers are an emerging area of intense research activity and not an available technology.

Conclusion

Dendrimers are one of the most important and exciting contributions in synthetic chemical and pharmaceutical areas preceding the 21st century. The application of this unique macromolecular structure as means of gene and drug delivery is promising. Following optimization, these supermolecules whose properties can be made to order and easy and rapid to perform could launch a significant new industry in medicine. We look forward to an extensive exploration of the study of this unique drug delivery system.

OTHER OCULAR DRUG DELIVERY SYSTEMS

Pumps

Pumps are small devices that deliver drugs to the eye via a tube for extended periods of time. These devices are usually designed small enough to be implanted in the subcutaneous space and do not need an external power source or battery. The tube is passed from the pump to the eye through a subcutaneous tunnel. The distal end of the tube can be located in the conjunctival sac, corneal stroma, anterior chamber, or vitreous.

Various types of pumps have been tested or are being invented. Pumps can be made to fit different tissue structures and for different durations of drug delivery. The following are a few examples.

Two-chamber Pump

One chamber contains the drug in aqueous solution and the other a charging solution. The charging fluid is in liquid-gas equilibrium that expands at body temperature driving the drug at a constant flow rate. An example is *Infusaid* pump (Metal Bellows Corporation, Sharon, MA).

Osmotic Pump

Such a pump is driven by osmotic imbibition of extracellular water. This pump can deliver fluid for up to 7 days. An example is *Alzet* osmotic minipump (Alza Corporation, Palo Alto, CA).

Adjustable Pump

Adjustable pump contains a miniaturized pump and a port for transcutaneous refilling. One unique feature of this pump is that if used in the clinic, the patient can release a preset quantity of intended drug by finger pressure on the modular miniature plunger as required. An example is *TI-DDS (totally implantable drug delivery system,* Micro Infusions Systeme GmbH, Bruhlstr, Germany).

Although a variety of pumps have been studied in animal models for their possible applications in ocular drug delivery systems, and some promising results have been obtained (i.e. sustained, high concentrations of drugs in targeted tissues),[114-119] pumps have not gained wide acceptance in practical clinical ophthalmology. The surgical procedure required for their insertion and potential problems with infection and extrusion limit their usefulness.

Ocular Inserts

Ocular inserts are unique devices made for extended duration of drug delivery and maintenance of an effective drug concentration in the target tissues.[120] Usually they are small enough to be inserted into the cul-de-sac of the conjunctiva or vitreous. Corneal collagen shields that have been described earlier in this chapter are considered to be ocular inserts. The ocular pump may be considered as a form of ocular insert. The general characteristics of ocular inserts are listed and some specific types of inserts are described.

Criteria for Successful Ocular Inserts

- Comfort and noninterference with vision
- Sufficient oxygen permeability
- Biocompatibility and stability
- Reproducibility of release kinetics
- Applicability to a variety of drugs
- Ease of sterility and nontoxicity
- Ease of handling (insertion and removal)
- Ease of manufacture and low cost.

Although most of the above features are not unique to ocular drug delivery systems, a few of them are required by all controlled-release devices.[120]

In general, ocular inserts can be made erodible or nonerodible. Compared to erodible ocular inserts, the advantages of nonerodible ocular inserts are: (i) better release kinetics of drug; (ii) ease of detection when they are expelled, and (iii) greater reliability. The disadvantage is that the nonerodible insert has to be removed after the intended drug delivery period.

Some marketed nonerodible ocular inserts include contact lenses and the ocusert®. Erodible ocular inserts include the Lacrisert®, the SODI (soluble ocular drug insert) and collagen shield. These devices are currently being used in ophthalmic clinics and they are reviewed in a variety of articles.[120-122]

Another development of ocular inserts is the minidisk, which is made like a miniature contact lens. The diameter of the minidisk is between 4 and 5 mm, which allows the device to be easily placed behind the lower or upper eyelid without compromising comfort, vision, or oxygen permeability. Minidisks can also be prepared from erodible or nonerodible polymers, and the nonerodible minidisk has hydrophilic and hydrophobic types.

In summary, ocular inserts have shown some efficacy for prolonged-release ocular drug delivery. However, some of the devices are not accepted universally by all patients due to discomfort and high dosing frequencies. To completely meet the criteria of successful ocular inserts, there are still many experimental and clinical studies that need to be done. The physical and chemical design of the ocular inserts have to be refined in order to optimize the device and eliminate current problems.

Particulate Polymers

Particulate polymeric drug delivery system refers to nano- (< 1 µm) and microparticles (≥ 1 µm), which are designed to be used to reduce the precorneal elimination rate from the eye and hence increase the extent of ocular absorption.[123-126] The upper size limit for microparticles for ophthalmic administration is about 5 to 10 mm. Above this size, a scratching feeling will occur after topical application, which causes the microparticles not to be suitable for ophthalmic use.

Nanoparticles are produced by emulsion polymerization. Polyalkylcyanoacrylates are the most frequently used ophthalmologic nanoparticles.[123] The binding of drugs depends on the physicochemical properties of the drugs as well as of the nano- or microparticle polymer and also on the manufacturing process for these vehicles. In most experimental studies, the drug absorption in the eye is enhanced significantly in comparison with conventional eyedrops owing to the much slower ocular elimination rates of the particles from the cul-de-sac. For instance, several antiglaucoma drugs have been successfully loaded onto nanoparticles for testing the drug delivery efficacy.[77,123-129]

Because smaller particles are better tolerated by patients, nanoparticles may become very comfortable ophthalmic prolonged-action drug delivery systems. However, more clinical trials of a variety of drugs need to be done for optimization of this unique ocular drug delivery system.

Mucoadhesive Polymers

Mucoadhesive (bioadhesive) ocular drug delivery system refers to applying natural or synthesized polymers to the corneal surface, where the dosage form adheres to the precorneal mucus and resides in the eye until the polymer dissolves or the mucin replaces itself. One obvious advantage of the mucoadhesive device is prolongation of drug release for ocular tissues, hence increasing the drug bioavailability.

A number of studies have been done regarding the issues of chemical structure and biophysical properties of mucoadhesive polymers relevant to their ocular drug delivery ability. Some representative mucoadhesives with good mucoadhesive performance include carboxymethylcellulose, carbopol, polymethylmethacrylate, acrylic acid, polycarbophil and sodium alginate. So far, mucoadhesives have shown some promising and beneficial properties as a unique ocular drug delivery system.[77,130,131]

Since the potential of a mucoadhesive agent is determined by a number of parameters, such as chain length, configuration, and molecular weight and electronic charges, the research on mucoadhesives is still in its early stages and further advances in understanding and manipulation of the dosage form are necessary to translate this unique drug delivery system into practical application in controlled drug delivery.

Penetration Enhances

One of the principal problems in ocular drug delivery is relatively low permeability of a drug across the ocular surface. Enhancement of drug penetration through intercellular junctions or the cell membrane is one solution.

Substances used to enhance corneal penetration of ophthalmic drugs include surfactants, bile acids, fatty acid, preservatives, and chelating agents. The mechanisms of action of enhancers include: (i) cytoskeletal modulation of corneal permeability; (ii) alteration of tight cellular junctions by promoting glucose or amino acid with sodium cotransport; and (iii) change of drug charge type or charge density for enhanced absorption, etc.[40,132]

Penetration enhancers have not been extensively studied to date. Since the eye is very sensitive to most penetration enhancers and these compounds are required to be pharmacologically inert, chemically stable, specific and nonsensitizing, more research is needed to develop new penetration enhancers with a high specificity of action and minimal local and systemic toxicity.

CONCLUSIONS AND NEW PERSPECTIVES

For over a century ophthalmologists and pharmacologists have been searching for the best ocular drug delivery system that can provide a sustained therapeutic concentration of a drug at targeted tissue in a safe and highly efficient way. Although only very few ophthalmic drug delivery systems have been commercialized and are currently available in clinic, research on new drug delivery systems has definitely provided an important dynamism as never before, with the promise of new and exciting directions. With further research on the understanding of the physiological and biochemical constraints that determine the relatively low ocular bioavailability of many drugs, we look forward to the development of new, unique ocular drug delivery systems that can eventually be widely used in clinic to benefit patients.

REFERENCES

1. Schoenwald RD. Ocular drug delivery. Clin Pharmacokinet 1990;18:255-69.
2. Mitra AK. Ophthalmic Drug Delivery Systems. Marcel Dekker: New York, 1993.

3. Klyce SD, Beuerman RW. Structure and function of the cornea. In Kaufman HE, Barron BM, McDonald MB (Eds): The Cornea (2nd edn) Butterworth-Heinemann: Boston, 1998;3-50.
4. Reidy JJ, Limberg M, Kaufman HE. Delivery of fluorescein to the anterior chamber using the corneal collagen shield. Ophthalmology 1990;97:1201-03.
5. Taravella M, Stepp P, Young D. Collagen shield delivery of tobramycin to the human eye. CLAO J 1998;24:166-68.
6. Mahlberg K, Krootila K, Uusitalo R. Compatibility of corticosteroids and antibiotics in combination. J Cataract Refract Surg 1997;23:878-82.
7. Chen CC, Takruri H, Duzman E. Enhancement of the ocular bioavailability of topical tobramycin with use of a collagen shield. J Cataract Refract Surg 1993;19:242-45.
8. Clinch TE, Hobden JA, Hill JM, et al. Collagen shields containing tobramycin for sustained therapy (24 hours) of experimental Pseudomonas keratitis. CLAO J 1992;18:245-47.
9. Assil KK, Zarnegar SR, Fouraker BD, et al. Efficacy of tobramycin-soaked collagen shields vs. tobramycin eyedrop loading dose for sustained treatment of experimental Pseudomonas aeruginosa-induced keratitis in rabbits. Am J Ophthalmol 1992;113:418-23.
10. Unterman SR, Rootman DS, Hill JM, et al. Collagen shield drug delivery: Therapeutic concentrations of tobramycin in the rabbit cornea and aqueous humor. J Cataract Refract Surg 1988;14:500-4.
11. Poland DE, Kaufman HE. Clinical uses of collagen shields. J Cataract Refract Surg 1988;14:489-91.
12. Sawusch MR, O'Brien TP, Dick JD, et al. Use of collagen corneal shields in the treatment of bacterial keratitis. Am J Ophthalmol 1988;106:279-81.
13. O'Brien TP, Sawusch MR, Dick JD, et al. Use of collagen corneal shields versus soft contact lenses to enhance penetration of topical tobramycin. J Cataract Refract Surg 1988;14:505-07.
14. Milani JK, Verbukh I, Pleyer U, et al. Collagen shields impregnated with gentamicin-dexamethasone as a potential drug delivery device. Am J Ophthalmol 1993;116:622-27.
15. Renard G, Bennani N, Lutaj P, et al. Comparative study of a collagen corneal shield and a subconjunctival injection at the end of cataract surgery. J Cataract Refract Surg 1993;19:48-51.
16. Silbiger J, Stern GA. Evaluation of corneal collagen shields as a drug delivery device for the treatment of experimental Pseudomonas keratitis. Ophthalmology 1992;99:889-92.
17. Liang FQ, Viola RS, del Cerro M, et al. Noncross-linked collagen discs and cross-linked collagen shields in the delovery of gentamicin to rabbit eyes. Invest Ophthalmol Vis Sci 1992;33:2194-98.
18. Baziuk N, Gremillion CM Jr, Peyman GA, et al. Colagen shields and intraocular drug delivery: Concentration of gentamicin in the aqueous and vitreous of a rabbit eye after lensectomy and vitrectomy. Int Ophthalmol 1992;16:101-07.
19. Phinney RB, Schwartz SD, Lee DA, et al. Collagen-shield delivery of gentamicin and vancomycin. Arch Ophthalmol 1988;106:1599-604.
20. Taravella MJ, Balentine J, Young DA, et al. Collagen shield delivery of ofloxacin to the human eye. J Cataract Refract Surg 1999;25:562-65.

21. Kuwano M, Horibe Y, Kawashima Y. Effect of collagen cross-linking in collagen corneal shields on ocular drug delivery. J Ocul Pharmacol Ther 1997;13:31-40.
22. Pleyer U, Legmann A, Mondino BJ, et al. Use of collagen shields containing amphotericin B in the treatment of experimental *Candida albicans*-induced keratomycosis in rabbits. Am J Ophthalmol 1992;113:303-08.
23. Schwartz SD, Harrison SA, Engstrom RE Jr, et al. Collagen shield delivery of amphotericin B. Am J Ophthalmol 1990;109:701-04.
24. Kuster P, Taravella M, Gelinas M, et al. Delivery of trifluridine to human cornea and aqueous humor using collagen shields. CLAO J 1998;24:122-24.
25. Gussler JR, Ashton P, van Meter WS, et al. Collagen shield delivery of trifluorothymidine. J Cataract Refract Surg 1990;16:719-22.
26. Hwang DG, Stern WH, Hwang PH, et al. Collagen shield enhancement of topical dexamethasone penetration. Arch Ophthalmol 1989;107:1375-80.
27. Sawusch MR, O'Brien TP, Updegraff SA. Collagen corneal shields enhance penetration of topical prednisolone acetate. J Cataract Refract Surg 1989;15: 625-28.
28. Murray TG, Stern WH, Chin DH, et al. Collagen shield heparin delivery for prevention of postoperative fibrin. Arch Ophthalmol 1990;108:104-06.
29. Kanpolat A, Batioglu F, Yilmaz M, et al. Penetration of cyclosporin A into the rabbit cornea and aqueous humor after topical drop and collagen shield administration. CLAO J 1994;20:119-22.
30. Kaufman HE. New approaches in topical drug administration and treatment of the dry eye. Klinische Monatsblatter fur Augenheilkunde 1993;202:195-98.
31. Reidy JJ, Gebhardt BM, Kaufman HE. The collagen shield. A new vehicle for delivery of cyclosporin A to the eye. Cornea 1990;9:196-99.
32. Chen YF, Gebhardt BM, Reidy JJ, et al. Cyclosporine-containing collagen shields suppress corneal allograft rejection. Am J Ophthalmol 1990;109:132-37.
33. Callizo J, Cervello I, Mayayo E, et al. Inefficacy of collagen shield in the rabbit corneal wound-healing process. Cornea 1996;15(258):262.
34. Hill JM, O'Callaghan RJ, Hobden JA, et al. Corneal collagen shields for ocular delivery. In Mitra AK (Ed). Ophthalmic Drug Delivery Systems. Marcel Dekker: New York, 1993;261-73.
35. Shofner RS, Kaufman HE, Hill JM. New horizons in ocular drug delivery. Ophthalmol Clin North Am 1989;2:15-24.
36. Kaufman HE, Steinemann TL, Thompson HW, et al. Collagen-based drug delivery and artificial tear. J Ocul Pharmacol 1994;10:17-27.
37. Wirtz R. Die ionentherapie in der augenheilkunde. Klin Monatsbl Augenheilkd 1908;46:543-79.
38. Hill JM, O'Callaghan RJ, Hobden JA. Ocular iontophoresis. In Mitra AK (Ed): Ophthalmic Drug Delivery Systems. Marcel Dekker: New York, 331-54, 1993 .
39. Zheng X, Marquart ME, Loutsch JM, et al. HSV-1 migration in latently infected and naive rabbits after penetrating keratoplasty. Invest Ophthalmol Vis Sci 1999;40:2490-97.
40. Gangarosa LP Sr, Ozawa A, Ohkido M, et al. Iontophoresis for enhancing penetration of dermatologic and antiviral drugs. J Dermatol 1995;22:865-75.
41. Rootman DS, Haruta Y, Hill JM. Reactivation of HSV-1 in primates by transcorneal iontophoresis of adrenergic agents. Invest Ophthalmol Vis Sci 1990;31:597-600.
42. Hill JM, Haruta Y, Rootman DS. Adrenergically induced recurrent HSV-1 corneal epithelial lesions. Curr Eye Res 1987;6:1065-71.

43. Hill JM, Rayfield MA, Haruta Y. Strain specificity of spontaneous and adrenergically induced HSV-1 ocular reactivation in latently infected rabbits. Curr Eye Res 1987;6:91-97.
44. Willey DE, Trousdale MD, Newburn AB. Reactivation of murine latent HSV infection by epinephrine iontophoresis. Invest Ophthalmol Vis Sci 1984;25: 945-50.
45. Pillai O, Nair V, Poduri R, et al. Transdermal iontophoresis. Part II: Peptide and protein delivery. Methods Find.Exp.Clin Pharmacol 1999;21(3):229-40.
46. Sasaki H, Yamamura K, Mukai T, et al. Enhancement of ocular drug penetration. Crit Rev Ther Drug Carrier Syst 1999;16:85-146.
47. Sarraf D, Lee DA. The role of iontophoresis in ocular drug delivery. J Ocular Pharm 1994;10:69-81.
48. Callegan MC, O'Callaghan RJ, Hill JM. Pharmacokinetic considerations in the treatment of bacterial keratitis. Clin Pharmacokinet 1994;27:129-49.
49. Frucht-Pery J, Solomon A Doron R, Ever-Hadani P, et al. Efficacy of iontophoresis in the rat cornea. Graefe's Arch Clin Exp Ophthalmol 1996;234:765-69.
50. Yoshizumi MO, Lee DA, Sarraf DA, et al. Ocular toxicity of iontophoretic foscarnet in rabbits. J Ocul Pharmacol Ther 1995;11:183-89.
51. Frucht-Pery J, Goren D, Solomon A, et al. The distribution of gentamicin in the rabbit cornea following iontophoresis to the central cornea. J Ocular Pharm Therapeut 1999;15(3):251-56.
52. Rieger G, Winkler R, Buchberger W, et al. Iodine distribution in a porcine eye model following iontophoresis. Ophthalmologica 1995;209:84-87.
53. Behar-Cohen FF, Parel JM, Pouliquen Y, et al. Iontophoresis of dexamethasone in the treatment of endotoxin-induced-uveitis in rats. Exp Eye Res 1997;65: 533-45.
54. Yoshizumi MO, Dessouki A, Lee DA, et al. Determination of ocular toxicity in multiple applications of Foscarnet iontophoresis. J Ocular Pharmcol Therapeut 1997;13(6):529-36.
55. Grossman RE, Sarraf D, Lee DA. Iontophoresis of methylene blue for gonioscopic pulsed dye laser sclerostomy. J Ocul Pharmacol 1993;9:277-85.
56. Melamed S, Solomon A, Neumann D, et al. Internal sclerostomy using laser ablation of dyed sclera in glaucoma patients: A pilot study. Br J Ophthalmol 1993;77:139-44.
57. Sarraf D, Lee DA. Iontophoresis of reactive black 5 for pulsed dye laser sclerostomy. J Ocul Pharmacol Ther 1993;9:25-33.
58. Jones RF, Maurice DM. New methods of measuring the rate of aqueous flow in man with fluorescein. Exp Eye Res 1966;5:208-20.
59. Starr PAJ. Changes in aqueous flow determined by fluorophotometry. Tans Ophthalmol Soc UK 1966;86:639-46.
60. Holm O. A photogrammetric method for estimation of the pupillary aqueous flow from the living human eye. Acta Ophthalmol 1968;46:254-77.
61. Kitazawa Y, Horie T. Denervation supersensitivity induced by chemical sympathectomy with 6-hydroxydopamine. Jpn J Ophthalmol 1974;18:109-18.
62. Kitazawa Y, Nose H, Horie T. Chemical sympathectomy with 6-hydroxy-dopamine in the treatment of primary open-angle glaucoma. Am J Ophthalmol 1975;79:98-103.
63. Watanabe H, Levene RZ, Bernstein MR. 6-hydroxydopamine therapy in glaucoma. Trans Am Acad Ophthalmol Otolaryngol 1977;83:69-77.

64. Colasanti BK, Trotter RR. Enhanced ocular penetration of the methyl ester of alpha-methyl-para-tyrosine after iontophoresis. Arch Int Pharmacodyn Ther 1977;228:171-76.
65. Kondo M, Araie M. Iontophoresis of 5-fluorouracil into the conjunctiva and sclera. Invest Ophthalmol Vis Sci 1989;30:583-85.
66. Sisler HA. Iontophoretic local anesthesia for conjunctival surgery. Ann Ophthalmol 1978;10:597-98.
67. Meyer DR, Lindberg JV, Vasquez RJ. Iontophoresis for eyelid anesthesia. Ophthalmic Surg 1990;21:845-48.
68. Rootman DS, Jantzen JA, Gonzalez JR, et al. Pharmacokinetics and safety of transcorneal iontophoresis of tobramycin in the rabbit. Invest Ophthalmol Vis Sci 1988;29:1397-1401.
69. Hodben JA, Reidy JJ, O'Callaghan RJ, et al. Ciprofloxacin iontophoresis for aminoglycoside-resistant Pseudomonas keratitis. Invest Ophthalmol Vis Sci accepted, 1990.
70. Choi TB, Lee DA. Transscleral and transcorneal iontophoresis of vancomycin in rabbit eyes. J Ocular Pharmacol 1988;4:153-64.
71. Barza MM, Peckman C, Baum J. Transcleral iontophoresis of gentamicin in monkeys. Invest Ophthalmol Vis Sci 1987;28:1033-36.
72. Church AL, Barza M, Baum J. An improved apparatus for transcleral iontophoresis of gentamicin. Invest Ophthalmol Vis Sci 1992;33:3543-45.
73. Lachaud JP. Considerations on the use of corticosteroids by ionization in certain ocular diseases. Bull des Societes D'Ophthalmologie de France 1965;65:84-89.
74. Lam TT, Edward DP, Zhu X, et al. Transcleral iontophoresis of dexamethasone. Arch Ophthalmol 1989;107:1368-71.
75. Asahara T, Shinomiya K, Naito T, et al. Induction of genes into the rabbit eye by iontophoresis. Acta Soc Ophthalmol Jpn 1999;103:178-85.
76. Shimomura Y. Iontophoresis for postherpetic neuralgia. Folia Ophthalmol Jpn 1987;38:175-82.
77. Bourlais CL, Liliane A, Hosein Z, et al. Ophthalmic drug delivery system—recent advances. Prog Retin Eye Res 1998;17:33-58.
78. Reimer K, Fleischer W, Brogmann B, et al. Povidone-iodine liposomes—an overview. Dermatology 1997;195(Suppl 2):93-99.
79. Desmettre T, Mordon S, Soulie S, et al. Liposome in ophthalmology. Review of the literature. J Francais d Ophthalmol 1996;19:716-31.
80. Niesman MR. The use of liposomes as drug carriers in ophthalmology. Crit Rev Ther Drug Carrier Syst 1992;9:1-38.
81. Langer R. New methods of drug delivery. Science 1990;249:1527-33.
82. Pleyer U, Elkins B, Ruckert D, et al. Ocular absorption of cyclosporine A from liposomes incorporated into collagen shields. Curr Eye Res 1994;13:177-81.
83. Velpandian T, Gupta SK, Gupta YK, et al. Ocular drug targeting by liposomes and their corneal interactions. J Microencapsulation 1999;16(2):243-50.
84. Whitcup SM, Pleyer U, Lai JC, et al. Topical liposome-encapsulated FK506 for the treatment of endotoxin-induced uveitis. Ocul Immunol Inflamm 1998;6: 51-56.
85. Milani JK, Pleyer U, Dukes A, et al. Prolongation of corneal allograft survival with liposome-encapsulated cyclosporine in the rat eye. Ophthalmology 1993; 100:890-96.

86. Van der Veen G, Broersma L, Dijkstra CD, et al. Prevention of corneal allograft rejection in rats treated with subconjunctival injections of liposomes containing dichloromethylene diphosphonate. Invest Ophthalmol Vis Sci 1994;35:305-15.
87. Assil KK, Frucht-Perry J, Ziegler E, et al. Tobramycin liposomes. Single subconjunctival therapy of pseudomonal keratitis. Invest Ophthalmol Vis Sci 1991;32: 3216-20.
88. Wiechens B, Grammer JB, Johannsen U, et al. Experimental intravitreal application of ciprofloxacin in rabbits. Ophthalmologica 1999;213:120-28.
89. Garcia-Arumi J, Pascual R, Fonseca MJ, et al. Pharmacokinetics and retinal toxicity of intravitreal liposome-encapsulated 5-fluorouridine. Ophthalmologica 1997;211: 344-50.
90. Akula SK, Ma PE, Peyman GA, et al. Treatment of cytomegalovirus retinitis with intravitreal injection of liposome encapsulated ganciclovir in a patient with AIDS. Br J Ophthalmol 1994;78:677-80.
91. Salah-Eldin M, Peyman GA, el-Aswad M, et al. Evaluation of toxicity and efficacy of a combination of antineoplastic agents in the prevention of PVR. Int Ophthalmol 1994;18:53-60.
92. Norley SG, Sendele D, Huang L, et al. Inhibition of herpes simplex virus replication in the mouse cornea by drug containing immunoliposomes. Invest Ophthalmol Vis Sci 1987;28:591-95.
93. Norley SG, Huang L, Rouse BT. Targeting of drug loaded immunoliposomes to herpes simples virus infected corneal cells: An effective means of inhibiting virus replication *in vitro*. J Immunol 1986;136:681-85.
94. Desmettre TJ, Soulie-Begu S, Devoisselle JM, et al. Diode laser-induced thermal damage evaluation on the retina with a liposome dye system. Lasers Surg Med 1999;24: 61-68.
95. Guran T, Zeimer RC, Shahidi M, et al. Quantitative analysis of retinal hemodynamics using targeted dye delivery. Invest Ophthalmol Vis Sci 1990;31: 2300-06.
96. Zeimer RC, Khoobehi B, Niesman MR, et al. A potential method for local drug and dye delivery in the ocular vasculature. Invest Ophthalmol Vis Sci 1988;29: 1179-83.
97. Khoobehi B, Peyman GA, Niesman MR, et al. Hyperthermia and temperature-sensitive liposomes: Selective delivery of drugs into the eye. Jpn J Ophthalmol 1989;33: 405-12.
98. Khoobehi B, Peyman GA, McTurnan WG, et al. Externally triggered release of dye and drugs from liposomes into the eye. An *in vitro* and *in vivo* study. Ophthalmology 1988;95: 950-55.
99. Singh K, Mezei M. Liposomal ophthalmic drug delivery system. I. Triamcinolone acetonide. Int J Pharm 1983;16: 339-44.
100. Singh K, Mezei M. Liposomal ophthalmic drug delivery system. II. Dihydrostreptomycin sulfate. Int J Pharm 1984;16: 263-69.
101. Lee VHL. Application of liposomes in ocular drug delivery. In Pleyer D, Schmidt K, Tiel HJ, (Eds): Liposomes in Ophthalmology and Dermatology. Hippokrates: Stuttart, 1993;53-59.
102. Tomalia DA, Esfand R. Dendrons, dendrimers, and dendrigrafts. Chemistry and Industry 1997;416-20.
103. Veprek P, Jezek J. Peptide and glycopeptide dendrimers. Part II. J Pept Sci 1999;5: 203-20.

104. Tomalia DA, Naylor AM, Goddard WAI. Starburst dendrimers: molecular-level control of size, shape, surface chemistry, topology, and flexibility from atoms to macroscopic matter. Angew Chem Int Ed Engl 1990;29:138-75.
105. Tomalia DA. Dendrimer molecules. Scientific Am 1995;42-46.
106. Bielinska A, Kukowska-Latallo JF, Johnson J, et al. Regulation of *in vitro* gene expression using antisense oligonucleotides or antisense expression plasmids transfected using starburst PAMAM dendrimers. Nucleic Acids Res 1996;24(11): 2176-82.
107. Hudde T, Rayner SA, Comer RM, et al. Activated polyamidoamine dendrimers, a non-viral vector for gene transfer to the corneal endothelium. Gene Therapy 1999;6: 939-43.
108. Qin L, Pahud DR, Ding Y, et al. Efficient transfer of genes into murine cardiac grafts by Starburst polyamidoamine dendrimers. Hum Gene Ther 1998;9:553-60.
109. Kukowska-Latallo JF, Bielinska AU, Johnson J, et al. Efficient transfer of genetic material into mammalian cells using Starburst polyamidoamine dendrimers. Proc Natl Acad Sci USA 1996;93: 4897-902.
110. Tang MX, Redemann CT, Szoka FC Jr: *In vitro* gene delivery by degraded polyamidoamine dendrimers. Bioconjug Chem 1996;7: 703-14.
111. Esfand R, Beezer AE, Mitchell JC. An investigation of synthesis and potential application of tetra-directional cascade dendrimers as drug delivery systems. 96 AD; London, 1996.
112. Sakthivel T, Toth I, Florence AT. Distribution of a lipidic 2.5 nm diameter dendrimer carrier after oral administration. Int J Pharm 1999;183: 51-55.
113. Attia SA, Shepherd VE, Rosenblatt MN, et al. Interaction of oligodeoxynucleotides with mycobacteria: Implications for new therapeutic strategies. Antisense Nucleic Acid Drug Dev 1998;8: 207-14.
114. Reidy JJ, Mondino BJ, Brown SI, et al. A long-term implantable aqueous delivery system for the external rabbit eye. Invest Ophthalmol Vis Sci 1980;19:428-30.
115. Michelson JB, Nozik RA. Experimental endophthalmitis treated with an implantable osmotic minipump. Arch Ophthalmol 1979;97:1345-46.
116. Roussel TJ, Osato MS, Wilhelmus KR. Cyclosporine and experimental corneal transplantation. Transplant Proc 2000;15: 3081-83.
117. Eliason JA, Maurice DM. An ocular perfusion system. Invest Ophthalmol Vis Sci 1980;19:102-05.
118. Ishibashi T, Miki K, Patterson R, et al. An intravitreal cannula system: Long-term follow-up study. Int Ophthalmol 1986;9: 5-9.
119. Miki K, Patterson R, Ryan SJ. An indwelling cannula system for the primate eye. J Neurosci Methods 1985;13: 267-79.
120. Bawa R. Ocular inserts. In Mitra AK (Ed): Ophthalmic Drug Delivery Systems. Marcel Dekker: New York: 1993;223-60.
121. Lee VH, Robinson JR. Topical ocular drug delivery: Recent developments and future challenges. J Ocul Pharmacol 1986;2:67-108.
122. Sieradzki E. Bioavailability of drugs applied to the eye externally. Klinika Oczna 1991;93: 34-36.
123. Calvo P, Vila-Jato JL, Alonso MJ. Comparative *in vitro* evaluation of several colloidal systems, nanoparticles, nanocapsules, and nanoemulsions, as ocular drug carriers. J Pharm Sci 1996;85: 530-36.

124. Das SK, Tucker IG, Hill DJ, et al. Evaluation of poly (isobutylcyanoacrylate) nanoparticles for mucoadhesive ocular drug delivery. I. Effect of formulation variables on physiochemical characteristics of nanoparticles. Pharm Res 1995;12: 534-40.
125. Joshi A. Microparticulates for ophthalmic drug delivery. J Ocul Pharmacol 1994;10: 29-45.
126. Kreuter J. Particulates (nanoparticles and microparticles). In Mitra AK (Ed): Ophthalmic Drug Delivery Systems. Marcel Dekker; New York: 1993;275-87.
127. Calvo P, Alonso MJ, Vila-Jato JL, et al. Improved ocular bioavailability of indomethacin by novel ocular drug carriers. J Pharm Pharmacol 1996;48: 1147-52.
128. Zimmer A, Mutschler E, Lambrecht G, et al. Pharmacokinetic and pharmacodynamic aspects of an ophthalmic pilocarpine nanoparticle-delivery system. Pharm Res 1994;11:1435-42.
129. Harmia T, Speiser P, Kreuter J. A solid colloidal drug delivery system for the eye: Encapsulation of pilocarpine in nanoparticles. J Microencapsul 1986;3: 3-12.
130. Krishnamoorthy R, Mitra AK. Mucoadhesive polymers in ocular drug delivery. In Mitra AK (Ed): Ophthalmic Drug Delivery Systems. Marcel Dekker: New York: 1993;199-221.
131. Robinson JR, Longer MA, Veillard M. Bioadhesive polymers for controlled drug delivery. Ann NY Acad Sci 1987;507: 307-14.
132. Liaw J, Robinson JR. Ocular penetration enhancers. In Mitra AK, (Ed): Ophthalmic Drug Delivery Systems. Marcel Dekker: New York 1993;369-81.

Chapter 6

Drug Permeability

Sunita Agarwal (India)

INTRODUCTION

When we apply a topically acting drug in the eye, its efficacy depends on the permeability of the cornea to the drug. The permeability of these drugs is contingent primarily on their lipid or water solubility. The epithelium and endothelium have hundred times the lipid content of the stroma and fat-soluble drugs readily penetrate these cellular layers. However, only water-soluble drugs can penetrate the stroma. Therefore, a drug should be amphipathic, i.e., it should have both lipophilic and hydrophilic characteristics to penetrate all layers of the cornea.

FACTORS

There are several factors that contribute to drug permeability.

Lipid Solubility

The drug should be lipid-soluble to penetrate the epithelium and endothelium.

Water Solubility

The drug should be water soluble to penetrate the stroma.

Molecular Size and Structure

Lipid soluble molecules pass through the phospholipid portion of the cell membrane by dissolving in it and diffusing through it irrespective of molecular size and shape. Water soluble molecules on the other hand are restricted to size 4A and filter through pores that may exist in or around the globular protein molecules in the cell membrane. The size of the pore restricts the flow of water soluble molecules. Substances with molecular weights of less than hundred pass readily through cell membranes and those of more than 500 do not. To overcome this limitation in molecular size, some ophthalmic drugs are prepared in high concentration so that by laws of mass action, a small percentage will reach the anterior chamber and an effect will be obtained.

Ionic Charge

Ions even with small molecular weights have difficulty in passing through the cell membrane because of their ionic charge. Both attracting and repulsing forces in the membrane block its passage. Only nonionized drugs can penetrate the lipid cellular layers, whereas ionized drugs readily traverse the water soluble stroma. Therefore, a drug should be able to exist in both an ionized and non-ionized form to penetrate the cornea. Such a model is therefore the alkaloid homatropine. In the epithelium, the non-ionized free base will readily penetrate and enter the stroma where it reionizes. The ionized homatropine freely traverses the stroma to the endothelium, where again only the nonionized form will pass through. In the aqueous, reionization occurs (Fig. 6.1). At each step, homatropine can penetrate each layer because of the different solubility characteristics of the ionized and nonionized forms. The process is not limited by the exhaustion of the homatropine supply, since equilibrium between the ionized and non-ionized forms is reestablished as soon as it passes through each layer. Substances that are exclusively electrolytes or nonelectrolytes will not pass through the cornea.

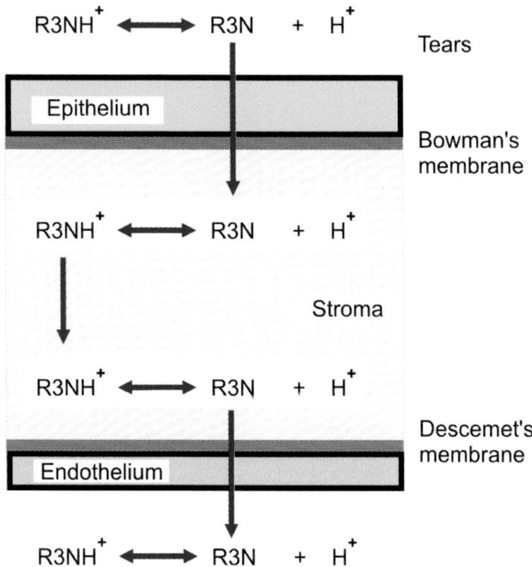

Fig. 6.1: Transfer of homatropine in the cornea

Fluorescein, a negatively charged ion will not penetrate the epithelium. This is the basis of the fluorescein dye test. If the epithelium is intact, fluorescein will not stain the cornea. Whereas if the epithelium is damaged or absent, fluorescein will stain the stroma.

Altering the Permeability Characteristics of the Eye

Hypotonic solutions will increase the permeability of the epithelium and surface active agents reduce the surface tension and so increase epithelial permeability.

Drug Contact Time

This also has an effect upon the absorption and penetration of drugs into the cornea. Increased contact time has been achieved with pilocarpine solutions of water soluble polymers. Pilocarpine in such a polymer penetrates the cornea three times as well as the same dose in a saline vehicle.

SECTION TWO

Classification of Antibiotics and their Clinical and Surgical Applications in Ophthalmology

Chapter 7

Update on Antibacterial Therapy

Ashok Garg (India)

Principles in antibiotic therapy remains the same in all medical specialities. The rational selection of anti-microbial drugs depends upon the diagnosis, senstivity and assay of bactericidal activity. Diagnosis can be made on the basis of clinical impression. In most infections the relationship between causative agent and clinical picture is not constant. It is therefore, important to obtain proper specimens for bacteriological identification of causative agent. Then chemotherapy can be started on the basis 'Suitable drug'. The suitable drug of a causative organism is based on the following:

1. The site of infection.
2. The age of the patient.
3. The place where the infection was acquired.
4. Mechanical predisposing factors.
5. Predisposing host factors.

The eye is particularly suitable for local application of antibiotics. The use of systemic antibiotics is limited by relatively poor penetration of antibiotics into the eye through the blood-eye barrier is reduced when the eye is inflamed.

The general principles to the management of infection elsewhere in the body also apply to the ocular antibiotic therapy. An accurate diagnosis confirmed by the culture and senstivity from the samples (corneal scraping in corneal ulcers, conjunctival swab in conjunctivitis and vitreous tap in endophthalmitis etc.) is necessary before selecting the most effective antibiotic.

External ocular infections have the advantage of being treatable with more toxic antibiotics that cannot be safely used systimatically. Such topical use of toxic antibiotic has the advantage of slowing down the development of bacterial resistance to the safer antibiotics and the individual advantage of prescribing a less commonly used antibiotic to which fewer organisms are already resistant. Inspite of relative delicacy of ocular surface, toxic effects like epithelial healing defect are not clinically significant with the use of commercially available ophthalmic antibiotics.

Unique to the eye is lipoidal barrier that resist penetration by the most antibiotics. The blood eye barrier is a significant obstacle to the treatment of the vitreous and aqueous cavities. The sclera and uveal tract are external to the blood eye barrier. When large protein molecules leak freely into the eye, so do antibiotic molecules. The clinically significant problem arise when minimal damage has been done by the organism entered into the eye via trauma, surgery or metastatic entry. At this early stage microorganism is relatively safe from systemic or topical antibiotics yet this is critical time for effective therapy. The routes of administration of antibiotics to achieve intraocular penetration are subconjunctival, sub-Tenon and intravitreal injections.

Subconjunctival antibiotic injection produces a constant and prolonged depot of medication supplying effective conc in the anterior segment. The main route for subconjunctival antibiotic injection is through the tear film and the cornea. The vitreous cavity is the most difficult area to be penetrated by topical and sub-conjunctival routes. Therefore, direct intravitreal injection of antibiotic is recommended in desperate situation like endophthalmitis.

The goal of achieving high antibiotic conc in anterior segment can be achieved by frequent instillation of antibiotic drops into the conjunctival sac.

The rational for prophylactic topical antibiotic before surgery is debatable. Organisms that may otherwise be considered normal flora such as Staph epidermidis are potential pathogens to the eye. The use of pre-operative topical antibiotic may decrease or eliminate bacterial flora from the conjunctiva that their use will not prevent intra-operative contamination of wound or anterior chamber.

Antibiotics are chemical substances produced by microorganisms that have the capacity to inhibit growth of or even destroy bacteria and other micro-organisms in dilute solution. The chemical structures of most therapeutic antibiotics have been identified.

The best per-requisite for the correct choice of an antimicrobial which at the same time will be fully active, safe and well tolerated is an exact clinical and bacteriological diagnosis.

The choice of an antimicrobial is not only influenced by the type of and susceptibility of the infecting organisms but also by mode of action and pharmacokinetics of the antibiotics, the severity and localization of infection, liver and kidney functions and age of the patient.

When more than one antibiotic is used, apart from the spectrum of the individual antibiotic, synergism and antagonism must be kept in mind, mechanism of action of antibiotics is some what variable. Generally, they achieve their effects by disturbing the metabolic activities of the bacteria.

Most antibiotics disturb cell wall synthesis of the bacteria, some interfere with protein synthesis, other produce alterations in bacterial membrane permeability. Antibacterial drugs that cause cell wall dysfunction by inhibiting peptidoglycan synthesis or by alteration of the osmotic barrier drugs while the other drugs cause inhibition of nucleic acid synthesis.

Antibiotics may be either bactericidal (those which kill organisms) or bacteriostatic (which inhibit bacterial multiplication). Certain Antibacterial drugs are designated as bacteriostatic or bactericidal dependent on the concentration of drug. Many bacteriostatic drugs become bactericidal when used in higher concentration as may occur with ophthalmic topical applications.

In preparation of therapy plan, the pharmacokinetics of the antibiotics must be taken into consideration. Absorption and blood levels, tissue diffusion and distribution, intra ocular penetration, protein binding, metabolism and excretion differ from each antimicrobial agent.

Because of tear flow, topically instilled antibiotics have a limited life span in the conjunctival sac and only a fraction of their volume penetrates the eyeball across the cornea. Drug penetration may be improved by frequent instillation, increasing the viscosity of the drug, by employing the vehicle or by altering the pH of the drug or by the use of fortified drops.

Topical antibiotics should be selected depending upon the severity of infection and the suspected Ocular pathogen. Preferably use less potent antibiotics in common ocular infection and reverse mega spectrum and high conc antibiotics for more severe infections or fulminant infections.

INDICATIONS FOR ANTI-MICROBIAL THERAPY

1. Significant infection of the eye proven bacteriologically and clinically. Topically instilled drugs are mostly useful in external ocular infections namely conjunctivitis, keratitis, keratoconjunctivitis, dacroycystitis, stye Chlazion and to a varying extent in anterior segment infections.
2. Prophylaxis to
   a. Prevent secondary bacterial infection in patients who are ill with other diseases.
   b. To protect healthy persons from the acquisition or invasion by specific infection to which they are exposed.
3. Confirmation of suspected diagnosis of significant bacterial infection by observing clinical response.

The commercially available antibiotics drops and Oint are marketed in Strength from 0.3 to 1%. However, in severe infections of the eye in addition to systemic therapy, high potency fortified drops are freshly prepared and used. However, these fortified eye drops have a very short life span.

However, indiscriminate use of antibiotics should be checked as it leads to:

a. Widespread sensitization resulting in hypersentivity anaphylaxis.
b. Changes in the normal flora of tear resulting in superinfection due to overgrowth of resistant organisms.

c. Direct drug toxicity due to prolong use.
d. Masking serious infections without eradicating it.
e. Development of drug resistances.

MECHANISMS OF RESISTANCE OF ANTIBIOTICS

a. Production of enzymes that cause inactivation of the drug e.g. β-lactamase which inactivate penicillin, acetyltransferases which inactivate Chloramphenicol, Kinases and other enzymes which inactivate aminoglycosides.
b. Alteration of drug binding sites. It occurs specially with aminoglycosides, erythromycin and penicillin.
c. Reduction of drug uptake by the bacteria e.g. Tetracycline.
d. Alternation of enzymes e.g. dihydrofolate reductase becomes insenstive to Trimethoprim.
e. Some strains of staphylococci have multiple resistance to practi-cally almost all current antibiotics involving the above mechanisms,resistance being transferred by transposons or plasmids.

In order to avoid resistance to topical antibiotics frequently try to follow following principles to limit the resistance development.

1. Limit antibiotic use to diagnosed infections caused by susceptible organisms. It is unnecessary to use broad spectrum antibiotics in condition like viral conjunctivitis.
2. Avoid chronic use of antibiotics. Ask the patient to follow strictly the ophthalmologist advice regarding the duration of antibiotics use.
3. Use newer antibiotics only when necessary for treatment of infections resistant to traditional therapy.
4. Completely treat all clinical infections and consider using a second therapeutic agent to prevent emergence of resistant organisms.

In ophthalmic infections there is tendency to use combination of antimicrobial agents by Ophthalmologists.

Indications

1. To give prompt treatment to the patient.
2. To delay the emergence of microbial mutants resistant to one drug on chronic use.
3. To treat mixed infections.
4. To achieve bactericidal Synergism.

Disadvantages

1. The more drugs are used, the greater the chances for drug reaction to occur.
2. The cost is unnecessarily high.

3. The relax in attitude of clinician of the effort to establish a specific diagnosis.
4. Antimicrobial combinations may accomplish no more than an effective single drug.
5. Increased incidence and variety of adverse effect.
6. Superinfection chances are high.

Most common pathogens seen in Ocular infective conditions are:

a. Gram-positive cocci:
   - *Staphylococcus aureus*
   - Staphylococcus epidermidis
   - *Streptococcus pneumoniae*
   - *Streptococcus faecalis*
   - α and β hemolytic streptococci.
b. Gram-negative cocci:
   - *Neisseria gonorrhea*
   - *Neisseria meningitidis*
   - *Branhamella and N.sicca, mucosa and flavescens.*
c. Gram-negative rods:
   - Acinetobacter
   - Enterobacter
   - *Escherichia coli*
   - *Haemophilus* species (*influenzae* and *aegyptius*)
   - *Klebsiella* species (*pneumoniae* and *oxytoca*)
   - *Moraxella* species (*Lacunata, bovis* and *non-liquefaciens*)
   - *Proteus* (*merabilis* and *vulgaris species*)
   - *Pseudomonas aeuroginosa* and *cepacia*
   - *Serratia* species (*marcescens* and *flexneri*)
   - *Brucella* species (*abortus, suis* and *Melitensis*)
   - *Shigella* species (*sonnei* and *flexneri*)
d. Gram-positive rods:
   - *Cl. tetani*
   - *Cl. welchi*
   - *C. diphtherial*
   - *C. Anthracis, cereus* and *subtilis*
   - *Corynebacteria* species (*diphtheria, xerosis* and *hemolyticus*)
   - *Listeria monocytogenes.*

The broad spectrum antibiotics are variable effective against both rods and cocci.

CLASSIFICATION OF ANTIBACTERIAL DRUGS

1. Beta-Lactams:
   - Penicillin (Natural and Semi-synthetic)
   - Cephalosporins (First, Second and Third Generations).
   - Cephamycins.

2. **Aminoglycosides** (Group of antibiotics and semisynthetic antibiotic derivatives)
3. Tetracyclines
4. Sulphonamides
5. Chloramphenicol
6. Macro lides including Erythromycin, Clindamycin, Roxithromycin and Spiramycin, Vancomycin.
7. Polypeptides including polymixin B, Bacitracin
8. Anti-microbial peptides
9. Fluoroquinolones including
   - Norfloxacin
   - Ciprofloxacin
   - Ofloxacin
   - Pefloxacin
   - Lomefloxacin
   - Sparfloxacin
   - Levofloxacin
   - Gatifloxacin
   - Moxifloxacin
10. Imidazoles derivatives
11. Cotrimoxazole
12. Miscellaneous

BETA-LACTAMS

These are so called because they contain β-lactam ring in their structure. It includes:

a. Penicillins
b. Cephalosporins
c. Cephamycins

Penicillins

Penicillin G is the first antibiotic produced by a fungus *Penicillin chrysogenum*.

It acts by interference with synthesis of peptidoglycan layer of cell wall penicillins are bactericidal and only effective against multiplying organisms.

Penicillins are classified into following groups :-

Natural Penicillins

Benzyl Penicillin (Penicillin G) is active against gram +ve organisms, gram -ve cocci, spirochaetes. It can be given orally, as drops, S/conjunctivally, Parenteral IV or IM. It is one of the most effective bactericidal antibiotic although many Staphylococci have developed resistance to it.

Dosage: Parenteral IM/IV adults
4-30 million units/24 divides doses 4-6 hourly.
Topically it is given in fortified drops form with conc of 100000 units/ml (Shelf life - 24 hours). Subconjunctival injection dose is 0.5-100000 units/ml.

It is drug of choice for streptococcal, pneumococcal and gonococcal infections.

Semi-synthetic Penicillin

Phenoxy methyl penicillin It is semisynthetic Acid resistant Penicillin alternative to Penicillin G.

It acts by inhibition of cell wall synthesis.

Dosage
It is given orally 250-500 mgm 6 hourly. It is equally effective like penicillin G against micro-organisms.

Penicillinase resistant penicillins have been developed.
There are:
1. Methicillin:
   It is a penicillinase resistant penicillin specially reserved for Staphylococcal infections. It is suitable for subconjunctival injection in cases of endophthalmitis.

Dosage:
Parenteral IM/IV: 1-2 G 4 hourly, subconjunctival injection conc is 150-200 mg/ml.
2. Cloxacillin:
   It is given orally is dose of 250-500 mgm 6 hourly.
   Highly effective against staphylococcal, penumococcus and streptococcus.
3. Flucloxacillin, Oxacillin and Dicloxacillin are effective against gram +ve organisms.
   a. Carboxy Penicillin include
      Carbenicillin and Ticarcillin are specially effective against *Pseudomonas, Proteus enterobacter, Klebsiella* and *E.coli.*

Dosage
Parenteral 400-500 mg/kg/day 4 hourly topically in conc of 4 mg/ml/ (fortified drops)
   b. Amino Penicillins are bactericidal for both gram +ve and gram -ve bacteria. Amino penicillins are susceptible to penicillinase and so ineffective against staphylococcus.
      1. Ampicillin: given orally 250-500 mg 4-6 hourly or by parenteral route. For SC concentration in injection 100-200/ml
         Intravitreal injection concentration 500 mg/ml, 10mg/ml (fortified drops).
      2. **Amoxycillin:** It is given orally in dose of 250-500 mgms
         4-6 hourly:

Broad spectrum penicillin derivatives, e.g. ampicillin and Amoxycillin are effective against a wide range of organisms but are inactivated by penicillinase.

ADVERSE REACTIONS OF PENICILLINS

Hypersensitivity reactions (Minor rash to Anaphylaxis)

- Rash, itching, urticaria, fever, Asthma, Serum sickness
- Exfoliative dermatitis
- Anaphylaxis
- Cross senstivity with the Cephalosporins.

Cephalosporins

Cephalosporins are obtained from a fugus Cephalosporium. These are derivatives of Cephalosporin.C produced by fungus Cephalosporium acromonium. Molecular structure is closely related to that of Pencillins. Mode of action is similar to pencillins since both group posses B lactam ring. Cephalosphorins bind to the bacterial enzymes that are necessary for the formation of the cell wall and cause inhibition of mucopeptide synthesis hence bactericidal. Classification by Generation is based on general features of antimicrobial activity and pharmacological properties.

First Generation Cephalosporins

They have good activity against gram-positive bacteria and relatively modest activity against gram-negative microorganisms. Most gram-positive cocci except enterococci are susceptible.

These are:

1. **Cefazolin**:
   - Parenteral dose : 1-6 gm/day 6-8 hourly
   - SC dose : 100 mg/ml
   - IV dose (Intravitreal dose) : 2000 ug/ml
   - Fortified eye drops : 50 mg/ml (Shelf life - 1 week)
2. Cephalothin:
   - Parenteral dose : 2-12 gm/day 6-8 hourly
   - SC dose : 50-100 mg/ml
3. **Cephapirin:**
   - Parenteral : 1-2 gm every 4 hour
4. **Cephaloridine:**
   - Parenteral : 2-4 gm/day 6 hourly
   - SC dose : 100 mg/ml
   - Intravitreal dose : 250 mg/ml
5. **Cephadrine:**
   - Oral, IM or IV : 0.5 - 1 gm every 6 hours.

6. **Cephalexin:**
   Oral : 0.5 gm-1 g every 6 hours
7. **Cefadroxyl:**
   Oral : 1 gm every 12 hours
8. **Cefaclor:**
   Oral : 0.5-1 gm every 8 hours

SECOND GENERATION CEPHALOSPORINS

These have excellent activity against gram-positive organism Staphylococcus and Streptococcus except *S. Faecalis*, more active than Ist generation against gram-negative microorganisms e.g. *E. coli*, *Klebsiella*, *H. influenzae* but not active against *Bacteroides* and *Pseudomonas*.

1. Cefamandole:
   Parenteral : 1 gm every 4 hours
   Fortified drops : 50 gm/ml (Shelf life 7 days)
2. **Cefoxitin:**
   It is more active against anaerobes Sp. *B. fragilis* 1-2 gm every 4 hourly.
3. **Cefuroxime :**
   750 mgm - 1.5 gm every 8 hours
4. **Cefonicid :**
   1-2 gm every 24 hours
5. **Cefaranide :**
   1 gm every 12 hours.
6. **Cefotiam :**
   1 gm every 12 hours.
7. **Cefotetan :**
   1 gm every 12 hours.

THIRD GENERATION CEPHALOSPORINS

These agents are mainly effective against gram-negative organisms but not against staphylococci.These are:

1. Cefotaxime:
   Parenteral : 1-2 gm every 4-6 hours
   Fortified eye drops : 50 mg/ml (shelf life 7 days)
2. Cefoparazone :
   1-4 gm every 4-8 hours.
3. **Cefixime :**
   200-400 mg/day
4. **Cefsulodin :**
   0.5 - 1gm 6-12 hourly.
5. **Ceftazidime :**
   1-2 gm every 8-12 hours.

The other third generation Cephalosporins used are :-

- Moxalactam
- Ceftizoxime (1-2 gm every 8-12 hours)
- Ceftriaxone (1-2 gm once a day)
- Cefpiramide

Cephalosporins should not ordinarily be used for infections proven be due to *Staph. aureus.*

Intra ocular Cephalosporin levels with systemic administration are shown in the Table 7.1.

Table 7.1: Cephalosporin dosage and conc in aqueous and vitreous

Drug	*Dose*	*Aqueous(ug/ml)*	*Dose*	*Vitreous (ug/ml)*
Cephalothin	1 g (IV)	0.55	2g IV	0.83
Cephalexin	2 g (oral)	1.2	2g(IV)	1.19
Cefoxitin	2 g (IV)	3.1	–	–
Ceftazidime	2 g (IV)	3.39	–	–
Cefuoroxime	1.5 g	2.7-6.2	–	–
Moxalactam	2 g (IV)	2.4-9.6	–	–

Certazidime, Moxa Lactam, Cefotaxime and Cefuroxime attain aqueous levels in the bactericidal range for most enterobacteriaceae except *P.aeruginosa*. Only Ceftazidime levels are in a range that inhbit a high Percentage of *P. aeruginosa*.

Vitreous Penetration of Cephalosporins

Vitreous levels of Ceftriaxone after IV administration achieve levels that exceed the MIC for 90 percents of *S. aureus* as well as many gram-negative rods excluding *P. aeruginosa* and *S.epidermidis*. Rest of other Cephalosporins do not achieve vitreous levels in the bactericidal range. Therefore, systemic Cephalosporins play a limited role in the treatment of endophthalmitis.

Subconjunctival Cephalosporins may be useful in enhancing surgical prophylaxis as an adjunct to sub-conjunctival aminoglycosides.

Intravitreal Cephalosporins provide excellent adjunct to aminoglycosides in the treatment of infectious endophthalmitis. Ceftazidime with Vancomycin or Cefazolin with Amikacin provide broadspectrum coverage on intravitreal administration.

Topical Cephalosporins are an excellent adjunct to topical aminoglycosides in the treatment of severe infectious keratitis. Cefazolin in a dosage of 50 mg/ml alternating with aminoglycosides every half hour round the clock for severe bacterial corneal ulcer is a most commonly used formulation.

Adverse reactions of Cephalosporins

Pain after IM injection specially Cephalothin and Cephapirin.

- Disulfiram like reactions.
- Hypersensitivity reactions similar to penicillin
- Nephrotoxicity.
- *Pseudomembranous colitis* and Vitamin K deficiency.
- False positive test results for eleveted creatinine (by systemic Cephalosporins by killing intestinal flora).

Aminoglycosides

These are produced by soil-actinomycetes. These are bactericidal agents which act inside the cell be binding irreversibly to the 30 S ribosome sub-units in such a way that incorrect amino acid sequences are entered into peptide chains. The abnormal proteins are fatal to microbes. Aminoglycosides are one of the most commonly used group of antibiotic drugs in ophthalmic practice. They contain one or two aminosugars glycosidally linked to an amino-cyclitol.

Spectrum They are bactericidal against a broad range of gram-negative bacilli and *Staphylococcus aureus*. They are not effective against streptococci, pneumococci, anaerobes and spirochaetes. They are given either topically or systemically only parenterally due to poor absorption from GI tract.

Adverse reactions
- Ototoxicity
- Nephrotoxicity
- Neurotoxicity - vague feelings of lips, headache, Lassitude, dizziness.
- Drug fever with eosinophilia
- Hematological abnormalities.

They comprise a group of antibiotics and semisynthetic antibiotic derivatives.

The various aminoglycosides used in Ophthalmology are:

1. Gentamicin:
   It is one of the most commonly used aminoglycoside for acute infections. It is obtained from cultures of *Micromonospora purpura*. It is effective against aerobic gram-negative bacilli inciuding *E. coli*, *Enterobacter*, *K. pneumoniae*, *Proteus* and Ps *aeruginosa*. Moderately active against streptococci and inactive against anaerobes.

Dosage:
- Parenteral - 3.5 mg/kg/day 8 hours (IM or IV)
- Vials 40 mg/ml
- Ophthalmic eye drops in conc. of 0.3%
- Fortified drops : 20 mg/ml/(shelf life 30 days)
- Ophthalmic ointment : 0.3 %
- SC dose : 20-80 mg/ml
- Intravitreal dose : 200-400 ug/ml.

The systemic use of gentamicin is recommended for endophthalmitis, ocular injuries with retained Foreign bodies. Synergism between β lactam antiobiotics and aminoglycosides has been shown. Topical gentamicin is more effective at decreasing bacterial counts and eliminating bacteria from the eye before surgery.

Aqueous levels of Gentamicin as high as 0.8 ml can be achieved by SC injection of 0.5 ml of 0.3% solution and 1.6 mg/ml by topical use of 0.3% solution. Topical drops achieve sufficent conc. to treat ocular surface injections while Fortified drops may be necessary to achieve therapeutic levels consistently in the anterior chamber.

Intra vitreal injection of 200-400 mg is recommended for severe ocular injections like endophthalmitis. Gentamicin is more toxic to retina than Amikacin. Fortified drops can be formulated from intravenous preparations. Fortified gentamicin in combination with a Cephalosporin or Vancomycin is recommended as the initial emperic treatment in bacterial corneal ulcers. Toxicity due to subconjunctival Gentamicin may be observed in form of pupillary mydriasis, conjunctival paresthesias and delay in corenal wound healing.

Tobramycin

It is obtained from cultures of *Streptomyces tenebrainus*. Its bacterial spectrum and pharmacokinetics are similar to Gentamicin. It is active against 90% of *P. aeruginosa* compared to 77% percent activity of Gentamicin. Tobramycin use should be restricted to those injections not responding to Gentamicin or antibacterial senstivity showing resistance to Gentamicin. It may also be used in the case of life thereatning or sight threatening infection that has a high probability of being caused by *P.aeruginosa* because of the differential senstivities of two drugs and importance of optimum intial emperic drug selection.

Dosage:

- Parenteral : 3.5 mg/kg/day 8 hourly
- Ophthalmic solution : 0.3%
- Ophthalmic ointment : 0.3%
- SC dose : 2.5-40 mg in 0.5 ml isotonic sodium chloride or sterile water
- Fortified drops : 20 mg/ml (Shelf life 30 days)
- Intravitreal dose : 150-200 ug/ml.

Amikacin

Amikacin is acetylate Kanamicin. This semi-synthetic additive prevents enzymatic destruction except by the acetyl transferase bacterial enzyme.

It is active against many enteric gram-negative bacilli that are resistant to Gentamicin. Amikacin has lowest frequency of resistant strains reported so far. It acts by inhibiting microbial protein synthesis. Amikacin is ineffective orally and is given IV/IM route.

Dosage:

- Parenteral : 15 mg/kg/day 8-12 hourly.
- Ophthalmic drops : 0.3 % (10-50 mg/ml).
- Fortified drops : 20 mg/ml (shelf life 30 days)
- SC dose : 20 mg/ml
- IV dose : 400 mg in 0.10 ml of solution

The subconjunctival delivery gives bactericidal anterior chamber conc without subjecting the patient to systemic toxicity. Although Amikacin is the aminoglycoside least frequently inactivated by bacterial enzymes, principle of good antibiotic usage is applied to reduce the rate of development of resistant organisms.

Amikacin is used as intravitreal antibiotic for the treatment of postoperative bacterial endophthalmitis. Intravitreal Amikacin is recommended in combination with Vancomycin or Cephalosporin. Intravitreal conc of 400 mg in 0.10 ml of solution has been shown to be non-toxic to the retina. Retinal toxicity is found with a dose of 1500 mg of Amikacin. Compared with 400 mg of Gentamicin or 800 mg of Tobramycin. Therefore, in sight threatening endophthalmitis, Amikacin offers a broader spectrum of action alongwith lower toxicity.

Topical use of Amikacin in the treatment of bacterial Keratitis should be restructed to culture proven organisms resistant to Gentamicin and Tobramycin.

Sisomicin

It has antibacterial activity similar to Gentamicin. It is effective in Gentamicin and Tobramycin resistant strains.

Dosage:

- Ophthalmic solution : 0.3%
- Fortified drops : 20 mg/ml (shelf life 30 days)
- Ophthalmic ointment : 0.3%
- SC dose : 20-80 mg/ml

Neomycin

It is obtained from *Streptomyces fradiae*. It acts by inhibition of micriobial protein synthesis, and is-bactericidal for many gram-positive and gram-negative organisms.

It is used in combination with Polymixin B and Gramicidin as broad spectrum antibacterial combination solution. Neomycin is also used in combination with Polymixin B and Bacitracin as an ointment.

Dosage:

- Parenteral dose : 4-12 gm/day 6 hourly
- Ophthalmic solution : 0.17 %
- Ointment : 5 mg/gm
- Fortified drops : 30-40 mg/ml/ (shelf life 7 days)
- SC dose : 250-500 mg/ml

Various Combination

a. Neomycin/Polymixin B/Bacitracin Combination :
   Topical ophthalmic Oint : 5000 units/gm Polymixin B, 500 units/gm bacitracin and 5 mg/gm neomycin.
b. Neomycin/Polymixin B Combination :
   Ophthalmic Oint : 6000 units/gm Polymixin B and 5 mg/gm neomycin.
c. Neomycin/Polymixin B/Gramicidin Combination :
   Topical ophthalmic solution : 1.75 mg neomycin, 10000 units of Polymixin B and 0.025 mg gramicidin/ml (Fig. 7.1)

Netilmycin

It is N-ethyl derivative of Sisomicin and has antibacterial activity similar to that of tobramycin.

Dosage:

Parenteral dose : 3-6.5 mg/kg/day 8 hourly.
SC dose : 20-40 mg/ml

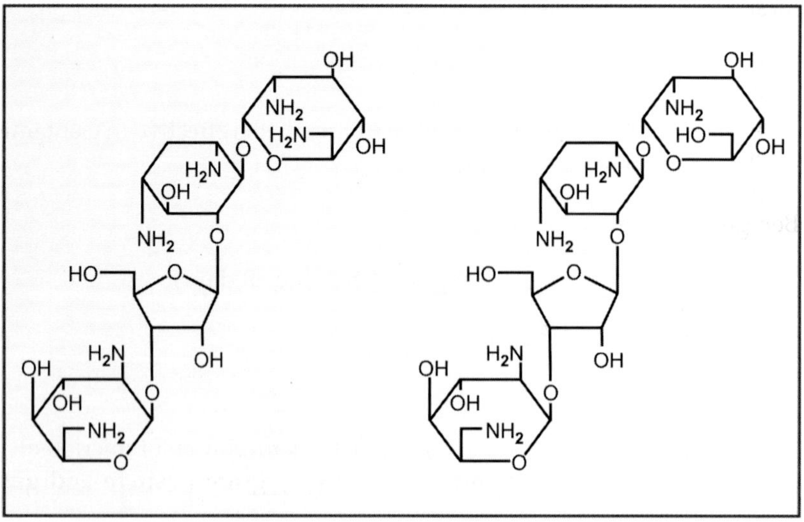

Fig. 7.1: Molecular structures of aminoglycosides [Neomycin (L) and paromomycin (R)]

Kanamycin

It is used for streptomycin resistant gram-negative bacillary infections and resistant tuberculosis. But not active against *Pseudomonas.*

Parenteral dosage	15 mg/kg/day 8 hourly
Fortified drops	10 mg/ml

Framycetin

Its antibacterial activity is similar to that of neomycin.

Dosage:
- Ophthalmic drops 0.5%
- Ophthalmic ointment 0.5 and 1.0%

Streptomycin

It is active against *E.coli, Proteus, P. aeruginosa, K. pneumoniae* and *H. influenzae.* It is obtained from *Streptomyces griseus.* It has limited bacterial spectrum and is not commonly used in ophthalmic practice.

Tetracyclines: Tetracyclines have a Broad spectrum bacteriostatic activity against gram-positive organisms, gram-negative bacilli, anaerobes, mycoplasma. Actenomyces, rickettsia, *Chlamydia spirochaetes,* however they are resistant to *Proteus, Serratia* and *P. aeruginosa* species.

They act by inhibiting protein synthesis at ribosome in both gram- positive gram-negative, microorganisms (Fig. 7.2).

Adverse Reactions

- GI disturbances - nausea, vomiting and diarrhea.
- Rashes
- Yellow discoloration of teeth in children
- Photosensitization.
- Nephrotoxicity
- Benign intracranial hypertension.

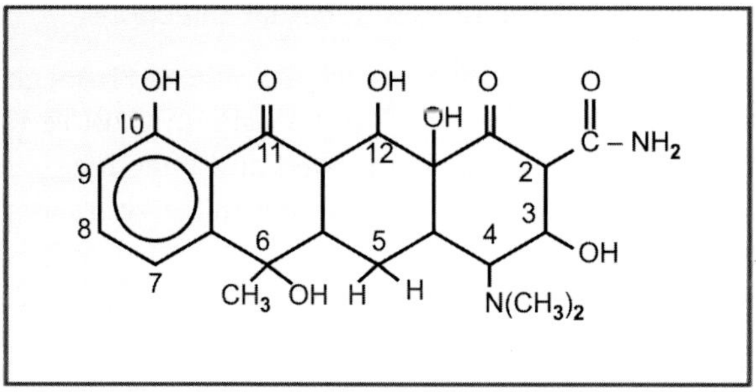

Fig. 7.2: Molecular structures of tetracycline

Classification

1. Short Acting (1-2 g dosage)
   - Chlor etracycline
   - Oxytetracycline
2. Intermediate acting (300 mg IBD dosage)
   - Methacycline
   - Demeclocycline
3. Long Acting : (100-200 mg IBD dosage)
   - Doxycyline
   - Minocycline
1. Tetracycline oral dose : 250-500 mg 6 hrly
   - Ophthalmic drops - 1%
   - Ophthalmic ointment - 1%
   - Chlorcyline and oxycyclin are also used with the same dosage.
2. Doxycycline :
   It is well absorbed from the gut highly effective against gram- positive and gram-negative microorganisms.

Dosage : 100-200 mg/dose 2-24 hourly

3. Chlotetracycline hydrocholorate.
   Dosage: 250-500 mg/dose 6 hourly
4. Methacycline :
   Dosage: 150-300 mg/ dose 6-12 hourly
5. Minocycline :
   Dosage: 200 mg/dose I/V.
6. Oxytetracycline :
   Dosage: 500 mg 6 hourly

- Ophthalmic ointment 1%

Therapy of Ocular Infections (Tetracyclines)

Surface ocular infections caused by susceptible microorganisms respond well to topical tetracycline. Although intraocular penetration of tetracycline is poor. Large oral dosage (6-8 gm/day) produce demonstrable aqueous conc and may be advised for the treatment of intraocular infections.

Chlamydial disease Adult inclusion conjunctivitis aquired from genital contract. Systemic tetracycline is recommended for the patient. A three week course of Tetracycline or Minocycline is recommended and effective.

- A prophylactic use of Topical tetracycline in newborn is very effective against ophthalmia neonatorum.
- Acute trachoma may be cured by topical and systemic tetracycline. Treatment should be continued for 2-4 weeks.

Phlyctenular keratoconjunctivitis Phlyctenular conjunctivitis responds well to Systemic tetracycline because phlyctenular. Keratoconjunctivitis is considered to be a non-specific hypersensitive reaction to bacterial proteins.

Toxoplasmosis A combination therapy with Minocycline and sulfadiazine is effective for treatment of active toxoplasmic retinochoroiditis.

Ocular rosacea Ocular rosacea treatment include one gm of tetracycline per day for 4-6 weeks followed by a slow taper to 250 mg every 1-2 days. The clinical improvement results from reduced lipase production by Staphylococci as well as reduction in Microflora.

Spirochaetal infection Tetracycline or Doxycycline is recommended for the treatment of Lyme disease. Tetracycline is acceptable alternative in the treatment of syphilis.

Persistent epithelial defects Persistent epithelial defects are caused by tissue and leucocytic collagenases. Tetracyclines have an anti collagenolytic effect independent of their antimicrobial properties. Systemic tetracyclines have been useful in healing persistent epithelial defects.

Identification of Neoplasms

Oxytetracycline is preferentially concentrated in rapidly growing neoplastic tissue. The presence of oxytetracycline in tissue can be detected at the time of surgery by examination under UV light which causes a brilliant yellow fluorescence. This method of tumor detection is applicable to surgery of orbital neoplasms. The dose of oxytetracycline for the Fluorescent detection of a neoplasms is 15 mg/kg/day for three days.

Sulphonamides

The sulphonamides have played a major role in the treatment and prophylaxis of bacterial eye infections but now have been susperceded by the newer anti-microbial agents.

Sulphonamides are bacteriostatic against Gram positive and gram negative bacteries. These are structural analogue of PABA competively inhibit bacterial folate synthetase. Sulphonamides are rapidly absorbed from G.I. tract and are well distributed through all body compartments including eye. It is highly soluble and are of value in the treatment of trachoma systemic treatment with Sulphonamides is not without side effects (Figs 7.3 and 7.4).

Sulphonamides used are:

- Sulfacetamide
- Sulfadiazine
- Sulfalene
- Sulfamethoxazole

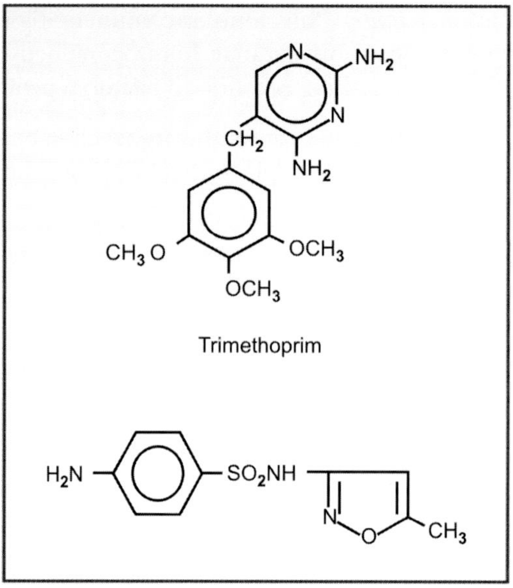

Trimethoprim

Fig. 7.3: Molecular structures of trimethoprim and sulfamethoxazole

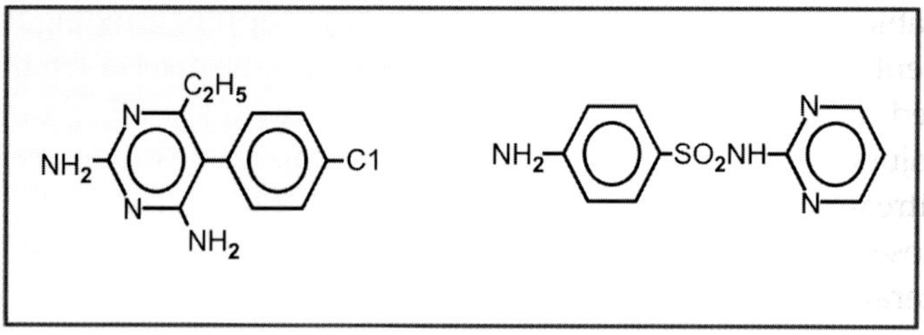

Fig. 7.4: Molecular structures of pyrimethamine and sulfadiazine

- Sulfisoxazole (Sulfafurazole)
- Sulfinpyrazone

Out of these Sulfacetamide is commonly used in eye as topical eye drops in conc of 10%, 20% and 30% and ophthalmic oint. in conc of 10 and 30%.

Systemic Doses of Sulphonamides

Oral dose : 2-4 gm/day 6 hourly
Parenteral dose : 100 mg/kg/day 6-8 hourly

Systemic Sulfonamide is an important supplement to pyrimethamine in the treatment of toxoplasmic retinochoroiditis.

Sulfisoxazole topical solution or ointment in conc of 4% is also used.

Adverse Reactions

Systemic administration may cause rashes, blood dyscrasias, GI disturbances like nausea, vomiting and diarrhea, urticaria and Hypersensitivity reactions.

Local administration is relatively free of side effect except of Hypersensitivity reactions in suspected cases.

Chloramphenicol

It is one of the most widely used broad spectrum antibiotic in the treatment of Ocular infections.

It is effective against a wide range of both gram-positive and gram-negative organisms (except *P. aeruginosa*), anaerobes.

It is bacteriostatic and interfers with protein synthesis.

Chloramphenicol is ideally suited for local application as it has little tendency to produce an allergic reaction and it is highly fat soluble which allows good corneal and intraocular penetration.

Systemic chloramphenicol is a very effective antibacterial agent. It penetrates into the aqueous following systemic administration. But systemic chloramphenicol has a number of side effect.

Dosage:

It is available as topical solution in strength of 0.4 to 1%.

- Ointment : 0.5%
- Fortified drops : 5-10 mg/ml
- Subconjunctival Injection dose : 50-100 mg/ml
- Intravitreal dose : 2 mg/ml
- Oral dose : 30-50 mg/kg/day 6 hourly
- Parenteral dose : 30-100 mg/kg/day 6 hourly
- Intracameral/Intravitreal dosage : 1-2 mg in 0.2-0.5 ml of isotonic sodium chloride solution.

Adverse Reactions

- On systemic administration most common is reversible dose-dependent bone marrow depression.
- Aplastic anemia
- Superinfections
- Agranulocytosis
- In infants cause Gray baby syndrome (abdominal distension pallid cyanosis, vasomotor collapse and death).

  Local application of chloramphenicol is relatively free of side effects.

Microlides

It includes:

Erythromycin It is bacteriostatic but in high doses, It is bactericidal. It is effective against gram-positive cocci, *H. influenzae*, *Mycoplasma*, *E.coli*, *Salmonella*, *Legionella* and *Chlamydia*. Streptococcal and Staphylococcal infections and *Mycoplasma* and *B. pertusis*. It acts by inhibiting protein synthesis by binding to the ribosome.

Dosage:
- Fortified drops - 5 mg/ml
- Ointment - 0.5%
- Subconjunctival dose - 100 mg/ml in isotonic Sodium Chloride solution.
- Intravitreal dose - 500 ug/ml
- Oral dose - 1-2 gm/day 6 hourly
- Parenteral dose - 1-4 gm/day continuous drip.

Adverse Reaction

In systemic use GI disturbance like epigastric distress, cholestatic jaundice, thrombophlebitis and allergic reactions.

Roxithromycin It is new second generation macrolide with improved pharmacokinetics, its antimicrobial spectrum is similar to that of erythromycin but has better penetration into bacterial cell and has bactericidal action and enhance host defence mechanism.

Dosage:

Orally 150 mg BD before food intake
Subconjunctival dose 50-100 mg/ml of isotonic sodium chloride solution.
- Fortified drops - 10 mg/ml
- Intravitreal dose - 50 ug/ml

Adverse Reactions

On systemic use it may cause nausea, abdominal distress, diarrhea, malaise, anorexia, constipation and hypersenstivity reactions, Dyspepsia, Dizziness, tinnitis, Headache and Vertigo.

Clindamycin

It is bacteriostatic agent but in higher doses it is bactericidal. It acts by inhibition of protein synthesis. It is active against gram-positive organisms, Actinomyces species, *B. fragilis* and *toxoplasmoses* (Fig. 7.5).

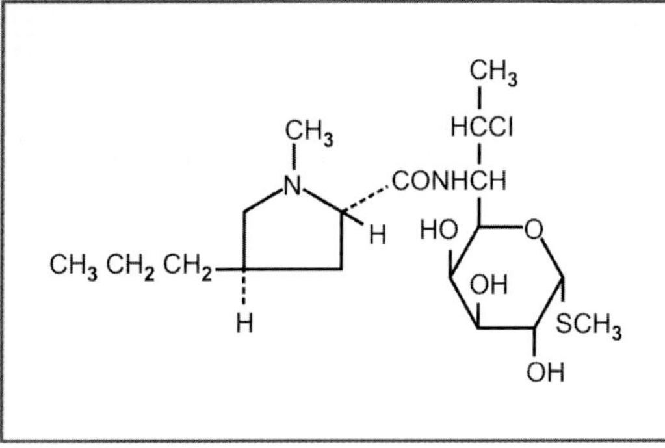

Fig. 7.5: Molecular structures of clindamycin

Dosage:

Subconjunctival doses : 15-40 mg/ml
Oral doses : 600 mg-1.8 gm/day 6 hourly
Parenteral dose : 1-3 gm/day 6 hourly

Adverse Reactions

Hypersenstivity reactions, GI disturbances.

Vancomycin

It is derived from cultures of *Nocardia orientalis.*

It is bactericidal for most gram-positive organisms staphylococci and *Clostridium*, enterococcal infections.

It acts by inhibition of bacterial cell wall synthesis. (Inhibition of glycopeptide depolymerization in the cell wall). It is useful for treatment of staphylococcal infection non-responsive to Cephalosporins, Methicillin resistant *Staphylococci* and *Streptococcus viridans.*

Dosage:

- Fortified drops : 50 mg/ml
- Subconjunctival dose : 25 mg/ml
- Intravitreal dose : 1.0 mg/ml
- Parenteral dose : 2 gm/day 6-12 hourly.

Intravitreal vancomycin with an aminoglycoside has been recommended as initial emperic therapy for exogenous endophthalmitis. A dose of 1 mg in 0.1ml intravitreally Establishes intraocular levels significantly higher than the MIC for most gram-positive organisms.

Adverse Reactions

On systemic use—Thrombophlebitis, allergic reactions, ototoxicity and nephrotoxicity and hypersensitivity rashes.

Spiramycin

It is latest generation macrolide antibiotic.

It is bacteriostatic by inhibition of bacterial protein synthesis. Suceptible organisms include Staphylococci, Streptococci, Bordetella, Diphtheria, Branhamella, Listeria, anaerobes. Gram-negative aerobic bacteria are not susceptible. Has potential synergistic action with metronidazole against organisms.

Dosage:

Oral dose 6-9 million IU/day in 2-3 divided doses for 5 days.

- Fortified drops : 10 mg/ml
- Subconjunctival dose : 50-100 mg/ml

Adverse Reactions

Hypersensitivity reaction, nausea, vomiting, abdominal pain, Diarrhea urticaria, macular rashes, benign hepatitis.

Azithromycin

It is macrolide antimicrobial as active as erythromycin against gram-positive organisms, but is more active against several gram-negative organisms. High conc are achieved in tissues and in macrophages and polymorphs. This makes azithromycin highly effective against intracellular pathogens such as *Mycoplasma*, *Chlamydia* and *Legionella*. The most exciting application for ophthalmic infection is in the treatment of *Chlamydia trachomatis*. Azithromycin is not active against *Pseudomonas* mode of action is by inhibition of protein synthesis.

Dosage:

Oral dose: 500 mg-1 g once daily for three days in Chlamydial infections.

Azithromycin is a promising treatment for trachoma because of difficulty of patient compliance with conventional treatment.

Adverse Effects

Hypersenstivity reaction, Mild to moderate nausea, vomiting, abdominal pain, diarrhea, Angioedema and Photosensitivity reactions.

Clarithromycin

It is one of the latest macrolide antibiotic investigated for topical and systemic administration. Both topical and systemic clarithromycin administration is effective against infectious Keratitis due to a typical mycobacteria Mycobacteria *Chelonei* and *M. fortuitum*. Clarithromycin is 10-50 times more active than Erythromycin and 48 times more active than Azithromycin against 55 strains of *M. Chelonei*.

The 14-hydroxymetabolite is also active and act synergestically. *Pseudomonas* and enterobacteriaceae are not susceptible to clarithromycin.

Oral dosage : 200-500 mg bid for a week.

Adverse Reactions

Pseudomembranous colitis, Anaphylaxis, Stevens-Johnson syndrome, GI. upset, headache, Hallucinations, rash, urticaria.

Another compound of Macrolide group Josamycin is under investigation for ophthalmic application.

Polypeptides

Polymixin B: It is bactericidal against gram-negative organisms, *E. coli, Pseudomonas*, Enterobacter, *K.pneumoniae* and *H. influenzae.*

It acts by the lysis of lipoprotein in the cell membrane, *Proteus*, gram-negative cocci, *Neisseria* and fungi are resistant.

Dosage:

Ophthalmic drops 0-5 to 1- 0% (In combination with neomycin)

Fortified drops : 1-2 mg/ml (shelf life 7 days)

Ointment : 1 to 1.5 mg/gm

Due to greater nephrotoxicity it is not systemically given its use is restricted to topical use. Local Adverse effects, on Topical use can lead to Hypersensitivity, itching, redness and edema of conjunctiva and eyelid.

Bacitracin

It is bactericidal against gram-positive and gram-negative organisms, spirochaetes, *E. histolytica* and Actinomyces.

It acts by inhibition of cell wall synthesis.

Dosages:

- Fortified drops—10000 units/ml
- Subconjunctival dose—10000 units
- Ointment—10000 units/gm.

It is also not systemically given due to potential toxicity. It has few side effects, like itching, congestion, edema of conjunctiva and eyelids.

Antimicrobial Peptides

The antimicrobial peptide group of antibacterial agents have been isolated from the immune defence of organisms such as insects, amphibians and mammals. It is an exciting area for antimicrobial agent development for clinical use. The antimicrobials of this group are:

Defensins Defensins are a group of antimicrobial and cytotoxic peptides with three distinct peptide families of defensins - Classical, beta and Insect defensins determined both by source and chemical structure of defensin. The classical and beta defensins are derived mainly from mammalian source.

These are active against a number of organisms including gram-negative and gram-positive bacteria, mycobacteria, fungi and viruses. Insect defensins are active predominantly against gram-positive bacteria.

Classic and beta defensins are highly active against human isolates from ulcerative Keratitis. Organisms tested includes an alpha hemolytic *Streptococcus* sps, *S. pneumoniae, P. aeruginosa* and *Morganella*. At a concentration of 10 ug/ml there was a marked bactericidal effect.

Besides it classic and beta defensins have a possible application as a microbicide in corneal storage media.

A concentration of 200 ug/ml successfully kill 99.9% of all three main organisms namely *S. aureus, S. pneumoniae* and *P. aeruginosa* with in 30 minutes at all three temperatares (4°C, 23°C and 37°C). This bactericidal effect is impressive specially when the rapidity and low temperatures are considered. Conventional antibiotics do not have significant effect on lower temperatures.

Cecropins These are antimicrobial peptides produced by giant silk moth (Hyalophora cecropia) in response to bacterial challange. It is highly effective against various gram-positive and negative bacteria, enveloped virus, fungi and protozoa.

It has bactericidal effect against various organisms *S. pneumoniae, P. aeruginosa* and *S. aureus* isolated from ulcerative Keratitis.

A synthetic cecropin analog D5C and natural antimicrobial peptide have potential bactericidal effect at conc of 100 ug/ml at 4oc and 27oc. The cecropin D5C has also been investigated as a possible antimicrobial additive for contact lens disinfecting solutions. The addition of D5C to leading disinfecting solutions did enhance the bactericidal effect of solution for certain specific organisms.

Megainins

The megainins were isolated from the skin of the frog Xenopus laevis. They have broad spectrum activity against a wide range of organisms including gram-positive and negative bacteria, viruses, fungi and protozoa. Initial investigations into the antimicrobial activity into ocular infections is promising.

Another antimicrobial peptide discovered in rabbit aqueous humour is under investigation for bactericidal activity.)

Fluoroquinolones

So far the most significant new antibiotics in ophthalmology are of Fluoroquinolone group. In modern ophthalmic practice fluoroquinolone group antibiotics are most commonly prescribed world wide with excellent response. The Fluroquinolone constitute a family of anti-bacterial agents based on the original 4-quinolone Nalidixic acid a drug first marketed in 1962 for treating UTI. The current quinolones have Fluorine at position six of the four quinolone nucleus. The new generation fluoroquinolone derivatives have much wider spectrum of anti bacterial activity, better tissue penetration and are associated with a lower rate of development of resistant organisms.

The group includes Norfloxacin, Ciprofloxacin, Ofloxacin Pefloxacin, Lomefloxacin, Sparfloxacin, Levofloxacin, Gatifloxacin, Moxifloxacin. The mechanisms of action of the Fluoroquinolone is the inhibition of bacterial DNA gyrase an enzyme important for DNA. Supercoiling and protein synthesis. These are synthesized chemically.

Good Aqueous humour concentrations of fluoroquinolones have been demonstrated in uninflamed human eyes after systemic administration in addition to topical route. It has been shown that Fluoroquinolone ocular penetration after systemic administration is related to their relative degree of lipophilicity. Sparfloxacin the most lipophilic compound had excellent ocular penetration (55%) comparing vitreous and serum levels followed by Ofloxacin (30%), Pefloxacin (10%) and Ciprofloxacin (5.5%).

The various drugs of this group used in ophthalmic field are:

1. Norfloxacin:

   It is bactercidal against gram-negative organism, *E. coli*, *Klebsiella*, enterobacter, *Proteus* Cetobacter, *Acinetobacter* sp. *Pseudomonas* aeruginosa, *N. gonorrheae* and gram-positive organisms like staphylococci including methicillin resistant strains, Enterococci and Strep. agalactic. It acts by its specific bacterial DNA gyrase blocker action.

   Topically it is commonly used against superficial infections of the eye.

Dosage:

Ophthalmic soln	:	0.3%
Ointment	:	0.3%
Fortified drops	:	20 mg/ml (shelf life 14 days)
Orally	:	400 mg BD.
Parenteral	:	200-400 mg/day 12 hourly.

Adverse Reactions

Nausea, vomiting, heart burn, diarrhea, headache, dizziness, depression, insomnia and seizures, rash, Drymouth, fever, arthralgia, eosinophilia, neutropenia, etc.

On topical use, side effects are minimal. Topical Norfloxacin has corneal epithelial toxicity greater than Ciprofloxacin.

Ciprofloxacin

This is one of the most potent fluoroquinolone derivative. It is bactericidal and has extended broad spectrum against most of gram-negative aerobic bacteria including *Pseudomonas, Chlamydia trachomatis.* Hemophilus, *Neisseriae* and against gram-positive aerobic bacteria including penicillinase producing and methicillin resistant staphylococci. However many strains of streptococci are resistant to it. Streptococci pneumoniae is susceptible at higher concentration of Ciprofloxacin.

It act by inhibition of bacterial DNA gyrase an enzyme essential in DNA supercoiling and replication.

It can be given topically or systemically. In topical form it is commonly used to treat conjunctivitis, keratitis, keratoconjunctivitis, corneal ulcers, Blepharitis, Dacrocystitis and pre-operatively, etc.

Dosage:

Ophthalmic solution	:	0.3%	
Fortified drops	:	20 mg/ml (shelf life 15 days)	
Ophthalmic ointment	:	0.3%	
Subconjunctival injection	:	20-40 mg/ml	
Intravitreal dose	:	200 mg/ml	
Orally	:	500-1500 mg/day	6 hourly
Parenteral	:	5 -10 mg/kg/day	12 hourly.

Ciprofloxacin is available as topical, oral and intravenous forms. After systemic administration of Ciprofloxacin, intraocular penetration in uninflamed eyes occurs with levels of 10% of that achieved in the patients serum and can reach intravitreal MIC for 90 percent of bacteria. Therefore, intravenous Ciprofloxacin is recommended in infectious endophthalmitis.

Topical ophthalmic use has excellent activity against gram-positive and gram-negative organisms. Topical Ciprofloxacin (0.3%) is well tolerated with no significant corneal or conjunctival epithelial toxicity as compare to topical aminoglycosides which are significantly toxic to corneal and conjunctival epithelial toxicity as compare to topical aminoglycosides which are significantly toxic to corneal and conjunctival epithelium having the potential to cause conjunctival membrane formation. The most common untoward effect of topical Ciprofloxacin for corneal ulcers is formation of white precipitate on the cornea. This precipitate has the advantage of providing a depot of the drug at the site of infection but is potentially harmful as it sometimes decreases visualization of the corneal infiltrates deep to the precipitates. Topical Ciprofloxacin Ointment is well tolerated by the cornea and Conjunctiva.

Systemic Ciprofloxacin and other quinolones should be avoided in children owing to the potential risk of arthropathy.

Adverse Reactions

On Systemic administration, Anaphylactoid reaction, GI disturbance on systemic use and CNS disturbances, Hypersensitivity reactions. Rashes blurred vision, joint pains, Hematological, hepatic and renal disturbances.

On local use side effects are minimal.

Ofloxacin

It is a newer potent fluorinated quinolone that has a broad spectrum of antimicrobial activity.

Ofloxacin possesses the widest spectrum of activity against gram-positive and gram-negative organisms (including resistant strains) as compared to Ciprofloxacin and Norfloxacin.

It is potent bactericidal and acts by inhibiting the bacterial DNA gyrase an essential enzyme that is a critical catalyst in the duplication, transcription and repair of bacterial DNA.

It is effective even against bacterial strains resistant to Ciprofloxacin. It can be given topically or systemically. In topical form this is an excellant drug to treat various infective conditions of eye.

Oral Ofloxacin has a longer half life and oral doses achieve higher serum and aqueous humour concentrations than Ciprofloxacin Ofloxacin is highly effective against most of the pathogenic bacteria causing ocular infections.

Pharmacokinetic studies have shown that conc of Ofloxacin in the aqueous humour and tear fluids on topical administration are above its MIC90 for ocular isolates. After application of 0.3% ointment the conc of Ofloxacin in tear fluid are 300.0 + 58.7 mg/ml at half hour and in the cul-de-sac 0.62 + 0.14 mg/ml in aqueous humour at 60 minutes.

Dosage:

Ophthalmic solution	– 0.3%
Ophthalmic ointment	– 0.3%
Fortified drops	– 20 mg/ml (shelf life 15 days)
Subconjunctival dose	– 20-40 mg/ml
Intravitreal dose	– 200 mg/ml
Oral dose	– 200-400 mg6 hourly
Parenteral	– 100-200 mg/day 12 hourly.
IV infusion	– 200 mg infusion over 30 minutes bid

Adverse Reactions

On systemic use nausea, vomiting, abdominal pain, diarrhea, Headache, Leukopenia and eosinophilia.

On topical use it is free of adverse effect except for Mild transient burning sensation and itching may occur.

Pefloxacin

It is a piperazine carboxylic acid derivative belong to this promising class of fluoroquinolone antibacterials. It is bactericidal and exhibits action by inhibtion of bacterial enzyme DNA gyrase. It also inhibits RNA synthesis. This unique mode of action ensures, potent wide spectrum bactericidal action and negligible resistance.

It is highly effective against gram-positive and gram-negative organisms including difficult pathogens like *Pseudomonas* species and *Chlamydia trachomatis*, enterobacteriaceae, Methicillin resistant strains of staphylococci and streptococci, *Chlamydia* and *Mycoplasma*. It is not active against anaerobes. The facultative anaerobes are also resistant.

It is also very effective against multi-drug resistant strains like beta lactamase producing aminoglycoside modifying and penicillinase producing *N. gonorrhea*.

It is deep acting antibacterial agent which in topical use is highly effective against various infective conditions of the eye. It has good intraocular penetration and has an average level of 0.95 mg/ml of aqueous concentration.

Dosage:

Ophthalmic Solution	–	0.3%
Fortified drops	–	20 mg/ml (shelf life 15 days)
Subconjunctival dose	–	20-40 mg/ml
Oral dose	–	400 mg BD
IV infusion	–	400 mg in 100 ml of 5% Dextrose solution infusion over 1 hour.

Adverse Reactions

On systemic use nausea, vomiting, diarrhea. Dizziness, headache, allergic reactions. Pseudomembranous colitis, superinfections on topical use little adverse effects are reported except for transient burning and itching.

Lomefloxacin

It is one of the latest derivative of fluoroquinolone antimicrobial available for topical and systemic administration. Lomefloxacin is a difluorinated quinolone derivative.

It is bactericidal and is bacterial DNA gyrase inhibitor effective against a wide ranges of gram-positive and gram-negative bacteria including resistant strains to previous quinolone derivatives. It acts by inhibiting bacterial DNA gyrase and on RNA synthesis. The target molecule for lomefloxacin is the A subunit of bacterial enzyme gyrase (tapoisomerase II). Plasmid mediated transfer of resistance has not been observed. The frequency of development of spontaneous mutation is less than 10 -8 to 10 -9. No cross resistance has been reported with Lomefloxacin. Lomefloxacin inhibits bacterial DNA related processes like replication, transcription recombination, transposition, supercoiling and relaxation of DNA.

Lomefloxacin is very effective against multi drug resistant strains like beta Lactamase producing aminoglycoside modifying and penicillinase producing N. gonorrheae. If is also highly effective against difficult pathogens like *Pseudomonas* species and *Chlamydia trachomatis.*

It is deep acting anti-bacterial agent which in topical use is very effective against various infective conditions of the eye. It has good intraocular penetration and has an average level of 0.95 mg/ml of aqueous concentration. After oral administration it has good aqueous humour concentration due to its Lypophilic activity. Lomefloxacin is prescribed topically for external ocular infections of the eye.

Dosage:

- Ophthalmic solution : 0.3 percent
- Fortified drops : 20 mg/ml (Shelf Life 15 days)
- Subconjunctival dose : 20-30 mg/ml
- Intravitreal dose : 200 mg/ml
- Oral dose : 400 mg once daily

Adverse Reactions

On topical use adverse effects are very low except transient burning and itching sensation, occasional allergic reaction. Bacteriostatic ophthalmic antibiotics should not be used concomitantly with topical Lomefloxacin.

On systemic use it is generally tolerated with mild to moderate side effects. Adverse effects include gastrointestinal symptoms like nausea, Diarrhea, pain, discomfort. Other side effects are:

Stevens-Johnson syndrome, Headache, Dizziness,Dermatological, Hypersenstivity reactions and photosenstivity.

Sparfloxacin

It is one of the latest derivative of fluoroquinolone group. It has an excellant broad spectrum bactericidal effect on gram-negative and gram-positive organisms including anaerobes specially *Bacteroids fragilis* and multidrug resistant enterococci. It is more active than Ciprofloxacin against *Strep pneumoniae, Staph aureus* (including MRSA), *Staph. epidermidis* and *Staph saprophyticus*. It is also active against *Chlamydia trachomatis, Mycobacteria sps, Citrobacter, Aeromonas* and *Pseudomonas sps*. It acts by inhibiting the supercoiling activity of DNA replication. Sparfloxacin as mentioned earlier that in addition to topical administration, it has excellant aqueous humour concentrations after systemic administration (Figs 7.6A to C).

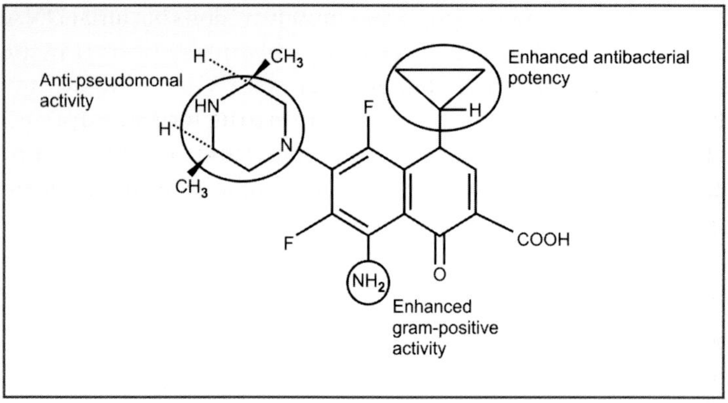

Anti-pseudomonal activity

Enhanced antibacterial potency

Enhanced gram-positive activity

$COOH$, NH_2, CH_3, F

Fig. 7.6A: Chemical structure of sparfloxacin

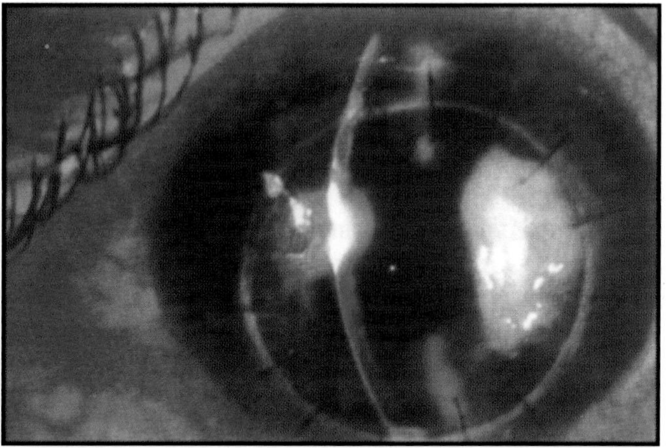

Fig. 7.6B: Bacterial keratitis *Streptococcus pneumonia* (*Courtesy*: FDC Limited)

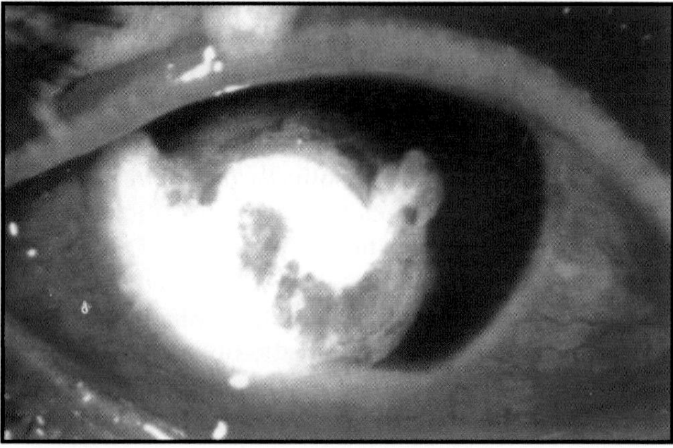

Fig. 7.6C: Bacterial keratitis *Pseudomonas aeruginosa* (*Courtesy*: FDC Limited)

Sparfloxacin is the most lipophilic compound tested and had excellaent ocular penetration (55%).

It is present at concentrations greater than 90% minimal inhibitory concentration (MIC90) for most gram-positive cocci for 18 hours.

Sparfloxacin is a promising new agent for its intravitreal and systemic applications in ophthalmology. Sparfloxacin is highly effective in the treatment of endophthalmitis due to the strain *G Streptoccus* sps and *S. aureus*.

Dosage:

Ophthalmic solution	– 0.3%
Oral dose	– 400 mg in divided doses
Intravitreal dose	– 20-60 ug/ml
Fortified drops	– 20 mg/ml (shelf life - 15 days)
Subconjunctival dose	– 20-40 mg/ml

Adverse Effects

On topical use no significant side effects has been reported except for transient burning and itching.

On systemic use diarrhea, abdominal pain, nausea, vomiting, stomatitis, renal failure, Anaphylactoid reaction, headache, dizziness etc.

Levofloxacin

It is one of recently introduced latest topical antibiotic of fluoroquinolone group. It is the pure(s) enantiomer of the recemic drug substance ofloxacin. Levofloxacin is a fluorinated 4-quinolone containing a six member (pyridobenzoxazine) ring from position 1 to 8 of the basic ring structure. It is L-isomer of the D, L-racemate ofloxacin.

It has highest bactericidal effect among all the fluoroquinolones effective against a broad spectrum of gram-positive and gram-negative micro-organisms. It is effective against *Corynebacterium* species, *Staphylococcus aureus, Staph epidermidis, Staph pneumoniae, Streptococcus, Acinetobacter iwolffi, Haemophilus influenzae, Serratia marcescens* and *Pseudomonas*. Its mechanisms of action includes inhibition of supercoiling activity of DNA replication.

It is highly lipophilic and has an excellent aqueous humor concentration on both topical and systemic administration. It is more soluble in water at neutral pH than ofloxacin. As compare to other topical quinolones levofloxacin is formulated at pH of 6.5.

Levofloxacin has an excellent clinical cure (82%) and eradication rates (90%). It has best solubility by far, i.e. 35.8 mg/ml. This leads to a high drug concentration at the site of infection after topical instillation. Due to highest bactericidal effect of Levofloxacin among fluoroquinolones results in rapid eradication of pathogens. Levofloxacin is transported across the cornea in patt by an active transport mechanisms. Currently levofloxacin is available as topical ophthalmic solution (0.5%) and is available at higher concentration than other fluoroquinolones and is indicated for the treatment of bacterial conjunctivitis caused by susceptible strains of gram-positive and gram-negative microorganisms and also for infection prophylaxis in ophthalmic surgical procedures.

Levofloxacin is safe and effective for use in pregnant ladies and in children. It has high antibacterial potency and good tolerability.

Adverse Effects

Levofloxacin has low incidence of adverse events (1-3%). The most frequently reported adverse effects on topical use are transient decrease in vision, fever, foreign body sensation, headache, transient ocular burning, ocular pain or discomfort, pharyngitis and photophobia.

Contraindications

Levofloxacin is contraindicated in patients with history of hypersensitivity to quinolones or to any of the components in this medication.

Gatifloxacin

Gatifloxacin is recently introduced Fourth generation Fluoroquinolone. This new generation antibiotic has the fluorine group in the sixth position and cyclopropyl group in the first position enhancing gram-positive coverage. The key difference between this new Fluoroquinolone and the older agents of this group is at the seventh position. The substitution here has decreased the propensity for resistance to occur in bacteria. This antibiotic is able to enter the bacterial cells and the cells efflux mechanism is blocked because of the large size of the C7 side chain. The cells are not able to pump out the antibiotic.

It has highest bactericidal effect against a broad spectrum of gram-positive and gram-negative microorganisms specially against Aerobic gram-positive bacteria like *Corynebacterium* propinquum, *Streptococcus mitis, Staphylococcus aureus, Streptococcus pneumoniae* and *Staphylococcus epidermidis*. It is highly effective also against Aerobic gram-negative bacteria like *Haemophilus influenzae.*

Its mechanism of action is similar to previous fluoroquinolones i.e. inhibition of supercoiling activity of DNA replication.

Based on ocular penetration and microbiological assay (MIC index) Gatifloxacin is highly lipophilic and has an excellent Aqueous humour concentration. Currently Gatifloxacin is available as Topical Ophthalmic Solution (0.3%) and is indicated for the treatment of bacterial infections of eye (Conjunctivitis, Keratitis etc.). For cataract prophylaxis (Therapy goals, infection prevention regimens) and for Reflactive Surgery Prophylaxis. Gatifloxacin has better Biocompatibility, better potency and therapeutic penetration and high anti-bacterial potency and good tolerability.

Dosage:

Ophthalmic solution	–	0.3 percent
Systemic dosage	–	400 mg in divided doses.
Intravitreal dose	–	200 mg/ml.
Fortified drops	–	20 mg/ml (shelf life 15 days)
Subconjunctival dose	–	20-40 mg/ml.
Ophthalmic ointments	–	0.3 percent

Adverse Effects

On topical use no significant side effects have been reported except for conjunctival irritation, Increased Lacrimation, Keratitis and Papillary Conjunctivitis.

Contraindications

It is contraindicated in patients with a history of hypersensitivity to Gatifloxacin, to other quinolones or to any of the components in this medication.

Moxifloxacin

Moxifloxacin is latest Fourth Generation Fluoroquinolone with 8 methoxy group. It has a bicyclic side chain which seems to increase resistance inhibition. Moxifloxacin has the ability to resist mutations much better than previous quinolones.

Moxifloxacin has better solubility and thus achieve higher therapeutic concentrations which is a positive characteristic because the mechanism of action against the bacteria is concentration dependent. The activity of Moxifloxacin is geater because of the methoxy group at the C-8 position which binds to both topoisomerase II and IV. In addition it has bulky side chain in the C-7 position. This side chain further increases activity and inhibits resistance. This side chain also inhibits the cells efflux pump which increases the drug stay with in the bacterial cells. This improves efficacy and minimizes resistance.

Moxifloxacin has superior potency and the broadest available spectrum of coverage against both gram-positive and negative microorganisms and even Fluroquinolone resistant pathogens. It eradicate pathogenes deep down where they live. It is highly effective against Methicillin resistant *S. aureus* (MRSA) and *Staphylococcus epidermidis* (MRSE). It is specially effective against aerobic gram-positive microorganisms like *Corynebacterium* species, *Micrococcus luteus*, *Streptococcus* and *Staphylococcus* species. It has high potency against Aerobic gram-negative microorganisms like *Acinetobacter livoffir*, Haemophilus species and the microorganisms.

It is highly Lipophilic and has an excellent aqueous humour penetration as shown by various MBC, MIC and MPC studies.

Moxifloxacin has an excellent clinical cure (96%) and eradication rate (95%). It has best solubility which leads to higher drug concentration at the site of infection after topical instillation. Currently Moxifloxacin is available as topical ophthalmic solution (0.5%) and is available at higher concentration than other Fluroquinolones. Clinically Moxifloxacin is indicated for various ocular bacterial infections, Pre and postoperative cataract prophylaxis and refractive surgery prophylaxis.

Moxifloxacin is safe and effective for use in pregnant ladies and in children.

Dosage:

Ophthalmic solution	–	0.5 percent
Oral dose	–	500 mg in divided doses
Intravitreal dose	–	200 mg/ml
Ophthalmic ointment	–	0.5 percent
Fortified drops	–	20 mg/ml (Shelf life 15 days)
Subconjunctival dose	–	20-40 mg/ml.

Adverse Effects

Moxifloxacin has low incidence of adverse effects (1-2%). The adverse effects reported over topical usage is conjunctivitis, decreased visual acuity, Dry Eye, ocular discomfort, pain and hypremia etc.

Contraindications

Moxifloxacin is contraindicated in patients with a history of hypersensitivity to it or other quinolones and to any of the components in this medication.

A number of other investigational fluoroquinolones are on the horizon. These includes:

- Tosufloxacin
- Trovafloxacin
- Gemifloxacin
- Clinafloxacin

Aqueous humor level studies of Levofloxacin, Moxifloxacin and Gemifloxacin have been conducted both in oral and topical (0.3%) prototype solution with encouraging results.

High performance liquid chromatographic studies have shown that Clinafloxacin and Gemifloxacin when given orally as well as topically achieved significant aqueous concentrations. Because of their excellent ocular penetration these fluoroquinolones may be considered as an alternative or additional choice for surgical prophylaxis and as an adjunctive therapy for endophthalmitis. Topical ophthalmic preparations of these new fluoroquinolones shall help in treating various ocular infective conditions in a better way in near future.

Clinafloxacin is a new fluoroquinolone that has been reported promising specially in ophthalmic use. It has been found effective *in vitro* against multi-drug resistant enterococci, *P.aeruginosa*, *Xanthomonas maltophilia* and other *Pseudomonas* species.

Another new Fluoroquinolone A-80556 is on the horizon. It has extended activity against gram-positive and gram-negitave organisms and is reported effective when given intravitreally in endophthalmitis due to *S. aureus* and *P.aeruginosa*.

Other derivatives Du-6859a, DV 7751a, BAY-Y3118 are on trials with excellent antibacterial activity against a broad spectrum of organisms including resistant species *in vitro.*

Imidazole Derivatives

It includes:

Metronidazoles

It is 5- nitro midazole derivative. It is potent bactericidal agent which interacts with DNA. It is effective against anaerobic bactreria like *B.fragilis*, clostridia, anaerobic streptococci, protozoa, *Entamoeba histolytica* and Guinea worm, *Fusobacterium* sps, *Clostridium* sps, *Peptococcus* and *Streptopeptococcus.*

Dosage:
Orally 400-800 mgm every 8 hourly.
IV onfusion : 15 mg/kg infusion over 30-60 minutes.

Adverse Reactions

Peripheral neuropathies, GI disturbances rash, seizures urticaria, pruritus, superinfection. CNS disturbances, metallic taste, Headache, dizziness and glossitis.

Cotrimoxazole

It is combination of Trimethoprim and sulfamethoxazole. It is bactericidal against all strains of *Strep. pneumoniae*, *C. diphtherial*, *N. meningitidis* 95%. Strains of *Strep aureus*, *E. coli*, *Klebsiella*, *Brucella*, Enterobacter and few strains of *Pseudomonas aeruginosa* and *Pneumocystis* carinii which is opportunistic pathogen in AIDS patients. They act by competing with PABA for synthesis of folic acid in the bacteria. It inhibit folic acid synthesis by the pathogen but at different stages which results in potentiation of action. It is given systemically.

Dosage:
Oral 1 tab (double strength) BD (Trimethoprim 160 mg and Sulphamethoxazole 800 mg).

Parenteral—20 mg TMP/kg/day 8 hourly.

In AIDS patients—T20+S100 mg in 3-4 divided doses for 14-21 days.

Adverse Reactions

Most frequent are skin rashes,GI disturbances, hypersensitivity reactions, blood dyscrasias and hepatocellular necrosis, Stevens-Johnson syndrome, diarrhea and vomiting, etc.

Miscellaneous

Use of Antibiotics in Irrigating Solutions for Intraocular Surgery

Antibiotics supplementation of intraocular infusions recently has been subject of discussion and possible widespread use.

Gentamicin (8ug/ml), Vancomycin (20 ug/ml) or gentamicin and Vancomycin combination (8 ug/ml and 20 ug/ml) are the most common anti-bacterial agents investigated in this manner. Scientists have reported a very low rate of endophthalmitis when gentamicin or vancomycin were added to the cataract infusion solution and the infusion solution was filtered. It is being depicted that antibiotic supplementation in infusion solution kills bacteria and prevents endophthalmitis. On examination of post cataract anterior chamber aspiration after surgery in which gentamicin (8 and 80 ug/ml) was used in the irrigating solution, no organisms were isolated. These results are encouraging, research is being conducted on *in vitro* model to evaluate the potential anti-microbial effects of piperacillin and tazobactam (512 ug and 64 ug/ml respectively) used in the combination in irrigating solution. Preliminary results are encouraging. Other antibiotic agents examined to determine their utility in intraocular infusions method of administration are Ofloxacilin and Sparfloxacilin.

Intracameral perfusion at (20-60 ug/ml) and infusion conc from 40-1280 ug/ml of Ofloxacilin have shown no toxic effects in rabbit model.

However, extreme caution should be taken by ophthalmologists against over use of antibiotics in irrigating solution from the potential for increasing antibiotic resistance which is becoming an increasingly common menance. The increasing prevalence of antibiotic resistance including the spectra of "superresistant" organisms is a very troublesome result of the inappropriate overuse of antibiotics.

Intravitreal Antibiotics

Intravitreal administration of antibiotics has many advantages in the treatment of localized ocular infection such as endophthalmitis. Higher concentration of antibiotics are immediately achieved without systemic exposure. Because of the advnatages of intravitreal administration. Research scientists recently have investigated some of the newer antibiotics for intravitreal application. Sparfloxacilin, Pefloxacilin, Ciprofloxacilin and imipenem have been reported as possible anti-bacterial agents for intravitreal administration from new generation of antibiotics with excellent response. These agents appear to have little toxicity when administered intravitreally. Further studies are being done to evaluate the antibacterial action of these agents at the levels achievable by intravitreal administration.

In ophthalmic practice the mode of administration is much more significant as intraocular penatration of antimicrobials differ considerably. Shelf life of the drugs must be kept in view for optimum therapeutic effect and convenience in their application specially for topical, subconjunctival and intraocular therapy.

BIBLIOGRAPHY

1. Agarwal Amar. Text book of ophthalmology, ed.1. New Delhi: Jaypee Medical Publishers, 2002.
2. Bartlett. JD. Clinical Ocular Pharmacology, ed.4. Boston: Butterworth-Heinemann, 2001
3. Bartlett. JD. Ophthalmic Drug facts: Lippincott—William and Wilkins, 2001.
4. Crick. RP, Trimble RB. Text book of clinical ophthalmology : Hodder and Stoughton, 1986.
5. Duane. TD. Clinical ophthalmology, ed. 4: Butterworth – Heinemann, 1999.
6. Duvall. Ophthalmic Medications and Pharmacology : Slack Inc, 1998.
7. Ellis. PP. Ocular Therapeutics and Pharmacology, ed. 7 : CV Mosby, 1985.
8. Fechner. Ocular Therapeutics : Slack Inc., 1998.
9. Fraunfelder. Current Ocular Therapy, ed. 5 : WB Saunders, 2000.
10. Garg Ashok. Current Trends in ophthalmology, ed. 1, New Delhi: Jaypee Medical Publishers, 1997.
11. Garg Ashok. Manual of Ocular Therapeutics, ed. 1, New Delhi: Jaypee Medical Publishers, 1996.
12. Garg Ashok Ready Reckoner of Ocular Therapeutics, ed.1, New Delhi 2002.
13. Goodman LS, Gilman A. Pharmacological basis of Therapeutics, ed.7, New York: Macmillan, 1985.
14. Havener's Ocular Pharmacology, ed. 6: CV Mosby, 1994.
15. Kanski. Clinical ophthalmology, ed. 4 : Butterworth – Heineman, 1999.
16. Kershner. Ophthalmic Medications and Pharmacology: Slack. Inc., 1994.
17. Kucers A, Bennett NM. The use of Antibiotics, ed.4, Philadelphia: JB Lippincott Company, 1987.
18. Olin BR et.al. Drugs Facts and Comparisons : Facts and Comparisons, St. Louis, 1997.
19. Onofrey. The Ocular Therapeutics; Lippincott-William and Wilkins, 1997.
20. Rhee. The Wills Eye drug Guide : Lippincott – William and Wilkins, 1998.
21. Seal. Ocular infection management and treatment : Martin – Dunitz, 1998.
22. Steven Podos. Text book of ophthalmology, New Delhi : Jaypee Medical Publishers, 2001.
23. Zimmerman. Text book of Ocular Pharmacology : Lippincott and William and Wilkins, 1997.

Chapter 8

PREOPERATIVE AND POST-OPERATIVE ANTIBIOTIC PROPHYLAXIS IN CATARACT SURGERY

NR Biswas, Srujana Mohanty, GK Das
Madhurjya Gogai (India)

Cataract extraction is one of the most commonly performed ophthalmic surgeries in the world. An infrequent but devastating complication is postoperative endophthalmitis, the reported prevalence in recent times being 0.04 to 0.26%.[1-3] Possible origins of infection include the ocular tear film, lids and adnexa; irrigating solutions and medications; surgical instruments including intraocular lenses; the respiratory and skin flora of the surgeon; and operating room air. Because sterile surgical techniques addresses many of these sources, it is now well established that the source of most infecting agents is the endogenous ocular flora.[4,5] The most commonly recovered organisms have been gram-positive bacteria (coagulase-negative staphylococci, *Staphylococcus aureus*, and streptococci) with gram-negative organisms making up a small proportion of the total.[6] Surface flora routinely gain entry to the anterior chamber during cataract surgery. In one study, 13 of 59 eyes (22%) grew gram-positive organisms from aqueous cultures taken at the time of wound closure after intraocular surgery, and 8 of these eyes (62%) had organisms isolated from the eyelids and conjunctiva before or after disinfection.[7] In the endophthalmitis vitrectomy study,[6] a randomized multicentered prospective clinical study, confirmed microbiologic growth was demonstrated in 69.3% of patients with clinically suspected endophthalmitis. Gram-positive organisms were isolated from 94.2% patients. Two hundred twenty-six of the 323 isolates obtained (70%) gram- positive coagulase-negative micrococci,32(9.9%) *Staphylococcus aureus*, 29 (9.0%) *Streptococcus species*, 7 (2.2%) *Enterococcus species*, 10 (3.1%) miscellaneous gram-positives) and 19 (5.9%) gram-negative species.[4]

Given the ability of surface flora to enter the eye during surgery, many of the prophylactic techniques to decrease the risk of endophthalmitis aim to suppress their number and to limit the growth of those organisms that do enter the eye before the development of frank endophthalmitis. Administration of an effective antimicrobial forms a part of such prophylactic measures. Although there are no sufficient data to support a definitive role of antibiotics in preventing endophthalmitis, studies do report a reduction in ophthalmic flora with antibiotic use.[8,9] Further, before perioperative prophylactic antibiotics (and before the modern methods of cataract surgery), the risk of endophthalmitis after a cataract operation was 0.21 to 1.0%.[10] Thus, although the consequences of bacterial endophthalmitis support the use of perioperative prophylactic antimicrobials, a particular choice of antimicrobial agents has not been agreed upon.[8] Since systemically administered antibiotics have not demonstrated good intraocular penetration, various routes of administration have been tried, including preoperative topical, intraoperative infusion, and sub-conjunctival routes.

ANTIBIOTIC PROPHYLAXIS

A variety of options are available for preoperative, intraoperative, and postoperative antibiotic prophylaxis in cataract surgery, but a direct comparative evaluation is often not available, with a review even suggesting that only preoperative antisepsis with 5% povidone iodine may provide some benefit, abit limited.[4]

The ideal prophylactic antibiotic for cataract surgery should be broad spectrum, effective prophylactically, preservative (benzalkonium chloride) free, nontoxic and convenient to use. Presently, fluoroquinolones are the dominant family of ophthalmic antibiotics. The recently introduced fourth generation topical ophthalmic fluoroquinolones, levofloxacin, gatifloxacin, and moxifloxacin-have shown enhanced spectrum and potency for gram-positive cocci and possibly atypical mycobacterium, improved penetration into the anterior segment, and reduced drug resistance as compared to the older fluoroquinolones (norfloxacin 0.3%, ciprofloxacin 0.3%, and ofloxacin 0.3%).

Antibiotic sensitivity varies, but in one series, more than 90% of bacterial isolates were susceptible to cephalothin, vancomycin, chloramphenicol, ofloxacin and gatifloxacin; 70 to 90% were susceptible to gentamicin, cefotaxime, oxacillin and ciprofloxacin; and less than 70% were susceptible to neomycin. There was increased resistance among coagulase-negative staphylococci to both ciprofloxacin (20-38%) and cefazolin (19-40%).[11] Resistance to bacitracin, trimethoprim-sulfamethoxazole, and vancomycin remained unchanged. Vancomycin retained *in-vitro* efficacy against more than 99% of gram-positive bacteria, and ceftazidime was effective against 100% of gram-negative bacteria tested, thus enabling their use in combination as reserve drugs (intravitreal injection) in the treatment of endophthalmitis.[12]

Preoperative prophylaxis for 3 days is effective in eliminating conjunctival microorganisms, and a number of antibiotics viz. fusidic acid, ofloxacin, gentamicin and cefmenoxime are useful.[13] Prophylactic preoperative antibiotics are most commonly used as eye drops. They are also used intraoperative intraocular (antibiotic infusion during surgery, intracamerally), intraoperative periocular [subconjunctivally (gentamicin, cefuroxime)], and postoperatively [aminoglycosides (neomycin, tobramycin, gentamicin) and fluoroquinolones].[14-16]

Intracameral bolus injection of cefazolin (1 mg in 0.1 ml solution), intracameral vancomycin (20 mg/ml), intracameral cefuroxime, and intracameral gentamicin (8 mg/ml) have been used at the time of cataract surgery with demonstrable efficacy and without apparent side effects.[17,18] Occasionally, the protective effect against postoperative endophthalmitis of intracameral prophylaxis is seen to be better with certain antibiotics (cefuroxime) as compared with topical antibiotics alone. Moxifloxacin 0.5% eye drop represents a first line antibiotic of choice for treating and preventing ophthalmic infections, but some have argued that it should be held in reserve (Table 8.1).

The ESCRS[19] endophthalmitis prophylaxis clinical trial is the latest and arguably the largest prospective European clinical study of antibiotic prophylaxis and the largest in ophthalmology on 35,000 cataract patients in 16 centers from 10 European countries. It showed a significant beneficial effect of cefuroxime injected intracamerally as compared to levofloxacin eye drops. Cefuroxime is a second generation bactericidal cephalosporin (β-lactam) antibiotic with activity against both gram-positive and gram-negative organisms, and is used only intracamerally.

Postoperatively, antibiotic may be used in combination with topical steroids as single preparation, without loss of efficacy, and it suffices in uneventful cataract surgeries. It reduces the number of eye drops to be used, possibly increasing compliance, but does not allow each constituent to be tapered

Table 8.1: Lists the antibiotics used commonly for prophylaxis in cataract surgery

Antibiotic	*Topical*	*Subconjunctival*	*Intracameral*
Ciprofloxacin	0.3%	—	—
Ofloxacin	0.3%	—	—
Gatifloxacin	0.3%	—	—
Moxifloxacin	0.5%	—	—
Cephazoline	5%	—	1 mg in 0.1 ml
Cefuroxime	—	—	1 mg
Vancomycin	2.5-5%	25 mg	Infusion=10-50 μg/ml Capsular bag = upto 1 μg/ml
Gentamicin	0.3-1.4%	20-40 mg	8 μg/ml
Amikacin		20-50 mg	—
Tobramycin	.3-1.4%	20-40 mg	—
Chloramphenicol	.5%	—	—

separately. The use of systemic antibiotics preoperatively, or postoperatively in uneventful surgeries, is no longer recommended. A preoperative conjunctival swab is no longer routine practice, with the possible exception of one eyed patients, and those with immunosuppression. Cost evaluation for the prophylactic use of intraocular intraoperative antibiosis in cataract surgery revealed an economically relevant decrease in direct endophthalmitis associated costs.[13] Cost and availability are important considerations in the Indian scenario.

Topical Antibiotics

Topical antibiotics are part of the typical regimen to prevent postoperative infections in patients receiving cataract surgery. These antibiotics have been shown to significantly reduce bacterial counts when given before surgery and also to alter the conjunctival flora. The degree of bacterial reduction depends on the antibiotic selected, the frequency and duration of antibiotic use, the bacterial species present, and the antibiotic sensitivities.

Gentamicin

One of the oldest antibiotics to be evaluated, gentamicin was found to be the most effective agent available for reducing the quantity of periocular organisms. Topical gentamicin can occasionally achieve significant aqueous and ocular tissue concentration, although intravitreal concentration remain variable. Fortified preparations lead to significant intraocular levels.

Trimethoprim-Polymyxin B Sulphate

Trimethoprim is synergistic when combined with polymixin B. Trimethoprim can be bacteriostatic or bactericidal depending upon its concentration and is effective against a wide variety of gram-positive and gram-negative organisms including *S. aureus* and *S. epidermidis*. Polymyxin B is effective against gram-negative organisms including *Pseudomonas*. The combination of trimethoprim and polymyxin B is effective against most of the gram-positive and gram-negative organisms.

Trimethoprim-polymyxin sulphate antibiotics have variable effect on conjunctival and lid organisms. One study by Bell et al[20] demonstrated that trimethoprim and polymyxin combination drugs have no demonstrable clinically significant antibacterial effect but another study by Osher et al[9] showed complete eradication of all organisms except *S. epidermidis* with these combination drugs. However, polymyxin – trimethoprim does not achieve significant concentration in the anterior chamber. Asley et al[21] showed that this combination is less effective than chloramphenicol or a combination of neomycin/polymyxin B/gramicidin and most effective against *Haemophilus influenzae*.

CHLORAMPHENICOL

Chloramphenicol, an antibiotic originally isolated from *Streptomyces venezuelae* but now produced synthetically was introduced into clinical practice in the year 1948. It is effective against both gram-positive and gram-negative organisms. But *Pseudomonas aeruginosa* and Mycobacteria are usually resistant. Seal et al [22] in a study involving 738 patients demonstrated 6 percent resistance to chloramphenicol, 9 percent resistance to tetracycline and around 20 percent resistance to aminoglycosides. Doona and Walsh [23] in a controversial article in British Medical Journal recommended that the use of chloramphenicol should be restricted as it may cause blood dyscrasias. However many subsequent studies by various ophthalmologists and hematologists countered this view. Walker et al [24] reported that the reversible marrow suppression occur in dose dependant manner with serum levels greater than 25 mg/l. They found that serum lever never reached 1 mg/l when the drug was administered topically at four times daily dose and concluded that chloramphenicol did not present any risk of inducing dose related bone marrow toxicity.

It is one of the ideal drug for topical use as its ocular toxicity is low, ocular penetration is excellent and has broad spectrum of activity.

TOPICAL FLUOROQUINOLONES

Fluoroquinolone eye drops have excellent broad spectrum activity, minimal toxicity and desirable kinetics. These agents nowadays are the most commonly used topical antibiotics as these agents achieve more antibiotic concentration in the anterior chamber as compared to other routinely used antibiotics including tobramycin. Within the fluoroquinolone group, different quinolone drugs achieve different antibiotic concentration within the anterior chamber. Topical ofloxacin 0.3% applied preoperatively achieve mean aqueous humor levels of 0.338 g/ml which is significant higher than those achieved with 0.3% ciprofloxacin and 0.3% norfloxcin.[8] Level of ofloxacin in the tear film 4 hours after topical application exceed MIC_{90} for wide range of ocular isolates. Again between ciprofloxacin and norfloxcin, ciprofloxacin has more antibacterial activity upon the ocular flora as compared to norfloxacin. Diamond et al[25] demonstrated that ciprofloxacin 0.3% was a patent perioperative prophylaxis of ocular infection.

Second and third generation fluoroquinolones which include ciprofloxcin and ofloxacin have broad spectrum of activity against gram-positive and gram-negative organisms. Ciprofloxcin 0.3% eye drugs is wide used clinically for the treatment of corneal upper and superficial infection of the eye and ocular adnexa caused by susceptible organisms. With topically used prophylacticals before cataract surgery, most of the susceptible organisms are inhibited. These drugs should be given only a few day before surgery at a dose of 4 times daily.

LOMEFLOXACIN

Lomefloxacin is specifically effective against superficial bacterial infections particularly acute bacterial conjunctivitis. Agius- Fernandez et al[26] compared the relative efficacy of lomefloxacin and chloramphenicol bacterial conjunctivitis patients and showed that both the drugs were equally well tolerated with no serious systemic or local adverse reactions. They concluded that lomefloxacin 0.3% eye drops instilled twice daily were as effective and well tolerated as chloramphenicol 0.5% eye drops instilled 5 times daily. Jauch et al[27] demonstrated that lomefloxacin eye drops used with a loading dose followed by a twice daily regimen proved as effective as other standard antibiotic drugs like gentamicin 0.3%, tobramycin 0.3% and norfloxacin 0.3%. Another advantage of lomefloxacin was that after the loading dose, lomefloxacin can be given in twice daily dose regimen.

Dosage: Ophthalmic solution 0.3% fortified drugs, 20 mg/ml subconjunctival dose, 20-30 mg/ml intravitreal, 200 mg/ml oral dose 400 mg OD.

Sparfloxacin: It has an excellent broad spectrum activity against both gram-positive and gram-negative organisms including anaerobes specially *Bacteroides fragilis* and multidrug resistant enterococci. It is more effective than ciprofloxacin against *Streptococcus pneumoniae, Staphylococcus aureus* and *Staphylococcus epidermidis.*

Dosage: Ophthalmic solutions 0.3%
Intravitreal dose – 20-60 mg/ml
Fortified drugs – 20 mg/ml
Subconjunctival Dose – 20-40 mg.

Ofloxacin

Ofloxacin has broad spectrum activity against both gram-positive and gram-negative organisms. It can be effective against bacterial strains which are resistant to ciprofloxacin. It is commonly used as 0.3% ophthalmic solution.

FOURTH GENERATION FLUOROQUINOLONES

The fourth generation fluoroquinolones include gatifloxacin and moxifloxacin and were approved by the US Food and Drug Administration (FDA) in 2003.

Both these antibiotics bound more strongly to topoisomerase II as compared to older generation fluoroquinolones. With the addition of methoxy group on carbon 8, the newer fluoroquinolone bind more effectively to topoisomerase II and IV, giving these drugs better clinical activities against gram-positive organisms. As these drugs act at two different sites these drugs have less chance of inducing drug resistance as the susceptible bacteria has to develop two mechanisms for development of resistance.

Both gatifloxacin and moxifloxacin have a lower MIC 90 against gram-positive bacteria than the 2nd and third generation fluoroquinolones. Both these drugs are effective against coagulase-negative *Staphylococcus* and *Streptococcus viridans,* two of the most common causes of postoperative endophthalmitis. The efficacy rate against gram-negative organisms are more or less same as seen with older fluoroquinolones.

Following topical use, the concentration of both gatifloxacin and moxifloxacin in the anterior chamber reach levels in excess of the MIC_{90} for most pathogenic organisms. Solomon et al[28] investigated cataract patients who received moxifloxacin 0.5%, gatifloxacin 0.3%, or ciprofloxacin 0.3% four times a day for 3 days before surgery and then every 15 minutes 3 times 1 hour before surgery. Anterior chamber drug levels were significantly higher in patients receiving moxifloxacin than in patients taking gatifloxacin.

Subconjunctival Antibiotics

Most of the topically used antibiotics can be given subconjunctivally. The ocular penetration following this route is diffusion through corneal stroma rather than through tear film. The therapeutic level may remain for more than 12 hours and because of longer duration of action antibiotics injected through subconjunctival route may be more effective in preventing postoperative endophthalmitis. The intravitreal concentration of most of the antibiotics given through subconjunctival route is extremely low. So once endophthalmitis has developed, subconjunctival antibiotics are of no value. Ideally the subconjunctival antibiotics should be given preoperatively so that effective concentration of antibiotic is present in the anterior chamber at the time the organisms are introduced.[8] Subconjunctival antibiotics have decreased the incidence of experimental endophthalmitis in animal models; animal models in which cataract extraction was followed by intentional inoculation of bacteria into the vitreous cavity.

Routinely the antibiotics used for subconjunctival route include gentamicin, tobramicin, cefazoline , vancomycin.

INTRACAMERAL ANTIBIOTICS

Intracameral antibiotics involve the use of antibiotics directly into anterior chamber either through direct injection into anterior chamber or through irrigating solution. Gills[28] reported low rate of postoperative endophthalmitis when the antibiotics were given through irrigating solutions. Gimbel et al[29] used 8 g/ml gentamicin in the irrigating solution and 1 mg vancomycin into the capsular bag at the end of the surgery with no cases of endophthalmitis in 11,748 procedures.

The spectrum of pathogens causing postcataract endophthalmitis changes over time, as also resistance to antibiotics used for its prophylaxis. In many instances, current routine practices of antibiotic prophylaxis reflect personal preferences, are empirical, and in a strict sense, not evidence-based. While recent studies suggest a beneficial role of antibiotic prophylaxis, such benefit is not yet unequivocally proven, the limitations being the relatively low prevalence of endophthalmitis that makes controlled studies with a large cohort difficult, and often, the non-availability of microbiological facilities where cataract surgeries are performed in large numbers. Presurgical antibiotic prophylaxis must be combined with additional measures such as topical preoperative 5% povidone-iodine, the use of an adhesive foil, and surgical technique. Rational antibiotics usage demands that a reserve bactericidal drug(s) be available. In the majority of situations, it is a combination of vancomycin (for gram-positive), and ceftazidime or amikacin (for gram-negative), used intravitreally for the treatment of endophthalmitis. Prevention of post-cataract surgery endophthalmitis is of utmost importance, and future prospective studies based on human clinical trials and microbiological studies will be required to continually provide updated information necessary to guide patient care.

REFERENCES

1. McCulley JP. Low acute endophthalmitis rate: Possible explanations. J Cataract Refract Surg 2005;31:1074-75.
2. Eifrig CWG, Flynn HW Jr, Scott IU, Newton J. Acute-onset postoperative endophthalmitis: Review of incidence and visual outcomes (1995-2001). Ophthalmic Surg Lasers 2002;33:37-38; erratum, 34:80.
3. Montan PG, Koranyi G, Setterquist H, et al. Endophthalmitis after cataract surgery: Risk factors relating to technique and events of the operation and patient history: A retrospective case-control study. Ophthalmology 1998;105:2171-77.
4. Ciulla TA, Starr MB, Masket S. Bacterial endophthalmitis prophylaxis for cataract surgery: An evidence based update. Ophthalmology 2002;109:13-26.
5. Bannerman TL, Rhoden DL, McAllister SK, et al. The source of coagulase-negative staphylococci in the endophthalmitis vitrectomy study. A comparison of eyelid and intraocular isolates using pulsed-field gel electrophoresis. Arch Ophthalmol 1997;115:357-61.
6. Han DP, Wisniewski SR, Wilson LA, et al. Spectrum and susceptibilities of microbiologic isolates in the endophthalmitis vitrectomy study. Am J Ophthalmol 1996;122:1-17;erratum, 920.
7. Ariyasu RG, Nakamura T, Trousdale MD, Smith RE. Intraoperative bacterial contamination of the aqueous humor. Ophthalmic Surg 1993;24:367-73;discussion 373-74.
8. Liesegang TJ. Perioperative antibiotic prophylaxis in cataract surgery. Cornea 1999;18:383-402.
9. Osher RH, Amdahl LD, Cheetham JK. Antimicrobial efficacy and aqueous humor penetration of preoperative and postoperative topical trimethoprim/polymyxin B sulfate versus tobramycin. J Cataract Refract Surg 1994;20:3-8.
10. Allen HF, Mangiaracine AB. Bacterial endophthalmitis after cataract extraction. Arch Ophthalmol 1964;72:454-62.
11. Arantes TE, Cavalcanti RF, Diniz Mde F, Severo MS, Lins Neto J, Castro CM. Conjunctival bacterial flora and antibiotic resistance pattern in patients undergoing cataract surgery. Arq Bras Oftalmol 2006;69: 33-6. Epub 2006, Feb 10.

12. Recchia FM, Busbee BG, Pearlman RB, Carvalho-Recchia CA, Ho AC. Changing trends in the microbiologic aspects of postcataract endophthalmitis. Arch Ophthalmol 2005;123:341-46.
13. Wejde G, Samolov B,Seregard S, Koranyi G, Montan PG. Risk factors for endophthalmitis following cartaract surgery: A retrospective case-control study. J Hosp Infect 2005;61:251-56.
14. Krummenauer F, Kurz S, Dick HB. Epidemiological evaluation of intraoperative antibiosis as a protective agent against endophthalmitis after cataract surgery. Pharmacoepidemiol Drug Saf 2006;15:662-66.
15. Rosha DS, Ng JQ, Morlet N, Boekelaar M, Wilson S, Hendrie D, Semmens JB. Cataract surgery practice and endophthalmitis prevention by Australian and New Zealand ophthalmologists. Clin Experiment Ophthalmol 2006;34:535-44.
16. Kim DH, Stark WJ, O'Brien TP, Dick JD. Aqqueous penetration and biological activity of moxifloxacin 0.5% ophthalmic solution and gatifloxacin 0.3% solution in cataract surgery patients. Ophthalmology 2005; 112: 1992-96. Epub 2005 Sep 23.
17. Romero P, Mendez I, Salvat M, Fernandez J, Almena M. Intracameral cefazolin as prophylaxis against endophthalmitis in cataract surgery. J Cataract Refract Surg 2006;32:438-41.
18. Ball JL, Barrett GD. Prospective randomized controlled trial of the effect of intracameral vancomycin and gentamicin on macular retinal thickness and visual function following cataract surgery. J Cataract Refract Surg 2006;32:789-94.
19. ESCRS endophthalmitis prophylaxis clinical trial. ESCRS office at escrs@escrs.org
20. Bell TA, Slack M, Harvey SG, Gibson JR. The effect of trimethoprim-polymyxin B sulphate ophthalmic ointment and chloramphenicol ophthalmic ointment on the bacterial flora of the eye when administered to the operated and unoperated eyes of patients undergoing cataract surgery. Eye 1988;2:324-29.
21. Ashley KC. The anti-bacterial activity of topical anti-infective eye preparations. Med Lab Sci 1986;43:157-62.
22. Seal DV, Barrett SP, McGill JI. Aetiology and treatment of acute bacterial infection of the external eye. Br J Ophthalmol 1982;66:357-60.
23. Doona M, Walsh JB. Use of chloramphenicol as topical eye medication: Time to cry halt? BMJ 1995;310:1217-18.
24. Walker S, Diaper CJM, Bowman R, Sweeney G, Seal DV, Krikness CM. Lack of evidence for systemic toxicity following systemic chloramphenicol use. Eye 1998;12:875-79.
25. Diamond JP, White L, Leeming JP, Bing Ho H, Easty DL. Topical 0.3% ciprofloxacin, norfloxacin, and ofloxacin in treatment of bacterial keratitis: A new method for comparative evaluation of ocular drug penetration. Br J Ophthalmol 1995;79:606-09.
26. Agius-Fernandez A, Patterson A, Fsadni M, Jauch A, Sunder Raj P. Topical lomefloxacin versus topical chloramphenicol in the treatment of acute bacterial conjunctivitis.Clin Drug Invest 1998;15:263-69.
27. Jauch A, Esadni M, Gamba G. Meta-analysis of six clinical phase III studies comparing lomefloxacin 0.3% eye drops twice daily to five standard antibiotics in patients with acute bacterial conjunctivitis. Graefes Arch Clin Exp Ophthalmol 1999;237:705-13.
28. Gills JP. Filters and antibiotics in irrigating solution for cataract surgery [Letter]. J Cataract Refract Surg1991;17:385.
29. Gimbel HV, Sun R, DeBroff BM. Prophylactic intracameral antibiotics during cataract surgery: The incidence of endophthalmitis and corneal endothelial loss. Eur J Implant Refract Surg 1994;6:280-85.

Chapter 9

Topical Ophthalmic Antibiotics

Renee Solomon, Eric Donnenfeld (USA)

FLUOROQUINOLONES

Chemistry, Ophthalmic Preparation and Pharmacologic Action

The fluoroquinolones, the newest class of available ophthalmic agents to be developed, are based on the prototype, nalidixic acid (1,8-naphthyridine), which was synthesized in 1962.[1] In the 1980s, the fluoroquinolones were created from nalidixic acid by adding a fluorine atom to position 6 of the molecule (Fig. 9.1). This addition widened the antibacterial spectrum of activity and resulted in

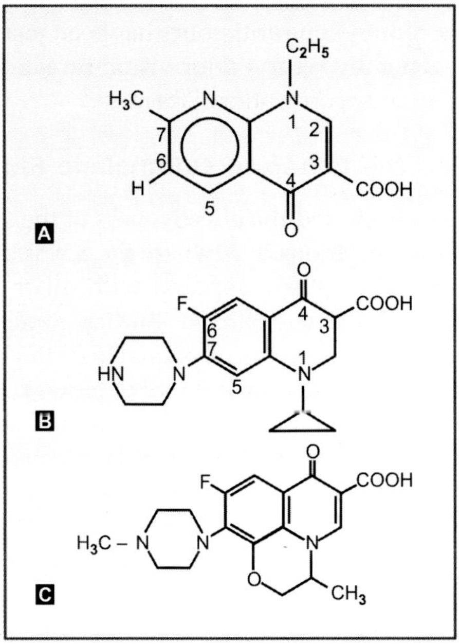

Fig. 9.1: Chemical structure of the nalidixic acid (A) from which the fluoroquinolones, including ciprofloxacin (B) and ofloxacin (C), were derived

decreased development of resistant organisms. Four fluoroquinolones available for ophthalmic use are ofloxacin 0.3% (Ocuflox, Allergan, Inc, Irvine, CA), ciprofloxacin 0.3% (Ciloxan, Alcon Laboratories, Inc, Fort Worth, TX), gatifloxacin 0.3% (Zymar, Allergan, Inc, Irvine, CA), and moxifloxacin 0.5% (Vigamox, Alcon Laboratories, Inc, Fort Worth, TX).

The fluoroquinolones are bactericidal and work by inhibiting bacterial DNA gyrase (bacterial topoisomerase II), the enzyme responsible for maintaining the superficial twists in bacterial DNA.[2] They provide broad-spectrum activity against gram-positive and gram-negative bacteria *in vivo* and *in vitro*. Moxifloxacin and gatifloxacin have additional activity against gram-positive bacteria due to their dual activity against DNA gyrase and topoisomerase. They have less predictable activity against anaerobes and streptococci.[3]

The fluoroquinolones are also available for systemic use, but clinical profiles of the ophthalmic and systemic formulations are distinctly different. For example, topical ophthalmic fluoroquinolones are approved in children as young as one year of age whereas systemic formulations are approved only for use in older children and adults because of concerns about the potential risk of drug deposition in cartilage and arthropathy. In addition, the prevalence of fluoroquinolone-resistant bacteria is much higher among systemic pathogens than among the ocular pathogens commonly associated with conjunctivitis and keratitis. Moreover, although the use of systemic fluoroquinolones must be carefully considered to prevent further induction of resistant strains, this is of much less concern in ophthalmic use, because the strains of bacteria affected are much lower. Although resistance has been less of a concern in ophthalmic use, resistance to fluoroquinolone antibiotics has been increasing, and for this reason, their use is generally reserved for vision-threatening infections and infections not responding to conventional therapy.[4]

Generalizations on the Group of Ophthalmic Fluoroquinolones

Multiple articles have supported the effectiveness of the fluoroquinolones in treating ocular bacterial infections.[5-7]What are the advantages and disadvantages of the fluoroquinolones as compared with other, so-called fortified antibiotics? The aforementioned clinical studies conclusively show that ciprofloxacin and ofloxacin are statistically equal to fortified antibiotics in time to heal and cure rate of infectious corneal ulcers. However, other parameters should be analyzed. The acute management of bacterial corneal ulcers requires rapid access to therapy. In addition, the cost and toxicity of antibiotic therapy must be considered. Fortified antibiotics are not commercially available and must be prepared on request. The fluoroquinolones are superior with respect to accessibility, cost, and low toxicity. The fluoroquinolones perform at least as well as, and often better than, the aminoglycosides in the treatment of gram-negative corneal ulcers. One of the main advantages of the fluoroquinolones is their high intrinsic solubility.[8]

EXTEMPORANEOUSLY COMPOUNDED FORTIFIED ANTIBIOTICS

Extemporaneously compounded fortified antibiotic eyedrop preparations contain high concentrations that are usually prepared from products formulated for intravenous use. A typical treatment regimen might consist of a combination of a cephalosporin (e.g. 50 mg/mL cefazolin) for gram-positive bacteria coverage and an aminoglycoside (e.g. 13 mg/mL tobramycin or gentamicin) for gram-negative bacteria coverage. However, these agents are not compatible when combined in the same solution and must be formulated separately and administered from different bottles. Another common extemporaneously fortified antibiotic is vancomycin 50 mg/mL. Most need to be refrigerated after dispensing to the patient, because, being derived from intravenous products, they do not contain a preservative. Instillation of the two agents must be separated by intervals of several minutes or more (e.g. 15 minutes might be ideal) to prevent washout of the first agent by the second. The high concentrations used in these preparations exacerbate their epithelial toxic potential. This is a special concern for the aminoglycosides.

In the treatment of bacterial keratitis, fortified cefazolin-aminoglycoside preparations are as effective as the fluoroquinolones ofloxacin and ciprofloxacin, but are more difficult to obtain and use. Not all pharmacies are equipped to formulate extemporaneously compounded agents and not all pharmacists are familiar with the procedures.

There has been some debate in the literature as to the efficacy of using a collagen shield as a vehicle to absorb and deliver drugs. Advocates argue that collagen shields soak up antibiotics and continuously deliver them to the cornea for several hours, enabling higher concentrations to be delivered for longer periods of time. However, some studies have found that collagen shields are not more efficacious than using fortified antibiotics alone.[9,10] According to several other studies, collagen shields are labor intensive yet as effective in treating bacterial keratitis, as frequent dosages of drops.[10,11]

AMINOGLYCOSIDES

Chemistry, Ophthalmic Preparation, and Pharmacologic Action

The two most commonly used aminoglycosides are tobramycin sulfate available as a 0.3% solution or ointment (AKTOB [Acorn, Inc, Buffalo Grove, IL], Defy, Tobrex [Alcon Laboratories, Fort Worth, TX]) and gentamicin sulfate (Fig. 9.2) available as a 0.3% solution (Garamycin, Genoptic [Allergan, Inc, Irvine, CA], Gentacidin, Gentak [Akorn, Inc, Buffalo Grove, IL], Ocu-mycin) and ointment (Garamycin, Genoptic). Neomycin [Bausch & Lomb Pharmaceutical, Inc, Tampa, FL] is also used, but is only available as a component of combination products, not as a single agent. The basic structure of aminoglycosides consists of two or more amino sugars connected by glycosidic bonds to a hexose nucleus. The individual characteristics of an aminoglycoside are determined by differences in the amino sugars attached to the nucleus.

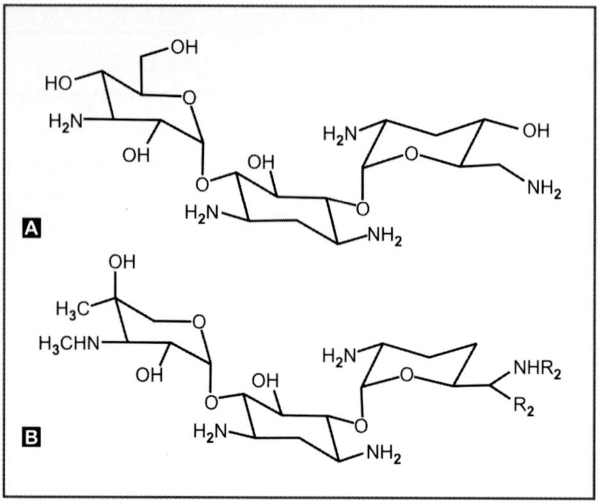

Fig. 9.2: The aminoglycosides, with some of the more commonly used ophthalmic formulations pictured, tobramycin (A), and gentamicin (B), which contain the characteristic two or more amino sugars connected by glycosidic bonds to a hexose nucleus

The aminoglycosides cause bacterial cell death by irreversibly binding to 30S ribosomes and causing misreading of the genetic code and decreased or abnormal protein synthesis.[12] Aminoglycosides are valued in the treatment of external ocular infections because they are active against aerobic gram-negative organisms, including *Pseudomonas* species, *Proteus* species, *Klebsiella* species, *Escherichia coli*, *Salmonella* species, *Shigella* species, *S. marcescens*, *Haemophilus* species and many gram-positive staphylococci.[13] *In vitro*, tobramycin is three times as effective as gentamicin against *Pseudomonas*.[14] The aminoglycosides have limited use as broad-spectrum agents because of resistance caused by aminoglycoside-modifying enzymes. This occurs at an unacceptably high frequency (29%–41%).[15] Of particular concern is their lack of relative efficacy against *S. epidermidis* and *S. pneumoniae*.

Clinical Experience and Ophthalmic Uses

Gentamicin and tobramycin have been shown to be effective in the treatment of conjunctivitis, blepharoconjunctivitis, and bacterial keratitis.[16] The commercially available concentrations are acceptable for the treatment of bacterial conjunctivitis, but the highly concentrated, fortified preparations are preferred for bacterial keratitis and are best used in conjunction with an antibiotic more active against gram-positive bacteria.

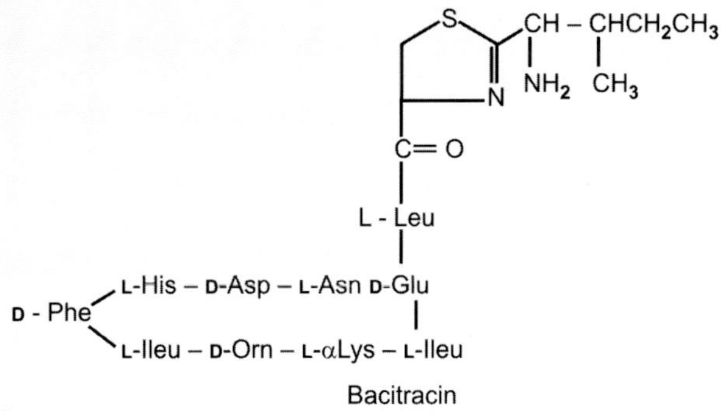

Fig. 9.3: Structural formula of bacitracin, the polypeptide antibiotic that contains a thiazolidine ring

BACITRACIN

Chemistry, Ophthalmic Preparation and Pharmacologic

Bacitracin is a polypeptide antibiotic that contains a thiazolidine ring structure (Fig. 9.3). Bacitracin is bactericidal by binding to cell membrane[17] and is commercially produced as a topical ophthalmic ointment (AK-Tracin, Akorn, Inc, Buffalo Grove, IL) or in combination with polymyxin B (AK-poly-bac [Akorn, Inc, Buffalo Grove, IL], Polysporin, Polytracin [Medical Ophthalmics, Tarpon Springs, FL]) or with polymyxin B and neomycin (AK-Spore [Akorn, Inc, Buffalo Grove, IL], Neosporin [Monarch Pharmaceuticals, Bristol, TN], Ocu-spor B). All these preparations contain bacitracin in a concentration of 500 U per gram of ointment. Unlike most of the other antibacterial agents discussed in this chapter, bacitracin is only available for topical use because of its systemic toxicity and poor solubility.

Clinical Experience and Ophthalmic Uses

Bacitracin is efficacious against most gram-positive organisms and select gram-negative organisms, including penicillinase-producing staphylococci, Neisseria species, Haemophilus species, and Actinomyces species. Bacitracin penetrates an intact cornea poorly, but its penetration may be increased by a corneal epithelial defect.[18]

BETA-LACTAM ANTIBIOTICS

Chemistry, Ophthalmic Preparation and Pharmacologic Action

This class of antibiotics includes the penicillins and cephalosporins. Penicillins (Fig. 9.4) are composed of a thiazolidine ring connected to a beta-lactam ring to which a side chain is connected. The side chain is responsible for the individual

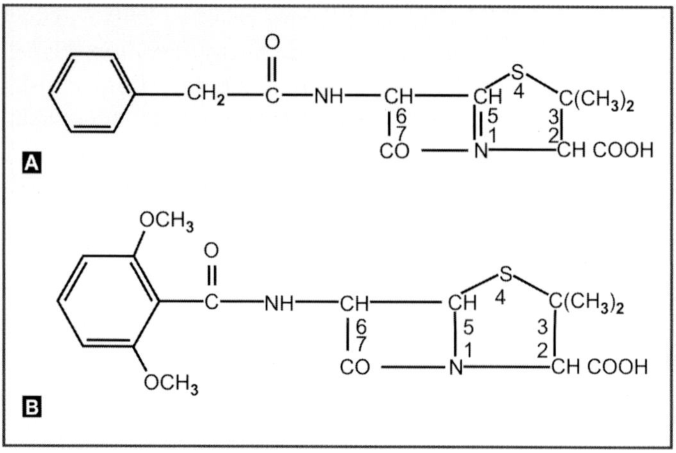

Fig. 9.4: Chemical formulas of the penicillin agents, which contain beta-lactam rings attached to thiazolidine rings [e.g. penicillin (A) and methicillin (B)]

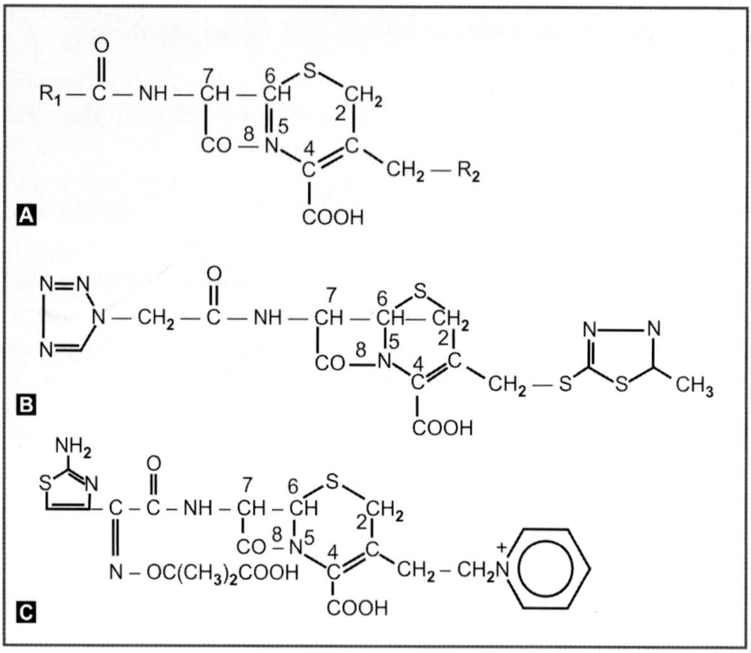

Fig. 9.5: Illustrations of the cephalosporins, which contain modifications to positions of the beta-lactam ring of cephalosporin (A), to create cefazolin (B), and ceftazidime (C)

characteristics of the penicillins. Like the penicillins, the cephalosporins (Fig. 9.5) contain a beta-lactam ring, are bactericidal, and inhibit cell wall synthesis. By preventing the synthesis of polysaccharides needed for bacterial cell wall structure, they cause bacterial death. They tend to be more active against gram-positive organisms, with increased gram-negative activity in the extended-spectrum penicillins and the second- and third-generation cephalosporins. Bacteria become resistant to penicillins by producing beta-lactamase; cephalosporins tend to be resistant to degradation by beta-lactamase. All methicillin-resistant *S. aureus* and enterococci are also resistant to cephalosporins. Approximately 10% of patients allergic to penicillin will also be allergic to cephalosporins.

Clinical Experience and Ophthalmic Uses

The beta-lactam antibiotics are not available in pharmaceutically manufactured topical ophthalmic preparations because of their poor stability. The most commonly used topical agent in this class is a first-generation cephalosporin, cefazolin 50 mg/mL, and is made from a parenteral preparation. As mentioned, cefazolin is used with a topical aminoglycoside in the treatment of bacterial keratitis. However, ceftazidime alone or in combination with an aminoglycoside or vancomycin has also been explored as an initial agent for topical therapy of bacterial keratitis. A third-generation cephalosporin, ceftazidime, was found to be as effective as cefazolin in treating rabbit corneal ulcers caused by *S. aureus* and *S. pneumoniae* and as effective as tobramycin against *P. aeruginosa*.[19]

CHLORAMPHENICOL

Chemistry, Ophthalmic Preparation and Pharmacologic Action

Chloramphenicol, a nitrobenzene derivative (Fig. 9.6), available as a 1% ointment or a 0.5% solution (AK-Chlor, Chlormycetin [Monarch Pharmaceuticals, Bristol, TN], Chloroptic [Allergan, Inc, Irvine, CA], Ocu-Chlor), was the first broad-spectrum antibiotic with gram-positive and gram-negative coverage. It has been widely used in ointment form for the treatment of external ocular infection.

Chloramphenicol inhibits bacterial protein synthesis by binding to the 50S ribosomal subunit. It is primarily bacteriostatic but may be bactericidal to some organisms (e.g. *H. influenzae*).

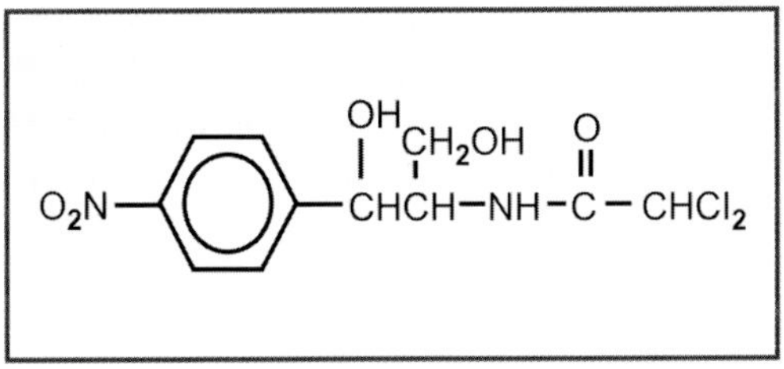

Fig. 9.6: Structure of chloramphenicol, a derivative of nitrobenzene

Clinical Experience and Ophthalmic Uses

Chloramphenicol has good antimicrobial activity against most gram-positive ocular isolates and limited gram-negative coverage. Chloramphenicol should not be used to treat infections in which gram-negative bacteria, especially *Pseudomonas* or *Serratia* species[21] are suspected. Because it is usually bacteriostatic, not bacteriocidal, and because of its limited spectrum, chloramphenicol should not be used in vision-threatening circumstances.

ERYTHROMYCIN

Chemistry, Ophthalmic Preparation and Pharmacologic Action

Erythromycin 0.5% is a macrolide antibiotic (Fig. 9.7) that inhibits bacterial protein synthesis by irreversibly binding to the 50S ribosomal subunit.[22] It is bacteriostatic in low concentrations but can be bactericidal in high concentrations. Other determinants of its bactericidal activity include organism susceptibility, growth rate of the bacteria, and pH.[23] Erythromycin is available in ointment form (0.5%) for topical ophthalmic use (Ak-mycin, Ilotycin).

Clinical Experience and Ophthalmic Uses

Erythromycin is used as prophylaxis against neonatal conjunctivitis caused by *C. trachomatis* and *N. gonorrheae*. It is also used to treat mild bacterial conjunctivitis. It has a broad spectrum of antibacterial activity[24] and is well tolerated by the ocular surface, but many resistant strains have developed. For example, several strains of *H. influenzae*, one of the most common pathogens in pediatric conjunctivitis, are resistant to erythromycin. Therefore, its usefulness in the treatment of external ocular infections is limited

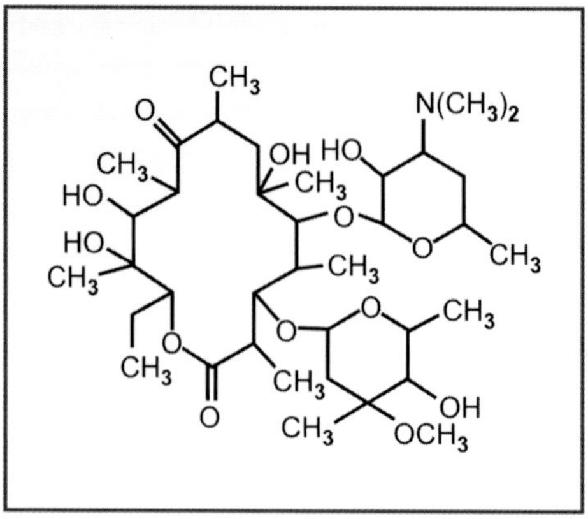

Fig. 9.7: Chemical structure of the macrolide antibiotic, erythromycin

POLYMYXIN AND COMBINATION PRODUCTS

Chemistry, Ophthalmic Preparation and Pharmacologic Action

Many of the combination products currently available in the United States contain polymyxin B sulfate (Fig. 9.8). It provides efficacy against commonly encountered gram-negative pathogens such as *H. influenzae*. Polymyxin is a bactericidal polypeptide antibiotic that interferes with cell wall synthesis and forms false pores in bacterial cell membranes. It is less effective against *Proteus*, *Providencia*, *Serratia*, and *Brucella* species. It came into use in ophthalmology in the 1950s, when it was shown that polymyxin was effective in treating *Pseudomonas* corneal ulcers in rabbits.[25] The effectiveness of this agent was then shown in treating human corneal ulcers infected with *Pseudomonas* species.[26,27]

Combinations of polymyxin B with neomycin and gramicidin or trimethoprim are available as solutions, and combinations with bacitracin, neomycin, and bacitracin, or oxytetracycline are available as ointments only. The ointments contain 10,000 U per gram of polymyxin B.

Two antibiotics commonly combined with polymyxin are gramicidin and trimethoprim. Gramicidin alters bacterial cell wall permeability. Like bacitracin, it is only used topically because of systemic toxicity. Trimethoprim is a competitive inhibitor of bacterial dihydrofolate reductase, an enzyme that is necessary for purine synthesis.[28] The other compounds that polymyxin B are combined with are addressed elsewhere in this chapter.

Clinical Experience and Ophthalmic Uses

All polymyxin combination products have shown efficacy against bacterial conjunctivitis,[29] but no clinical studies of their use in the treatment of bacterial keratitis have been conducted. Clinical studies have shown that polymyxin B-trimethoprim and polymyxin B-neomycin-gramicidin are as effective as each other[30] and gentamicin sulfate, sodium sulfacetamide, and chloramphenicol in the treatment of bacterial conjunctivitis.

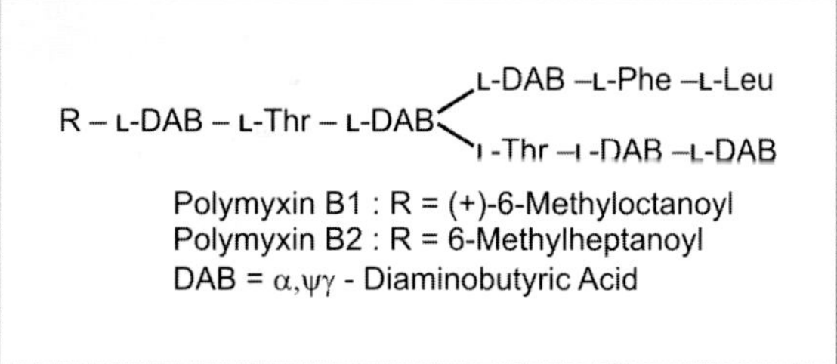

Fig. 9.8: Polymyxin B sulfate, a polypeptide antibiotic, which is the most common polymyxin in clinical use

SULFACETAMIDE

Chemistry, Ophthalmic Preparation and Pharmacologic Action

Sulfacetamide (Fig. 9.9) 10% ointment (AK-Sulf, Cetamide, Sulamyd Sodium) and sulfacetamide 10% to 30% solutions (10% AK Sulf [Akorn, Inc, Buffalo Grove, IL], Bleph-10 [Allergan, Inc, Irvine, CA], Ophthacet, Ocusulf, Sulf-10 [CIBA Vision, Duluth, GA], Sulamyd Sodium, and Isopto Cetamide) act by preventing the incorporation of para-aminobenzoic acid into folic acid, thus inhibiting bacterial purine biosynthesis. Sulphonamides are bacteriostatic.

Clinical Experience and Ophthalmic Uses

Sulphonamides were used in the treatment of external ocular infections before the need to perform efficacy studies. It is difficult to find documentation of their value in the medical literature. In a study of 158 cases of culture-positive pediatric conjunctivitis, topical sulfacetamide was found to be equivalent in efficacy to trimethoprim-polymyxin B and gentamicin sulfate solutions.[31] Like erythromycin, sulfacetamides have a broad spectrum of antibacterial activity, but many strains of resistant bacteria have developed. Sulfacetamide is still effective against *H. influenzae* but is ineffective against many staphylococcal isolates, *S. marcescens*, and *P. aeruginosa*, which makes it a poor choice as a first-line treatment for bacterial keratitis. It remains a drug of choice for the treatment of *Nocardia* species.[32]

TETRACYCLINES

Chemistry, Ophthalmic Preparation and Pharmacologic Action

Tetracycline (Fig. 9.10) inhibits bacterial protein synthesis by binding to the 30S ribosome, and it is among the broadest spectrum agents available. For most organisms, tetracycline is bacteriostatic.

Clinical Experience and Ophthalmic Uses

Systemic and topical (ointment) tetracyclin are used concurrently to treat *C. trachomatis* conjunctivitis. Tetracycline can also be used for prophylaxis against ophthalmia neonatorum from *N. gonorrhoeae* [32] gonorrheae or chlamydial

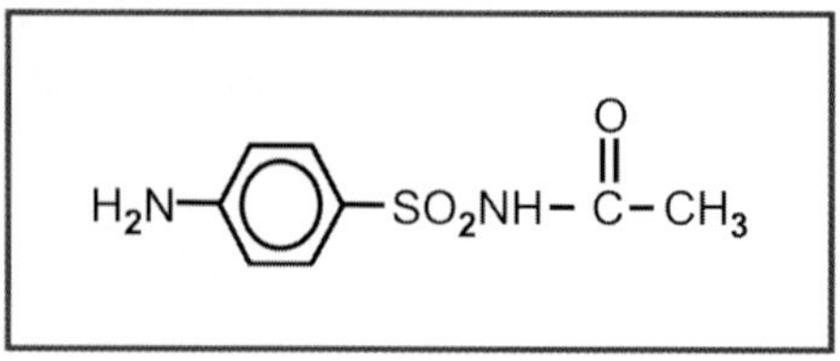

$$H_2N-C_6H_4-SO_2NH-\overset{O}{\overset{\|}{C}}-CH_3$$

Fig. 9.9: Chemical structure of sulfacetamide one of the more commonly used sulfonamides in ophthalmic preparations

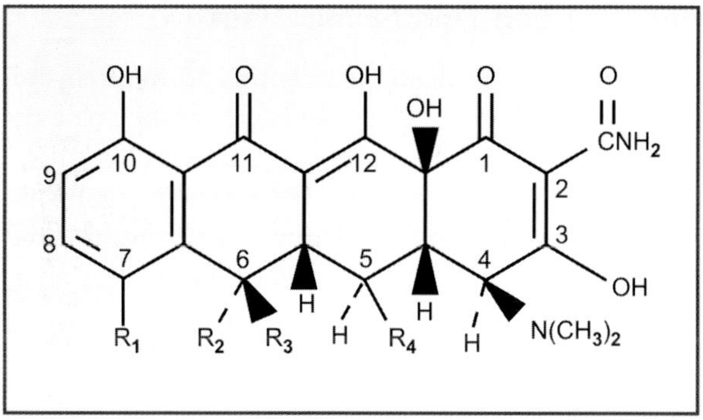

Fig. 9.10: The basis of the tetracyclines, shown above, is a four-ring naphthacencecarboxamide

infections.[160,161] In newborns developing ophthalmia neonatorum, coexisting oropharyngeal involvement usually requires more than topical drug use.

Adverse Effects

Adverse reactions from tetracyclines, including deposition in the teeth and bones, may be seen with both systemic use and topical application.

VANCOMYCIN

Chemistry, Ophthalmic Preparation and Pharmacologic Action

Vancomycin is a complex bactericidal tricyclic glycopeptide (Fig. 9.11) that inhibits bacterial cell wall synthesis. It is active primarily against gram-positive bacteria, including methicillin-resistant *S. aureus*, *S. epidermidis*, and *Enterococcus* species.

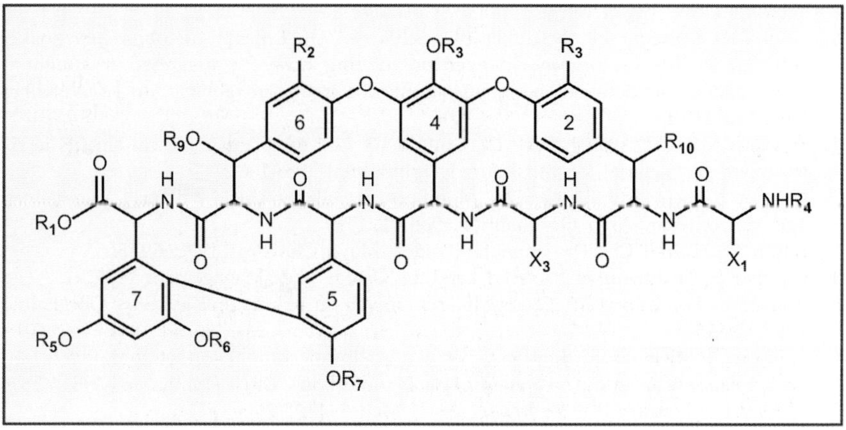

Fig. 9.11: Vancomycin is a complex bactericidal tricyclic glycopeptide

Clinical Experience and Ophthalmic Uses

Topical vancomycin has been used successfully to treat chronic methicillin-resistant *S. aureus* in institutionalized patients. Vancomycin has not been tested against other antibiotics in the treatment of bacterial keratitis, but there are numerous reported cases of keratitis caused by resistant organisms that resolved with topical vancomycin therapy. Vancomycin 50 mg/mL has been tested against ciprofloxacin 0.3% in a rabbit model of methicillin-resistant *S. aureus* keratitis; ciprofloxacin was found to be more effective in that study. These results have not been verified in clinical studies. Vancomycin should be considered as a first-line therapy in severe cases of keratitis in patients at high risk for infection by methicillin-resistant organisms, such as healthcare workers or institutionalized patients.

REFERENCES

1. Lesher GY, Froelich ED, Gruet MD, et al. 1,8 Naphthyridine derivatives. A new class of chemotherapeutic agents. J Med Pharm Chem 1962;5:1063.
2. Smith JT. The mode of action of 4-quinolones and possible mechanisms of resistance. J Antimicrob Chemother 1986;18:21.
3. Wolfson JS, Hooper DC. The fluoroquinolones: structures, mechanisms of action and resistance, and spectra of activity in vitro. Antimicrob Agents Chemother 1985;28:581.
4. Snyder ME, Katz HR. Ciprofloxacin-resistant bacterial keratitis. Am J Ophthalmol 1992;114:336.
5. Cutarelli PE, Kass JH, Lazarus IM, et al. Topical fluoroquinolones: antimicrobial activity and in vitro corneal epithelial toxicity. Curr Eye Research 1991;10:557.
6. Serdarevic ON. Role of the fluoroquinolones in ophthalmology. Int Ophthalmol Clin 1993;33:163.
7. Veights SA, Dick JD, O'Brien TP, et al. Comparative in vitro activities of fluoroquinolones vs aminoglycoside against human ocular isolates [abstract]. Invest Ophthalmol Vis Sci 1992;33:S936.
8. Donnenfeld ED, Perry HW, Snyder RW, et al. Intracorneal, aqueous humor, and vitreous humor penetration of topical and oral ofloxacin. Arch Ophthalmol 1997;115:173.
9. Finkelstein I, Trope GE, Menon IA, et al. Potential value of collagen shields as subconjunctival depot release system. Curr Eye Res 1990;9:653.
10. Assil KK, Zarnegar SR, Fouraker BD, Schanzlin DJ. Efficacy of tobramycin-soaked collagen shields vs tobramycin eyedrop loading dose for sustained treatment of experimental Pseudomonas aeruginosa-induced keratitis in rabbits. Am J Ophthalmol 1992;113:418.
11. Sawusch MR, O'Brien TP, Dick JD, Gottsch JD. Use of collagen corneal shields in the treatment of bacterial keratitis. Am J Ophthalmol 1988;106:27.
12. Phinney RB Schwartz SD, Lee DA, Mondino BJ. Collagen-shield delivery of gentamicin and vancomycin. Arch Ophthalmol 1988;106:1599.
13. Edson RS, Terrell CL: The aminoglycosides. Mayo Clin Proc 1991;66:1158.
14. Gardner S. Treatment of bacterial keratitis. Ocular Ther Management 1990;3:1.
15. Wilhelmus KR, Gilbert Ml, Osato MS. Tobramycin in ophthalmology. Surv Ophthalmol 1987;32:111.
16. Laibson P, Michaud R, Smolin G, et al. A clinical comparison of tobramycin and gentamicin sulfate in the treatment of ocular infections. Am J Ophthalmol 1981;92:836.
17. Meleny FL, Johnson BA. Bacitracin. Am J Med 1949;7:794.

18. Bellows JG, Farmer CJ. Use of bacitracin in ocular infections; tolerance and permeability in rabbit eye. Am J Ophth 1948;31:1070.
19. Kremer I, Robinson A, Braffman M, et al. The effect of topical ceftazidime on pseudomonas keratitis in rabbits. Cornea 1994;13:360.
20. Bower KS, Kowalski RP, Gordon YJ. Fluoroquinolones in the treatment of bacterial keratitis. Am J Ophthalmol 1996;121:712.
21. Jensen HG, Felix C. In vitro antibiotic susceptibilities of ocular isolates in North and South America. In Vitro Antibiotic Testing Group. Cornea 1998;17:79.
22. Mao JC Putterman M, Wiegand RG. Biochemical basis for the selective toxicity of erythromycin. Biochem Pharmacol 1970;19:391.
23. Sabath LD, Lorian V, Gerstein D, et al. Enhancing effect on alkalinization of the medium on the activity of erythromycin against gram-negative bacteria. Appl Microbiol 1968;16:1228.
24. Washington JA, Wilson WR. Erythromycin: a microbial and clinical perspective after 30 years of clinical use. Mayo Clin Proc 1985;60:271.
25. Wiggins RL. Experimental studies on eyes with polymyxin B. Am J Ophth 1952;35:83.
26. Moorman LT. Treatment of pseudomonas corneal ulcers. Arch Ophth 1955;53:345.
27. McNeel JW, Wood RM, Senterfit LB. Effect of polymyxin B sulfate on Pseudomonas corneal ulcers. Arch Ophthalmol 1961;66:646.
28. Van Rensburg SF, Gibson JR, Harvey SG, Burke CA. Trimethoprim-polymyxin ophthalmic solution versus chloramphenicol ophthalmic solution in the treatment of bacterial conjunctivitis. Pharmatherapeutica 1982;3:274.
29. The Trimethoprim-Polymyxin B Sulphate Ophthalmic Ointment Study Group: Trimethoprim-polymyxin B sulphate ophthalmic ointment versus chloramphenicol ophthalmic ointment in the treatment of bacterial conjunctivitis—a review of four clinical studies. J Antimicrob Chemother 1989;23:261.
30. Gibson JR. Trimethoprim-polymyxin B ophthalmic solution in the treatment of presumptive bacterial conjunctivitis—a multicenter trial of its efficacy versus neomycin-polymyxin B-gramicidin and chloramphenicol ophthalmic solutions. J Antimicrob Chemother 1983;11:217.
31. Lohr JA, Austin RD, Grossman M, et al. Comparison of three topical antimicrobials for acute bacterial conjunctivitis. Pediatr Infect Dis J 1988;7:626.
32. Sridhar MS, Sharma S, Reddy MC, et al. Clinicomicrobiological review of Nocardia keratitis. Cornea 1998;17:17.
33. American Academy of Pediatrics Committee. Prophylaxis and treatment of neonatal gonococcal infections. Pediatrics 1980;65:1047.

Chapter 10

Clinical Applications of Antibiotics in the Eye

NR Biswas, Srujana Mohanty, GK Das, Madhurjya Gogai (India)

The term antibiotic – meaning "against life" in Greece was coined by Selman Waksman, who along with Albert Sehatz discovered streptomycin. The word is commonly used to signify antibacterials. The search for newer, stronger and safer antibacterials has been continuing since the time Dr. Carl Crede in the 1880s first advocated silver nitrate prophylaxis for protection against neonatal gonococcal conjunctivitis.[1]

Antibiotics are either bactericidal (that cause death of the bacteria) or bacteriostatic (that retard the growth of bacteria). Bactericidal drugs include the β-lactam family (penicillins and cephalosporins), aminoglycosides, and fluroquinolones. Examples of bacteriostatic drugs include tetracyclines and sulfonamides. It is important to note that bacteriostatic and bactericidal are relative terms. Some drugs that are bacteriostatic become bactericidal after extended exposure, whereas some bactericidal drugs may be less effective against particular strains of bacteria. Further, once a static drug is removed from the system, the microbe may resume its growth and spread.

Administration of Ocular Antibiotics

Antibiotics for eye infection can be given topically as drops or ointments, by subconjunctival or intravitreous injection, or systemically.[2]

Eyedrops are easily instilled, rapidly effective and best used when the eyes are to remain uncovered. Since the conjunctival sac can hold a volume of less than one drop, it is wasteful to instill more than one drop at a time. When two different eyedrops are required at the same time, dilution and overflow may occur when one immediately follows the other; an interval of 10-15 minutes should be allowed between the two applications. It is important that the patient does not squeeze the eye shut after administration of the drop, as this will eliminate the fluid from the conjunctival sac. If necessary, the lid should be gently held open for 1 to 2 minutes after a drop has been administered. Systemic absorption, which may occur after topical application of eyedrops, can be minimized by using the finger to compress the lacrimal sac at the medial canthus for at least one minute after instillation of the drops. This helps block the passage of the drops through the nasolacrimal duct.

Eye ointments are applied similarly; the ointment melts rapidly and blinking helps to spread it. Eye ointments are retained for a longer period in the conjunctival sac, resulting in a more sustained absorption. After application, if blurring of vision is a problem, the ointment may be used overnight or when the eye is to be covered with an eye patch.

Subconjunctival injection is a useful form of drug delivery, particularly in serious corneal and intraocular infections. The drug diffuses mainly through the cornea of the eye and higher intraocular concentrations may be achieved than with topical drops or ointments. The maximum volume of injected drug is usually restricted to 1 ml.

An ideal topical antibiotic should not be related to an oral drug and should be restricted to topical use only. It should not demonstrate cross-resistance or multiple resistance to unrelated antibiotics and it should have a broad enough spectrum of activity to be used as a single agent. Topical antibiotics are used to treat bacterial conjunctivitis, blepharitis, keratitis (corneal ulcers) and external hordeola (styes). They are also used as adjunctive treatment in cases of endophthalmitis and prophylactically to prevent infection before and after ophthalmic surgery. Treatment is usually empirical and topical agents should have activity against the common etiological agents namely, *Staphylococcus aureus*, coagulase negative staphylococci, Streptococcus species, *Haemophilus influenzae*, and coliforms. Although most cases of acute bacterial conjunctivitis may resolve spontaneously, anti-infective treatment shortens the infectious process and prevents complications. Acute infective conjunctivitis is treated with antibacterial eyedrops by day and eye ointment applied at night.

Pharmacokinetics of Topical Medications

Less than 5% of medication instilled via eyedrops enters the systemic circulation. Topical administration of antimicrobials has the advantage of applying the medication directly to the site of infection. The relative degree of water and lipid solubility determines the penetration of eyedrops. Absorption through the corneal epithelium requires fat solubility, and water solubility is required for diffusion through the corneal stroma into the anterior chamber.[3]

The minimum inhibitory concentration (MIC) is defined as the lowest concentration of an antimicrobial that will inhibit visible growth of an organism.[4] The MIC for antibiotics is often expressed as the MIC_{90} – the concentration of antibiotic needed to inhibit 90% of a bacterial isolate. Generally, bacteria are considered to be sensitive to an antibiotic if the achievable serum level is four times the MIC. However, bacteria reported as resistant because of lower achievable concentrations in serum may be susceptible when the medication is used topically because of the higher achievable concentration with frequent topical dosing.

Bacteria can develop resistance to antibiotics by four main methods. They can alter the composition of their cell walls, thus creating a barrier to entrance of the medication. Second, the bacteria can upregulate active transport mechanisms to remove pharmacologic agents from the cell. Third, the bacterial target enzyme can be altered to prevent the action of the antimicrobial and a final method is induction of or de novo development of a bacterial enzyme that can deactivate or neutralize the drug.

Aminoglycosides

Aminoglycosides are potent bactericidal agents that are particularly useful against aerobic gram-negative bacteria. They have no useful activity against streptococci, anaerobes, or intracellular bacteria. They inhibit bacterial protein synthesis through interference with translation of mRNA at the ribosomal level, especially, by inhibiting formation of the ribosomal initiation complex and by causing misreading of mRNA. Clinically important aminoglycosides include gentamicin, tobramycin, neomycin, amikacin, netilmicin, kanamycin, and streptomycin. Of these, tobramycin, gentamicin and neomycin are by far the ones most commonly used in ophthalmology. Streptomycin, the first aminoglycoside which was derived from *Streptomyces griseus*, has no significant clinical use in ophthalmology. Neomycin is produced by a different species of *Streptomyces*. Gentamicin and netilmicin are derived from *Micromonospora purpurea*. Amikacin and netilmicin are semisynthetic aminoglycoside preparations. Resistance to aminoglycosides occurs when the drugs fail to penetrate the cytoplasm of the organism. Since penetration of the bacterial cytoplasmic membrane is an oxygen-dependent, active process, strictly anaerobic bacteria and facultative bacteria under anaerobic conditions are highly resistant. Bacteria can also become resistant to aminoglycosides by the production of aminoglycoside-modifying enzymes that inactivate or destroy these agents or by mutations that result in configurational change of the aminoglycoside-ribosomal receptor site.

Aminoglycosides are used topically for treatment of bacterial conjunctivitis, bacterial keratitis and infections of the external eye and its adnexa caused by susceptible gram-negative bacteria and pseudomonas. They have little activity against anaerobic organisms and gram-positive bacteria. Most gram-negative organisms that possess plasmid-mediated aminoglycoside-modifying enzymes will be resistant to both gentamicin and tobramycin. However, bacterial susceptibility studies demonstrate that in some cases, microorganisms resistant to gentamicin retain susceptibility to tobramycin. Because of a chemical modification, amikacin is protected from aminoglycoside inactivating enzymes and thus is the preferred drug for treatment of gram-negative infections in which resistance to both gentamicin and tobramycin occurs.[5] In cases of bacterial conjunctivitis, commercially available gentamicin, tobramycin or amikacin eyedrops (available as 0.3% solution) may be instilled four times daily. However, bacterial corneal ulcers require significantly higher concentrations of topical drops than are commercially available alongwith frequent dosing every 30 to 60 minutes. Highly concentrated, fortified preparations (20 mg/ml) can be prepared, from intravenous preparations, soon before use, due to a limited shelf-life.

When the responsible bacterial agent is unknown, these concentrated preparations of aminoglycosides are usually alternated with a fortified preparation of cephalosporin (such as cefazolin 100 mg/ml or cephamandole 50 mg/ml).[5] The fortified aminoglycosides are used primarily for a broad gram-negative coverage along with the fortified cephalosporin to cover potential gram-positive pathogens. Once the etiological agent has been isolated by culture, the topical regimen can be modified according to the sensitivity results. Frequent dosing of fortified aminoglycoside preparations can result in severe corneal epithelial toxicity, including near total epithelial defect, eyelid skin erythema and even cicatrical changes in the eyelids. Occurrence of pseudomembranous conjunctivitis is common with fortified topical gentamicin and occasionally with fortified topical tobramycin.

Neomycin, the oldest of the ocular aminoglycosides, is rarely used alone, but is widely used as prophylaxis in combination with corticosteroids following ocular surgery. Neomycin possess antiprotozoal activity and is normally used in combination with other agents in the treatment of *Acanthamoeba* keratitis. When neomycin is combined with a diamidine, it has an additive effect.[6,7] Prolonged and intensive antiamoebic therapy consisting of topical neomycin-polymyxin B-gramacidin, propamidine and miconazole has shown promise in treating patients with documented *Acanthamoeba* keratitis. Topical ocular application of neomycin frequently results in sensitization to the drug, which can lead to contact dermatitis in approximately 4% of patients.

Chloramphenicol

Chloramphenicol, a broad spectrum bacteriostatic antibiotic was introduced into clinical use in 1948. Originally isolated from *Streptomyces venezuelae*, it is now mainly produced synthetically. It is highly active against most gram-negative and gram-positive pathogens, Rickettsia and Mycoplasma. Enterobacteriaceae show variable resistance and *Pseudomonas aeruginosa* and mycobacteria are usually resistant.[8] Chloramphenicol inhibits protein synthesis by reversibly binding to the 50S ribosomal subunit of bacteria, and, to a lesser degree, to mammalian cells. Chloramphenicol appears to prevent the binding of the amino acid containing tRNA to the acceptor site on the 50S ribosome. Due to the reversible binding, chloramphenicol is bacteriostatic.

Chloramphenicol is an ideal drug for topical use. It penetrates well into the aqueous humor after topical application, has low ocular surface toxicity, and relatively low rates of development of resistance.[8] It is the gold standard for the treatment of conjunctivitis against which other topical treatments are tested. Bone marrow hypoplasia including aplastic anemia and death has been reported following systemic administration, but topical chloramphenicol does not appear to present such a substantial risk of inducing dose-related bone marrow toxicity.[9,10] Chloramphenicol is particularly effective against *Haemophilus influenzae* and topical preparations are used to treat infections caused by *H. influenzae*, *S. aureus*, *Streptococcus* species including *S. pneumoniae*, *E. coli*, *Klebsiella*, *Enterobacter*, *Neisseria* and *Moraxella* species. The usual dose of chloramphenicol solution is 1% drop to the affected eye 2 to 4 times a day or as often as advised or 1% ointment placed in the lower conjunctival sac every 3 hours or less.[11]

Polymixin B Sulfate

Polymixin B sulfate is a polypeptide antibiotic derived from *B. polymyxa*. It has a bactericidal action against almost all gram-negative bacilli except the proteus group and *Serratia*. All gram-positive bacteria, fungi, and gram-negative cocci including *N. gonorrhoae* and *N. meningitidis* are resistant. Polymixins increase the permeability of bacterial cell membranes. Topical or subconjunctival administration of polymixin B is useful for treating acute infections caused by susceptible strains of *Pseudomonas aeruginosa*. Topical solutions are prepared by dissolving 500,000 units polymixin-B sulfate in 20-50 ml sterile distilled water or sterile physiologic saline for 10,000-25,000 units per ml concentration. For the treatment of *Pseudomonas aeruginosa* infections of the eye, a concentration of 0.1% to 0.25% (10,000 to 25,000 units per ml) is administered 1-3 drops every hour, increasing the intervals as response indicates.[12] The drug is contraindicated in persons with a prior history of hypersensitivity reactions to the polymixin.

Bacitracin

Bacitracin is a bactericidal antibiotic with a range of activity closely resembling that of penicillin. It acts by interfering with bacterial cell wall synthesis. In contrast to polymixin, it is active chiefly against gram-positive organisms but also affects spirochetes, gonococci, and actinomyces. Bacitracin is ineffective against most gram-negative bacilli. Most gram-positive organisms are inhibited by 0.001 to 0.5 unit/ml of the drug.[12] Although the antibacterial spectrum of bacitracin is comparable to that of penicillin, for topical ocular use, bacitracin is preferable to penicillin, because fewer strains of organisms are resistant, allergy is less frequent and sensitization that prevents future use of penicillin is avoided. Bacitracin does not penetrate the cornea in therapeutic amounts. Concentrations of 500 to 1000 units/g are nonirritating to the eye and other tissues and cause no undesirable systemic effects.

Chlortetracycline

Since the discontinuation of tetracycline eyedrops and ointment, chlortetracycline eye ointment is the only tetracycline available for topical ocular use. Derived from *Streptomyces aureofaciens*, chlortetracycline is a broad spectrum, bacteriostatic antibiotic effective against a wide range of bacteria. Amongst the gram-positive organisms, *Streptococcus pneumoniae* is susceptible to chlortetracycline. It also inhibits coliforms, *Haemophilus* species, *Neisseria* species and most other gram-negative organisms except *Pseudomonas aeruginosa*. Since it is actively concentrated within phagocytes, chlortetracycline is useful against intracellular pathogens such as Chlamydia and is used in the treatment of trachoma (in conjunction with oral therapy).[13] For topical use, the ointment (1%) is applied to the affected eye every 2 hours or more frequently as indicated by the severity of infection and the degree of the response. Tetracycline (1%) is also included as an acceptable and effective prophylaxis of ophthalmia neonatorum due to *N. gonorrhoeae* or *Chlamydia trachomatis*.[14]

Fluoroquinolones

In 1963, nalidixic acid was discovered during chloroquine synthesis and was noted to have antibacterial properties, but it was excreted too quickly to have any significant systemic antibacterial effects. This problem was solved in 1967, however, by fluorinating the quinolones, which gave these compounds far greater antibacterial activity, therapeutic blood levels, and low toxicity.[3] Fluoroquinolones are bactericidal and inhibit bacterial DNA synthesis by blocking the action of two of the topoisomerase enzymes, which are present only in bacteria. Topoisomerase II, also known as DNA gyrase, allows the uncoiling and supercoiling of double-stranded DNA, and topoisomearse IV cleaves the doubled DNA of replicating DNA, allowing daughter cell formation. Bacteria can develop resistance to fluoroquinolones by altering their target enzymes, altering the permeability of the drug into the organism, increasing efflux pumps, and upregulating a gene conferring quinolone resistance.

Second- and Third-Generation Fluoroquinolones

The second-generation fluoroquinolones include ciprofloxacin and ofloxacin, which have broad-spectrum coverage against gram-positive and gram-negative bacteria. The initial ophthalmic use of the fluoroquinolones was to treat corneal and conjunctival infections; however, they have also gained wide acceptance in the prophylaxis of bacterial endophthalmitis after intraocular surgery.

Ciprofloxacin, a second-generation fluoroquinolone, was approved in 1990 and is a solution of ciprofloxacin 0.3% with 0.006% BAK as a preservative and a pH of 4.5. Ofloxacin, a second-generation fluoroquinolone, contains ofloxacin 0.3% and 0.005% BAK and has a pH of 6.4.[3] Ofloxacin has a greater solubility at neutral pH than ciprofloxacin allowing it to be constituted at a more physiologic pH and permitting less drug precipitation. Because ofloxacin is more lipophilic than ciprofloxacin, it has greater penetration through the corneal epithelium. Ciprofloxacin has a lower solubility at neutral pH, which can lead to corneal precipitates.

Levofloxacin, the L-isomer of ofloxacin, is considered a third-generation fluoroquinolone. It has a higher solubility at neutral pH, allowing for a higher concentration of medication, 0.5%. It has a pH of 6.5 and is preserved with 0.005% BAK. Adverse reactions to topical second-and third-generation fluoroquinolones are mild and include discomfort, chemosis, hyperemia, eyelid edema, and punctate epithelial keratitis.

Ciprofloxacin and ofloxacin are both indicated for treatment of corneal ulcers and bacterial conjunctivitis as follows:

Corneal Ulcers

Ciprofloxacin Two drops every 15 minutes for the first 6 hours and then two drops into the affected eye every 30 minutes for the rest of the first day. On the second day, use two drops every hour and then use 2 drops every 4 hours for the consecutive days of treatment.

Ofloxacin One to two drops every 30 minutes while awake and one to two drops once during the night for 2 days. For days 3 through 7 of treatment, use drops hourly, and then four times a day for the remainder of the treatment.

Bacterial Conjunctivitis

Ciprofloxacin—one to two drops every 2 to 4 hours for 2 days and then every 4 hours for 5 days.

Ofloxacin—one to two drops every 2 to 4 hours for 2 days and then every 4 hours for 5 days.

Different studies investigating the aqueous humor penetration of ofloxacin and ciprofloxacin in various clinical settings have shown that ofloxacin has a consistently higher penetration into the aqueous humor as compared to ciprofloxacin, although the difference was not always statistically significant.[15,16] Despite the greater penetration of ofloxacin, ciprofloxacin has higher antimicrobial activity (lower MIC_{90}) than ofloxacin for most pathogens. Ciprofloxacin has also been shown to reduce the bacterial flora on human conjunctiva severely within 15 minutes, with an antimicrobial effect lasting at least 2 hours, whereas ofloxacin did not result in a significant reduction in bacterial flora.[15]

Fourth-Generation Fluoroquinolones

The recently introduced fourth-generation fluoroquinolones, gatifloxacin and moxifloxacin, have shown enhanced spectrum and potency for gram-positive bacteria in addition to retaining an equal efficacy against gram-negative bacteria as the earlier fluoroquinolones. This is because the fourth-generation fluoroquinolones bind effectively to both topoisomerases II and IV, in contrast to the older fluoroquinolones which bind more strongly to topoisomerase II, an enzyme more important for gram-negative bacteria. Moxifloxacin and gatifloxacin penetrate well into the anterior chamber and achieve levels in excess of the MIC_{90} for most pathogenic organisms. For topical use, they are available as moxifloxacin 0.5% and gatifloxacin 0.3% solution.[17] They play an important role in the treatment of bacterial conjunctivitis and keratitis and in the perioperative prophylaxis against endophthalmitis.

REFERENCES

1. Dunn PM. Dr Carl Crede (1819-1892) and the prevention of ophthalmia neonatorum. Arch Dis Child Fetal Neonatal Ed 2000;83:F158-9.
2. McCloskey RV. Topical antimicrobial agents and antibiotics for the eye. Med Clin North Am 1988;72:717-22.
3. Levinson BA, Rutzen AR. New antimicrobials in ophthalmology. Ophthalmol Clin North Am 2005;18:493-509.
4. Miles RS, Amyes SGV. Laboratory control of antimicrobial therapy. In: Collee JG, Duguid JP, Fraser AG, Marmion BP. Mackie and McCartney Practical Medical Microbiology. 14th edn. London: Churchill Livingstone; 1996;151-78.
5. Patalano SM, Hyndiuk RA. Aminoglycosides in ophthalmology. In: Zimmerman TJ, Kooner KS, Sharir M, Fechtner RD (Eds). Textbook of Ocular Pharmacology. New York: Lippincot Raven; 1997;531-35.
6. Burger ST, Mondino BJ, Hoft RH, et al. Successful medical management of *Acanthamoeba* keratitis. Am J Ophthalmology 1990;110:395-403.
7. Hay J, Kirkness CM, Seal DV, Wright P. Drug resistance and Acanthamoeba keratitis: The quest for alternative antiprotozoal chemotherapy. Eye 1994;8: 555-63.
8. Lam RF, Lai JS, Ng JS, Rao SK, Law RW, Lam DS. Topical chloramphenicol for eye infections. Hong Kong Med J 2002;8:44-47.
9. Walker S, Diaper CJM, Bowman R, Sweeny G, Seal DV, Kirkness CM. Lack of evidence for systemic toxicity following topical chloramphenicol use. Eye 1998; 12:875-9.
10. Lancaster T, Swart AM, Jick H. Risk of serious hematological toxicity with use of chloramphenicol eye-drops in a British general practice database. BMJ 1998; 316;667.

11. Karp CL, Gussler JR, Alfonso EC. Chloramphenicol. In: Zimmerman TJ, Kooner KS, Sharir M, Fechtner RD (Eds). Textbook of Ocular Pharmacology. New York: Lippincott Raven; 1997;525-29.
12. Biswas NR, Gupta V. Antibacterials. Ocular Therapeutics, 2nd ed. New Delhi: CBS Publishers; 2004;1-21.
13. Barrettt S. Tetracyclines: Their role today in general practice. Prescriber 1994;5: 41-46.
14. Periodic Health Examination, 1992 update: 4. Prophylaxis for gonococcal and chlamydial ophthalmia neonatorum. Canadian Task Force on the Periodic Health Examination. Can Med Assoc J 1992; 147: 1449-54.
15. Snyder-Perlmutter LS, Katz HR, Melina M. Effect of topical ciprofloxacin 0.3% and ofloxacin 0.3% on the reduction of bacterial flora on the human conjunctiva. J Cataract Refractive Surg 2000; 26: 1620-25.
16. Yalvac IS, Basci NE, Bozkurt A, et al. Penetration of topically applied ciprofloxacin and ofloxacin into the aqueous humor and vitreous. J Cataract Refractive Surg 2003;29:487-91.
17. Solomon R, Donnenfeld ED, Perry HD, et al. Penetration of topically applied gatifloxacin 0.3%, moxifloxacin 0.5%, and ciprofloxacin 0.3% into the aqueous humor. Ophthalmology 2005;112:466-69.

Chapter 11

The Next Generation of Fluoroquinolone Antibiotics

John D Sheppard (USA)

Can we really better prevent postoperative ocular infections with the next generation of fluoroquinolone antibiotics?

TRUE OPHTHALMOLOGIC EMERGENCIES

There are a handful of acute infectious ocular emergencies that truly threaten vision. Coupled with extreme time sensitivity, these afflictions send fear through the heart of every ophthalmic surgeon on the planet. Ocular infections considered to be truly emergent include:

- Postoperative endophthalmitis
- Post-traumatic endophthalmitis
- Endogenous endophthalmitis
- Infectious keratitis
- Post-LASIK interface keratitis
- Post-trabeculectomy blebitis
- Hyperacute gonococcal conjunctivitis
- Acute retinal necrosis syndrome
- Macular toxoplasmosis
- Severe toxoplasmosis vitritis
- Orbital cellulitis
- Sphenoid sinus thrombosis.

Despite common clinical practice, it has been exceedingly difficult to unequivocally establish the efficacy of modern topical antibiotics as preventive agents in our crusade for complication free elective surgery, at least with a squeaky clean prospective, randomized clinical study. Due to the fortunately low incidence of blinding corneal and vitreous disease, statistical significance would require exorbitantly expensive trials enrolling thousands of subjects. Thus, in the best interest of our patients, we must decide what is truly best for surgical candidates within the context of our own practice. We remain vigilant for vision threatening infections. Bacterial keratitis and endophthalmitis are the most emergent.

IS THERE A TRUE NEED FOR PERIOPERATIVE ANTIMICROBIAL PROPHYLAXIS?

The vast majority of ophthalmic surgeons agree that perioperative antibiotics can prevent postoperative infections. This sentiment is also shared, at least somewhat, but other surgical specialties. In 1974, Allen reported a remarkable 23-fold decrease in postoperative endophthalmitis following extracapsular cataract surgery when perioperative topical chloramphenicol was prescribed.[1] This landmark study truly convinced most surgeons that antibiotics were necessary for all of their elective surgery patients. Prospective studies have been few and far between. Gills[2] and Gimbel[3] collected data on thousands of postoperative cataract surgery patients in the phacoemulsification era demonstrating a trend towards endophthalmitis prevention with intra-operative irrigating solution antibiotic administration. Ciulla[4] showed that the only demonstrably effective method for endophthalmitis prevention in the phacoemulsification population was the traditional preoperative povidone iodide scrub. Nevertheless, an emerging trend towards increased incidence of endophthalmitis with clear corneal incisions strongly implicates a role for prophylactic topical antimicrobials.

IS THE RISING INCIDENCE OF POST-INFECTIOUS ENDOPHTHALMITIS REVERSIBLE?

A recent landmark retrospective review of over 9000 phacoemulsification patients at Utah's Moran Eye Center unveiled a shockingly significant 3-fold higher rate of endophthalmitis in patients treated with perioperative ciprofloxacin drops when compared to those treated with topical ofloxacin.[5] These sequential cases were largely performed by resident physicians, but within the context of the same institution, surgical facility, and attending faculty. Nagaki[6] in Japan has found a 6-fold increase in endophthalmitis with the switch from scleral tunnel to clear corneal incisions. This data also suggests that continuously therapeutic aqueous levels of antimicrobial are important in controlling bacterial introduction into the anterior chamber after surgery has been completed, likely through paroxysmal communications between the anterior chamber the and ocular surface through a sutureless temporal corneal incision. Thus, although sterilization of the ocular surface and meticulous sterile technique are clearly required of the cataract surgeon, the role of topical antibiotics has not definitively been proven essential. This proof would be prohibitively expensive considering the costs of prospective randomized clinical trials, and the exceedingly rare incidence of endophthalmitis.

Nonetheless, there is alarming new data suggesting that the risk of postoperative endophthalmitis has risen, perhaps as a result of the significant move to clear corneal temporal incision by many surgeons.

DO SURGEONS REALLY NEED NEXT GENERATION FLUOROQUINOLONE ANTIBIOTICS FOR SURGICAL PROPHYLAXIS?

The current ophthalmic media is teeming with reports of new generation topical ophthalmic antibiotics. Clinicians anticipate even better protection with even less toxicity. Despite remarkable improvements in the spectrum and efficacy of systemic antibiotics, these innovations may not necessarily translate into benefits for patients at risk for ocular infection. Nevertheless, ophthalmology has always taken leads from colleagues in the infectious disease community, bringing established systemic antibiotics into the topical ophthalmic market place. The newest agents approved for topical ophthalmic use include Levofloxacin 0.5% (Quixin, Santen, Napa), Gatifloxacin 0.3% (Zymar, Allergan, Irvine), and Moxifloxacin 0.5% preservative free multi-dose (Vigamox, Alcon, Fort Worth). The introduction of Levofloxacin 1.5% (IQuix, Vistakon, Jacksonville) preservative free multi-dose drop further congests the market place in the United States. As a result of these introductions as well as patent expirations, ofloxacin 0.3% (Ocuflox, Allergan) and Ciloxan 0.3% (Ciloxan, Alcon) have become available as generic preparations, undoubtedly raising important questions about such issues as vehicle quality, preservatives, efficacy and cost savings.

A now broader spectrum of activity is assumed to provide superior protection with the development of newer fluoroquinolone molecules, be they fourth generation, next generation, new age or whatever. Clearly, these newer drugs have significantly lower MICs for gram-positive organisms as well as some additional classes of pathogens, including mycobacteria, chlamydia, and anerobes. Gram-negative activity, however, has remained universally vigorous among all of the available topical fluoroquinolones. As resistance develops to currently popular agents, treatment failures, and even prophylaxis failures will ensue. Because the majority of emergent ocular infections are gram-positive, particularly postoperative endophthalmitis, the enhanced coverage and broadened spectrum is welcomed.

HOW IMPORTANT ARE SOLUBILITY AND PENETRATION?

Antibiotic levels and MICs on the ocular surface, intracamerally, and in the serum can be confused. Mean Inhibitory Concentrations (MICs) are established by the NCCLS (National Committee of Clinical Laboratory Standards) and are derived from *in vitro* data obtained under strictly standardized conditions. These standards are based upon concentrations of antibiotic in the serum: there are no standards for topical ocular therapy that represent the concentrations of antibiotics in ocular tissues. Thus, ocular surface concentrations from a single drop may exceed several fold the maximum achievable serum concentration. Furthermore, interactions between the tear film, the ocular surface, and sustained release capacitance effects created by absorbed drug in the conjunctiva and uvea may also affect peak and trough bioavailability. Surface kill curves may be more relevant to conjunctivitis or preoperative sterilization, intrastromal corneal levels more applicable to refractive surgery, while aqueous humor levels may be more important during postoperative cataract healing. These levels may differ in potency from tissue to tissue, from drug to drug, and from bug to bug. As a result, detailed analyses of target tissue bioavailability with respect to each pathogen is necessary in order to make any conclusions about the best fluoroquinolone for a given indication.

As ophthalmologists we must consider once again the best solution to ophthalmic infections and prophylaxis for our patients within the plethora of pharmaceutical change. Given current and anticipated data regarding sensitivity, kill curves, inhibitory quotient, and penetration, we can make intelligent assumptions about antimicrobial activity on the ocular surface as well as within the eye. Genuine improvements in anticipated treatment success should clearly reward our patients. New fluoroquinolones, the next generation, hopefully will provide this added reassurance.

Orally administered fluoroquinolones can generally provide effective intravitreal concentrations, even in the absence of inflammation. Sparfloxacin, trovafloxacin, gatifloxacin,[7] moxifloxacin and levofloxacin[8] all reach effective MICs within the vitreous when given by mouth. There are no human studies to evaluate this strategy for either the prevention or treatment of endophthalmitis, however.[9]

Most ophthalmic microbiology experts agree that ocular surface and lid organisms cause the lion's share of postoperative endophthalmitis. It is also likely that organisms can be introduced intracamerally not only at the time of surgery, but also afterwards through the cataract wound, particularly with clear corneal incisions. Thus, antibiotics with rapid kill curves but poor penetration into the aqueous humor will only prevent intraoperative inoculation of surface flora. Topical agents with excellent solubility and penetration will also prevent postoperative contamination of the anterior chamber by providing continuous inhibitory concentrations despite momentary gaping of the unhealed wound due to rubbing, blinking, or unusual nocturnal positions. Once the wound has sealed, certainly by postoperative day 10, the risk of inoculation should decrease markedly.

Highly soluble molecules achieve effective intracameral concentrations,[10] as suggested by comparative data indicating effective intraocular MICs following topical administration of levofloxacin. Thus, an agent with higher albeit effective MICs on the ocular surface may in fact achieve much lower concentrations below the effective MICs in the eye compared to a more soluble agent with lower MICs on the surface. Thus has been the case of ciprofloxacin drops compared to more soluble, commercially available agents. This phenomenon of potency at the intended target tissue is described by the Inhibitory Quotient, or IQ: the ultimate concentration of antibiotic at the site of action. The IQ = Concentration of drug at active site ÷ MIC_{90}. Thus an adequate IQ is equal to or greater than 1. Although directly comparative human studies are now in progress with the recent approval and release of topical gatifloxacin and moxifloxacin, initial animal data demonstrates the superior penetration and aqueous concentrations attained with topical levofloxacin and moxifloxacin when compared to gatifloxacin, ofloxacin, and ciprofloxacin.[11]

WHO IS THE UNIVERSALLY ACCEPTED DECISION MAKER FOR ANTIBIOTIC GENERATION NOMENCLATURE?

There remains considerable confusion regarding the current generation nomenclature system, particularly for fluoroquinolones. Nalidixic acid, first synthesized in 1962, is considered by most to represent the first generation, even though it is not a fluorinated molecule. Ofloxacin and ciprofloxacin are generally considered to be second generation. Thereafter, opinions unfortunately vary. Several articles describe a reasonable criterion for classification, but prove contradictory with one another.

Antibiotics can be classified in several ways, the most commonly accepted being spectrum of anti-microbial activity, as utilized with the cephalosporins. This system of course relies upon *in vitro* data. Another viable method utilizes instead the chemical structure or more specifically, the molecular structural activity relationships, relying upon chemical data. Finally, variations of this theme might include both characteristics as well as penetration into selected body compartments or tissues, thereby relying upon clinical efficacy data. The nomenclature for antibiotic generation assignment clearly falls within the realm of systemic applications, and has never been determined by ophthalmology. Thus, our specialty is dependent upon the wisdom of our infectious disease and pharmacology colleagues to provide us with useful classification guidelines. An authoritative text dedicated to fluoroquinolones[12] describes moxifloxacin as a fourth generation antibiotic, with gatifloxacin as a third generation and levofloxacin as a second-generation fluoroquinolone. The author recalls separating fluoroquinolones into generations in a manner similar to the cephalosporin generations, based upon broadened spectrum of action, while acknowledging the fact that the system of nomenclature remains clearly arbitrary. The patent for moxifloxacin, interestingly enough, deems it a third generation drug. Thus even more confusion to decipher. Some sources describe both gatifloxacin and moxifloxacin as 4th generation fluoroquinolones, while others classify them both with levofloxacin as 3rd generation, with trovafloxacin deemed the only agent with sufficient spectrum of action worthy of the 4th generation moniker.[13]

OPHTHALMOLOGISTS CAN COMBAT ANTIBIOTIC RESISTANCE EVERYDAY

Clinicians and specifically ophthalmologists and optometrists can effectively battle resistance in the office setting. The bottom line, regardless of nomenclature synthesized in the universe of human imagination, is killing pathogens. Since the time of sulfonamides and Alexander Fleming, antibiotic resistance has proven itself a universal nemesis. Physicians prescribing systemic antibiotics are the chief creative engine behind antibiotic resistance, particularly in congested, crowded, or high pathology environments like nursing homes or intensive care units. Improper use by patients or erroneous prescriptions by doctors also contribute. In addition, over the counter availability of numerous antibiotics in countries without vigorous prescription regulation also contributes to resistance, as well as massive use by the agriculture and veterinarian industries. Topical ocular use is unlikely, however, to contribute to the overall worldwide problem with antibiotic resistance, due to the relatively miniscule numbers of organisms exposed on the ocular surface. Nevertheless, exposure of the nasopharynx to topical ophthalmics through nasolacrimal drainage raises ongoing questions regarding systemic resistance.

There is a wide variety in risk profiles for the development of resistance, since some antibiotic classes are more likely to allow antibiotic resistance to develop. Pneumococci, for example, become resistant to fluoroquinolones and macrolides more rapidly than to ceftriaxone, a third generation cephalosporin, in an *in vitro* model.[14] Whether or not this is applicable to clinical situations, let alone ocular disease remains to be established. Nevertheless, eye care professionals prescribing antibiotics should beware that fluoroquinolone resistance is developing in the community, and furthermore, that improper topical administration of antibiotics can create resistant flora. Thus, less that QID dosing, administration lasting less than the recommended 7 days or longer than 3 weeks, and dilution with other concomitant medications can create resistance during treatment for conjunctivitis or prior to surgery. Sound advice, therefore, would include switching antibiotics prior to elective surgery if either a resistant organism is identified upon preoperative culture, or if the particular patient was known to have self administered the intended prophylactic antibiotic improperly prior to surgery.

EACH SURGEON MUST MAKE INDIVIDUALIZED DECISIONS

Ophthalmic topical antibiotics can provide outstanding surface sterilization and therapeutic intracameral and intrastromal bactericidal concentrations. Improved protection with next generation topical fluoroquinolones against peri-operative infections or conjunctivitis[15] has already been documented *in vitro* and in animal models. Fluoroquinolones are firmly established as the drug class of choice for these indications, due to superlative spectrum and toxicity profiles when compared to other available topical agents. Topical prophylactic antibiotic use, even though never unequivocally proven to prevent postcataract endophthalmitis, has become an integral part of the perioperative regimen for most surgeons. Although this is not an established community standard for care, continuous pressure to provide this added protection comes from numerous fronts: colleagues, patients, pharmaceutical companies, risk management underwriters, and a growing body of scientific evidence. Therefore, selection of the most appropriate and effective agent is central to providing the best possible care for our patients. This intense concern for better outcomes and fewer complications applies not only to cataract surgery, but also to refractive surgery patients as well as patients suffering from bacterial conjunctivitis. Newer fluoroquinolone agents offer improved spectrum, better solubility, greater penetration, and thereby superior efficacy. One matter is certain, and that is that resistance will emerge.[16] The quest for new antimicrobials and better therapeutic and prophylactic strategies follows.

Fourth generation, or better the next generation of fluoroquinolones, regardless of numerical assignment, raises expectations even higher, hopefully to the ultimate benefit of our patients. Clinical data directly comparing the next generation, levofloxacin, gatifloxacin and moxifloxacin, is growing. As clinicians, we await unbiased *in vivo* human clinical data collection and purposeful scientific analysis, the essence of the annual ARVO meeting each spring. Newer medications including topical azithromycin [17] are entering the market regularly. With each new antibiotic introduced into the market place, into the systemic therapeutic milieu, and into ophthalmic clinical practice, new resistance issues arise.[17] As always we as surgeons can be pleased that continuous pharmaceutical advances have been made to hopefully counter the rising tide of endophthalmitis, avoid the tragedy of blinding infection after elective refractive surgery, and provide truly efficacious broad spectrum coverage for bacterial keratitis and contagious bacterial conjunctivitis.

REFERENCES

1. Allen HF. Margiaracine AB. Bacterial Endophthalmitis after Cataract Extraction: Incidence in 36,000 Consecutive Operations with Special Attention to Preoperative Topical Antibiotics. Arch Ophthalmol 1974;91:3-6.
2. Gills JP. Filters and antibiotics in irrigating solutions for cataract surgery. J Cataract and Refract Surg 1991;17(3):385.
3. Gimbel HV. Letter to the Editor, Ophthalmology 2000;107:1614-15.
4. Ciulla TA, Starr MB, Masket S. Bacterial endophthalmitis prophylaxis for cataract surgery: an evidence based update. Ophthalmology 2002;109:13-24.
5. Jensen MK, Fiscella RG, Olsen RP. Comparison of Endophthalmitis Rates Over Four Years Associated with Topical Ofloxacin Vs. Ciprofloxacin: Moran Eye Center Retrospective Post-Cataract Endophthalmitis Study. ARVO 2002.
6. Nagaki. Bacterial endophthalmitis after small incision cataract surgery. JCRS 2003.
7. Hariprasad SM, Mieler WF, Holz ER. Vitreous and aqueous penetration of orally administered gatifloxacin in humans. Arch Ophthalmol 2003;121(3):345-50.

8. Garcia-Saenz MC, Arias-Puente A, Fresnadillo-Martinez MJ, Carrasco-Font C. Human aqueous humor levels of oral ciprofloxacin, levofloxacin and gatifloxacin. J Cataract Refract Surg 2001;27(12):1969-74.
9. Ng EW, Samiy N, Ruoff KL, et al. Treatment of experimental *Staphylococcus epidermidis* endophthalmitis with oral trovafloxacin. Am J Ophthalmol 1998; 126(2):278-87.
10. Bucci FA. An *in vivo* comparison of the ocular absorption of levofloxacin versus ciprofloxacin prior to phacoemulsification. ARVO: B589, 2002.
11. Levine JM, Noecker RJ, Snyder RW, et al. Comparative Penetration of the Fluoroquinolone Antibiotics Gatifloxacin and Levofloxacin into the Rabbit Aqueous Humor after Topical Dosing: ARVO B729, 2002.
12. Andriole VT (Ed). The Quinolones. 3rd edition. London: Academic Press; 2000; 477-91.
13. King DE, Malone R, Lilley SH. New classification system and update on the quinolone antibiotics. Am Fam Physician 2002:16(9):2741-48.
14. Browne, FA, Clark C, Bozdogan B, et al. Single and multi-step resistance selection in *Streptococcus pneumoniae* comparing ceftriaxone with levofloxacin, gatifloxacin, and moxifloxacin; Int J Antimicrobial Agents 2002;93-99.
15. Graves A, Henry M, O'Brien TP, et al. *In vitro* susceptibilities of bacterial ocular isolates to fluoroquinolones. Cornea 2001;20(3):301-05.
16. Williams PB, Crouch ER Jr, Sheppard JD Jr, Lattanzio FA Jr, Parker TA, Mitrev PV. The birth of ocular pharmacology in the 20th century. The Journal of Clinical Pharmacology, 2000;40:990-1006.
17. Gaynor BD, Chidambaram JD, Cevallos V, Miao Y, Miller K, Jha HC, et al. Topical ocular antibiotics induce bacterial resistance at extraocular sites. British Journal of Ophthalmology 2005;89:1097-99.

Chapter 12

Management of Corneal Ulcers

Marta Calatayud, José L Güell, Oscar Gris (Spain)

INTRODUCTION

Despite the fact that many pathogens can cause infectious corneal lesions, and that many corneal ulcers are secondary to noninfectious processes we generally use the term corneal ulcer in the context of bacterial infectious keratitis. Strictly speaking, we will consider a corneal ulcer as any loss of superficial corneal tissue due to necrosis secondary to an infectious process.[10]

Any pathological process of the cornea that can produce irregularities or opacification of the cornea may result in a decrease in visual acuity to a greater, or lesser degree, depending on the location and extension of the lesion. The complications of corneal disease quite often arise through incorrect management, so it is important to be aware of the etiology and treatment of corneal ulcers.

CLASSIFICATION

There are various clinical classifications of corneal ulcers, but at a practical level the most useful is that based on the site of the lesion, distinguishing between two major groups:[7]

1. Central corneal ulcers
   These are typically infectious ulcers (Figs 12.1 to 12.5). The most frequent causal agents are:
   Staphylococcus aureus, Streptococcus epidermidis, Streptococcus pneumoniae, Group D Streptococcus and Bacillus species. Gram-negative bacteria include: *Haemophilus, Pseudomonas, Moraxella,* Enterobacterias (Proteus, *E.coli, Klebsiella sp*).
2. Marginal ulcers
   These are usually associated with autoimmune diseases and are caused by *Staphylococcus* or *Moraxella* species either directly or indirectly, via immune responses.

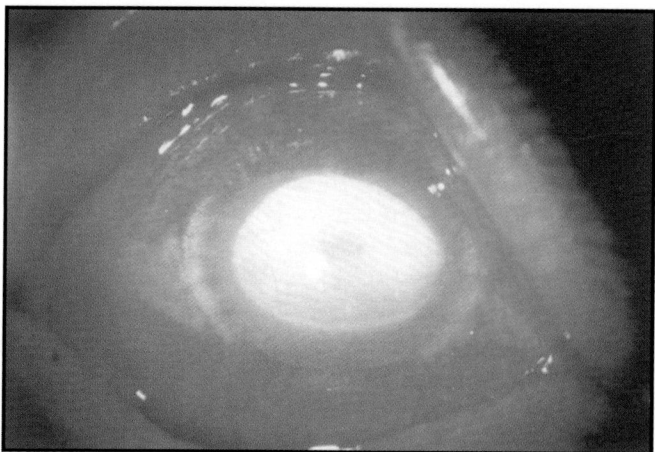

Fig. 12.1: Bacterial ulcer

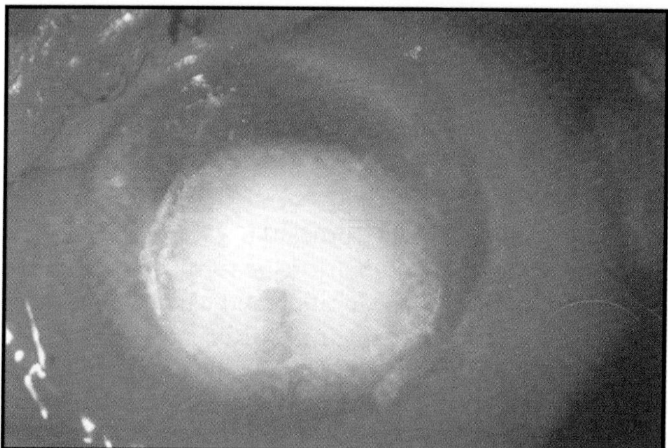

Fig. 12.2: Fulminating corneal ulcer

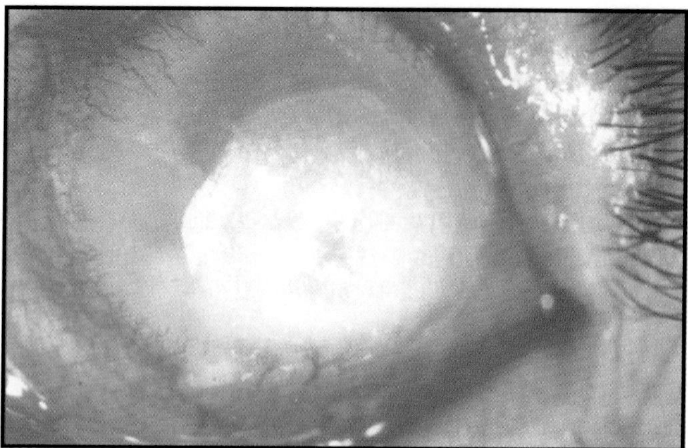

Fig. 12.3: Corneal ulcer

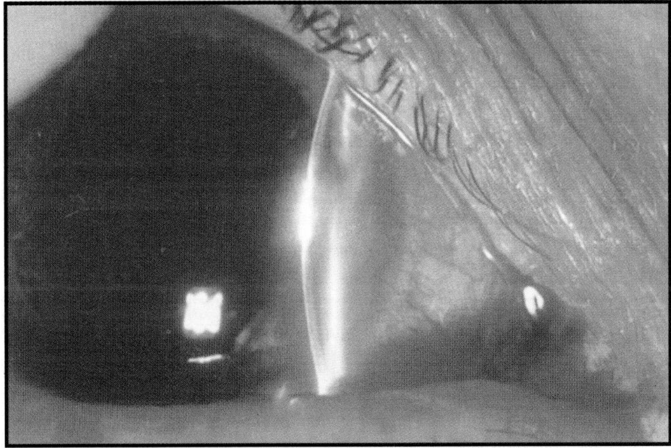

Fig. 12.4: Corneal ulcer

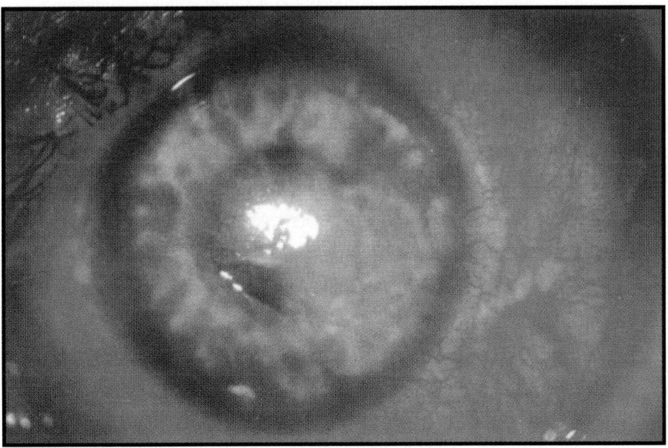

Fig. 12.5: Corneal ulcer

Fortunately, as long as the cornea is healthy, the majority of bacteria are unable to cross or adhere to the corneal epithelium. However, there are a few species that are capable of penetrating an intact epithelium, for example, *Neisseria gonorrhoea, Haemophilus, Aegyptus, Corynebacterium diphtheriae* and *Lysteria* species. The bacteria multiply and proliferate within the stroma, liberating enzymes and toxins which provoke an initial polymorphonuclear cell infiltrate with phagocytosis of the bacteria. The enzymes liberated by the bacteria and leukocytes produce necrosis of the stroma with epithelial loss.

PREDISPOSING FACTORS

The most common predisposing factor that facilitates bacterial infection, primarily through lesions of the corneal epithelium, is that of contact lens use, being most frequent in previously healthy eyes in industrialized countries. The most prevalent organism isolated is *Pseudomonas aeruginosa*.[20-22] Other factors that can contribute towards the formation of corneal ulcers include diseases of the ocular surface that either, in a direct or indirect manner, affect the defense mechanisms of the eye and consequently the integrity of the epithelium. These include especially herpetic corneal disease, dry eye syndrome, exposure keratitis, bullous keratopathy among others.

CLINICAL PRESENTATION

Although there are specific presentations depending on the bacteria involved, there exists a series of symptoms and signs common to all that allow for a rapid diagnosis, and therefore early treatment of corneal ulcers. The most important symptoms are pain, conjunctival injection, photophobia, and decreased visual acuity.[6-9]

In general, on biomicroscopic examination a localized epithelial deficit is observed surrounded by an area of epithelial edema which produces the elevated edges typical of infectious ulcers. This is accompanied by a central area of dense stromal inflammation with subsequent opacification of the corneal tissues.[7-10] Other associated signs include endothelial lesions in the form of plaques, anterior chamber inflammatory reaction and hypopyon.

There are clinical signs characteristic of specific organisms, for example, *Pseudomonas aeruginosa* produces large ulcers with irregular edges due to stromal necrosis accompanied by an adherent whitish-yellow exudate, *Streptococcus* and *Staphylococcus* species produce round or oval yellow plaques surrounded by relatively normal stroma and, enterobacteria produce ulcers with a more greyish appearance.[6-11] Other slower growing organisms, like anaerobes or mycobacteria frequently produce stromal suppuration with an intact epithelium.

Crystalline infectious keratopathy is an uncommon condition.[10] It is often wrongly diagnosed in cases of secondary infectious keratitis, which in the majority of cases, are in fact due to infection with *Streptococcus viridans*. Ramificated crystal-like opacifications can be observed within the superficial and medial stroma which appear typically in patients receiving intense topical steroid treatment and, more especially, after penetrating keratoplasty. Acanthamoeba (Fig. 12.6) is another infrequent causative organism, and characteristically proliferates in certain preservative medias, and is therefore more common in soft contact lens wearers. It produces mostly central ulcers, accompanied with white satellite lesions. Typically the pain experienced is extremely intense, which at first presentation of the ulcer can be dispropor-tionate with respect to the biomicroscopic findings.[7,8] Fungal keratitis (Figs 12.7 and 12.8) is much less frequent; cases of Candida infection can be found in patients with predisposing pathology, such as in the prolonged use of steroids,

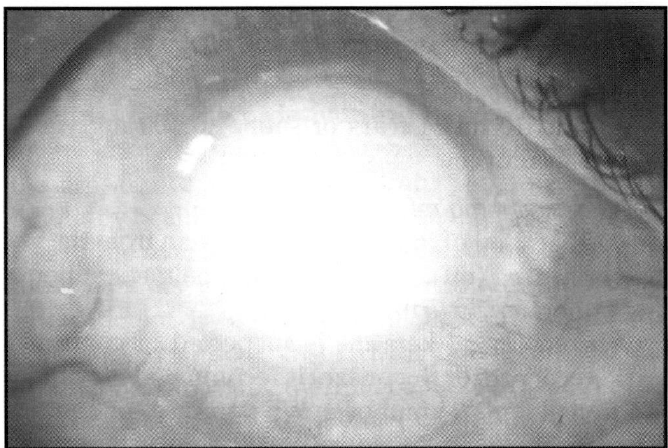

Fig. 12.6: Acanthamoeba corneal ulcer

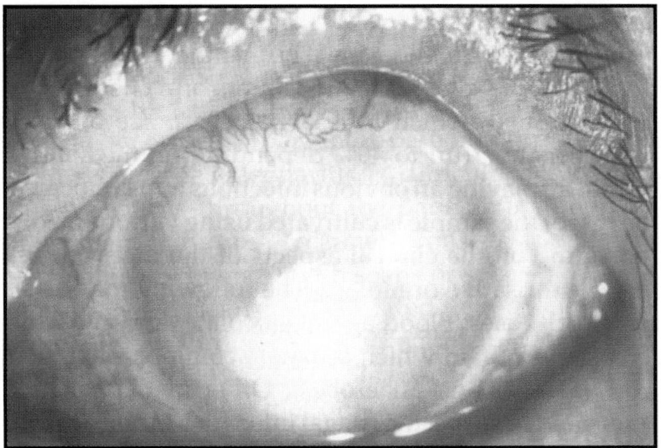

Fig. 12.7: Fungal corneal ulcer (Candida)

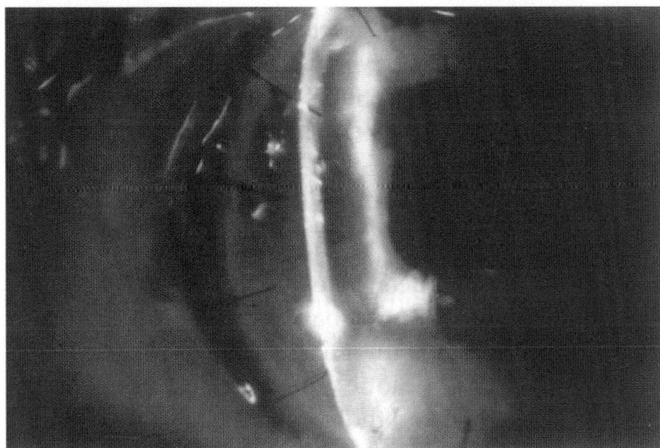

Fig. 12.8: Fungal corneal ulcer (Candida)

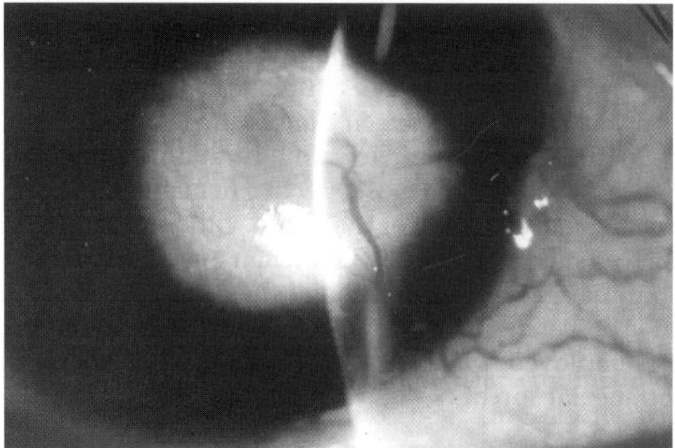

Fig. 12.9: Post-herpetic lipid deposits

in cases of dry eye syndrome, exposure keratopathy, *Herpes simplex* keratopathy (Fig. 12.9), or with previous keratoplasia. The filamentous fungi, *Fusarium* or *Aspergillus* have also been identified as causative agents of infectious keratitis. These ulcers are poorly circumscribed, often surrounded by infiltrative satellite lesions and follow a more chronic course.

DIAGNOSIS

A microbiological diagnosis is always advisable before initiating any specific treatment if an infectious origin is suspected. Before the use of topical anesthesia the maximum amount of material must be obtained both from the ulcer base and edges. An initial Gram and Giemsa stain are performed, which in a large percentage of ulcers prove negative (up to 40% depending on the source), despite displaying an obvious infectious appearance.[12-14] The rest of the sample is cultivated using various medias depending on the clinical aspects of the ulcer and the possible causative organism. The following medias are used in all cases: Blood agar, Chocolate agar and Thioglycolate broth, in which the most common pathogens grow (aerobes and anaerobes). Other medias include: Sabouraud in suspected fungal infections in both sporing and filamentous type, and nonnutrient agar with *E. coli* overlay in suspected cases of Acanthamoeba infection.[7,8] Impression cytology can also be a useful diagnostic tool. Despite correct handling and processing of the sample there are a high percentage of culture-negative results, between 30-40 percent of cases, which means that in many of our patients empirical treatment is continued and modified according to the clinical response.[14-17,19]

TREATMENT

Once the sample has been taken for culture, it is a priority to start antibiotic treatment based on the clinical impression and Gram stain, if this has proved positive. In reality there is no single antibiotic which is effective against all corneal pathogens, and the appearance of resistance is a constant problem. However, recent studies suggest that the fluoroquinolones, administered frequently (for example every 15 minutes at the start of treatment), work in 90 percent of cases, being equally as effective as fortified topical antibiotics and less toxic.

It is interesting to point out that there is no clear and direct correlation between antibiotic sensitivity *in vitro* and *in vivo*, or with respect to antibiotic resistance.

With regards to means of administration of antibiotics, topical therapy is the most effective in maintaining concentrations at the site of the lesion. Other local options such as subconjunctival or subTenon injections produce an initial peak concentration at the ocular level which later descends to very low levels.[8] Systemic antibiotics are employed when there is a suspicion of scleral or intra-ocular spread.

MYDRIATIC

Mydriatic agents, especially cyclopentolate, must be used in all cases of infectious keratitis in order to prevent posterior synechiae forming in miosis and to decrease the pain induced by ciliary spasm. The use of steroids is more controversial. Topical steroid treatment should only be commenced when active infection is controlled and when the benefits of its anti-inflammatory properties, that decrease the amount of stromal necrosis, outweigh the potential risks of perforation. We prescribe prednisolone acetate or prednisolone sulphate at low doses (every 4-6 hours) and monitor the patient every 24-48 hours, although every case must be evaluated individually.

Choice of Antibiotic

An adequate antibiotic is chosen whilst awaiting the results of the culture based on the appearance of the ulcer, the associated clinical signs and possible risk factors involved (e.g. contact lens use). However, considering the frequency with which the cultures prove negative, and the lack of correlation between antibiotic response *in vitro* and *in vivo* we believe that as long as the clinical response is adequate, the result of the culture has limited value, and is not the only factor to be taken into account when modifying the treatment strategy.

In general, antibiotic combinations are employed, for instance a cephalosporin with an aminoglycoside, being active against both gram-positive and gram-negative organisms, and also effective in cases where no organism is isolated or indeed when multiple organisms are found.[23-24] The fluoroquinolones are also active against gram-negative bacilli[18] and vancomycin is useful in cases of cephalosporin-resistant staphylococcus infections.

Fortified Topical Antibiotic Preparation[7]

Cefazolin 50 mg/ml

- Dissolve one vial of cefazolin (containing 1 g) in 9.2 ml of tears.
- Take 5 ml of the solution and add 5 ml of tears.

Ceftazidime 50 mg/ml

- Dissolve one vial of ceftazidime (containing 1 g) in 9.2 ml of tears.
- Take 5 ml of the solution and add 5 ml of tears.

Vancomycin 50 mg/ml

- Add 10 ml of tears or saline to 500 mg vial of vancomycin.

Tobramycin 14 mg/ml

- Take 2 ml of injectable vancomycin from the vial of 40 mg/ml and add to an ophthalmic solution of tobramycin (5 ml).

When a fungal keratitis is suspected or confirmed oral ketoconazol or fluconazol is recommended with the addition of topical amphotericin B in cases of Candida or Aspergillus keratitis. However, although in these types of keratitis drug penetrance of the cornea is poor, so in many cases a penetrating keratoplasty is required. Acanthamoeba keratitis is treated, with regards to choice of antibiotic, with either topical neomycin-polymyxin or cotrimoxazole 1 percent, accompanied, in some cases by oral ketoconazol. Propamidine and the biguanides are by far the most useful drugs. Propamidine, in drops or ointment form, appears to be more effective in association with topical polymyxin B-neomycin, and is prescribed at high dosages, initially every 30 minutes for the first 3-4 days (this medication is not available in the USA). Disinfectants, such as those of the biguanide family, are the alternative option. We use chlorhexidine at 0.02 percent, initially every hour or every half hour, reducing the dose gradually, depending on the clinical response, over several months with the intention to perform a keratoplasty, if necessary, when infection becomes inactive. Either of the two options alone are effective, although based on our experience, the indolent course of the ulcers, the long treatment that they require and the frequency with which resistances arise we always associate a topical antibiotic with a topical antiseptic.

Penetrating keratoplasty when infection is still active is generally indicated in cases of progressive disease despite medical treatment (especially in fungal keratitis when fungus can spread to the anterior chamber, and in cases of Acanthamoeba, although recurrences of infection and intraocular invasion have been described after keratoplasty). In cases of descematocele or perforation, lamellar or penetrating keratoplasty is carried out when infection is inactive in order to correct leukomas that have appeared after satisfactory medical treatment.[23,24]

MARGINAL ULCERS

Here reference is made to peripheral corneal ulcers that result from a hypersensitivity reaction to bacterial antigens (proteins). In our experience they are mainly seen in cases of meibomitis or chronic blepharitis where a hypersensitivity against the staphylococci, that habitually colonize the palpebral borders, occurs in these patients. Primarily these cases are identified as stromal keratitis, in other words, with an intact epithelium, with the superior and inferior zones being most affected with the appearance of corneal infiltrates separated from the limbus by healthy cornea. However, later on, breaks and loss of the overlying epithelium can occur. In many of these patients the picture is also complicated by the association of dry eye syndrome of a multicausal nature which makes these cases difficult to control. Tear production, especially the lipid component, is affected in meibomitis, but also, staphylococci produce a variety of lipases and other enzymes that further alter the lipid composition affecting the stability of the tear film (this is known as the SSS syndrome, *Staphylococcus*-Seborreia-Sicca).[7] Topical steroids are the treatment of choice in these cases, once the possible diagnosis of a bacterial infection has been excluded, although it is a priority to treat the underlying palpebral pathology in order to avoid recurrence. Blepharitis is difficult to cure, and usually persists throughout the patients lifetime with intermittent flare ups. Treatment consists of adequate daily palpebral hygiene with soaps or specific preparations for eyelid cleansing associated with the antibiotic ointments, erythromycin and bacitracin which have shown to be effective against *Staphylococcus aureus* when applied twice daily to the corneal surface.

Noninfectious Peripheral Corneal Ulcers

There are a series of systemic diseases where thinning and peripheral stromal necrosis can be associated with an epithelial defect that can lead, in severe cases, to perforation of the eye. Such examples include the collagen diseases, rheumatoid arthritis, Wegener´s granulomatosis, systemic lupus erythematosus, relapsing polychondritis, scleroderma and giant cell arteritis. The mechanisms behind the corneal ulceration are immune, mediated by immunocomplexes, although not identical in all examples as vasculitic processes also play an important role in the manifestation of ocular disease. Although less common, peripheral corneal ulceration has also been described in other diseases such as infections with hepatitis C virus, acute leukemia and lethal midline granuloma.[7-10]

Treatment of these ulcers basically involves the initial use of topical steroid, accompanied with lubricants, ocular occlusion and therapeutic contact lenses in order to aid wound re-epithelialization, however, therapeutic contact lenses should never be employed with steroids. Despite the poor predictability of conjunctival peritomy it can produce favorable results in some cases (probably due to the elimination of the source of inflammatory cells and chemical mediators that serve to maintain the inflammation), overweighing the later risk of losing an important extent of limbus. Other therapeutic options include the use of systemic immunosuppressive agents like cyclophosphamide or cyclosporin A. Either a rheumatologist, or another specialist familiar with this type of treatment, should always be consulted for a pretreatment evaluation in view of the potential side effects with cyclosporin A, such as myelosuppression, nephrotoxicity, or hepatotoxicity. Corneal lesions when associated with rheumatoid arthritis respond very well to cyclosporin at doses of 10-20 mg/kg/day in order to reach plasma levels of 100-400 ng/ml, later reducing gradually to a maintenance doses of 4-8 mg/kg/day.

Mooren´s Ulcer

Mooren´s ulcer is a peripheral noninfectious ulcerative keratitis. It is usually painless, follows a chronic course, and most probably has a immune origin (cellular reaction mediated by antibodies).

The clinical picture is of a peripheral corneal ulcer that extends both in a circumferential and centripetal manner, but rarely towards the sclera. It has an active margin that progresses, leaving behind areas of scarring with thinning, vascularization and opacification of the cornea, where the eye can perforate with minimal trauma.

Two types of Mooren´s ulcer have been described based on the clinical evolution. Type 1, the most frequent in our experience, is usually unilateral (75% of cases) and slow growing, with an acceptable response to conservative treatment. It is more common in older patients, with no differences between sexes, and is characterized by the moderate pain or indeed absence of pain experienced.

Type 2 appears in young, black male adults. Some of these patients have been found to be infected with the Hepatitis C virus, and have responded well to treatment with interferon-alpha, which is also used to treat the hepatitis associated with this infection. Type 2, in contrast to the Type 1, is usually bilateral (75%), evolves rapidly, and has a poor response to any kind of medical or surgical treatment.

There are many therapeutic options for the treatment of Mooren´s ulcer, none of which are totally effective. In view of the probable immune origin of this pathology, topical steroids are indicated, along with topical antibiotics and immunosuppressive agents such as cyclosporin A. Systemic immunosuppressive drugs are employed when topical treatment fails. Cyclosporin A is far more effective via systemic administration, despite the possible side effects which, nevertheless, are dose dependent and reversible once treatment has been stopped. In our experience we have obtained favorable results using 3-5 mg/kg/day of cyclosporin A in two divided doses.

Other more aggressive treatments include: limbal conjunctival peritomy, which can be repeated a number of times, and is indicated where no response to treatment has occurred after 4-5 days or if there is a risk of perforation; cryotherapy of the conjunctiva adjacent to the affected cornea (with similar results as with conjunctival excision); lamellar keratoplasty with the view to slowing the process and conserving visual acuity where possible, solving perforations, curing the ulcer in some cases, and avoiding recurrences; lastly phototherapeutic keratopathy of the central cornea with the excimer laser.[6-11]

Exposure Keratopathy

This pathology is included in this chapter on corneal ulcers as extensive ulceration can occur in some cases, which can even lead to perforation. However, it should be emphasized that in the majority of cases of exposure keratitis no worse than punctate epithelial defects are observed.[7]

Any condition that affects the correct functioning of the eyelids can result in an exposure keratopathy, more or less severe, depending on the causative pathology. Examples include ectropion of whatever cause, palpebral lesions, facial paralysis, lagophthalmous or proptosis.

The clinical picture is usually mild, with punctate, fluorescein positive lesions of the inferior third of the cornea. In more severe cases there is epithelial loss that can coalesce to form large areas of ulceration with stromal necrosis or perforation. The symptoms, although somewhat dependent on the extent of the lesions consist of photophobia, foreign-body sensation and excess tearing.

In mild cases treatment simply involves the administration of topical lubricants. Artificial tears are used as drops during the day, and as ointment during the night with occlusion if lagophthalmos or any other pathology that compromises nocturnal closure is present. In cases of facial paralysis either temporal or definitive tarsorrhaphy, or eyelid gold-weight implants should be considered.

NEUROTROPHIC KERATOPATHY

The diagnosis of neurotrophic keratopathy is made when any corneal lesion is produced from a partial or total, complete or incomplete dysfunction of the ophthalmic branch of the trigeminal nerve. There are many possible causes, however, the most important, listed in order of frequency are: Ophthalmic *Herpes zoster* (neurotrophic keratopathy complicating up to 25% of infections), *Herpes simplex*, surgical trauma of the trigeminal nerve, cerebrovascular accidents, aneurysms, multiple sclerosis and tumors, and also systemic diseases like diabetes mellitus, especially Type 1.[25,27,28,34,35] Sensorial hereditary neuropathy, an autosomal recessive disease, is another less frequent cause,[29,33] which consists of a selective reduction of the small myelinated nerve fibers, with or without the addition of an autonomic nervous system dysfunction.

Neurotrophic keratopathy presents with persistent epithelial defects in the more mild cases, mostly in a central or paracentral inferior location with elevated borders, that can lead to symptomless secondary stromal necrosis and perforation, due to diminished corneal sensitivity, in addition to loss of the lacrimonasal reflex and a decrease in tear film production.[26,30,31]

There is little difference in treatment from that of dry eye syndrome, with the use of topical lubricants in drop or ointment form, occlusions, and in some cases therapeutic contact lenses in order to repair the neurotrophic ulcers. Hyperosmotic agents are also used for their action in decreasing the edema at the edges of the lesion and favoring epithelialization;[29,32] and the amniotic membrane graft has been shown, based on previous experience with animals, to be indicated in specific cases. Lee and Tseng were the first to recommend the use of the amniotic membrane graft in the treatment of epithelial defects and corneal ulcers, and Kruse proposed the so called multilayered transplant in neurotrophic corneal ulcers. The amniotic tissue has an anti-inflammatory action regulating the production of mediators, such as interleukin 8 or gro-alpha,[6] it also allows for rapid epithelialization and produces a stable corneal surface in the long-term.[1-5] The possible treatment options are symptomatic only, since the underlying etiologies are untreatable. Tarsorrhaphy prevents large ulcerations, as in addition to occluding the cornea with the eyelid, it also avoids the evaporation of the tear film.[7,8]

Lamellar or penetrating keratoplasty have poor outcomes in these cases as epithelial reparation processes are affected and they are therefore used mainly to treat residual central scarring that interferes with the visual acuity of the patient.[7]

REFERENCES

1. Scheffer CG, Tseng et al. Amniotic membrane transplantation with or without limbal allografts for corneal surface reconstruction in patients with limbal stem cell deficiency. Arch Ophthalmol 1998;116: 431-41.
2. Jun Shimakazi, Hao-Yung Yang, Kazuo Tsubota. Amniotic membrane transplantation for ocular surface reconstruction in patients with chemical and thermal burns. Ophthalmol 1997; 104: 2068-76.
3. Shwu-Huey L, Scheffer CG. Amniotic membrane transplantation for persistent epithelial defects with ulceration. Am J Ophthalmol 1997; 123: 303-12.
4. Kruse MD, Klaus R, Hans EV. Multilayer amniotic membrane transplantation for reconstruction of deep corneal ulcers. Ophthalmol 1999; 106: 1504-11.
5. Augusto Azuara-Blanco, Pillai CT, Dua HS. Amniotic membrane transplantation for ocular surface reconstruction. Br J Ophthalmol 1999; 83: 399-402.
6. Grayson. Diseases of the cornea. Mosby Year-Book, 1997.
7. Basic and Clinical Science Course: American Academy of Ophthalmology. External Disease and Cornea 1995-1996.
8. Manual of Ocular Diagnosis and Therapy (4th ed). Deborah Pavan-Langston.
9. Rafael I Barraquer, et al. Imagenes Diagnosticas en Oftalmologia. Espax SA: Barcelona, 1998.

10. Tomas Marti Huguet. Signos clinicos en patologia de la Cornray de la Superficie Ocular. AlconCusi SA: Barcelona.
11. David J, Roger A, Paul A. Atlas of Clinical Ophthalmology (2nd ed). Mosby Year-Book Europe Limited, 1995.
12. Baum J. Diagnosing and treating bacterial corneal ulcers. Ophthalmol 1996; 103(3): 479-84.
13. Morlet N, Dart J. Routine antibiotic sensitivity testing for corneal ulcers. Arch Ophthalmol 1997; 115(4): 462-65.
14. Empirical or culture-guided therapy for microbial keratitis? A plea of data. Arch Ophthalmol 1996; 114(1): 84-87.
15. McLeod SD. The role of cultures in the management of ulcerative keratitis. Cornea 1997; 16(4): 383-86.
16. The importance of initial management in the treatment of severe infectious corneal ulcers. Ophthalmol 1995; 102(12): 1943-48.
17. Comparison of techniques for culturing corneal ulcers. Ophthalmol 1992; 99(5): 800-04.
18. Fluoroquinolones in the treatment of bacterial keratitis. Am J Ophthalmol 1996; 121(6): 712-15.
19. Limberg MB. A review of bacterial keratitis and bacterial conjunctivitis. Am J Ophthalmol 1991; 112(suppl 4): 2S-9S.
20. Pseudomonas keratitis and contact lens wear. The lens/eye is at fault. Cornea 1990; 9 (suppl 1): S36-8; S39-40.
21. Liesegang TJ. Contact lens-related microbial keratitis: Part I: Epidemiology. Cornea 1997; 16(2): 125-31.
22. Liesegang TJ. Contact lens-related microbial keratitis: Part II: (Pathophysiology). Cornea 1997; 16(3): 265-73.
23. Pineda R, Dohlman CH. Adjunctive therapy and surgical considerations in the management of bacterial ulcerative keratitis. Int Ophthalmol Clin 1996;36(3):37-48.
24. Clinical Ophthalmology—A Systematic Approach Butterworth-Heineman Ltd, 1994.
25. Johnson SM. Neurotrophic corneal defects after diode laser cycloablation. Am J Ophthalmol 1998; 126(5): 725-27.
26. Heigle TJ, Pflugfelder SC. Aqueous tear production in patients with neurotrophic keratitis. Cornea 1996; 15(2): 135-38.
27. Ocular manifestations of Lyme disease. Am J Med 1995; 98(4a): 60S-62S.
28. Neurotrophic keratitis presenting in infancy with involvement of the motor component of the trigeminal nerve. Br J Ophthalmol 1993; 77(10): 679-80.
29. Saini JS, Sharma A, Grewal SP. Chronic corneal perforations. Ophthalmic Surg 1992; 23(6): 399-402.
30. Treatment of persistent epithelial defects in neurotrophic keratitis with epidermal growth factor. A preliminary open study. Graefes Arch Clin Exp Ophthalmol 1992; 230(4): 314-17.
31. Cavanagh HD, Colley AM. The molecular basis of neurotrophic keratitis. Acta Ophthalmol 1989; 192: 115-34.
32. Management of noninfectious corneal ulcers. Surv Ophthalmol 1987; 32(2): 94-110.
33. Donaghy M, Hakin RN, Bamford JM, et al. Hereditary sensory neuropathy with neurotrophic keratitis. Description of an autosomal recessive disorder with a selective reduction of small myelinated nerve fibers and a discussion of hereditary sensory neuropathies. Brain 1987; 110(Pt3): 563-83.
34. Liesegang TJ. Corneal complications from Herpes zoster ophthalmicus. Ophthalmol 1985; 92(3): 316-24.
35. Hyndiuk RA, Kazarian EL, Schultz RO, et al. Neurotrophic corneal ulcers in diabetes mellitus. Arch Ophthalmol 1977; 95(12): 2193-96.

Chapter 13

Bacterial Keratitis and Management

Mary E Marquart (USA), Emma BH Hume (Australia), Xiadong Zheng (Japan), Armando Caballero, James M Hill, Richard J O'Callaghan (USA)

INTRODUCTION

Keratitis is an inflammatory disease of the cornea that can be infectious or non-infectious. Microbial keratitis is infectious keratitis that can be caused by a variety of microorganisms including bacteria, fungi, viruses, and parasites. Microbial keratitis is associated with hyperemia of the conjunctiva, pain, photophobia, corneal infiltration by white blood cells, a corneal epithelial break, and localized epithelial and stromal edema. *Pseudomonas, Staphylococcus,* and *Streptococcus* represent the largest percentage of species isolated from bacterial keratitis. A number of different cocci and bacilli—gram-negative or gram-positive, aerobic or anaerobic—can cause infections of the cornea. Species once thought not to cause keratitis are now emerging as corneal pathogens because of the wide use of general antibiotics and newer risk factors for bacterial keratitis such as contact lens wear. Bacterial infections of the cornea usually begin at the epithelial layer of the cornea and rapidly invade the stroma.

NORMAL FLORA OF THE EYE

The normal flora of the conjunctiva include *Staphylococcus epidermidis, Staphylococcus aureus, Micrococcus, Corynebacterium, Streptococcus*[1-6] and *Propionibacterium* species.[3,5,6] The antimicrobial action of tears[7] and the mechanical process of blinking maintain the resident bacteria at limited numbers in the tear film.[8] The evasion of host defense mechanisms by bacteria is an initial event in the development of keratitis.

NATURAL HOST DEFENSES

The body possesses mechanisms for safeguarding against eye infections. Eyelids and eyelashes are the first barriers that bacteria must pass to get into the eye.

The eye itself routinely washes away bacteria and other particles by producing tears and blinking. Tears also contain natural antimicrobial proteins such as lactoferrin, lysozyme, betalysins, vitronectin, cystatin S, lipocalin, complement, and lymphocytes. These proteins inhibit bacterial proliferation or attack and destroy bacteria. Secretory IgA and other immunoglobulins are also important in the inhibition of bacterial adhesion.[7,9-11] Natural antimicrobial peptides called defensins and phospholipase A have also been suggested to act against bacteria in the tears.[12]

Behind the tears, basal corneal cells are tightly bound by junctions preventing the invasion of bacteria while superficial wing cells are continually sloughed off, releasing those cells that may have bacteria attached. Bacteria such as *Pseudomonas aeruginosa* also have difficulty adhering to the cornea due to the glycocalyx of the corneal epithelial cells,[13] and a layer of mucin adds to the inhibitory effect of the glycocalyx.[7,14] Growth factors, cytokines, and chemokines produced by the corneal stroma help facilitate corneal wound healing and thus decrease its vulnerability to pathogens.[14]

RISK FACTORS

Factors that place one at a higher risk of corneal infection include local ocular dysfunctions, trauma to the eye (Fig. 13.1),[15-17] dry eye,[15] prolonged eyelid closure,[18] and preexisting viral eye infections (Fig. 13.2).[17,19-23] Dry eye problems can result in keratoconjunctivitis sicca, which is a keratoconjunctivitis that directly results from dry eye irritation, but dry eye can also make the eye susceptible to microbial keratitis. Defects in the eyelid such as ectropion (turning outward), entropion (turning inward),[17] cicatrical pemphigoid (conjunctival

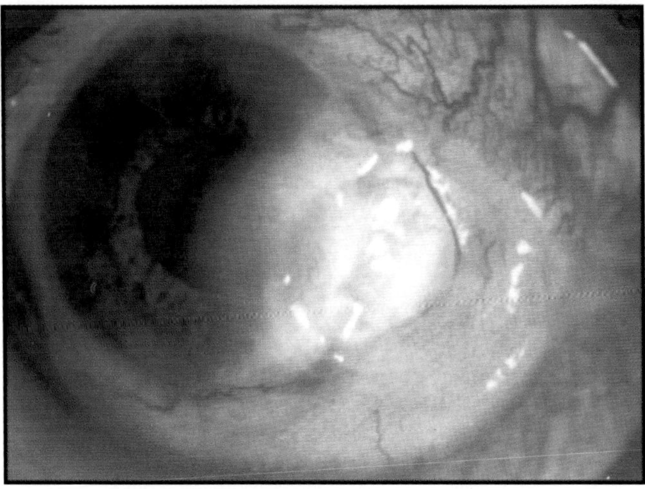

Fig. 13.1: *Bacillus* sclerokeratitis with trauma to the eye as a predisposing factor

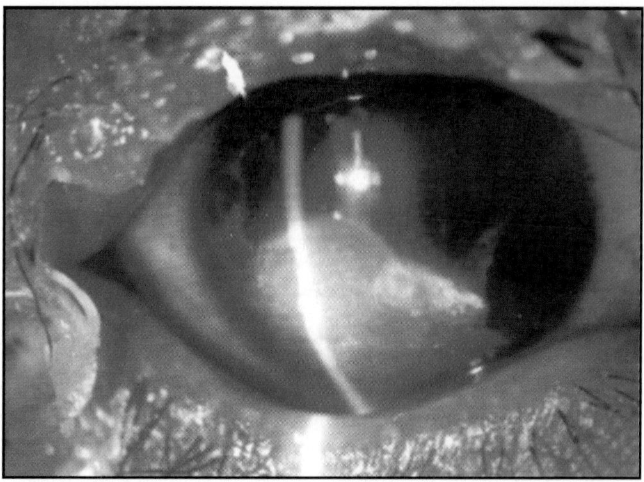

Fig. 13.2: *Moraxella* ulcer and lateral tarsorrhaphy in the inferior third of eye with lagopthalmos and herpes zoster ophthalmicus as predisposing factors

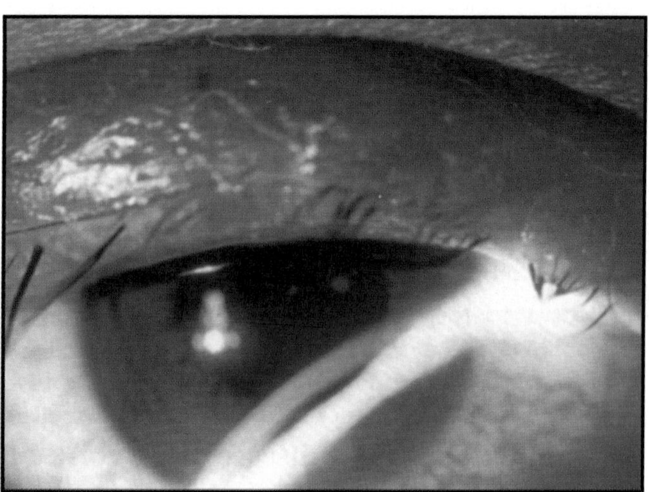

Fig. 13.3: Ulcerative blepharitis. The eyelid is edematous and eyelashes have been shed. Note the limbal infiltrates at lower right

blisters), blepharitis (inflammation) (Fig. 13.3)[16,24] and meibomianitis (sebaceous gland inflammation) (Fig. 13.4) [24,25] can also increase corneal vulnerability to bacterial infection. Trichiasis, or the turning inward of the eyelashes, is often a problem associated with entropion, and abrasion of the cornea by the eyelashes can cause infection. Inflammation of the lacrimal gland, or dacryocystitis, is also a common risk factor (Fig. 13.5).

Local ocular conditions are not the only possible risk factors for bacterial keratitis. Systemic conditions such as HIV/AIDS,[26-28] diabetes,[16,17,29]

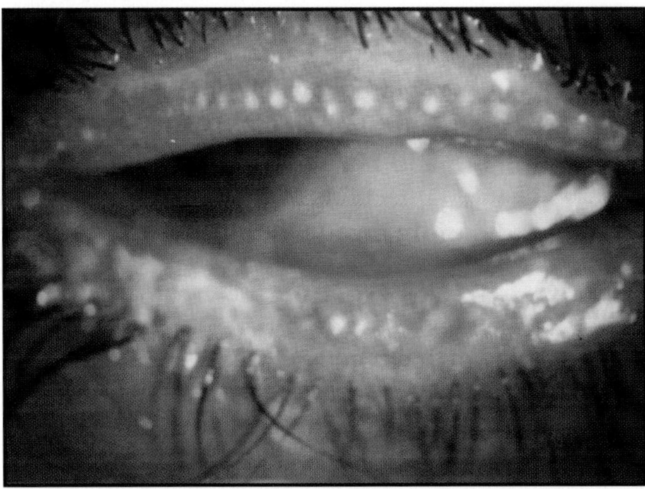

Fig. 13.4: Severe meibomianitis. Inflammation of the meibomian orifices can be seen

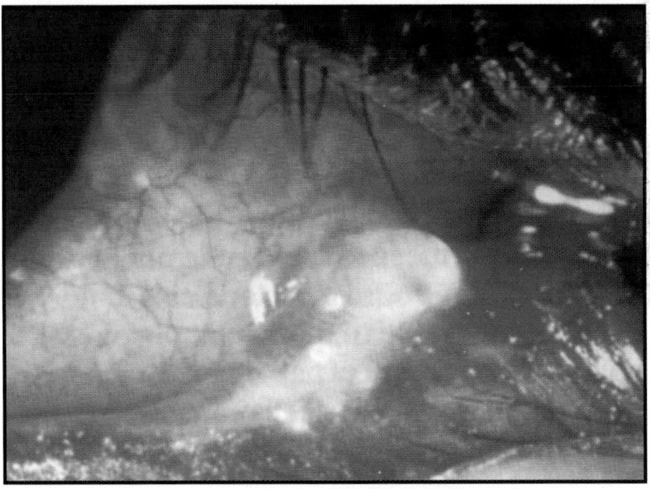

Fig. 13.5: Dacryocystitis. The lower punctum produces purulent discharge with pressure

malnutrition,[30,31] and alcoholism,[30,31] can increase susceptibility to bacterial keratitis (Table 13.1). Mucosal scarring or lesion disorders like Stevens-Johnson syndrome (erythema multiforme) and Sjögren's syndrome will predispose patients to eye infections.[20,25] Certain risk factors, such as old age and previous ocular surgery, complicate cases of bacterial keratitis and thus promote the need for more radical interventions (e.g. penetrating keratoplasty).[32] Ocular surgeries, including radial keratotomy (Figs 13.6 and 13.7), penetrating keratoplasty (Fig. 13.8), and laser *in situ* keratomileusis (LASIK), can also be risk factors for keratitis.[16,17,33-44]

Table 13.1: Susceptibility factors for bacterial keratitis

Type	*Examples*
Local ocular factors	
Trauma or corneal disease	Foreign bodies[16,17]
	Edema[15,24]
	Epithelial erosions[36]
	Abrasions[45]
	Exposure[20,29]
	Bullous keratopathy[20,23,31,46,47]
	Previous or preexisting eye infection (e.g., *Herpes simplex* virus keratitis)[17,19-23]
Abnormal tear function	Dry eye (sicca)[15,17,22,23]
	Dacryocystitis (lacrimal inflammation)[25,48]
Abnormal lid function	Blepharitis (inflammation)[16,24]
	Cicatrical pemphigoid (blisters)[25]
	Entropion or ectropion (turning in or out)[17]
	Lagophthalmos (incomplete eyelid closure)[24,25]
	Meibomianitis (sebaceous inflammation)[24,25]
	Trichiasis (lashes turned in)[17,25]
Cosmetic	Contact lens wear[16,17,22,23,49]
	Cosmetic eye makeup[50]
Drugs and treatments	Topical corticosteroids[17,19,21,25,35,36,47]
	Bandage contact lens wear[25,47,51]
	Ocular surgery/surgical sutures[17,20,22,23,25,33-44]
	Cyanoacrylate adhesive (alternative to sutures)[52]
Systemic factors	
Drugs and treatments	Systemic immunosuppression treatment[25,53]
Systemic conditions	Alcoholism[30,31]
	Body burns[53]
	Coma[54]
	Diabetes[16,17,22,29]
	AIDS[26-28]
	Malnutrition[30,31]
	Cancer[29]
	Rheumatoid arthritis[24]
	Sjögren's syndrome[20,25]
	Stevens-Johnson syndrome (erythema multiforme)[20,25]

Contact Lens Use

Contact lens wear has become the most common risk factor leading to bacterial keratitis.[49] Ulcerative keratitis, the most serious complication of bacterial keratitis, is 80 times more likely to occur in infections following contact lens wear than in non-contact lens wear.[55] In contact lens-associated microbial keratitis, use of extended wear lenses accounts for 79 percent of the keratitis cases.[56] The likelihood of developing ulcerative keratitis with overnight wearing

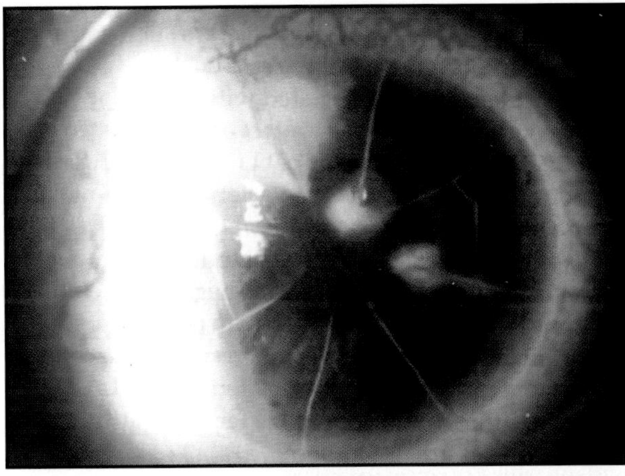

Fig. 13.6: Multifocal *Streptococcus pneu-moniae* keratitis one day after radial keratotomy

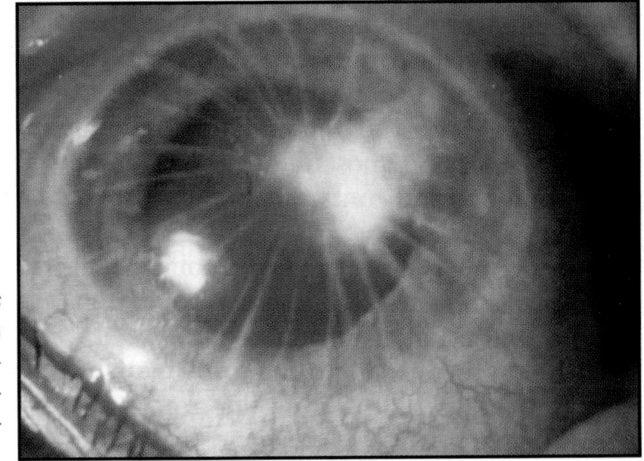

Fig. 13.7: *Staphylococcus epidermidis* keratitis ten years after radial keratotomy. No other predisposing factor was apparent

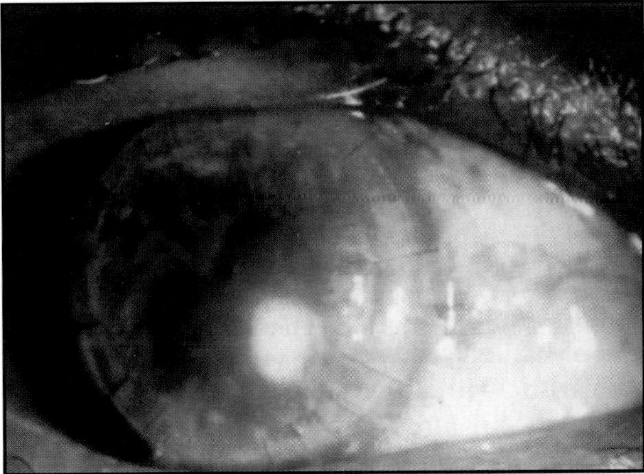

Fig. 13.8: Alpha-hemolytic (Viridans group) *Streptococcus* graft infiltrate after penetrating keratoplasty (PKP)

of lenses is 8-15 times higher than the daily wear of contact lenses.[57,58] The lowest incidence of keratitis with contact lenses involves the use of rigid gas permeable lenses.[59]

Prolonged wearing of contact lenses reduces the thickness of the epithelium and stroma and impedes oxygen uptake by epithelial cells. Contact lenses also induce epithelial microcysts and cause endothelial cell polymegathism (cells of various sizes).[60] The reduction in oxygen uptake by epithelial cells can compromise the epithelium and leave it more susceptible to infection.[60] The negative effects that contact lenses have on the eye have been well described:

Contact lens use compromises multiple specific functions of the tear film. Such compromised tear functions could include the flushing action, preventing desiccation of the tissue, lubricating ocular surfaces, serving as a vehicle for oxygen and carbon dioxide, and providing a soluble defense against infection.[61]

Contact lenses can cause epithelial defect, a major predisposing event leading to bacterial keratitis.[62] *P. aeruginosa* has been repeatedly reported to be the most common pathogen implicated in contact lens-related keratitis,[16,17,62-69] however, a wide range of other gram-negative bacterial species such as *Serratia* and *Haemophilus*,[68,70,71] as well as some gram-positive bacterial species such as *Staphylococcus aureus*[56,68,72,73] and *Streptococcus pneumoniae*,[68,74] have caused contact lens-associated keratitis.

There have been contradictory findings regarding the effect of contact lens wear on the normal flora of the eye. There have been reports that the use of contact lenses does not alter the normal microbial flora,[75,76] that it reduces the normal flora,[77] and that it increases the normal flora with both rigid gas permeable and soft contact lenses.[5,8,78] Hart *et al*[79] and Sankaridurg *et al*[74] found that the majority of lens contamination was due to *Staphylococcus epidermidis,* which is considered to be an organism of the normal conjunctival flora. Lens contamination was associated with a statistically significant increase in colony forming units per lens in extended lens wearers as compared to daily wearers.[79] Potentially pathogenic bacteria have also been found to be reduced in contact lens wear in some reports,[77] unchanged,[78] and increased in others[5,74,80] Høvding[81] reported that contact lens wear changed the spectrum of microorganisms, with a decrease in gram-positive bacteria and an increase in numbers of gram-negative species. Stapleton *et al*[8] found an increase in the amount of pathogenic organisms in the overnight use of contact lenses as compared to the daily wear of contact lenses. Overnight use of contact lenses was hypothesized to only temporarily increase the numbers of pathogenic organisms associated with the cornea.[8] Variations in the findings of these studies could be due to different lens types studied, length of lens wear, and the disinfection regimes used by the lens wearer, or perhaps less obvious factors such as climate differences that could affect the results.

Contact lens use is associated with an ocular inflammatory condition known as contact lens-associated acute red eye (CLARE). The eyes of patients with

CLARE have been found to harbor any of a variety of gram-negative bacteria such as *Pseudomonas, Serratia*, or *Klebsiella*, but can also harbor gram-positive bacteria such as *Staphylococcus* and *Pneumococcus*.[74] Gram-negative bacteria are eight times more likely to be present in the eyes of CLARE patients than in the eyes of normal contact lens wearers.[1] The pathogenic processes associated with CLARE and how they differ from those of bacterial keratitis caused by these species are not known.

The source of bacterial contamination of contact lenses has not been elucidated. Hygiene regimen is a possible source of corneal contamination.[67,82,83] Contact lens solutions (preserved and unpreserved) have been found to be contaminated with bacteria.[84-88] *P. aeruginosa* has been cultured from the cornea and in unpreserved homemade saline solutions in patients with contact lens related corneal ulcers.[89] Mayo *et al*[90] reported that contamination by *S. marcescens* occurred most frequently in commercially prepared solutions and contamination by *P. aeruginosa* in homemade saline.

Another organism associated with contact lens use is *Serratia. S. marcescens* and *S. liquefaciens* have been found to persist in a variety of disinfecting solutions.[91] *S. marcescens* has the ability to adapt to and grow in disinfecting solutions containing chlorhexidine that are used for rigid gas permeable lenses.[92-94] Marrie and Costerton[95] also found that *S. marcescens* could survive in chlorhexidine handwashes in concentrations up to 20 mg/mL (2.0%). This concentration of chlorhexidine is much higher than in lens disinfecting solutions. *S. marcescens* is also more resistant to lens disinfectants than both *P. aeruginosa* and *Staphylococcus epidermidis*.[96] In a more recent study with newer disinfecting solutions, *S. marcescens* was killed after six hours in the majority of solutions.[97] One strain of the bacterium was used in this study, therefore the results may not be indicative of the efficacy of lens solutions against all strains of *S. marcescens*.

Contact lens cases have also been found to be a favorable environment for bacterial contamination.[98-100] *S. marcescens* was cultured from 31 percent of storage cases in one study,[101] and appears to thrive in cases where preserved solutions are used. The percentage of *S. marcescens* isolates found in contact lens cases in which preserved solutions had been used was 34 percent, while the percentage in cases that had previously contained preservative-free solutions was only 10 percent.[102] Moreover, 84 percent of contact lens cases that had contained disinfectants but had not been dried were culture-positive for *S. marcescens*.[96] Patients with CLARE caused by *Pseudomonas aeruginosa, Serratia liquefaciens*, and *Aeromonas hydrophila* also had contact lens cases that grew the same organisms.[103] Use of disposable contact lenses avoids the need for storage cases and lens storage solutions, but lessening contact with cases and solutions does not guarantee protection from bacterial infection. In fact, two studies found that disposable lenses had the highest risk of microbial keratitis relative to all types of contact lenses.[104,105] Several other cases of bacterial keratitis related to disposable contact lens wear have been summarized by John.[106]

Body sites, in particular the fingertips, are more likely to be a source of contamination as they are used to manipulate contact lenses. The ability of bacteria to persist on the hands is a concern for contact lens wearers. Finger and hand contamination in hospital infections is well known.[107-110] Studies have shown that handling of contact lenses is a predominant source of lens contamination.[111,112] However, these studies have not typed the strains and therefore have not proven that the same bacteria on the fingers were the same strains as those on the lens.

Other potential body sites that could cause contamination of contact lenses include the throat, ears and nose. An example of contamination by these means is *Haemophilus influenzae,* an organism that colonizes the nasopharynx of the asymptomatic population and from this site contaminates contact lenses.[113] One of the most common environmental sources of bacteria that contaminates contact lenses is tap water (from showering or washing). Tap water can contribute highly pathogenic bacteria such as *S. marcescens, S. liquefaciens, P. aeruginosa, Aeromonas hydrophilia,* or *Stenotrophomonas maltophilia*. These species of bacteria have been implicated in ocular infection associated with contact lens wear and can be found in contaminated water supplies.[114-118]

EPIDEMIOLOGY

Bacterial keratitis is an important health problem because it can cause significant and often irreversible damage to the cornea, resulting in decreased vision or blindness. Bacterial corneal infections are not limited to any one particular group of people. They occur worldwide and in all groups, regardless of age, ethnicity, status, or sex. Table 13.2 lists the species of bacteria responsible for keratitis in various geographic locations. The three most common bacteria isolated from infected corneas in each study are listed as a percentage of the total cases of microbial (including fungal and parasitic) keratitis. Climate has been suggested to influence the species of bacteria most commonly responsible for keratitis,[119] however, *Staphylococcus, Streptococcus,* and *Pseudomonas* species are the most frequently isolated organisms in cases of bacterial keratitis all over the world (Table 13.2).

In summary, bacterial keratitis appears to have the ability to occur in anyone, and no particular climate or geographical location can assure protection from this disease. The human eye naturally harbors some bacterial species, and has defense mechanisms that protect it from overproliferation of the normal flora or infection by pathogens introduced to the eye. Any change in the condition of the corneal epithelium, and many systemic conditions, can cause the eye to become vulnerable to potentially hazardous pathogenic microbes.

FREQUENT CAUSES OF BACTERIAL KERATITIS

A variety of bacterial species have been shown to cause keratitis (Table 13.3), however the majority of bacterial keratitis incidences are caused by

Table 13.2: Geographic distribution of bacterial keratitis isolates

Country	*Bacterium*	*Incidence**	*Reference(s)*
Africa			
Soweto, S. Africa	Coagulase-negative staphylococci	32%	120
	Staphylococcus aureus	29%	
	Streptococcus pneumoniae	16%	
Australia			
Adelaide, SA	*S. aureus*	23%	20
	Staphylococcus epidermidis	14%	
	Pseudomonas aeruginosa	10%	
Perth, WA	*Staphylococcus* sp.	42%	23
	Pseudomonas sp.	12%	
	not provided		
Sydney, NSW	*S. epidermidis*	23%	22
	Corynebacterium sp.	20%	
	S. aureus	15%	
Bangladesh	*S. pneumoniae*	17[a]-20[b]%	[a]121; [b]122
	P. aeruginosa	12[b]-13[a]%	
	S. epidermidis	12[b]%	
Ghana	*P. aeruginosa*	13%	123
	S. epidermidis	11%	
	S. pneumoniae	6%	
India			
Hyderabad			
Children	*S. epidermidis*	23%	124
	S. aureus	20%	
	S. pneumoniae	15%	
Adults	*S. pneumoniae*	35%	48
	S. epidermidis	17%	
	Pseudomonas sp.	13%	
Madurai	*S. pneumoniae*	25%	125
	Pseudomonas sp.	8%	
	Corynebacterium xerosis	7%	
Kuwait	*S. epidermidis*	64%	126
	S. aureus	12%	
	Pseudomonas sp.	7%	
Nepal	*S. pneumoniae*	31%	127
	Corynebacterium xerosis	12%	
	S. epidermidis	11%	
Singapore	*P. aeruginosa*	59%	16
	S. pneumoniae	8%	
	S. aureus, Klebsiella, and coagulase-negative staphylococci	4% each	
Sri Lanka	*S. pneumoniae* and *P. aeruginosa*	3% each	128
	unidentified beta-hemolytic coccus	2%	
	not provided		
Taiwan (Taipei)	*P. aeruginosa*	33%	17
	coagulase-negative staphylococci	18%	
	Acinetobacter sp.	7%	

contd..

Table 13.2 contd..

Country	*Bacterium*	*Incidence**	*Reference(s)*
United States			
Atlanta, GA	*P. aeruginosa*	39%	129
	Streptococcus sp.	16%	
	Staphylococcus sp.	14%	
Baltimore, MD	*S. epidermidis*	28[a]-47[b]%	[a]130; [b]131
	P. aeruginosa	16[a]-21[b]%	
	S. aureus	13[b]-16[a]%	
Boston, MA	*S. aureus*	27%	132
	coagulase-negative staphylococci, diphtheroids, and *P. aeruginosa*	14% each	
	S. pneumoniae	12%	
Los Angeles, CA	Coagulase-negative staphylococci	29%	46
	S. aureus	22%	
	P. aeruginosa	19%	
Miami, FL	*P. aeruginosa*	31[a]-34[b]%	[a]133; [b]134
	S. aureus	21%[a,b]	
	S. epidermidis or *S. pneumoniae*	8%[a]/17%[b]	
New York City, NY	*Staphylococcus* sp.	48%	30
	Moraxella sp.	16%	
	P. aeruginosa and *S. pneumoniae*	8% each	
Philadelphia, PA	*S. epidermidis*	31%	135
	Streptococcus viridans	15%	
	S. pneumoniae, Bacillus sp. *Haemophilus aegyptius,* and *Haemophilus influenzae*	8% each	
Pittsburgh, PA	*Staphylococcus* sp. other than *S. aureus*	37%	136
	S. aureus	24%	
	Streptococcus sp.	11%	

Incidence indicates the percentage of microbial keratitis patients from whom that particular bacterium was isolated of the total number of patients who had microbial keratitis, including fungal keratitis.

Staphylococcus aureus, Streptococcus pneumoniae (pneumococcus), and *Pseudomonas aeruginosa.* Enterobacteria comprise the fourth most common bacteria that cause keratitis, and of this group, *Serratia marcescens* is probably the most frequently isolated pathogen because it is a common etiologic agent of contact lens-related bacterial keratitis.[53]

Staphylococcus Aureus

Corneal infection by *Staphylococcus aureus* is a major cause of bacterial keratitis in children and adults in India[124,172] and the United States.[134,135,172] *Staphylococcus aureus* corneal infections occur primarily in patients with defects in their ocular immunity and contact lens wearers.[208-210] *Staphylococcus* is a gram-positive bacterium that populates the normal flora of the skin and nasopharynx, and in low numbers can be cultured from the tear film of normal

Table 13.3: Bacteria that cause keratitis

Gram stain identification and morphology	*Bacterium*
Gram-positive coccus	*Enterococcus faecalis*[123]
	Micrococcus[27,137]
	Peptococcus[45,138]
	Peptostreptococcus[20,139]
	Staphylococcus
	S. aureus[20,22,36,137]
	S. epidermidis[19,20,36,123,137]
	S. hemolyticus[36]
	S. warneri[135]
	Streptococcus
	S. faecalis[120]
	S. mitis[22,32,135,140]
	S. mutans[34]
	S. pneumoniae (pneumococcus)[15,20,22,135,137,141]
	S. pyogenes[36,137]
	S. sanguis[32,142]
	S. viridans[15,36,72,135,143-148]
Gram-positive bacillus	*Bacillus*[36,120,134,135,137,149]
	Clostridium perfringens[33]
	Corynebacterium
	C. diphtheriae[150]
	C. hofmannii[137]
	C. pyogenes[137]
	C. striatus[137,151]
	C. xerosis[137,152]
	Listeria monocytogenes[153,154]
	Mycobacterium
	M. asiaticum[155]
	M. avium-intracellulare[155,156]
	M. chelonae[19,43,137,157-161]
	M. flavescens[162]
	M. fortuitum[137,159,163-165]
	M. gordonae[166]
	M. leprae[167,168]
	M. marinum[169,170]
	M. nonchromogenicum[155]
	M. smegmatis[159]
	M. triviale[155]
	Propionibacterium acnes[32,36,45,137,171]
Gram-negative coccus	*Veillonella*[172]
Gram-negative bacillus	*Acinetobacter calcoaceticus-A. baumannii*[25,29,137]
	Alcaligenes xylosoxidans[173,174]
	Azotobacter[53,172,175]
	Bacteroides[172,176,177]
	Capnocytophaga[26-28,178-180]
	Eikenella corrodens[46,181]

contd..

Table 13.3 contd..

Gram stain identification and morphology	*Bacterium*
	Enterobacteria
	Aeromonas hydrophila[120,137]
	Citrobacter[46,182]
	Enterobacter
	E. aerogenes[182]
	E. cloacae[19,123]
	Erwinia[172,183]
	Escherichia coli[46,121,137]
	Klebsiella
	K. pneumoniae[21,137,184]
	K. oxytoca[19,20]
	Morganella morganii[22]
	Proteus mirabilis[16,19,20,68,120]
	Salmonella[185-188]
	Serratia
	S. liquefaciens[174]
	S. marcescens[19,20,22,174]
	Shigella
	S. flexneri[120,189]
	S. sonnei[190]
	Flavobacterium
	F. indologenes[191]
	F. meningosepticum[192]
	Fusobacterium[172]
	Pseudomonas aeruginosa[16,20-22,46,67,120,123,131,135,137,193,194]
	Stenotrophomonas maltophilia[70,182,195]
	Vibrio
	V. metschnikovii[123]
	V. vulnificus[196,197]
Gram-negative coccobacillus	*Haemophilus*
	H. aegyptius[135]
	H. haemoglobinophilus[137]
	H. influenzae[20,22,46,52,68,120,123,134,135,137]
	H. parainfluenzae[25]
Gram-negative diplococcus	*Neisseria*[22,120,123,137]
Gram-negative diplobacillus	*Moraxella*
	M. catarrhalis[30,31]
	M. lacunata[24,134,137,198]
	M. nonliquefaciens[198]
Gram-positive filamentous	*Actinomyces*[22,45]
	Nocardia
	N. asteroides[22,44,137,199]
	N. caviae[137,200]
Spirochetes	*Borrelia*[135,201-205]
	Leptospira[206]
	Treponema[172,207]

eyes. *S. aureus* can cause infections when epithelial cells are compromised (Figs 13.9A to and 13.10). Keratitis caused by *Staphylococcus* can result in corneal edema, rapid loss of the corneal epithelium, and the infiltration of neutrophils at the infection site and in the tear film. Those pathologic effects have been attributed to the toxicity of *S. aureus* alpha-toxin,[211] a cytolytic exoprotein produced by about 75 percent of *S. aureus* strains.[212-216] Bacterial mutants deficient in alpha-toxin have been shown to cause significantly less corneal erosion, iritis, and inflammation than their wild type parent strains.[212;213] Purified alpha-toxin injected into the stroma induces iritis, corneal erosion,

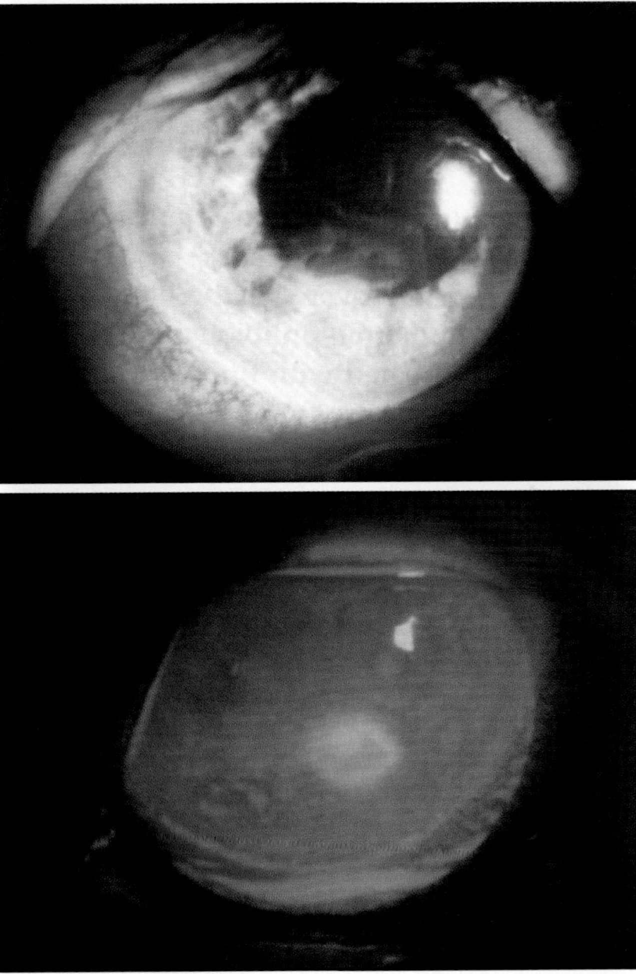

Figs 13.9A and B: *Staphylococcus aureus* paracentral corneal ulcer without (A) and with (B) fluorescein staining

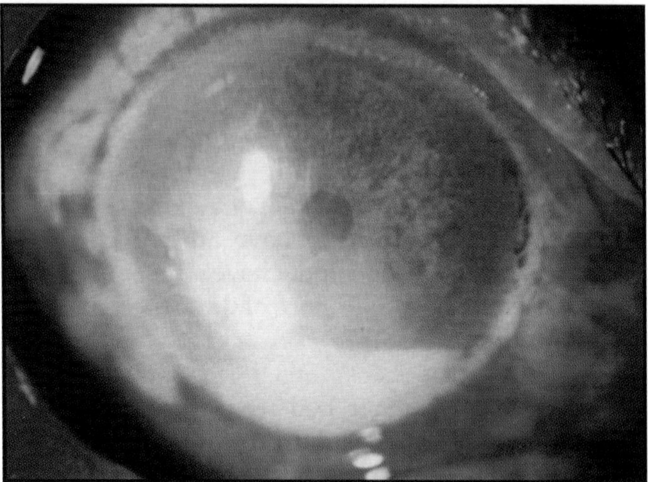

Fig. 13.10: Hypopyon and ulcer caused by *Staphylococcus aureus* keratitis

and inflammation within three hours.[213] Purified alpha-toxin has also been shown to mediate cell death in rabbit corneas by necrosis and apoptosis and to induce corneal epithelial sloughing and edema.[217] Inactivation of alpha-toxin by heat eliminates its pathological effects in the rabbit eye demonstrating that the toxin is important for virulence.[213] Other proteins include beta-toxin and gamma-toxin, which are involved in virulence to a lesser extent than alpha-toxin,[213,218] and protein A and coagulase, which do not contribute to corneal virulence in a rabbit model of infection.[211,212] Some of major virulence factors are represented in Table 13.4.

Strains of methicillin-resistant *S. aureus* (MRSA) are significant nosocomial pathogens.[219-221] These MRSA strains, which were discovered in the 1960s, were found to be resistant to numerous antibiotics.[219] MRSA strains were successfully treated with fluoroquinolones when the fluoroquinolones were first introduced in the early 1980s. Now these dangerous hospital-acquired strains are resistant to the fluoroquinolones,[219,220,222-227] as are *S. aureus* strains as a whole.[136] MRSA strains are also showing resistance to vancomycin,[228-231] which has been a successful alternative to the fluoroquinolones.[220,232-240]

Pseudomonas Aeruginosa

Pseudomonas aeruginosa is a ubiquitous gram-negative, aerobic rod. *Pseudomonas* can also conduct anaerobic respiration using a variety of nitrogen compounds as the final electron acceptor. Cultures of *Pseudomonas* are recognized by their characteristic grape-like odor, and by their distinctive coloration, which result from the production of at least 4 types of pigments, of which pyocyanin is the most commonly described.[249] Most strains are motile, exhibiting a single polar

Table 13.4: Major virulence factors

Bacterium	*Virulence factor*	*Function*
Staphylococcus aureus[211-213,218,241,242]	alpha-toxin	cytotoxicity, inflammation
	beta-toxin	inflammation
	gamma-toxin	inflammation
Pseudomonas aeruginosa[53,211,243-247]	alkaline protease	metalloproteases; degrades host gamma-interferon
	capsule	adherence, protection
	cytotoxin	pore formation
	elastase	metalloprotease
	elastase A	metalloprotease
	elastase D	unknown
	exoenzyme S	cytotoxicity
	exoenzyme T	phagocytosis inhibitor
	exoenzyme U	cytotoxicity
	exotoxin A	inhibits protein synthesis in human cells
	flagella	motility
	pili	adherence
	lipopolysaccharide (LPS)	endotoxicity
	phospholipase C	degrades host cell membrane
	protease IV	serine protease
Streptococcus pneumoniae[248]	autolysin	releases pneumolysin
	capsule	survival in the host
	cell wall polysaccharide	attachment and
	pneumococcal surface	inflammation
	protein A (PspA)	unknown
	pneumolysin	cytotoxicity

flagellum, and can also produce pili of the type IV variety, which contain N-methyl-phenylalanine.[250] This organism is very tough, being resistant to many chemical agents, and can also grow well at 42°C.[249]

Pseudomonas aeruginosa is an opportunistic human pathogen that infects patients with burns, cystic fibrosis, urinary tract infections, pneumonia, skin infections, cancer, and acquired immunodeficiency syndrome.[249,251-260] *P. aeruginosa* is also the leading cause of contact lens-associated bacterial keratitis.[16,49,53] The incidence of bacterial keratitis among this otherwise healthy population is estimated to be 21 cases per 10,000 users of extended wear soft contact lenses.[261,262] Prolonged eyelid closure associated with contact lens wear increases the risk for *Pseudomonas* keratitis due to hypoxia and the ability of *Pseudomonas* to adhere to contact lenses.[18] Corneal infections with this pathogen are often devastating and can cause very large ulcers (Figs 13.11 to 13.13) leading to corneal perforation, scleral suppuration, and phthisis bulbi.[53,172,258,263-265]

Pseudomonas produces multiple potential virulence factors, including flagella, pili, alginate capsular material, lipopolysaccharide (LPS), several phospholipases, multiple proteases, ribosylating toxins, cytotoxic proteins, and

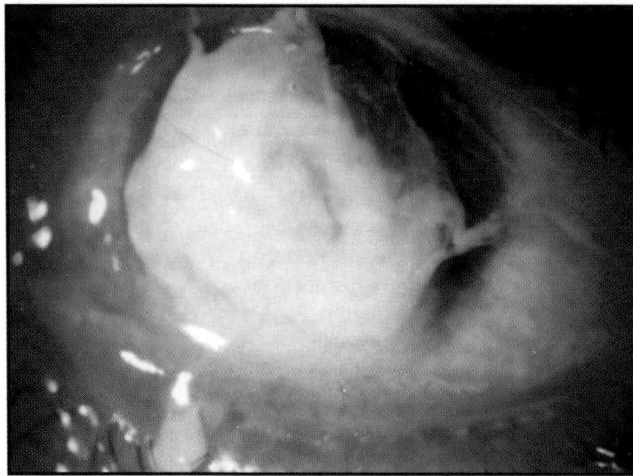

Fig. 13.11: *Pseudomonas aeruginosa* keratitis with copious green purulent discharge

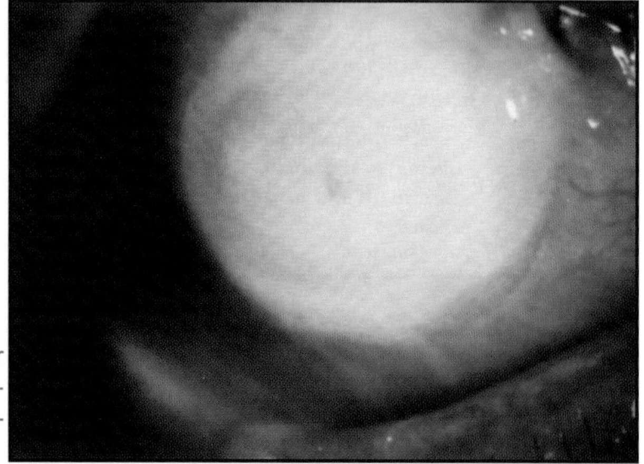

Fig. 13.12: Corneal ulcer and central corneal thinning caused by *Pseudomonas aeruginosa*

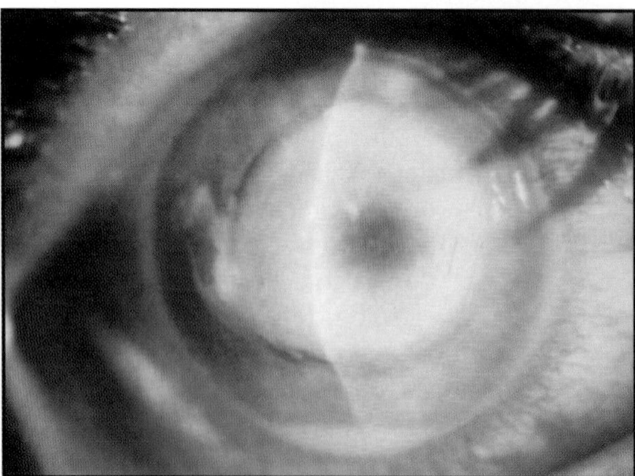

Fig. 13.13: Hypopyon and ring infiltrates caused by *Pseudomonas aeruginosa*

proteins for invasiveness (Table 13.4). The role of any specific factor in keratitis is difficult to determine. The factors that seem to be important in these *Pseudomonas* infections include adherence to contact lenses followed by transfer and adherence to the cornea, invasiveness, cytotoxicity, protease activity, and the immune response to the organism.

Pseudomonas has been shown capable of binding to the inert surface of contact lenses.[266-273] Adherence of *Pseudomonas* to corneal epithelial cells seems to involve a loose binding of bacteria by flagella and pili and then a more intimate binding by LPS or other mechanisms.[274-281] *Pseudomonas* binding to epithelial cells is inhibited by host mucus.[13]

The next event in infection involves the movement of bacteria through the epithelium to the corneal stroma, a process that is not fully understood. *Pseudomonas* can invade the basolateral surface of epithelial cells in a process that is mediated by genes of the exoenzyme S operon. The invasive strains inject exoenzyme S (exo S) into the cell and thus induce the cell to phagocytize the bacteria. Once intracellular, the invasive strain can replicate for hours.[269,282-284] Genes in this same operon code for two proteins (Exo U and Exo T) that cause cellular cytotoxicity. These proteins, like exo S, are thought to be delivered to target cells by a micro-injection process designated as type III secretion.[283-288] About half of the strains analyzed can be shown in culture to have an active invasive mechanism, while the remainder have an active cytotoxic activity. The relative importance of these mechanisms to keratitis is not yet resolved.

Once in the corneal stroma *Pseudomonas* mediates extensive corneal damage that seems to correlate with the production of extracellular proteases. Alkaline protease, the elastases and protease IV have been shown to degrade components of the complement system, cytokines, IgG, and IgA *in vitro*. Furthermore, *in vivo* experiments have shown that injection of these proteases into the cornea produces significant pathology.[246,289-302] Recent work with mutants, however, seems to minimize the role of elastase and alkaline protease as major ocular virulence factors, although they may still be responsible for some of the corneal damage once the infection is established (Dr. Jeff Hobden, personal communication).[303] Protease IV, on the other hand, could play an important role in the initiation and maintenance of the infection, and could possibly be responsible for the corneal damage seen in *Pseudomonas* keratitis.[301,302,304,305] Proof of protease IV as the major virulence factor, however, has yet to be obtained.

Finally, damage to the cornea as a result of *Pseudomonas* infection can also result from activation of host derived products, such as those associated with PMN infiltration (Fig. 13.13) and corneal matrix metalloproteinases, which have been shown to degrade collagen in the cornea.[306]

Streptococcus Pneumoniae

The most frequent streptococcal species involved in bacterial keratitis is *Streptococcus pneumoniae*, or *pneumococcus*. *S. pneumoniae* is a typical upper respiratory tract pathogen, but can be a very harmful corneal pathogen, causing severe corneal ulcers (Figs 13.6, 13.14, and 13.15). Corneal scarring and decreased visual acuity[34] or loss of the eye[46,307] can result from pneumococcus keratitis. Recent observations of an increase in penicillin-resistant *S. pneumoniae*, in addition to its resistance to many other drugs, have heightened concern regarding this pathogen.[141,308] *Pneumococcus* is also a common cause of infectious crystalline keratopathy, a keratitis that presents crystal-like infiltrates in the cornea.[36,182,309]

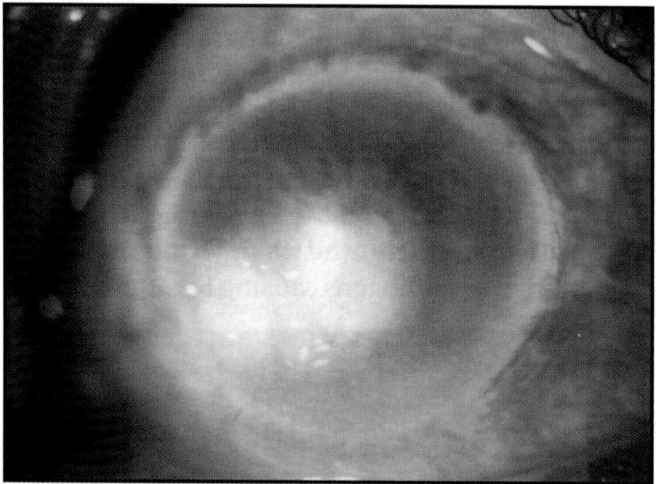

Fig. 13.14: *Streptococcus pneumoniae* ulcers with spheroidal degeneration

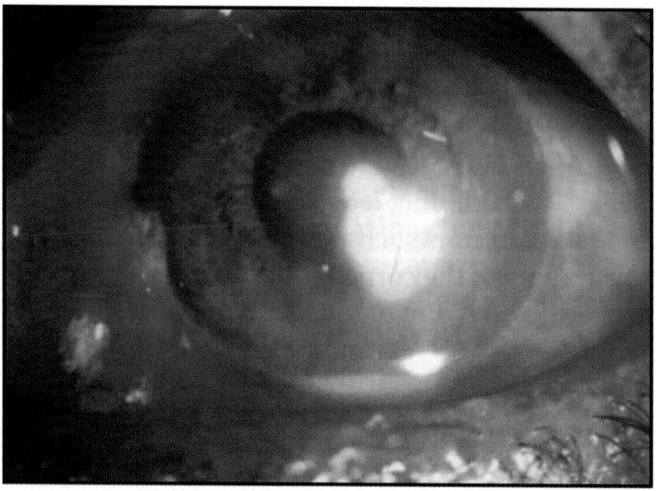

Fig. 13.15: *Streptococcus pneumoniae* keratitis ulcer and hypopyon

Corneal virulence of *Pneumococcus* has been correlated with pneumolysin (Table 13.4).[248] Pneumolysin's corneal virulence relates to its complement activating domain and not to its lytic domain. Pneumolysin is released not by secretion, but by another pneumococcal protein, autolysin.[248] Pneumococcal surface protein A (PspA) is also an important virulence factor, but its precise mechanism of action is not clear. Alonso deVelasco and colleagues[248] suggest that one of PspA's functions is inhibition of complement activation.

S. pneumoniae is not commonly isolated as the causative agent of contact lens-associated bacterial keratitis, but does have the ability to infiltrate the corneas of contact lens wearers and cause an inflammation reaction called contact lens-associated acute red eye (CLARE).[74] CLARE cases rarely need antibiotic treatment to resolve.[74] A predisposing factor that has been correlated with pneumococcal keratitis is dacryocystitis, a condition in which the lacrimal sac is inflamed or infected and prevents the drainage of tears (Fig. 13.5).[48] If *S. pneumoniae* is the organism infecting the lacrimal sac, it can spread to the cornea and cause keratitis, especially if the cornea has been traumatized.[48] *Pneumococcus* keratitis appears to be decreasing as *Pseudomonas* keratitis is increasing, but *S. pneumoniae* remains a significant etiologic agent in keratitis in Bangladesh,[121] India,[48,124,125] and Nepal.[127]

Serratia Marcescens

Serratia marcescens, a gram-negative enteric bacterium, can cause a variety of nosocomial infections such as urinary tract infections and endocarditis[310] and has been reported as the etiologic agent of keratitis in at least fifteen studies.[19,22,56,62,65,71,311-319] Ormerod and Smith[65] found that 8 percent of contact lens associated microbial keratitis incidents were due to *S. marcescens*, and that it was the fourth most frequently isolated pathogen after *Pseudomonas*, *Staphylococcus*, and *Streptococcus* species. One recent study showed *S. marcescens* to be the most common gram-negative bacterium isolated as the etiologic agent of contact lens related microbial keratitis.[319] This bacterium is a common cause of contact lens-induced acute red eye (CLARE), a condition that usually occurs with overnight wear of soft contact lenses and causes pain, redness, and photophobia (Fig. 13.16),[103,320] however, the strains of *S. marcescens* that cause CLARE might not be capable of also causing infectious keratitis.[321] *S. marcescens* was also recently found to be commonly isolated from nonulcerating keratitis cases associated with contact lens wear in which epithelial infiltrates and stromal inflammation were observed.[174] *Serratia* keratitis associated with contact lens wear can be aggravated by additional risk factors such as keratoconus, or the thinning and protrusion of the cornea.[322] *Serratia* virulence factors include adhesion (due to pili), LPS, hemolysin, motility and proteases.[310,323] Variations in the pathogenesis of *Serratia* strains have been observed.[324,325]

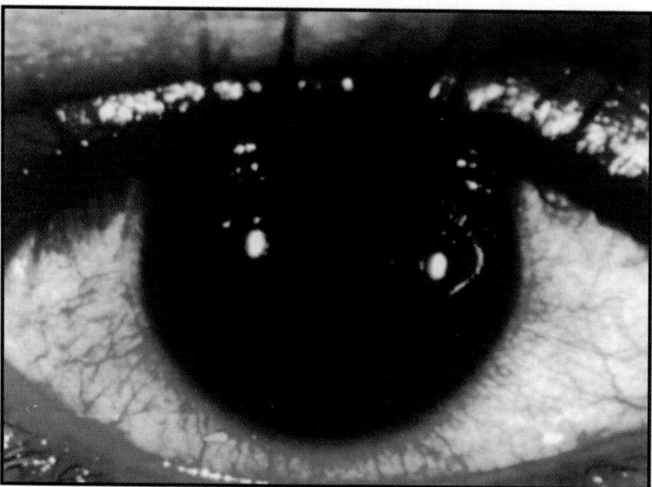

Fig. 13.16: Contact lens-associated acute red eye (CLARE) caused by *Serratia marcescens*

Serratia produces proteases that induce acute inflammation, descemetocele formation and liquefactive necrosis of the rabbit and guinea pig cornea.[326,327] The destruction of corneal stroma allows space for the further spreading of bacteria.[328] *S. marcescens* produces a 56 kilodalton protease that correlates with ulceration of the cornea and tissue destruction.[329] Both *Serratia*[330] and *Pseudomonas proteases*[245,331] are also able to degrade corneal proteins. Bacterial proteases can activate corneal proteinases, including the normally inactive corneal matrix metalloprotease-2, that could contribute to the degradation of the corneal matrix. Factors other than *Serratia* proteases contribute to corneal virulence, however, because different strains of *S. marcescens* that are similar in their production of several proteases, can exhibit different disease symptom severity.[324]

S. marcescens is a dangerous corneal pathogen because it can live and grow in minimal nutrient conditions.[310,332] This bacterium can adhere readily to soft contact lenses and can survive for long periods of time in a number of different contact lens solutions, especially those containing polyquaternium as the active ingredient.[90,332] *Serratia* can also contaminate topical ocular medications such as timolol maleate,[311] or the caps of bottles containing those medications,[333] and thereby cause keratitis. *S. marcescens* can be an ocular nosocomial pathogen and has been associated with radial keratotomy[315] and suture infection after penetrating keratoplasty.[35] Furthermore, *S. marcescens* can be resistant to numerous antibiotics such as ampicillin, beta-lactams, aminoglycosides, and fluoroquinolones.[310]

INFREQUENT CAUSES OF BACTERIAL KERATITIS

Gram-Positive Pathogens

Staphylococcus aureus, *Streptococcus pneumoniae*, and *Staphylococcus epidermidis* are the most commonly documented gram-positive bacteria that cause bacterial keratitis. *S. epidermidis* is normally found on the skin and ocular surface. Like *S. aureus*, *S. epidermidis* can become an opportunistic pathogen of the cornea (Fig. 13.7),[19,22] but information about its pathogenesis is limited. Other gram-positive pathogens, however, have been isolated as etiologic agents of the disease (Table 13.3). For example, other *Streptococcus* species such as *Streptococcus viridans* and *Streptococcus pyogenes* can cause keratitis, including post-surgical graft infiltrates (Fig. 13.8, caused by a *Streptococcus* of the Viridans group, and Fig. 13.17, caused by a group A *Streptococcus*) and interstitial ring keratitis characterized by ring abscesses in the cornea.[15] *Streptococcus viridans* has been shown to be associated with contact lens wear[72] and is a common cause of infectious crystalline keratopathy.[143-148]

Numerous gram-positive bacteria have been shown to cause keratitis. Atypical Mycobacteria, which are all species of *Mycobacterium* other than *M. tuberculosis*, have been identified as pathogens causing keratitis, including *M. chelonae* and *M. fortuitum*, the two most commonly described atypical Mycobacteria isolated from cases of keratitis.[43,155,157,158,160,161,163-165,334-338] *Nocardia* is a gram-positive filamentous bacterium that causes keratitis in people who work outside,[339] although *N. asteroides* has been shown to be involved in chronic keratitis induced by extended-wear soft contact lenses[199] and other undetermined causes (Fig. 13.18).[22] Diphtheroids are pleomorphic *Corynebacterium* and *Propionibacterium* species that have recently been implicated

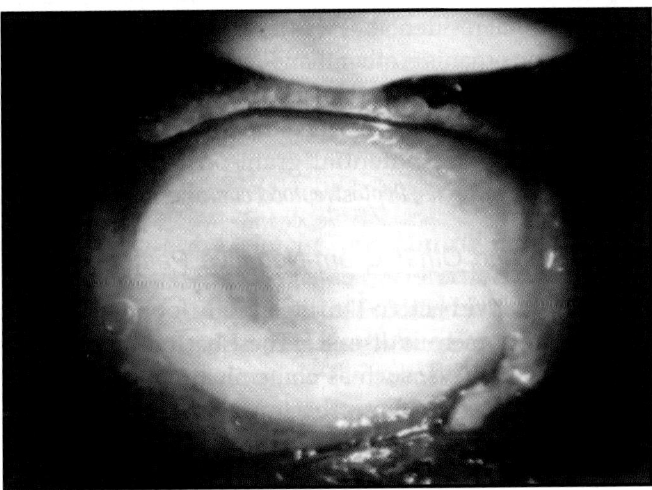

Fig. 13.17: Corneal ulcer caused by a group A *Streptococcus*. A corneal transplant was done because the ulcer did not resolve

CLINICAL MANIFESTATION

Patients with bacterial keratitis can have a variety of symptoms such as pain, photophobia, and/or a foreign body sensation. Their eyes may look normal at first glance, or show redness or ulcers. Ulcers can vary in color, size, shape, texture, and the amount of pus produced. The ulcers can also be centrally (Figs 13.11, 13.12, and 13.15) or peripherally located (Figs 13.9 and 13.19). Sometimes a hypopyon, which is an accumulation of white blood cells, will appear in the anterior chamber (Figs 13.10, 13.13, 13.15, and 13.18). Ring infiltrates or crystalline infiltrates may be present in the cornea, or a herniation of the Descemet's membrane, a descemetocele, may form (Fig. 13.20). No single specific symptom or presentation of bacterial keratitis can determine the identity of the etiologic agent, however, some clinicians have noticed characteristics that seem to gravitate to particular organisms. The presence of a shaggy green ulcer has been associated with *Pseudomonas* (Fig. 13.11),[53,172] although not all *Pseudomonas* keratitis cases will exhibit shaggy green ulcers. *Pseudomonas* might also cause a hypopyon (Fig. 13.13).[53] Crystalline infiltrates[36,182,309] or hypopyon (Fig. 13.15)[34,46,53,172] have been linked to pneumococcus, although gram-negative bacteria, including *P. aeruginosa,* have also been shown to cause crystalline keratopathy.[182] *Staphylococcus* often produces round ulcers with distinct edges (Figs 13.9 and 13.10).[53]

DIAGNOSIS

Proper diagnosis of suspected bacterial keratitis is crucial to effective treatment and cannot be based solely on clinical manifestation of the disease. Accurate laboratory culture and identification is essential for proper treatment. Proper

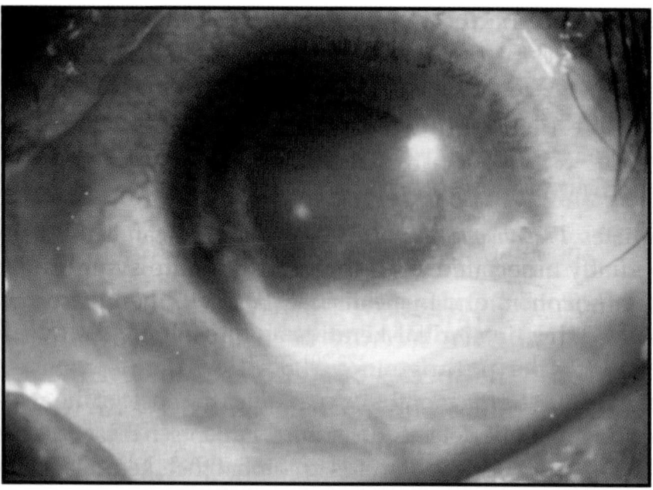

Fig. 13.19: Peripheral keratitis

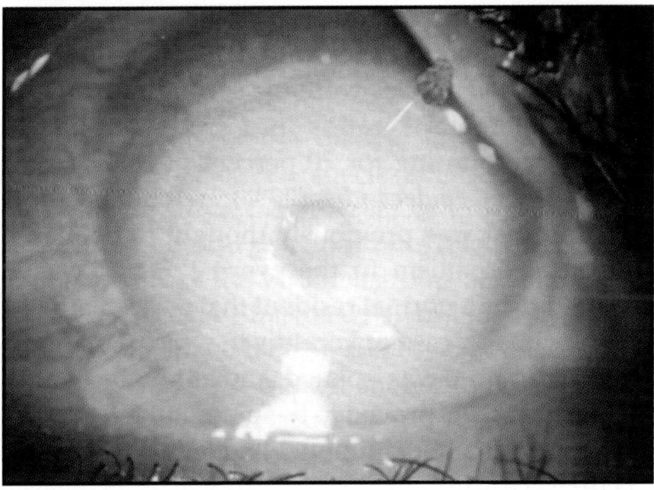

Fig. 13.20: Descemetocele

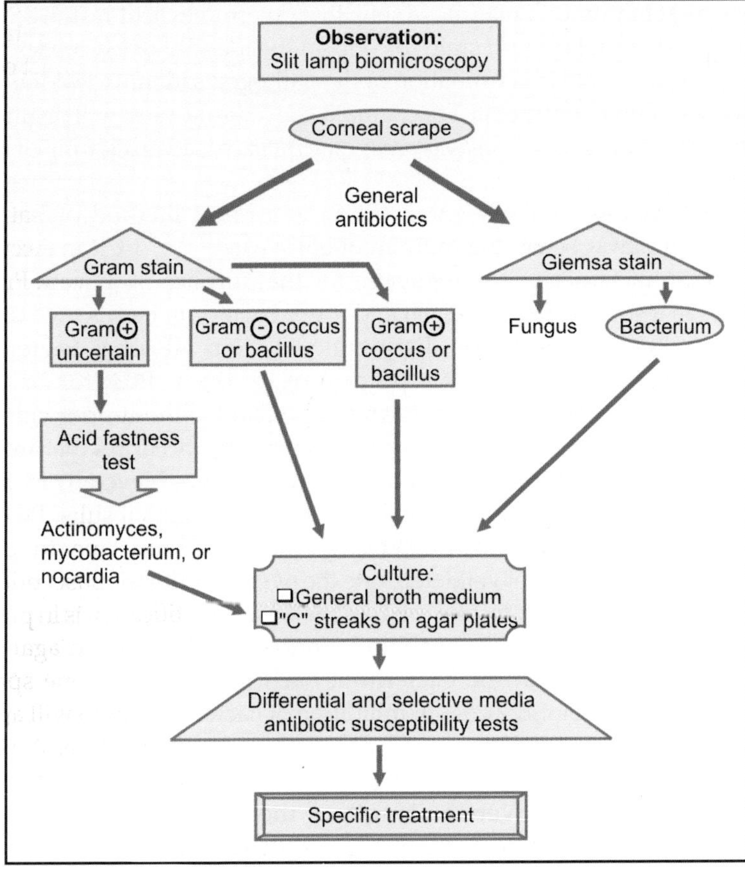

Fig. 13.21: Identification of an etiologic agent of bacterial keratitis

culture identification is often neglected even though it is a consensus among physicians that cultures are necessary for the diagnosis of bacterial keratitis.[350,351] A common procedure to identify the infecting agent in a case of suspected bacterial keratitis is outlined in Figure 13.21. The patient's cornea is usually scraped with a spatula in several places prior to treatment, and each specimen is cultured for identification and antibiotic susceptibility testing.[352] In the meantime, a general antibiotic or combination of drugs is administered in an attempt to treat the infection. The laboratory personnel do a Gram stain on each specimen. The Gram stain will distinguish the shape of the organism (coccus, bacillus, filamentous, or coccobacillus), how it is arranged (singly, in pairs, or in chains), and whether it is gram-positive or gram-negative. In cases in which there is difficulty determining whether the etiologic agent is bacterial or fungal, a Giemsa stain can be done. The specimen is then cultured using media that can grow a variety of organisms (for example, thioglycolate broth). Laboratory personnel will use broth cultures and agar plates containing several "C" streaks (for each scraping) to isolate and grow the pathogen. Such culturing separates pathogens in mixed culture cases of bacterial keratitis. Further staining can be done at this time. Sometimes a stain that determines acid-fastness will be used in addition to the Gram stain to confirm the identity of Mycobacteria or *Nocardia* isolates. Final determination of the pathogen's identity is done using selective and differential media. For example, the coagulase test will distinguish *Staphylococcus aureus* from *Staphylococcus epidermidis* based on clotting of rabbit plasma.

The polymerase chain reaction (PCR) is a rapid method of bacterial identification that is becoming more frequently used.[353-363] PCR involves the amplification of target DNA sequences for the purpose of detecting those sequences in a specific fashion. Each and every bacterium has its own unique genome and can therefore be distinguished from all other bacteria by amplification and detection of a portion of its DNA. PCR for bacterial identification can be done after culturing or possibly without prior culturing and thus eliminates several time-consuming culturing procedures that are done in the classical methods of identification. The accuracy achieved by PCR also decreases the ambiguity of differential and selective media results. PCR and other molecular methods can also determine a pathogen's resistance to specific antibiotics,[364-366] but cannot yet determine the overall antibiotic susceptibility.

Antibiotic susceptibility testing can be done while identification is in process, and usually consists of placing antibiotic-containing disks on an agar plate that was inoculated with the bacterium. Each disk contains one specific concentration of antibiotic. Zones of inhibition of bacterial growth will appear around the antibiotic disks to which the bacterium is sensitive. A newer procedure uses strips (called E strips) coated with antibiotic applied in a concentration gradient over the length of the strip. Minimal inhibitory concentrations (MICs) of the antibiotic can be determined by measuring the zone of inhibition around the E strip. E strips are becoming very popular because the MIC can be determined by merely observing the lowest concentration that causes growth inhibition.

TREATMENT

Antibiotics

The therapeutic strategy for patients with bacterial keratitis can be difficult in terms of the selection of antibiotics prior to the laboratory identification and antibiotic susceptibility tests of the infecting organisms. The infected eye is often treated with a general antibiotic, or combination of drugs, before the pathogen is identified. Not all bacteria will be susceptible to a general antibiotic, so initial treatment before diagnosis in some cases is not effective. On the other hand, waiting for culture results can delay the treatment of a cornea that is at risk of developing severe pathology that could cause permanent damage to the eye. An additional problem is that the use of topical anesthetics such as proparacaine and tetracaine during corneal scraping for bacterial culture can yield false negative results, as these agents temporarily inhibit the growth of *Pseudomonas aeruginosa* and *Staphylococcus aureus*.[367]

The drugs of choice for bacterial keratitis vary depending upon the etiologic agent (Table 13.5), and the doses and combination can vary depending upon personal preference of the physician and the individual reaction of the bacterium to the drug. Table 13.6 outlines topical dose suggestions for the treatment of bacterial keratitis. Cefazolin or vancomycin is commonly used for *Staphylococcus* infections whereas gentamicin or tobramycin is used for gram-negative infections.[234,235] Ciprofloxacin and ofloxacin are part of a newer class of antibiotics called fluoroquinolones and have been shown to be effective in treating *P. aeruginosa* or *S. aureus* keratitis.[368-370] Fleroxacin, another fluoroquinolone, appears to be extremely effective against *P. aeruginosa* and enterics.[371] Ciprofloxacin was found to be effective against methicillin-resistant *S. aureus* (MRSA),[236,372,373] however, more recently the susceptibility of *S. aureus* to the fluoroquinolones has declined dramatically.[136,220,225,237,374,375] Most *Staphylococcus* strains, including about 20 percent of MRSA strains, are susceptible to clarithromycin both *in vitro* and in a rabbit model of keratitis.[376] However, vancomycin is clearly the drug of choice for the great majority of MRSA infections.[220,232-240] Unfortunately, there are recent reports of vancomycin resistance.[228,231,377,378] Of concern also is the isolation of MRSA strains from outpatients; such strains were formerly referred to as "hospital strains" and were found exclusively in nosocomial infections.[219]

Resistance to antibiotics is found not only in *S. aureus*, but resistance to fluoroquinolones has also been found in *P. aeruginosa* and *S. marcescens* strains.[193;379;380] *P. aeruginosa* has also been found to be extremely resistant to chloramphenicol.[16] Consequently, there is a continuous search for new antibiotics and/or combination therapies.

Table 13.5: Treatment agents for bacterial keratitis

Organism	*Drug(s)*	*Possible resistance*
Common Causes		
Pseudomonas aeruginosa	ceftazidime,[172,382,383] cephazolin,[21] ciprofloxacin,[137,193,382,384] fleroxacin,[371] gentamicin,[16,22,382,383] ofloxacin,[21,382] piperacillin,[53,172] polymyxin B,[53] ticarcillin,[382] tobramycin,[21,53,172,382,383] trovafloxacin[385]	chloramphenicol,[16] ciprofloxacin,[137,193] fluoroquinolones[380]
Staphylococcus aureus	bacitracin,[172] cefazolin,[21,36,53,137,172] cefuroxime,[119] ciprofloxacin,[172] clarithromycin,[376] gentamicin,[22,119] lomefloxacin,[386] ofloxacin,[36,172,382,387] pefloxacin,[388] penicillin G,[53] tobramycin,[21] vancomycin[172]	fluoroquinolones,[136,220,225,237,374,375] oxacillin,[389] vancomycin[230,377,378]
Streptococcus pneumoniae	bacitracin,[172] cefazolin,[137,172] cefuroxime,[34] chloramphenicol,[137] gentamicin,[22] ofloxacin,[389] penicillin,[34,53,172,382] vancomycin[141,172]	chloramphenicol,[16] ciprofloxacin,[137] penicillin[141,308]
Serratia marcescens	aminoglycosides,[310] ampicillin,[53] gentamicin,[22] tobramycin[172]	ampicillin, carbapenem, cephalosporins, ciprofloxacin, gentamicin, netilmicin[310]
Uncommon Causes		
Acinetobacter calcoaceticus-A. baumannii complex	4-fluoroquinolones, gentamicin[29]	chloramphenicol, 4-fluoroquinolones, mezlocillin, penicillin, piperacillin[29]
Alcaligenes xylosoxidans	Bactrim,[173] ceftazidime,[131] imipenem, Timentin[173]	gentamicin,[131] among many[173]
Azotobacter	gentamicin[53]	
Bacillus	cefazolin,[36] chloramphenicol, gentamicin,[137] ofloxacin, tobrex[36]	
Capnocytophaga	ampicillin,[26,28,180] carbenicillin, cefamandole,[26,180] cefuroxime,[26] cephazolin,[28] chloramphenicol,[26,180] ciprofloxacin,[26] clindamycin,[28,179] erythromycin, penicillin,[26,28,180] tetracycline[26,180]	aminoglycosides,[26,28,179,180] cephalosporins,[28,179] semisynthetic penicillin, vancomycin[26,180]
Clostridium perfringens	chloramphenicol[33]	
Corynebacterium	bacitracin,[53] cefazolin,[36,137] ciprofloxacin,[157] erythromycin,[151] gentamicin,[22] tobramycin,[36] vancomycin[151]	ciprofloxacin[137]
Eikenella corrodens	cephalosporin, penicillin[181]	aminoglycosides, penicillinase-resistant penicillin[181]
Enterobacter	ciprofloxacin[137]	
Enterococcus faecalis	ofloxacin[389]	
Flavobacterium meningosepticum	trimethoprim-sulfamethoxazole[192]	amikacin, ampicillin, cephalosporin, chloramphenicol, piperacillin, tetracycline, ticarcillin, tobramycin[192]
Haemophilus influenzae	ampicillin[53]	
Klebsiella pneumoniae	cefazolin, tobramycin[21]	
Listeria monocytogenes	ampicillin,[53] cephaloridine,[153] gentamicin,[153,154] penicillin[154]	

Contd...

Table 13.5 contd...

Organism	*Drug(s)*	*Possible resistance*
Moraxella	aminoglycoside,[390] bacitracin,[30] cefazolin,[31] cephalosporin,[390] chloramphenicol,[30] ciprofloxacin,[24,137] erythromycin,[31] gentamicin,[30,53] neomycin, penicillin, polymyxin,[30] tetracycline, tobramycin, vancomycin[31]	cefazolin,[24] clindamycin,[31] gentamicin,[24] nafcillin,[31] norfloxacin,[24] penicillin G[390]
Mycobacterium chelonae	amikacin,[19,157] cefoxitin,[158] ciprofloxacin[159]	many[159]
Mycobacterium fortuitum	ciprofloxacin[159]	many[159]
Neisseria	penicillin G[53]	
Nocardia	amikacin,[119] chloramphenicol (*N.* asteroides), gentamicin (*N.* asteroides),[137] trimethoprim, vancomycin[119]	
Peptococcus variabilis	chloramphenicol[45]	
Propionibacterium acnes	cefazolin,[36] cephapirin,[171] chloramphenicol[45] ciprofloxacin,[137] erythromycin,[171] ofloxacin[36]	
Proteus mirabilis		gentamicin[16]
Shigella flexneri	chloramphenicol, gentamicin[189]	
Shigella sonnei	gentamicin[190]	
Staphylococcus epidermidis	cefazolin,[36,131,137] cephalothin,[22] ciprofloxacin,[131,157] ofloxacin,[36] vancomycin[131]	cefazolin,[131] chloramphenicol,[22] ciprofloxacin,[131,137] gentamicin,[131] penicillin, sulfonamides, tetracycline[22]
Staphylococcus hemolyticus	sulfacetamide[36]	
Stenotrophomonas maltophilia	fluoroquinolones, sulfamethoxazole, trimethoprim[70]	aminoglycosides, beta-lactams, fluoroquinolones[70]
Streptococcus pyogenes	penicillin[391]	
Streptococcus sanguis	cefazolin[36]	
Streptococcus viridans	cefazolin[36,72] vancomycin[131]	
Vibrio vulnificus	ciprofloxacin, neosporin, vancomycin[196]	

S. pneumoniae has exhibited less antibiotic resistance than *P. aeruginosa* and *S. aureus* but remains a significant threat to the cornea, and it is showing resistance to many antibiotics, including penicillin,[141] chloramphenicol,[16] and fluoroquinolones.[136] *S. pneumoniae* keratitis can be treated successfully with antibiotics such as gentamicin and vancomycin, but not without damage to the cornea since the bacterium is very destructive to the epithelium.[34,46,141] Previous use of beta-lactam antibiotics has been associated with antibiotic resistance of *Pneumococcus*.[381] The inflammatory response to *S. pneumoniae* has been implicated in destruction of the corneal epithelium; early administration of topical steroids such as prednisolone and dexamethasone can quicken the healing process.[34]

Table 13.6: Topical treatment doses for commonly used antibiotics

Identity of bacterium	*Topical treatment and dose*
Unknown	1. 0.3% ofloxacin[119,382] 2. 0.3% ciprofloxacin[119,382] 3. 5% cephalosporin[a] + 1.5% gentamicin[119,382] 4. 5% cephalosporin + 1.5%[382] or 1.4%[53,172] tobramycin
Staphylococcus aureus	1. 0.3% ofloxacin[382] 2. 5% cefazolin[53,172,392] or 5% vancomycin or 10,000 U/ml bacitracin or 0.3% fluoroquinolone[b] if penicillin-resistant[172] 3. 5% vancomycin or 10,000 U/ml bacitracin or 0.3% fluoroquinolone if methicillin-resistant[172,392] 4. 100,000 U/ml penicillin G if penicillin-sensitive[53]
Streptococcus pneumoniae	1. 5000 U/ml penicillin[382] 2. 100,000 U/ml penicillin G[53,172] 3. 5% cefazolin[172] 4. 5% vancomycin[172] 5. 10,000 U/ml bacitracin[172]
Pseudomonas aeruginosa	1. 0.3% ofloxacin or ciprofloxacin + 5% ceftazidime[382] 2. 0.3% ofloxacin or ciprofloxacin + 5% ticarcillin[382] 3. 0.3% ofloxacin or ciprofloxacin + 1.5% gentamicin[382] 4. 0.3% ofloxacin or ciprofloxacin + 1.5% tobramycin[382] 5. 1.4% tobramycin + 2% piperacillin[172] 6. 1.4% tobramycin + 5% ceftazidime[172,383] 7. 0.2% tobramycin + 0.2% polymyxin B or 0.7% piperacillin[53]
Serratia marcescens	1. 1.4% tobramycin[172]

[a]Cephalosporin = cephazolin, cefuroxime, or ceftazidime
[b]fluoroquinolone = ciprofloxacin, norfloxacin, or ofloxacin

Determining the proper treatment for uncommon causes of bacterial keratitis requires significant decision-making since specific therapy for keratitis caused by these bacteria is less documented. Table 13.5 lists these rare causes and their treatments based on available information. Some bacteria such as *Peptostreptococcus* or *Shigella flexneri* have not been isolated from cases of keratitis in years or even decades. By the same token, the potential for identifying a new bacterial cause of keratitis is likely. New patterns of antibiotic resistance among all species are being discovered. Therefore, the ophthalmologist cannot rely solely on the treatments in previous cases of keratitis for even the common causes.

Anti-inflammatory Agents

The use of steroids in combination with antibiotics in the treatment of bacterial keratitis remains an issue of debate but has appeared to be beneficial in certain circumstances.[34,209,392-399] Some cases of keratitis are accompanied by increased intraocular pressure, and corticosteroids might be used to decrease the pressure.[119] Other cases of keratitis, such as those elicited by Lyme disease and tertiary syphilis, are successfully treated with anti-inflammatory agents because the keratitis appears to be an immune response to the overall disease.[201,348] One suggestion for the use of steroids to treat inflammation caused by bacterial keratitis is to apply steroids after the pathogen has been identified and antibiotic treatment has begun to decrease bacterial numbers.[20]

The treatment of *P. aeruginosa* keratitis requires combination therapy that not only stops the microorganism from growing, but also inhibits the ensuing inflammatory response.[400,401] *S. aureus* also causes an inflammatory response of the eye during keratitis.[402] Several studies[370,403-405] have demonstrated that the effectiveness of an antibiotic-steroid combination is dependent upon the specific antibiotic and steroid being employed. Although not completely successful, the best anti-inflammatory results obtained to date in an animal model of *Pseudomonas* keratitis were with the use of prednisolone and tobramycin.[403]

The use of nonsteroidal anti-inflammatory drugs (NSAIDs) in combination with antibiotics is also important to limit the damage from the host response to the infection.[406-410] NSAIDs combined with antibiotics have been tested in animal models of bacterial keratitis. Reductions in pathology (inflammation) have been attributed to combined fluoroquinolone and NSAID administration, but the improvements were very limited.[410] Moreira *et al*[409] reported that therapy with either flurbiprofen or nordihydroguaiaretic acid produces only partial reductions in inflammation during *Pseudomonas* keratitis. As with steroids,[403] the efficacy of NSAID-antibiotic combinations could vary, and testing with a variety of specific antibiotics may be necessary to identify the most effective combination.[404,405]

Antibiotic Resistance

Keratitis is generally a community-acquired infection and, as such, typically involves antibiotic susceptible strains. Some rare community-acquired strains that cause keratitis are resistant to multiple antibiotics. Also, keratitis that develops as a postsurgical infection may involve hospital strains with significant antibiotic resistance. Among the bacteria that are noted for their resistance are the four most common agents of keratitis, that is, *Staphylococcus, Pseudomonas, Pneumococcus*, and *Serratia*. Methicillin-resistant strains of *Staphylococcus* are not only common as nosocomial isolates, but have now emerged as agents of community-acquired infection.[224,226,232,411-421] *Pseudomonas* and *Serratia* strains with broad resistance to antibiotics are a frequent cause of opportunistic nosocomial infections.[222,422-425] Highly resistant pneumococci have caused particularly stubborn infections in children, mainly as community-acquired infections.[381] In addition to these common causes of keratitis, Mycobacteria strains capable of causing keratitis have also demonstrated extreme antibiotic resistance. The AIDS-related Mycobacteria are particularly noted for their extensive antibiotic resistance.[426-430]

PROGNOSIS

The prognosis for bacterial keratitis can range from favorable to extremely tragic depending on response to treatment. A favorable outcome of bacterial keratitis includes a steady decline of symptoms and ulcers resulting in little or no irreversible scarring of the cornea. The patient experiencing such an outcome can fully recover his sight. Other cases of bacterial keratitis, however, might not recover as readily as this. The corneal scarring can be very severe and contribute to corneal opacity and decreased visual clarity. If visual loss is severe, more drastic procedures such as corneal transplantation might need to be done to restore vision.

CONCLUSION

Any bacterium in existence cannot be excluded as a potential pathogen of the cornea, as evidenced by continuously occurring cases of bacterial keratitis caused by bacteria not previously documented as etiologic agents of keratitis. As with any type of disease caused by bacteria, bacterial keratitis can be very dangerous to the afflicted person. Lack of successful treatment can cause the keratitis to progress to a point where the patient could lose his vision. Prerequisites for successful treatment and management of bacterial keratitis are awareness of what has been documented for previous cases and knowledge of antibiotic resistance patterns. The future of bacterial keratitis therapy could rely heavily on alternatives to antibiotics and combination therapy to reduce or eliminate irreversible scarring.

REFERENCES

1. Willcox MDP, Stapleton F. Ocular bacteriology. Rev Med Micro 1996; 7: 123-31.
2. Izquierdo N, Mendoza SD, Townsend W, et al. Prevalence of the microbiologic flora in contact lens wearers at the Puerto Rico medical center. Biol Assoc Med Puerto Rico 1991; 83: 96-98.
3. Singer TR, Isenberg SJ, Apt L. Conjunctival anaerobic and aerobic bacterial flora in paediatric versus adult subjects. Br J Ophthalmol 1988; 72: 448-51.

4. Smith CH: Bacteriology of the healthy conjunctiva. Br J Ophthalmol 1954;38: 719-26.
5. Fleiszig SMJ, Efron N. Conjunctival flora in extended wear of rigid gas permeable contact lenses. Optom Vis Sci 1992;69:354-7.
6. Perins RE, Kundsin RB, Prate MV et al: Bacteriology of normal and infected conjunctiva. J Clin Microbiol 1975; 1: 147-49.
7. Gachon AMF, Lacazette E. Tear lipocalin and the eye's front line of defence. Br J Ophthalmol 1998;82:453-55.
8. Stapleton F, Willcox MDP, Fleming CM, et al: Changes to the ocular biota with time in extended-and daily-wear disposable contact lens use. Infect Immun 1995; 63:4501-5.
9. Liesegang TJ: Bacterial keratitis. Infect Dis Clin N America 1992;6:815-29.
10. Limberg MB: A review of bacterial keratitis and bacterial conjunctivitis. Am J Ophthalmol 1991;112:2S-9S.
11. Russell MW, Sibley DA, Nikolova EB, et al. IgA antibody as a non-inflammatory regulator of immunity. Biochem Soc Trans 1997;25:466-70.
12. Haynes RJ, Tighe PJ, Dua HS: Innate defence of the eye by antimicrobial defensin peptides. Lancet 1998;352:451-52.
13. Fleiszig SMJ, Zaidi TS, Ramphal R et al. Modulation of Pseudomonas aeruginosa adherence to the corneal surface by mucus. Infect Immun 1994; 62: 1799-804.
14. Wheater MK, Kernacki KA, Hazlett LD: Corneal cell proteins and ocular surface pathology. Biotech Histochem 1999;74:146-59.
15. Liesegang TJ, Samples JR, Waller RR: Suppurative interstitial ring keratitis due to Streptococcus. Ann Ophthalmol 1984;16:392-96.
16. Tan DTH, Lee CPL, Lim ASM: Corneal ulcers in two institutions in Singapore: analysis of causative factors, organisms and antibiotic resistance. Ann Acad Med Singapore 1998;24:823-9.
17. Wang AG, Wu CC, Liu JH: Bacterial corneal ulcer: a multivariate study. Ophthalmologica 1998;212:126-32.
18. Baum JL: Prolonged eyelid closure is a risk to the cornea. Cornea 1997; 16: 602-11.
19. Boisjoly HM, Pavan-Langston D, Kenyon KR et al: Superinfections in herpes simplex keratitis. Am J Ophthalmol 1983;96:354-61.
20. Coster DJ, Badenoch PR: Host, microbial, and pharmacological factors affecting the outcome of suppurative keratitis. Br J Ophthalmol 1987;71:96-101.
21. Vajpayee RB, Sharma N, Chand M et al: Corneal superinfection in acute hemorrhagic conjunctivitis. Cornea 1998;17:614-7.
22. McClellan KA, Bernard PJ, Billson FA: Microbial investigations in keratitis at the Sydney Eye Hospital. Aust N Z J Ophthalmol 1989;17:413-6.
23. Gebauer A, McGhee CNJ, Crawford GJ: Severe microbial keratitis in temperate and tropical Western Australia. Eye 1996;10:575-80.
24. Garg P, Mathur U, Athmanathan S et al: Treatment outcome of Moraxella keratitis: our experience with 18 cases—a retrospective review. Cornea 1999;18:176-81.
25. Ormerod LD, Fong LP, Foster CS: Corneal infection in mucosal scarring disorders and Sjogren's syndrome. Am J Ophthalmol 1988;105:512-8.
26. Aristimuño B, Nirankari VS, Hemady RK et al: Spontaneous ulcerative keratitis in immunocompromised patients. Am J Ophthalmol 1993;115:202-8.
27. Hemady RK: Microbial keratitis in patients infected with the human immunodeficiency virus. Ophthalmol 1995;102:1026-30.

28. Ticho BH, Urban RC Jr, Safran MJ et al: Capnocytophaga keratitis associated with poor dentition and human immunodeficiency virus infection. Am J Ophthalmol 1990; 109: 352-3.
29. Marcovich A, Levartovsky S: Acinetobacter exposure keratitis. Br J Ophthalmol 1994; 78: 489-90.
30. Asbell P, Stenson S: Ulcerative keratitis. Survey of 30 years' laboratory experience. Arch Ophthalmol 1982; 100: 77-80.
31. Marioneaux SJ, Cohen EJ, Arentsen JJ et al: Moraxella keratitis. Cornea 1991; 10: 21-24.
32. Miedziak AI, Miller MR, Rapuano CJ et al: Risk factors in microbial keratitis leading to penetrating keratoplasty. Ophthalmol 1999; 106: 1166-71.
33. Badenoch PR, Aggarwal RK, Coster DJ: Clostridium perfringens keratitis after penetrating keratoplasty. Aust N Z J Ophthalmol 1995; 23 :245-6.
34. Charteris DG, Batterbury M, Armstrong M et al: Suppurative keratitis caused by Streptococcus pneumoniae after cataract surgery. Br J Ophthalmol 1994; 78: 847-9.
35. Leahey AB, Avery RL, Gottsch JD et al: Suture abscesses after penetrating keratoplasty. Cornea 1993; 12: 489-92.
36. Sutphin JE, Kantor AL, Mathers WD et al: Evaluation of infectious crystalline keratitis with confocal microscopy in a case series. Cornea 1997; 16: 21-26.
37. Webber SK, Lawless MA, Sutton GL et al: Staphylococcal infection under a LASIK flap. Cornea 1999; 18: 361-5.
38. Dada T, Sharma N, Dada VK et al: Pneumococcal keratitis after laser in situ keratomileusis. J Cataract Refract Surg 2000; 26: 460-1.
39. Quiros PA, Chuck RS, Smith RE et al: Infectious ulcerative keratitis after laser in situ keratomileusis. Arch Ophthalmol 1999; 117: 1423-7.
40. Hovanesian JA, Faktorovich EG, Hoffbauer JD et al: Bilateral bacterial keratitis after laser in situ keratomileusis in a patient with human immunodeficiency virus infection. Arch Ophthalmol 1999; 117: 968-70.
41. Al Reefy M: Bacterial keratitis following laser in situ keratomileusis for hyperopia. J Refract Surg 1999; 2(15): 216-7.
42. Kim HM, Song JS, Han HS et al: Streptococcal keratitis after myopic laser in situ keratomileusis. Kor J Ophthalmol 1998; 12: 108-11.
43. Reviglio V, Rodriguez ML, Picotti GS et al: Mycobacterium chelonae keratitis following laser in situ keratomileusis. J Refract Surg 1998; 14: 357-60.
44. Perez-Santonja JJ, Sakla HF, Abad JL et al: Nocardial keratitis after laser in situ keratomileusis. J Refract Surg 1997; 13: 314-17.
45. Jones DB, Robinson NM: Anaerobic ocular infections. Trans Am Acad Ophthalmol Otolaryngol 1977; 83: 309-31.
46. Ormerod LD, Hertzmark E, Gomez DS et al: Epidemiology of microbial keratitis in southern California. Ophthalmol 1987; 94: 1322-33.
47. Luchs JI, Cohen EJ, Rapuano CJ et al: Ulcerative keratitis in bullous keratopathy. Ophthalmol 1997; 104: 816-22.
48. Aasuri MK, Reddy MK, Sharma S et al: Co-occurrence of pneumococcal keratitis and dacryocystitis. Cornea 1999; 18: 273-6.
49. Liesegang TJ: Contact lens-related microbial keratitis: Part I: epidemiology. Cornea 1997; 16: 125-31.
50. Wilson LA, Kuehne JW, Hall SW et al: Microbial contamination in ocular cosmetics. Am J Ophthalmol 1971; 71: 1298-302.

51. Beatty S, Tyagi A, Kirkby GR: Klebsiella keratitis complicating bandage contact lens use [letter]. Acta Ophthalmol Scand 1998; 76 :757-8.
52. Cavanaugh TB, Gottsch JD: Infectious keratitis and cyanoacrylate adhesive. Am J Ophthalmol 1991; 111: 466-72.
53. Arffa RC: Infectious ulcerative keratitis: bacterial. Grayson's Diseases of the Cornea. Mosby-Year Book: St.Louis: 1991; 163-98.
54. Dua HS: Bacterial keratitis in the critically ill and comatose patient. Lancet 1998; 351: 387-8.
55. Dart JKG, Stapleton F, Minassian D: Contact lenses and other risk factors in microbial keratitis. Lancet 1991; 338: 650-3.
56. Schein OD, Omerod LD, Barraquer E et al: Microbiology of contact lens-related keratitis. Cornea 1989; 8: 281-85.
57. Schein OD, Glynn RJ, Poggio EG et al: The relative risk of ulcerative keratitis among users of daily-wear and extended wear soft contact lenses. A case-control study. New Eng J Med 1989; 321: 773-8.
58. Schein OD, Buehler PO, Stamler JF et al: The impact of overnight wear on the risk of contact-lens associated ulcerative keratitis. Arch Ophthalmol 1994; 112: 186-90.
59. Chalupa E, Swarbrick HA, Holden BA et al: Severe corneal infections associated with contact lens wear. Ophthalmol 1987; 94: 17-22.
60. Holden BA, Sweeney DF, Vannas A et al: Effects of long-term extended contact lens wear on the human cornea. Invest Ophthalmol Vis Sci 1985; 26: 1489-501.
61. Korb DR: Tear film-contact lens interactions. Adv Exp Med Biol 1994; 350: 403-10.
62. Cohen EJ, Laibson PR, Arentsen JJ et al: Corneal ulcers associated with cosmetic extended wear soft contact lenses. Ophthalmol 1987; 94: 109-14.
63. Seal DV: Contact-lens-associated microbial keratitis in The Netherlands and Scotland [letter]. Lancet 2000; 355: 143-4.
64. Tabbara KF, El Sheikh HF, Aabed B: Extended wear contact lens related bacterial keratitis [In Process Citation]. Br J Ophthalmol 2000; 84: 327-8.
65. Ormerod LD, Smith RE: Contact lens-associated microbial keratitis. Arch Ophthalmol 1986; 104: 79-83.
66. Glastonbury J, Crompton JL: Pseudomonas aeruginosa corneal infection associated with disposable contact lens use. Aust N Z J Ophthalmol 1989; 17: 451.
67. Dini LA, Cockinos C, Frean JA et al: Unusual case of Acanthamoeba polyphaga and Pseudomonas aeruginosa keratitis in a contact lens wearer from Gauteng, South Africa. J Clin Microbiol 2000; 38: 826-9.
68. Koidou-Tsiligianni A, Alfonso E, Forster RK: Ulcerative keratitis associated with contact lens wear. Am J Ophthalmol 1989; 108: 64-67.
69. Weissman BA, Mondino BJ, Pettit TH et al: Corneal ulcers associated with extended-wear soft contact lenses. Am J Ophthalmol 1984; 97: 476-81.
70. Penland RL, Wilhelmus KR: Stenotrophomonas maltophilia ocular infections. Arch Ophthalmol 1996; 114: 436.
71. Lemp MA, Blackman HJ, Wilson LA et al: Gram-negative corneal ulcers in elderly aphakic eyes with extended-wear lenses. Ophthalmol 1984; 91: 60-63.
72. Nauheim RC, Nauheim JS: Contact lens-related Streptococcus viridans keratitis presenting as an epithelial defect. Arch Ophthalmol 1991; 109: 1354.
73. Patrinely JR, Wilhelmus KR, Rubin JM et al: Bacterial keratitis associated with extended wear soft contact lenses. CLAO J 1998; 11: 234-36.

74. Sankaridurg PR, Sharma S, Willcox M et al: Colonization of hydrogel lenses with Streptococcus pneumoniae: risk of development of corneal infiltrates. Cornea 1999; 18: 289-95.
75. Tragakis MP, Brown SI, Pearce DB: Bacteriologic studies of contamination associated with contact lenses. Am J Ophthalmol 1973; 75: 496-9.
76. Elander TR, Goldberg MA, Salinger CL et al: Microbial changes in the ocular environment with contact lens wear. CLAO J 1992; 18: 53-55.
77. Herdė J, Wilhelms D, Paschold S et al: Conjunctival flora of soft lens wearers, and emmetropes in polluted environment. Contactalogica 1991; 13: 134-6.
78. Callender MG, Tse LSY, Charles AM et al: Bacterial flora of the eye and contact lens cases during hydrogel lens wear. Am J Physiol Optom 1985; 63: 177-80.
79. Hart DE, Reindel W, Proskin HM et al: Microbial contamination of hydrophilic contact lenses: quantitation and identification of microorganisms associated with contact lenses while on the eye. Optom Vis Sci 1993; 70: 185-91.
80. Fleiszig SMJ, Efron N: Microbial flora in eyes of current and former contact lens wearers. J Clin Microbiol 1992; 30: 1156-61.
81. Høvding G: The conjunctival and contact lens bacterial flora during lens wear. Acta Ophthalmol 1981; 59: 387-401.
82. Pitts RE, Krachmer JH: Evaluation of soft contact lens disinfection in the home environment. Arch Ophthalmol 1979; 97: 470-2.
83. Kapetansky FM, Suie T, Doswell Gracy A et al: Bacteriologic studies of patients who wear contact lenses. Am J Ophthalmol 196; 57: 255-58.
84. Donzis PB, Mondino BJ, Weissman BA et al: Microbial contamination of contact lens care systems. Am J Ophthalmol 1987; 104: 325-33.
85. Jenkins C, Phillips AJ: How sterile is unpreserved saline? Clin Exp Optom 1986; 69: 131-6.
86. Güler G, Bakici Z, Yuksel N et al: Bacterial contamination of soft contact lens solutions. Contactologica 1990; 12E:106-9.
87. Sweeney DF, Taylor P, Holden BA et al: Contamination of 500mL bottles of unpreserved saline. Clin Exp Optom 1992; 75: 67-75.
88. Mondino BJ, Weissman BA, Farb D et al: Corneal ulcers associated with daily-wear and extended-wear contact lenses. Am J Ophthalmol 1986; 102: 58-65.
89. Wilson LA, Schlitzer RL, Ahearn DG: Pseudomonas corneal ulcers associated with soft contact-lens wear. Am J Ophthalmol 1981; 92: 546-54.
90. Mayo MS, Schlitzer RL, Ward MA et al: Association of Pseudomonas and Serratia corneal ulcers with use of contaminated solutions. J Clin Microbiol 1987; 25: 1398-400.
91. Parment PA, Rönnerstam R, Walder M: Persistence of Serratia marcescens, Serratia liquefaciens and E.coli in solutions for contact lenses. Acta Ophthalmol 1986; 64: 456-62.
92. Gandhi PA, Sawant AD, Wilson LA et al: Adaption and growth of Serratia marcescens in contact lens disinfectant solutions containing chlorohexidine gluconate. Appl Environmental Microbiol 1993; 59: 183-88.
93. Vigeant P, Loo VG, Bertrand C et al: An outbreak of Serratia marcescens infections related to contaminated chlorhexidine. Infect Control Hosp Epidemiol 1998; 19: 791-4.
94. May LL, Gabriel MM, Simmons RB et al: Resistance of adhered bacteria to rigid gas permeable contact lens solutions. CLAO J 1995; 21: 242-46.

95. Marrie TJ, Costerton JW: Prolonged survival of Serratia marcescens in chlorhexidine. Appl Environmental Microbiol 1981; 42: 1093-102.
96. Wilson LA, Sawant AD, Ahearn DG: Comparative efficacies of soft contact lens disinfectant solutions against microbial films in lens cases. Arch Ophthalmol 1991; 109: 1155-57.
97. Parment PA, Colucci B, Nyström B: The efficacy of soft contact lenses disinfection solutions against Serratia marcescens and Pseudomonas aeruginosa. Acta Ophthalmologica Scand 1996; 74: 235-7.
98. Siwoff R, Haupt EJ: Bacterial growth on contact lens cases: do solutions make a difference. Contact Lens Forum 1986; 9: 47-52.
99. Larkin DFP, Kilvington S, Easty DL: Contamination of contact lens storage cases by Acanthamoeba and bacteria. Br J Ophthalmol 1990; 74: 133-35.
100. Kanpolat A, Kalayci D, Arman D et al: Contamination in contact lens care systems. CLAO J 1992; 18: 105-07.
101. Leluan P, Liotet S, Batellier L et al: Amoebic and bacterial contamination of contact lens storage cases—a study of 32 keratitis patients and 63 healthy lens wearers. Contactologica 1991; 13E: 137-41.
102. Wilson LA, Sawant AD, Simmons RB et al: Microbial contamination of contact lens storage cases and solutions. Am J Ophthalmol 1990; 110: 193-8.
103. Sankaridurg PR, Vuppala N, Sreedharan A et al: Gram negative bacteria and contact lens induced acute red eye. Ind J Ophthalmol 1996; 44: 29-32.
104. Matthews TD, Frazer DG, Minassian DC et al: Risks of keratitis and patterns of use with disposable contact lenses. Arch Ophthalmol 1992; 110: 1559-62.
105. Buehler PO, Schein OD, Stamler JF et al: The increased risk of ulcerative keratitis among disposable soft contact lens users. Arch Ophthalmol 1992; 110: 1555-8.
106. John T: How safe are disposable soft contact lenses? Am J Ophthalmol 1991; 111: 766-8.
107. Hu B: Lower respiratory tract flora in intubated patients. Chung-Hua-I-Hsueh-Tsa-Chih 1991; 71: 243-5.
108. Getchell-White SI, Donowitz LG, Groschel DH: The inanimate environment of an intensive care unit as a potential source of nosocomial bacteria: evidence for long survival of Acinetobacter calcoaceticus. Infect Cont Hosp Epidemiol 1989; 10: 402-7.
109. Kjolen H, Andersen BM: Handwashing and disinfection of heavily contaminated hands-effective or ineffective? J Hosp Infect 1992; 21: 61-71.
110. Speert DP, Campbell ME: Hospital epidemiology of Pseudomonas aeruginosa from patients with cystic fibrosis. J Hosp Infect 1987; 9: 11-21.
111. Mowrey-McKee MF, Sampson HJ, Proskin HM: Microbial contamination of hydrophilic contact lenses. Part II: Quantitation of microbes after patient handling and after aseptic removal from the eye. CLAO J 1992; 18: 240-44.
112. Hart DE, Shih KL: Surface interactions on hydrogel extended wear contact lenses: microflora and microfauna. Am J Physiol Optom 1987; 64: 739-48.
113. Kilian M, Biberstein EL: Haemophilus. In Krieg NR, Holt JG, (Eds): Bergeys Manual of Systematic Bacteriology. Williams and Wilkins: Baltimore 1984; 558-69.
114. Willcox MD, Power KN, Stapleton F et al: Potential sources of bacteria that are isolated from contact lenses during wear. Optom Vis Sci 1997; 74: 1030-8.
115. Palleroni NJ: Pseudomonas. In Krieg NR, Holt JG (Eds): Bergey's Manual of Systemic Bacteriology, Williams and Wilkins: Baltimore, 1984; 1: 141-99.

116. Grimont PAD, Grimont F: Serratia. In: Krieg NR, Holt JG (Eds). Bergey's Manual of Systematic Bacteriology. Williams and Wilkins: Baltimore, 1984; 1: 477-85.
117. Popoff M: Aeromonas. In Krieg NR, Holt JG (Eds): Bergey's Manual of Systematic Bacteriology. Williams and Wilkins: Baltimore, 1984; 545-8.
118. Power KN, Taylor J, Willocx MDP et al: Possible sources of gram negative contamination of extended wear contact lenses. Aust Microbiologist 1994; 15: A126.
119. Bennett HGB, Hay J, Kirkness CM et al: Antimicrobial management of presumed microbial keratitis: guidelines for treatment of central and peripheral ulcers. Br J Ophthalmol 1998; 82: 137-45.
120. Ormerod LD: Causation and management of microbial keratitis in subtropical Africa. Ophthalmol 1987; 94: 1662-68.
121. Dunlop AAS, Wright ED, Howlader SA et al: Suppurative corneal ulceration in Bangladesh. Aust N Z J Ophthalmol 1994; 22: 105-10.
122. Williams G, Billson F, Husain R et al: Microbiological diagnosis of suppurative keratitis in Bangladesh. Br J Ophthalmol 1987; 71: 315-21.
123. Hagan M, Wright E, Newman M et al: Causes of suppurative keratitis in Ghana. Br J Ophthalmol 1995; 79: 1024-8.
124. Kunimoto DY, Sharma S, Reddy MK et al: Microbial keratitis in children. Ophthalmol 1998; 105: 252-7.
125. Srinivasan M, Gonzales CA, George C et al: Epidemiology and aetiological diagnosis of corneal ulceration in Madurai, south India. Br J Ophthalmol 1997; 81: 965-71.
126. Al-Samarrai AR, Sunba MSN: Bacterial corneal ulcers among Arabs in Kuwait. Ophthalmic Res 1989; 21: 278-84.
127. Upadhyay MP, Karmacharya PCD, Koirala S et al: Epidemiologic characteristics, predisposing factors, and etiologic diagnosis of corneal ulceration in Nepal. Am J Ophthalmol 1991; 111: 92-99.
128. Gonawardena SAS, Ranasinghe KP, Arseculeratne SN et al: Survey of mycotic and bacterial keratitis in Sri Lanka. Mycopathologia 199; 127: 77-81.
129. Wilson LA: Acute bacterial infection of the eye: bacterial keratitis and endophthalmitis. Trans Ophthalmologic Soc U K 1986; 105: 43-60.
130. Wahl JC, Katz HR, Abrams DA: Infectious keratitis in Baltimore. Ann Ophthalmol 1991; 23: 234-37.
131. Levey SB, Katz HR, Abrams DA et al: The role of cultures in the managment of ulcerative keratitis. Cornea 1997; 16: 383-6.
132. Gudmundsson OG, Ormerod D, Kenyon KR et al: Factors influencing predilection and outcome in bacterial keratitis. Cornea 1989; 8: 115-21.
133. Liesegang TJ, Forster RK: Spectrum of microbial keratitis in south Florida. Am J Ophthalmol 1980; 90: 38-47.
134. Cruz OA, Sabir SM, Capo H et al: Microbial keratitis in childhood. Ophthalmol 1993; 100: 192-6.
135. Clinch TE, Palmon FE, Robinson MJ et al: Microbial keratitis in children. Am J Ophthalmol 1994; 117: 65-71.
136. Goldstein MH, Kowalski RP, Gordon YJ: Emerging fluoroquinolone resistance in bacterial keratitis. Ophthalmol 1999; 106: 1313-38.
137. Kunimoto DY, Sharma S, Garg P et al: In vitro susceptibility of bacterial keratitis pathogens to ciprofloxacin. Ophthalmol 1999; 106: 80-85.
138. Liu X: Culture of anaerobic bacteria and antibiotic sensitivity test in ocular infectious diseases. Chung Hua Yen Ko Tsa Chih 1991; 27: 80-83.

139. Eiferman RA, Ogden LL, Snyder J: Anaerobic peptostreptococcal keratitis. Am J Ophthalmol 1985; 100: 335-36.
140. McDonnell JM, Gritz DC, Hwang D et al: Infectious crystalline keratopathy with ring opacity. Cornea 1992; 11: 479-83.
141. Wilkins J, Whitcher JP, Margolis TP: Penicillin-resistant Streptococcus pneumoniae keratitis. Cornea 1993; 15: 99-100.
142. Salabert D, Robinet A, Colin J: Infectious crystalline keratopathy occurring after penetrating keratoplasty (Keratopathie cristalline infectieuse survenue apres keratoplastie transfixiante). J Fr Ophthalmol 1994; 17: 355-7.
143. Touzeau O, Borderie V, Razavi S et al: Use of topical cyclosporin in microcrystalline keratopathy due to Streptococcus. Utilisation topique de ciclosporine dans une keratopathie microcristalline a Streptocoque. J Fr Ophthalmol 1999; 22: 662-5.
144. Patitsas C, Rockwood EJ, Meisler DM et al: Infectious crystalline keratopathy occurring in an eye subsequent to glaucoma filtering surgery with postoperative subconjunctival 5-fluorouracil. Ophthalmic Surg 1991; 22: 412-13.
145. Ormerod LD, Ruoff KL, Meisler DM et al: Infectious crystalline keratopathy. Role of nutritionally variant streptococci and other bacterial factors. Ophthalmol 1991; 98: 159-69.
146. Kintner JC, Grossniklaus HE, Lass JH et al: Infectious crystalline keratopathy associated with topical anesthetic abuse. Cornea 1990; 9: 77-80.
147. Reiss GR, Campbell RJ, Bourne WM: Infectious crystalline keratopathy. Surv Ophthalmol 1986; 31: 69-72.
148. Meisler DM, Langston RH, Naab TJ et al: Infectious crystalline keratopathy. Am J Ophthalmol 1984; 97: 337-43.
149. Donzis PB, Mondino BJ, Weissman BA: Bacillus keratitis associated with contaminated contact lens care systems. Am J Ophthalmol 1988; 105: 195-7.
150. Chandler JW, Milam DF: Diphtheria corneal ulcers. Arch Ophthalmol 1978; 96: 53.
151. Heidemann DG, Dunn SP, Diskin JA et al: Corynebacterium striatus keratitis. Cornea 1991; 10: 81-82.
152. Rubinfeld RS, Cohen EJ, Arentsen JJ et al: Diphtheroids as ocular pathogens. Am J Ophthalmol 1989; 108: 251-4.
153. Holland S, Alfonso E, Gelender H et al: Corneal ulcer due to Listeria monocytogenes. Cornea 1987; 6: 144-6.
154. Zaidman GW, Coudron P, Piros J: Listeria monocytogenes keratitis. Am J Ophthalmol 1990; 109: 334-9.
155. Ford JG, Huang AJ, Pflugfelder SC et al: Nontuberculous mycobacterial keratitis in south Florida. Ophthalmol 1998; 105: 1652-8.
156. Knapp A, Stern GA, Hood CI: Mycobacterium avium-intracellulare corneal ulcer. Cornea 1987; 6: 175-80.
157. Garg P, Athmanathan S, Rao GN: Mycobacterium chelonei masquerading as Corynebacterium in a case of infectious keratitis: a diagnostic dilemma. Cornea 1998; 17: 230-2.
158. McClellan KA, Bernard PJ, Robinson LP et al: Atypical mycobacterial keratitis. Aust N Z J Ophthalmol 1989; 17: 103-5.
159. Lin R, Holland GN, Helm CJ et al: Comparative efficacy of topical ciprofloxacin for treating Mycobacterium fortuitum and Mycobacterium chelonae keratitis in an animal model. Am J Ophthalmol 1994; 117: 657-62.
160. Hu FR, Chang SC, Luh KT et al: The antimicrobial susceptibility of Mycobacterium chelonae isolated from corneal ulcer. Curr Eye Res 1997; 16: 1056-60.

161. Khooshabeh R, Grange JM, Yates MD et al: A case report of Mycobacterium chelonae keratitis and a review of mycobacterial infections of the eye and orbit. Tubercle Lung Dis 1994; 75: 377-82.
162. Bullington RH Jr, Lanier JD, Font RL: Nontuberculous mycobacterial keratitis. Report of two cases and review of the literature. Arch Ophthalmol 1992; 110: 519-24.
163. Dugel PU, Holland GN, Brown HH et al: Mycobacterium fortuitum keratitis. Am J Ophthalmol 1988; 105: 661-9.
164. Levenson DS, Harrison CH: Mycobacterium fortuitum corneal ulcer. Arch Ophthalmol 1966; 75: 189-91.
165. Turner L, Stinson I: Mycobacterium fortuitum as a cause of corneal ulcer. Am J Ophthalmol 1965; 60: 329.
166. Telahun A, Waring GO, Grossniklaus HE: Mycobacterium gordonae keratitis. Cornea 1992; 11: 77-82.
167. Messmer EM, Raizman MB, Foster CS: Lepromatous uveitis diagnosed by iris biopsy. Graefes Arch Clin Exp Ophthalmol 1998; 236: 717-9.
168. Poon A, MacLean H, McKelvie P: Recurrent scleritis in lepromatous leprosy. Aust N Z J Ophthalmol 1998; 26: 51-55.
169. Schonherr U, Naumann GO, Lang GK et al: Sclerokeratitis caused by Mycobacterium marinum. Am J Ophthalmol 1989; 108: 607-8.
170. David DB, Hirst LW, McMillen J et al: Mycobacterium marinum keratitis: pigmentation a clue to diagnosis [letter]. Eye 1999; 13(Pt 3a): 377-9.
171. Zaidman GW: Propionibacterium acnes keratitis. Am J Ophthalmol 1992; 113: 596-8.
172. Liesegang TJ: Bacterial keratitis. In Kaufman HE, Barron BA, McDonald MB (Eds): The Cornea (2nd ed). Butterworth-Heinemann: Boston, 1998; 159-218.
173. Lin A, Driebe WT Jr, Polack P: Alcaligenes xylosoxidans keratitis post penetrating keratoplasty in a rigid gas permeable lens wearer. CLAO J 1998; 24: 239-41.
174. McLeod SD, Goei SL, Taglia DP et al: Nonulcerating bacterial keratitis associated with soft and rigid contact lens wear. Ophthalmol 1998; 105: 517-21.
175. Liesegang TJ, Jones DR, Robinson NM: Azotobacter keratitis. Arch Ophthalmol 1981; 99: 1587-90.
176. Brook I: Recovery of anaerobic bacteria from clinical specimens in 12 years at two military hospitals. J Clin Microbiol 1988; 26: 1181-8.
177. Stern GA, Stock EL: Experimental Bacteroides fragilis keratitis. Arch Ophthalmol 1978; 96: 2264-6.
178. Ormerod LD, Foster CS, Paton BG et al: Ocular Capnocytophaga infection in an edentulous, immunocompetent host. Cornea 1988; 7: 218-22.
179. Heidemann DG, Pflugfelder SC, Kronish J et al: Necrotizing keratitis caused by Capnocytophaga ochracea. Am J Ophthalmol 1988; 105: 655-60.
180. Parenti DM, Snydman DR: Infections in nonimmunocompromised and immunocompromised hosts. J Infect Dis 1985; 151: 140.
181. Klein B, Couch J, Thompson J: Ocular infections associated with Eikenella corrodens. Am J Ophthalmol 1990; 109: 127-31.
182. Khater TT, Jones DB, Wilhelmus KR: Infectious crystalline keratopathy caused by Gram-negative bacteria. Am J Ophthalmol 1997; 124: 19-23.
183. Mason GI, Bottone EJ, Podos SM: Traumatic endophthalmitis caused by an Erwinia species. Am J Ophthalmol 1976; 82: 709-13.

184. Aung T, Chan TK: Nosocomial Klebsiella pneumoniae conjunctivitis resulting in infectious keratitis and bilateral corneal perforation. Cornea 1998; 17: 558-61.
185. Adamson PJW, Jang SS: Ulcerative keratitis associated with Salmonella arizonae infection in a horse. J Am Vet Med Assoc 1985; 186: 1219-20.
186. Lepage P, Bogaerts J, Nsengumuremyi F et al: Metastatic focal infections due to multiresistant Salmonella typhimurium in children: a 34 month experience in Rwanda. Eur J Epidemiol 1986; 2: 99-103.
187. Belfort R Jr., Toledo MR, Burnier M et al: Experimental guinea pig ocular infection by Salmonella typhimurium. Invest Ophthalmol Vis Sci 1985; 26: 591-4.
188. Voino-Iasenetskii MV, Ismailov EM, Dragunskaia EM et al: [Experimental salmonellosis conjunctivitis and keratitis in guinea pigs] Eksperimental'nyi sal'monelleznyi kon'iunktivit i keratit u morskikh svinok. Zh Mikrobiol Epidemiol Immunobiol 1977; 102-5.
189. Kelinske M, Poirier R: Corneal ulceration due to Shigella flexneri. J Ped Ophthalmol Strabismus 1980; 17: 48-51.
190. Tobias JD, Starke JR, Tosi MF: Shigella keratitis: a report of two cases and a review of the literature. Ped Infect Dis 1987; 6: 79-81.
191. Lu PC, Chan JC: Flavobacterium indologenes keratitis. Ophthalmologica 1997; 211: 98-100.
192. Bucci FA, Holland EJ: Flavobacterium meningosepticum keratitis successfully treated with topical trimethoprim-sulfamethoxazole. Am J Ophthalmol 1991; 111: 116-8.
193. Garg P, Sharma S, Rao GN: Ciprofloxacin-resistant Pseudomonas keratitis. Ophthalmol 1999; 106: 1319-23.
194. Forster RK: The management of infectious keratitis as we approach the 21st century. CLAO J 1998; 24: 175-80.
195. Cheng KH, Leung SL, Hoekman HW et al: Incidence of contact-lens-associated microbial keratitis and its related morbidity. Lancet 1999; 354: 181-5.
196. Massey EL, Weston BC: Vibrio vulnificus corneal ulcer: rapid resolution of a virulent pathogen. Cornea 2000; 19: 108-9.
197. Penland RL, Boniuk M, Wilhelmus KR: Vibrio ocular infections on the U.S. Gulf Coast. Cornea 2000; 19: 26-29.
198. Baum J, Fedukowicz HB, Jordan A: A survey of Moraxella corneal ulcers in a derelict population. Am J Ophthalmol 1980; 90: 476-80.
199. Parsons MR, Holland EJ, Agapitos PJ: Nocardia asteroides keratitis associated with extended wear soft contact lens. Can J Ophthalmol 1989; 24: 120-2.
200. Sridhar MS, Sharma S, Reddy MK et al: Clinicomicrobiological review of Nocardia keratitis. Cornea 1998; 17: 17-22.
201. Balcer LJ, Winterkorn JMS, Galetta SL: Neuro-ophthalmic manifestations of Lyme disease. J Neuro-Ophthalmol 1997; 17: 108-21.
202. Baum J, Barza M, Weinstein P et al: Bilateral keratitis as a manifestation of Lyme disease. Am J Ophthalmol 1988; 105: 75-77.
203. Orlin SE, Lauffer JL: Lyme disease keratitis. Am J Ophthalmol 1989; 107: 678-80.
204. Huppertz HI, Munchmeier D, Lieb W: Ocular manifestations in children and adolescents with Lyme arthritis. Br J Ophthalmol 1999; 83: 1149-52.
205. Miyashiro MJ, Yee RW, Patel G et al: Lyme disease associated with unilateral interstitial keratitis. Cornea 1999; 18: 115-6.
206. Mancel E, Merien F, Pesenti L et al: Clinical aspects of ocular leptospirosis in New Caledonia (South Pacific). Aust N Z J Ophthalmol 1999; 27: 380-6.

207. Schwartz GS, Harrison AR, Holland EJ: Etiology of immune stromal (interstitial) keratitis. Cornea 1998; 17: 278-81.
208. Kerr N, Stern GA: Bacterial keratitis associated with vernal keratoconjunctivitis. Cornea 1992; 11: 355-9.
209. Liesgang TJ: Bacterial and fungal keratitis. In: Kaufman HE, Barron BA, McDonald MB, Waltman SR (Eds). The Cornea. New York: Churchill Livingstone; 1988; 217-70.
210. Palmer ML, Hyndiuk MD: Contact lens-related infectious keratitis. Int Ophthalmol Clin 1993; 33: 23-49.
211. O'Callaghan RJ: Role of exoproteins in bacterial keratitis: the fourth annual Thygeson lecture, presented at the Ocular Microbiology and Immunology Group meeting, 1998. Cornea 18: 532-7, 1999.
212. Callegan MC, Engel LS, Hill JM et al: Corneal virulence of Staphylococcus aureus: roles of alpha-toxin and protein A in pathogenesis. Infect Immun 199; 62: 2478-82.
213. O'Callaghan RJ, Callegan MC, Moreau JM et al: Specific roles of alpha-toxin and beta-toxin during Staphylococcus aureus corneal infection. Infect Immun 1997; 65: 1571-8.
214. Arvidson SO: Extracellular enzymes from Staphylococcus aureus. In: Easmon CSF, Adlam C (Eds). Staphylococci and Staphylococcal Infections. Academic Press: London, 1983; 745-808.
215. Coia JE, Browning L, Haines L et al: Comparison of enterotoxins and haemolysins produced by methicillin-resistant (MRSA) and sensitive (MSSA) Staphylococcus aureus. J Med Microbiol 1992; 36: 164-74.
216. Seal D, Ficker L, Ramakrishnan M et al: Role of staphylococcal toxin production in blepharitis. Ophthalmol 1990; 97: 1684-88.
217. Moreau JM, Sloop GM, Engel LS et al: Histopathological studies of staphylococcal alpha-toxin: effects on rabbit corneas. Curr Eye Res 1997; 16: 1221-8.
218. Dajcs JJ, Hume EBH, Moreau JM et al: The role of Staphylococcus aureus gamma-toxin in corneal virulence. Invest Ophthalmol Vis Sci 2000.
219. Ayliffe GAJ: The progressive intercontinental spread of methicillin-resistant Staphylococcus aureus. Clin Infect Dis 1997; 24(1): S74-S79.
220. Aldridge KE, Gelfand MS, Schiro DD et al: The rapid emergence of fluoroquinolone-methicillin-resistant Staphylococcus aureus infections in a community hospital. Diag Microbiol Infect Dis 1992; 15: 601-08.
221. Edmond MB, Wallace SE, McClish DK et al: Nosocomial bloodstream infections in United States hospitals: a three-year analysis. Clin Infect Dis 1999; 29: 239-44.
222. Acar JF, Goldstein FW: Trends in bacterial resistance to fluoroquinolones. Clin Infect Dis 1997; 24 (Suppl 1): S67-S73.
223. Cruciani M, Bassetti D: The fluoroquinolones as treatment for infections caused by Gram-positive bacteria. J of Antimicrob Chemother 1994; 33: 403-17.
224. Durmaz B, Durmaz R, Sahin K: Methicillin-resistance among Turkish isolates of Staphylococcus aureus strains from nosocomial and community infections and their resistance patterns using various antimicrobial agents. J Hosp Infect 1997; 37: 325-9.
225. Harnet S, Brown S, Krishnar C: Emergence of quinolone-resistance among clinical isolates of methicillin-resistant Staphylococcus aureus in Ontario, Canada. Antimicrob Agents Chemother 1991; 35: 1911-3.

226. Hershow RC, Khayr WF, Schreckenberger PC: Ciprofloxacin resistance in methicillin-resistant Staphylococcus aureus: associated factors and resistance to other antibiotics. Am J Ther 1998; 5: 213-20.
227. Wise R, Andrews JM: The in vitro activity and tentative breakpoint of gemifloxacin, a new fluoroquinolone. J Antimicrob Chemother 1999; 44: 679-88.
228. Update: Staphylococcus aureus with reduced susceptibility to vancomycin-United States, 1997, published erratum appears in MMWR Morb Mortal Wkly Rep 46(36): 851, 1997. MMWR Morb Mortal Wkly Rep 1997; 46: 813-15.
229. Chiew YF: Vancomycin-resistant enterococci. Ann Acad Med Singapore 1997; 26: 808-14.
230. Kantzanou M, Tassios PT, Tseleni-Kotsovili A et al: Reduced susceptibility to vancomycin of nosocomial isolates of methicillin-resistant Staphylococcus aureus. J Antimicrob Chemother 1999; 43: 729-31.
231. Tenover FC: Implications of vancomycin-resistant Staphylococcus aureus. J Hosp Infect 43 (Suppl): 1999; S3-S7.
232. Berlet G, Richards RS, Roth JH: Clenched-fist injury complicated by methicillin-resistant Staphylococcus aureus. Can J Surg 1997; 40: 313-14.
233. Ross J, Abate MA: Topical vancomycin for the treatment of Staphylococcus epidermidis and methicillin-resistant Staphylococcus aureus conjunctivitis. DICP Ann Pharmacother 1990; 68: 636-42.
234. Hammond RW, Edmondson W: Treatment of ocular bacterial infections: an update. J Am Optom Assoc 1997; 79: 178-87.
235. Steinert RF: Current therapy for bacterial keratitis and bacterial conjunctivitis. Am J Ophthalmol 1991; 112: 10S-4S.
236. Callegan MC, Engel LS, Hill JM et al: Ciprofloxacin versus tobramycin for the treatment of Staphylococcal keratitis. Invest Ophthalmol Vis Sci 1994; 35: 1033-37.
237. Blumberg HM, Rimland D, Carroll DJ et al: Rapid development ciprofloxacin resistance in methicillin-susceptible and resistant Staphylococcus aureus. J Infect Dis 1991; 163: 1279-85.
238. Fleischer AB, Hoover DL, Khan JA et al: Topical vancomycin formulation for methicillin-resistant Staphylococcus epidermidis blepharoconjunctivitis. Am J Ophthalmol 1986; 101: 283-87.
239. Goodman DF, Gottsch JD: Methicillin-resistant Staphylococcus epidermidis keratitis treated with vancomycin. Arch Ophthalmol 1988; 106: 1570-1.
240. Maffett M, O'Cay DM: Ciprofloxacin-resistant bacterial keratitis. Am J Ophthalmol 1993; 115: 545-6.
241. Supersac G, Piemont Y, Kubina M et al: Assessment of the role of gamma-toxin in experimental endophthalmitis using a hlg-deficient mutant of Staphylococcus aureus. Microb Pathog 1998; 24: 241-51.
242. Siqueira JA, Speeg-Schatz C, Freitas FI et al: Channel-forming leucotoxins from Staphylococcus aureus cause severe inflammatory reactions in a rabbit eye model. J Med Microbiol 1997; 46: 486-94.
243. Fleiszig SMJ, Lee EJ, Wu C et al: Cytotoxic strains of Pseudomonas aeruginosa can damage the intact corneal surface in vitro. CLAO J 1998; 24: 41-47.
244. Kernacki KA, Fridman R, Hazlett LD et al: In vivo characterization of host and bacterial protease expression during Pseudomonas aeruginosa corneal infections in naive and immunized mice. Curr Eye Res 1997; 16: 289-97.

245. Twining SS, Kirschner SE, Mahnke LA et al: Effect of Pseudomonas aeruginosa elastase, alkaline protease, and exotoxin A on corneal proteinases and proteins. Invest Ophthalmol Vis Sci 1993; 34: 2699-712.
246. Horvat RT, Parmely MJ: Pseudomonas aeruginosa alkaline protease degrades human gamma interferon and inhibits its bioactivity. Infect Immun 1988; 56: 2925-32.
247. Van Delden C, Iglewski BH: Cell-to-cell signaling and Pseudomonas aeruginosa infections. Emerg Infect Dis 1998; 4: 551-60.
248. AlonsoDeVelasco E, Verheul AFM, Verhoef J et al: Streptococcus pneumoniae: virulence factors, pathogenesis, and vaccines. Microbiol Rev 1995; 59: 591-603.
249. Pollack M: Pseudomonas aeruginosa. In Mandell GL, Bennett JE, Dolin R (Eds): Principles and Practice of Infectious Diseases. Churchill Livingstone: Philadelphia, 2000.
250. Ottow JC: Ecology, physiology, and genetics of fimbriae and pili. Annu Rev Microbiol 1975; 29: 79-108.
251. Doring G: Virulence factors of Pseudomonas aeruginosa. In Campa M, Bendinelli M Freidman H (Eds): Pseudomonas aeruginosa as an Opportunistic Pathogen. Plenum Press: New York, 1993.
252. Strand CL, Bryant JK, Morgan JW et al: Nosocomial Pseudomonas aeruginosa urinary tract infections. JAMA 1982; 248: 1615-8.
253. Trueb RM, Gloor M, Wuthrich B: Recurrent Pseudomonas folliculitis. Pediatr Dermatol 1994; 11: 35-38.
254. Dart JK: The use of epidemiological techniques to assess risk: the epidemiology of microbial keratitis. Eye 1995; 9: 679-83.
255. Killingsworth DW, Stern GA: Pseudomonas keratitis associated with the use of disposable soft contact lenses. Case report. Arch Ophthalmol 1989; 107: 795-6.
256. Flanigan MJ, Hochstetler LA, Langholdt D et al: Continuous ambulatory peritoneal dialysis catheter infections: diagnosis and management. Perit Dial Int 199; 14: 248-54.
257. Aquino VM, Pappo A, Buchanan GR et al: The changing epidemiology of bacteremia in neutropenic children with cancer [see comments]. Pediatr Infect Dis J 1995; 14: 140-3.
258. Holland SP, Pulido JS, Shires TK et al: Pseudomonas aeruginosa ocular infections. In Fick RB Jr (Eds): Pseudomonas aeruginosa: the Opportunist. CRC Press: Inc Boca Raton, 1993; 159-76.
259. Rolston KV, Bodey GP: Pseudomonas aeruginosa infection in cancer patients. Cancer Invest 1992; 10: 43-59.
260. Flores G, Stavola JJ, Noel GJ: Bacteremia due to Pseudomonas aeruginosa in children with AIDS. Clin Infect Dis 1993; 16: 706-8.
261. Barza M: Use of quinolones for treatment of ear and eye infections. Eur J Clin Microbiol Infect Dis 1991; 10: 296-303.
262. Schein OD, Poggio EC: Ulcerative keratitis in contact lens wearers. Incidence and risk factors. Cornea 1990; 9(1): S55-S58.
263. Stern GA: Update on the medical management of corneal and external eye diseases, corneal transplantation, and keratorefractive surgery. Ophthalmol 1988; 95: 842-54.
264. Iglewski B: Probing Pseudomonas aeruginosa, an opportunistic pathogen. ASM News 1989; 55: 303-7.
265. Barza M: Antibacterial agents in the treatment of ocular infections. Infect Dis Clin N America 1989; 3: 533-51.

266. Aswad MI, John T, Barza M et al: Bacterial adherence to extended wear soft contact lenses. Ophthalmol 1990; 97: 296-302.
267. Baum J, Barza M: Pseudomonas keratitis and extended-wear soft contact lenses. Arch Ophthalmol 1990; 108: 663-4.
268. Fleiszig SMJ, Efron N, Pier GB: Extended contact lens wear enhances Pseudomonas aeruginosa adherence to human corneal epithelium. Invest Ophthalmol Vis Sci 1992; 33: 2908-16.
269. Fleiszig SMJ, Zaidi TS, Fletcher EL et al: Pseudomonas aeruginosa invades corneal epithelial cells during experimental infection. Infect Immun 1994; 62: 3485-93.
270. Fleiszig SMJ, Zaidi TS, Preston MJ et al: Relationship between cytotoxicity and corneal epithelial cell invasion by clinical isolates of Pseudomonas aeruginosa. Infect Immun 1996; 64: 2288-94.
271. Klotz SA, Misra RP, Butrus SI: Contact lens wear enhances adherence of Pseudomonas aeruginosa and binding of lectins to the cornea. Cornea 1990; 9: 266-70.
272. Miller MJ, Wilson LA, Ahearn DG: Adherence of Pseudomonas aeruginosa to rigid gas-permeable contact lenses. Arch Ophthalmol 1991; 109: 1447-8.
273. Stern GA: Pseudomonas keratitis and contact lens wear: the lens/eye is at fault. [Review] [11 refs]. Cornea 1990; 9(1): S36-S38.
274. Zaidi TS, Fleiszig SM, Preston MJ et al: Lipopolysaccharide outer core is a ligand for corneal cell binding and ingestion of Pseudomonas aeruginosa. Invest Ophthalmol Vis Sci 1996; 37: 976-86.
275. Fletcher EL, Weissman BA, Efron N et al: The role of pili in the attachment of Pseudomonas aeruginosa to unworn hydrogel contact lenses. Curr Eye Res 1993; 12: 1067-71.
276. Fletcher EL, Fleiszig SM, Brennan NA: Lipopolysaccharide in adherence of Pseudomonas aeruginosa to the cornea and contact lenses. Invest Ophthalmol Vis Sci 1993; 34: 1930-6.
277. Hazlett LD: Analysis of ocular microbial adhesion. Methods Enzymol 1995; 253: 53-66.
278. Hazlett LD, Moon MM, Singh A et al: Analysis of adhesion, piliation, protease production and ocular infectivity of several P. aeruginosa strains. Curr Eye Res 1991; 10: 351-62.
279. Hazlett LD, Rudner XL: Investigations on the role of flagella in adhesion of Pseudomonas aeruginosa to mouse and human corneal epithelium proteins. Ophthalmic Res 1994; 26: 375-79.
280. Hazlett L, Rudner X, Masinick S et al: In the immature mouse, Pseudomonas aeruginosa pili bind a 57-kd (alpha 206) sialylated corneal epithelial cell surface protein: a first step in infection. Invest Ophthalmol Vis Sci 1995; 36: 634-43.
281. Panjwani N, Zhao Z, Raizman MB et al: Pathogenesis of corneal infection: binding of Pseudomonas aeruginosa to specific phospholipids. Infect Immun 1996; 64: 1819-25.
282. Fleiszig SMJ, Zaidi TS, Pier GB: Pseudomonas aeruginosa invasion of and multiplication within corneal epithelial cells in vitro. Infect Immun 1995; 63: 4072-77.
283. Fleiszig SM, Wiener-Kronish JP, Miyazaki H et al: Pseudomonas aeruginosa-mediated cytotoxicity and invasion correlate with distinct genotypes at the loci encoding exoenzyme S. Infect Immun 1997; 65: 579-86.

284. Frank DW: The exoenzyme S regulon of Pseudomonas aeruginosa. Mol Microbiol 1997; 26: 621-29.
285. Cowell BA, Chen DY, Frank DW et al: ExoT of cytotoxic Pseudomonas aeruginosa prevents uptake by corneal epithelial cells. Infect Immun 2000; 68: 403-6.
286. Kang PJ, Hauser AR, Apodaca G et al: Identification of Pseudomonas aeruginosa genes required for epithelial cell injury. Mol Microbiol 1997; 24: 1249-62.
287. Finck-Barbancon V, Goranson J, Zhu L et al: ExoU expression by Pseudomonas aeruginosa correlates with acute cytotoxicity and epithelial injury. Mol Microbiol 1997; 25: 547-57.
288. Mlot C: Pseudomonas can thwart the eye's multitiered infection defenses. ASM News 2000; 66: 63-64.
289. Hong YQ, Ghebrehiwet B: Effect of Pseudomonas aeruginosa elastase and alkaline protease on serum complement and isolated components C1q and C3. Clin Immunol Immunopathol 1992; 62: 133-8.
290. Parmely M, Gale A, Clabaugh M et al: Proteolytic inactivation of cytokines by Pseudomonas aeruginosa. Infect Immun 1990; 58: 3009-14.
291. Fick RB Jr., Baltimore RS, Squier SU et al: IgG proteolytic activity of Pseudomonas aeruginosa in cystic fibrosis. J Infect Dis 1985; 151: 589-98.
292. Galloway DR: Pseudomonas aeruginosa elastase and elastolysis revisited: recent developments. Mol Microbiol 1991; 5: 2315-21.
293. Heck LW, Alarcon PG, Kulhavy RM et al: Degradation of IgA proteins by Pseudomonas aeruginosa elastase. J Immunol 1990; 144: 2253-57.
294. Heck LW, Morihara K, McRae WB et al: Specific cleavage of human type III and IV collagens by Pseudomonas aeruginosa elastase. Infect Immun 1986; 51: 115-8.
295. Kessler E, Kennah HE, Brown SI: Pseudomonas protease. Purification, partial characterization, and its effect on collagen, proteoglycan, and rabbit corneas. Invest Ophthalmol Vis Sci 1977; 16: 488-97.
296. Goldberg JB, Ohman DE: Activation of an elastase precursor by the LasA gene product of Pseudomonas aeruginosa. J Bacteriol 1987; 169: 4532-9.
297. Kessler E, Safrin M, Abrams WR et al: Inhibitors and specificity of Pseudomonas aeruginosa LasA. J Biol Chem 1997; 272: 9884-9.
298. Peters JE, Galloway DR: Purification and characterization of an active fragment of the LasA protein from Pseudomonas aeruginosa: enhancement of elastase activity. J Bacteriol 1990; 172: 2236-40.
299. Peters JE, Park SJ, Darzins A et al: Further studies on Pseudomonas aeruginosa LasA: analysis of specificity. Mol Microbiol 1992; 6: 1155-62.
300. Schad PA, Iglewski BH: Nucleotide sequence and expression in Escherichia coli of the Pseudomonas aeruginosa lasA gene. J Bacteriol 1988; 170: 2784-89.
301. Engel LS, Hill JM, Caballero AR et al: Protease IV, a unique extracellular protease and virulence factor from Pseudomonas aeruginosa. J Biol Chem 1998; 273: 16792-97.
302. Engel LS, Hill JM, Moreau JM et al: Pseudomonas aeruginosa protease IV produces corneal damage and contributes to bacterial virulence. Invest Ophthalmol Vis Sci 1998; 39: 662-5.
303. Kernacki KA, Hobden JA, Hazlett LD et al: In vivo bacterial protease production during Pseudomonas aeruginosa corneal infection [published erratum appears in Invest Ophthalmol Vis Sci 36(10):1947, 1995]. Invest Ophthalmol Vis Sci 1995; 36: 1371-78.
304. O'Callaghan RJ, Engel LS, Hobden JA et al: Pseudomonas keratitis. The role of an uncharacterized exoprotein, protease IV, in corneal virulence. Invest Ophthalmol Vis Sci 1996; 37: 534-43.

305. Engel LS, Hobden JA, Moreau JM et al: Pseudomonas deficient in protease IV has significantly reduced corneal virulence. Invest Ophthalmol Vis Sci 1997; 38: 1535-42.
306. Schultz G, Khaw PT, Oxford K et al: Growth factors and ocular wound healing. Eye 1994; 8: 184-7.
307. Santa Cruz C, Cohen EJ, Rapuano CJ et al: Microbial keratitis resulting in loss of the eye. Ophthalm Surg Lasers 1998; 29: 803-7.
308. Penland RL, Wilhelmus KR: Emergence of penicillin-resistant Streptococcus pneumoniae ocular infections. Cornea 1998; 17: 135-40.
309. Matoba AY, O'Brien TP, Wilhelmus KR et al: Infectious crystalline keratopathy due to Streptococcus pneumoniae. Ophthalmol 1994; 101: 1000-4.
310. Hejazi A, Falkiner FR: Serratia marcescens. (Review) (123 refs). J Med Microbiol 1997; 46: 903-12.
311. Schein OD, Wasson PJ, Boruchoff SA et al: Microbial keratitis associated with contaminated ocular medications. Am J Ophthalmol 1988; 105: 361-5.
312. Cooper RL, Constable IJ: Infective keratitis in soft contact lens wearers. Br J Ophthalmol 1977; 61: 250-54.
313. Parment PA, Rönnerstam RA: Soft contact lens keratitis associated with Serratia marcescens. Acta Ophthalmol 1981; 59: 560-5.
314. Hilton E, Adams AA, Uliss A et al: Nosocomial bacterial eye infections in intensive-care units. Lancet 1983; 8337: 1318-20.
315. Duffey RJ: Bilateral Serratia marcescens keratitis after simultaneous bilateral radial keratotomy. Am J Ophthalmol 1995; 119: 233-6.
316. Lazachek GW, Boyle GL, Schwartz AL et al: Serratia marcescens, an ocular pathogen; new considerations. Arch Ophthalmol 1971; 86: 599-603.
317. Simcock PR, Butcher JM, Armstrong M et al: Investigation of microbial keratitis: an audit from 1988-1992. Acta Ophthalmologica Scand 1996; 74: 183-6.
318. Knox CM, Dean D: PCR of ribosomal RNA and phylogenetic analysis as a method for identifying microorganisms in bacterial keratitis. Invest Ophthalmol Vis Sci 1996; 37(Suppl): S874.
319. Levine M, Serdarevic O, Mahar M et al: Microbial trends and fluoroquinolone resistance in contact lens related microbial keratitis. Invest Ophthalmol Vis Sci 1996; 37 (Suppl): 876.
320. Holden BA, LaHood D, Grant T et al: Gram-negative bacteria can induce contact lens related acute red eye (CLARE) responses. CLAO J 1996; 22: 47-52.
321. Willcox MD, Hume EB: Differences in the pathogenesis of bacteria isolated from contact-lens-induced infiltrative conditions. Aust N Z J Ophthalmol 1999; 27: 231-3.
322. Donnenfeld ED, Schrier A, Perry HD et al: Infectious keratitis with corneal perforation associated with corneal hydrops and contact lens wear in keratoconus. Br J Ophthalmol 1996; 80: 409-12.
323. Kreger A, Griffin O: Cornea damaging proteases of Serratia marcescens. Investigative Ophthalmol 1975; 14: 190-98.
324. Hume EB, Conerly LL, Moreau JM et al: Serratia marcescens keratitis: strain-specific corneal pathogenesis in rabbits. Curr Eye Res 1999; 19: 525-32.
325. Ang-Kucuker M, Buyukbaba-Boral O, Tolun V et al: Effect of some antibiotics on pigmentation in Serratia marcescens [In Process Citation]. Zentralbl Bakteriol 2000; 289: 781-85.
326. Lyerly D, Gray L, Kreger A: Characterization of rabbit corneal damage produced by Serratia keratitis and by a serratia protease. Infect Immun 1981; 33: 927-32.

327. Molla A, Matsumoto K, Oyamada I et al: Degradation of protease inhibitors, immunoglobulins, and other serum proteins by Serratia protease and its toxicity to fibroblast in culture. Infect Immun 1986; 53: 522-9.
328. Miyagawa S, Matsumoto K, Kamata R et al: Spreading of Serratia marcescens in experimental keratitis and growth suppression by chicken egg white ovomacroglobulin. Jpn J Ophthalmol 1991; 35: 402-10.
329. Kamata R, Matsumoto K, Okamura R et al: The Serratial 56K protease as a major pathogenic factor in serratial keratitis. Ophthalmol 1985; 92: 1452-9.
330. Matsumoto K, Miyajima S, Kimura A et al: Matrix metalloproteinase (MMP) in experimental Serratial keratitis in guinea pig. Invest Ophthalmol Vis Sci 1996; 37 (Suppl): S1014.
331. Matsumoto K, Shams NBK, Hanninen LA et al: Cleavage and activation of corneal matrix metalloproteases by Pseudomonas aeruginosa isolates. Invest Ophthalmol Vis Sci 1993; 34: 1945-53.
332. Parment PA: The role of Serratia marcescens in soft contact lens associated ocular infections. Acta Ophthalmologica Scand 1997; 75: 67-71.
333. Templeton WC III, Eiferman RA, Snyder JW et al: Serratia keratitis transmitted by contaminated eyedroppers. Am J Ophthalmol 1982; 93: 723-6.
334. Chang WJ, Tse DT, Rosa RH Jr et al: Periocular atypical mycobacterial infections. Ophthalmol 1999; 106: 86-90.
335. Mirate DJ, Hull DS, Steel JH Jr et al: Mycobacterium chelonei keratitis: a case report. Br J Ophthalmol 1983; 67: 324-6.
336. Meisler DM, Friedlaender MH, Okumoto M: Mycobacterium chelonei keratitis. Am J Ophthalmol 192; 94: 398-401.
337. Willis WE, Laibson PR: Intractable Mycobacterium fortuitum corneal ulcer in man. Am J Ophthalmol 1971; 71: 500-4.
338. Zimmerman LE, Turner L, McTigue JW: Mycobacterium fortuitum infection of the cornea. A report of two cases. Arch Ophthalmol 1969; 82: 596-601.
339. Hirst LW, Harrison GK, Merz WG et al: Nocardia asteroides keratitis. Br J Ophthalmol 1979; 63: 449-54.
340. van Bijesterveld OP: The incidence of moraxella on mucous membranes and the skin. Am J Ophthalmol 1972; 74: 72-76.
341. Park M: Ocular manifestations of Lyme disease. J Am Optom Assoc 1989; 60: 284-9.
342. Orlin SE, Lauffer JL: Lyme disease keratitis. Am J Ophthalmol 1989; 107: 678-80.
343. Kornmehl EW, Lesser RL, Jaros P et al: Bilateral keratitis in Lyme disease. Ophthalmol 1989; 96: 1194-97.
344. Flach AJ, Lavoie PE: Episcleritis, conjunctivitis, and keratitis as ocular manifestations of Lyme disease. Ophthalmol 1990; 97: 973-75.
345. Winterkorn JM: Lyme disease: neurologic and ophthalmic manifestations. Surv Ophthalmol 1990; 35: 191-204.
346. Karma A, Seppala I, Mikkila H et al: Diagnosis and clinical characteristics of ocular Lyme borreliosis [see comments]. Am J Ophthalmol 1995; 119: 127-35.
347. Lesser RL: Ocular manifestations of Lyme disease. Am J Med 1995; 98(4A): 60S-2S.
348. Deschenes J, Seamone C, Baines M: The ocular manifestations of sexually transmitted diseases. Can J Ophthalmol 1990; 25: 177-85.
349. Knox CM, Holsclaw DS: Interstitial keratitis. Int Ophthalmol Clin 1998; 38: 183-95.
350. Gritz DC, Whitcher JP: Topical issues in the treatment of bacterial keratitis. Int Ophthalmol Clin 1998; 38: 107-14.

351. Vajpayee RB, Dada T, Saxena R et al: Study of the first contact management profile of cases of infectious keratitis: a hospital-based study. Cornea 2000; 19: 52-56.
352. Diamond J, Leeming J, Coombs G et al: Corneal biopsy with tissue micro-homogenisation for isolation of organisms in bacterial keratitis. Eye 1999; 13: 545-49.
353. Lee SE, Kim SY, Kim SJ et al: Direct identification of Vibrio vulnificus in clinical specimens by nested PCR. J Clin Microbiol 1998; 36: 2887-92.
354. Knox CM, Cevellos V, Dean D: 16S ribosomal DNA typing for identification of pathogens in patients with bacterial keratitis. J Clin Microbiol 1998; 36: 3492-6.
355. Ikonomopoulos JA, Gorgoulis VG, Zacharatos PV et al: Multiplex PCR assay for the detection of mycobacterial DNA sequences directly from sputum. In Vivo 1998; 12: 547-52.
356. Towner KJ, Talbot DC, Curran R et al: Development and evaluation of a PCR-based immunoassay for the rapid detection of methicillin-resistant Staphylococcus aureus. J Med Microbiol 1998; 47: 607-13.
357. McCabe KM, Zhang YH, Huang BL et al: Bacterial species identification after DNA amplification with a universal primer pair. Mol Genet Metab 1999; 66: 205-11.
358. Winters DK, Maloney TP, Johnson MG: Rapid detection of Listeria monocytogenes by a PCR assay specific for an aminopeptidase. Mol Cell Probes 1999; 13: 127-31.
359. Gillespie SH: The role of the molecular laboratory in the investigation of Streptococcus pneumoniae infections. Semin Respir Infect 1999; 14: 269-75.
360. Ke D, Picard FJ, Martineau F et al: Development of a PCR assay for rapid detection of enterococci. J Clin Microbiol 1999; 37: 3497-503.
361. Morrison KE, Lake D, Crook J et al: Confirmation of psaA in all 90 serotypes of Streptococcus pneumoniae by PCR and potential of this assay for identification and diagnosis. J Clin Microbiol 2000; 38: 434-7.
362. Beggs ML, Stevanova R, Eisenach KD: Species identification of Mycobacterium avium complex isolates by a variety of molecular techniques. J Clin Microbiol 2000; 38: 508-12.
363. Ke D, Menard C, Picard FJ et al: Development of conventional and real-time PCR assays for the rapid detection of group B streptococci [In Process Citation]. Clin Chem 2000; 46: 324-31.
364. Speciale A, Musumeci R, Blandino G et al: Molecular mechanisms of resistance in Pseudomonas aeruginosa to fluoroquinolones. Int J Antimicrob Agents 2000; 14: 151-6
365. Watterson SA, Wilson SM, Yates MD et al: Comparison of three molecular assays for rapid detection of rifampin resistance in Mycobacterium tuberculosis. J Clin Microbiol 1998; 36: 1969-73.
366. Petrich AK, Luinstra KE, Groves D et al: Direct detection of vanA and vanB genes in clinical specimens for rapid identification of vancomycin resistant enterococci (VRE) using multiplex PCR. Mol Cell Probes 1999; 13: 275-81.
367. Mullin GS, Rubinfeld RS: The antibacterial activity of topical anesthetics. Cornea 1997; 16: 662-5.
368. Callegan MC, Hobden JA, Hill JM et al: Topical antibiotic therapy for the treatment of experimental Staphylococcus aureus keratitis. Invest Ophthalmol Vis Sci 1992; 33: 3017-23.
369. Engel LS, Callegan MC, Hill JM et al: The effectiveness of two ciprofloxacin formulations for experimental Pseudomonas and Staphylococcus keratitis. Jpn J Ophthalmol 1996; 40: 212-9.

370. Hobden JA, O'Callaghan RJ, Hill JM et al: Ciprofloxacin and prednisolone therapy for experimental Pseudomonas keratitis. Curr Eye Res 1992; 11: 259-66.
371. Araque M, Velazco E: In vitro activity of fleroxacin against multiresistant gram-negative bacilli isolated from patients with nosocomial infections. Intensive Care Med 1998; 24: 839-44.
372. Callegan MC, Hill JM, Insler MS et al: Methicillin-resistant Staphylococcus aureus keratitis in the rabbit: therapy with ciprofloxacin, vancomycin and cefazolin. Curr Eye Res 1992; 11: 1111-9.
373. Insler MS, Fish LA, Silbernagel J et al: Successful treatment of methicillin-resistant Staphylococcus aureus with topical ciprofloxacin. Ophthalmol 1991; 98: 1690-2.
374. Sanders CC, Sanders WE, Thomson KS: Fluoroquinolone resistance in Staphylococci: new challenges. Europ J Clin Microbiol and Infect Dis 1(Suppl): 1995; s6-s11.
375. Wilhelmus KR, Penland RL: Emerging resistance among ocular isolates of gram-positive cocci. Invest Ophthalmol Vis Sci 1996; 37 (Suppl): s877.
376. Hume EBH, Moreau JM, Conerly LL et al: Clarithromycin for experimental Staphylococcus aureus keratitis. Curr Eye Res 1999; 18: 358-62.
377. Hiramatsu K, Aritaka N, Hanaki H et al: Dissemination in Japanese hospitals of strains of Staphylococcus aureus heterogeneously resistant to vancomycin. Lancet 1997; 350: 1670-73.
378. Peterson DL: Vancomycin-resistant Staphylococcus aureus. Infect Med 1999; 16: 235-38.
379. Masecar BL, Robillard NJ: Spontaneous quinolone resistance in Serratia marcescens due to a mutation in gyrA. Antimicrob Agents and Chemother 1991; 35: 898-902.
380. Neu HC: Bacterial resistance to fluoroquinolones. Rev Infect Dis 10 (suppl): 1988; s57-s82.
381. Clavo-Sánchez AJ, Girón-González JA, López-Prieto D et al: Multivariate analysis of risk factors for infection due to penicillin-resistant and multidrug-resistant Streptococcus pneumoniae: a multicenter study. Clin Infect Dis 1997; 24: 1052-9.
382. Seal DV: Antibiotic management of presumed microbial keratitis. HKJ Ophthalmol 1998; 1: 129-38.
383. Robinson A, Kremer I, Avisar R et al: The combination of topical ceftazidime and aminoglycosides in the treatment of refractory pseudomonal keratitis. Graefes Arch Clin Exp Ophthalmol 1999; 237: 177-80.
384. Ogawa GSH, Hyndiuk RA: The fluoroquinolones: new antibiotics in ophthalmology. Int Ophthalmol Clin 1993; 33: 59-68.
385. Isenberg HD, Alperstein P, France K: In vitro activity of ciprofloxacin, levofloxacin, and trovafloxacin, alone and in combination with beta-lactams, against clinical isolates of Pseudomonas aeruginosa, Stenotrophomonas maltophilia, and Burkholderia cepacia. Diagn Microbiol Infect Dis 1999; 33: 81-86.
386. Velpandian T, Gupta SK, Gupta YK et al: Comparative studies on topical lomefloxacin and ciprofloxacin on ocular kinetic and experimental corneal ulcer. J Ocul Pharmacol Ther 1999; 15: 505-11.
387. Panda A, Ahuja R, Sastry SS: Comparison of topical 0.3% ofloxacin with fortified tobramycin plus cefazolin in the treatment of bacterial keratitis (In Process Citation). Eye 1999; 13:744-7.
388. Vajpayee RB, Sharma N, Verma B et al: Topical pefloxacin in bacterial keratitis. Int Ophthalmol 1998; 22: 47-51.
389. Jensen HG, Felix C: In vitro antibiotic susceptibilities of ocular isolates in North and South America. Cornea 1998; 17: 79-87.

390. Heidemann DG, Alfonso E, Forster RK et al: Branhamella catarrhalis keratitis. Am J Ophthalmol 1987; 103: 576-81.
391. Kaplan EL: Recent evaluation of antimicrobial resistance in ß-hemolytic streptococci. Clin Infect Dis 1997; 24 (suppl 1): S89-S92.
392. Callegan MC, O'Callaghan RJ, Hill JM: Pharmacokinetic considerations in the treatment of bacterial keratitis. Clin Pharmacokinet 1994; 27: 1-21.
393. Badenoch PR, Coster DJ: Antibiotics and corticosteroids: functions and interaction in ocular disease. In: Cavanagh HD (Ed). The Cornea: Transactions of the World Congress on the Cornea III. New York: Raven Press; 1988; 475-83.
394. Carmichael TR, Gelfand Y, Welsh NH: Topical steroids in the treatment of central and paracentral corneal ulcers. Br J Ophthalmol 1990; 74: 528-31.
395. Frangie JP, Leibowitz HM: Steroids. Int Ophthalmol Clin 1993; 33: 9-29.
396. Gritz DC, Kwitko S, Trousdale MD et al: Recurrence of microbial keratitis concomitant with antiinflammatory treatment in an animal model. Cornea 1992, 11: 404-8.
397. Stern GA, Buttross M: Use of corticosteroids in combination with antimicrobial drugs in the treatment of infectious corneal disease. Ophthalmol 1991; 98: 847-53.
398. Laibson PR: Pseudomonas aeruginosa. In Fraunfelder FT, Roy FH (Eds): Current Ocular Therapy. WB Saunders: Philadelphia, 1990; 35-37.
399. O'Day DM: Corticosteroids: an unresolved debate. Ophthalmol 1991; 98: 845-46.
400. Hobden JA, Engel LS, Callegan MC et al: Pseudomonas aeruginosa keratitis in leukopenic rabbits. Curr Eye Res 1993; 12: 469-73.
401. Kernacki KA, Barrett RP, Hobden JA, et al: Macrophage inflammatory protein-2 is a mediator of polymorphonuclear neutrophil influx in ocular bacterial infection. J Immunol 2000; 164: 1037-45.
402. Sloop GD, Moreau JM, Conerly LL et al: Acute inflammation of the eyelid and cornea in Staphylococcus keratitis in the rabbit. Invest Ophthalmol Vis Sci 1999; 40: 385-91.
403. Engel LS, Callegan MC, Hobden JA et al: Effectiveness of specific antibiotic/steroid combinations for therapy of experimental Pseudomonas aeruginosa keratitis. Curr Eye Res 1995; 14: 229-34.
404. Hobden JA, Engel LS, Hill JM et al: Prednisolone acetate or prednisolone phosphate concurrently administered with ciprofloxacin for the therapy of experimental Pseudomonas aeruginosa keratitis. Curr Eye Res 1993; 12: 469-73.
405. Hobden JA, Hill JM, Engel LS et al: The effect of age on the therapeutic outcome of experimental Pseudomonas aeruginosa keratitis treated with ciprofloxacin, prednisolone, and flurbiprofen. Antimicrob Agents Chemother 1993; 37: 1856-9.
406. Flach AJ: Nonsteroidal anti-inflammatory drugs in ophthalmology. In Smolin G, Friedlander MH (Eds): International Ophthalmology Clinics. Pharmacology. Little, Brown and Company: Boston, 1993; 1-7.
407. Gritz DC, Lee TY, Kwitko S et al: Topical antiinflammatory agents in an animal model of microbial keratitis. Arch Ophthalmol 1990; 108: 1001-5.
408. Leopold IH, Gaster RN: Ocular inflammation and antiinflammatory drugs. In Kaufman HE, Barron BA, McDonald MB, Waltman SR (Eds): The Cornea. Churchill Livingstone: New York, 1988; 67-84.
409. Moreira H, McDonnell PJ, Fasano AP et al: Treatment of experimental Pseudomonas keratitis with cyclo-oxygenase and lipoxygenase inhibitors. Ophthalmol 1991; 98: 1693-97.

410. Ohadi C, Litwin KL, Moreira H et al: Anti-inflammatory therapy and outcome in a guinea pig model of Pseudomonas keratitis. Cornea 1992; 11: 398-403.
411. Hartstein AI, LeMonte AM, Iwamoto PK: DNA typing and control of methicillin-resistant Staphylococcus aureus at two affiliated hospitals. Infect Control Hosp Epidemiol 1997; 18: 42-48.
412. Hoefnagels-Schuermans A, Borremans A, Peetermans W et al: Origin and transmission of methicillin-resistant Staphylococcus aureus in an endemic situation: differences between geriatric and intensive-care patients. J Hosp Infect 1997; 36: 209-22.
413. Flournoy DJ: Methicillin-resistant Staphylococcus aureus at a Veterans Affairs Medical Center (1986-96). J Okla State Med Assoc 1997; 90: 228-35.
414. Herold BC, Immergluck LC, Maranan MC et al: Community-acquired methicillin-resistant Staphylococcus aureus in children with no identified predisposing risk [see comments]. JAMA 1998; 279: 593-8.
415. Lindenmayer JM, Schoenfeld S, O'Grady R et al: Methicillin-resistant Staphylococcus aureus in a high school wrestling team and the surrounding community. Arch Intern Med 1998; 158: 895-9.
416. Maguire GP, Arthur AD, Boustead PJ et al: Clinical experience and outcomes of community-acquired and nosocomial methicillin-resistant Staphylococcus aureus in a northern Australian hospital. J Hosp Infect 1998; 38: 273-81.
417. Shahin R, Johnson IL, Jamieson F et al: Methicillin-resistant Staphylococcus aureus carriage in a child care center following a case of disease. Toronto Child Care Center Study Group. Arch Pediatr Adolesc Med 1999; 153: 864-8.
418. Frank AL, Marcinak JF, Mangat PD et al: Community-acquired and clindamycin-susceptible methicillin-resistant Staphylococcus aureus in children. Pediatr Infect Dis J 1999; 18: 993-1000.
419. Gorak EJ, Yamada SM, Brown JD: Community-acquired methicillin-resistant Staphylococcus aureus in hospitalized adults and children without known risk factors [see comments]. Clin Infect Dis 1999; 29: 797-800.
420. Morgan M, Evans-Williams D, Salmon R et al: The population impact of MRSA in a country: the national survey of MRSA in Wales, 1997. J Hosp Infect 2000; 44: 227-39.
421. File TM Jr: Overview of resistance in the 1990s. Chest 1999; 115(Suppl 3): 3S-8S.
422. Kirwan JF, Potamitis T, El-Kasaby H et al: Lesson of the week: microbial keratitis in intensive care. Br Med J 1997; 314: 433-4.
423. Edgeworth JD, Treacher DF, Eykyn SJ: A 25-year study of nosocomial bacteremia in an adult intensive care unit [see comments]. Crit Care Med 1999; 27: 1421-8.
424. Yu WL, Lin CW, Wang DY: Serratia marcescens bacteremia: clinical features and antimicrobial susceptibilities of the isolates. Chung Hua Min Kuo Wei Sheng Wu Chi Mien I.Hsueh Tsa Chih 1998; 31: 171-9.
425. Lu CH, Chang WN, Chuang YC et al: Gram-negative bacillary meningitis in adult post-neurosurgical patients. Surg Neurol 1999; 52: 438-43.
426. Matteelli A, Signorini L, Tebaldi A et al: Long term treatment with clarithromycin for cryptosporidiosis and emergence of drug resistant disseminated infection due to Mycobacterium avium: case report. J Chemother 1998; 10: 474-5.
427. Long R, Nobert E, Chomyc S et al: Transcontinental spread of multidrug-resistant Mycobacterium bovis. Am J Respir Crit Care Med 1999; 159: 2014-17.

428. Vernon A, Burman W, Benator D et al: Acquired rifamycin monoresistance in patients with HIV-related tuberculosis treated with once-weekly rifapentine and isoniazid. Tuberculosis Trials Consortium. Lancet 1999; 353: 1843-7.
429. Griffith DE: Risk-benefit assessment of therapies for Mycobacterium avium complex infections. Drug Saf 1999; 21: 137-52.
430. Salamina G, Sodano L, Mezzetti F et al: The threat of multidrug-resistant tuberculosis: results of 1 yr of surveillance in the Lombardy region of Italy. Monaldi Arch Chest Dis 1999; 54: 332-36.

Chapter 14

Recommended Antibiotic Dosages for Various Clinical Conditions of the Eye

Ashok Garg (India)

In this chapter I shall discuss important optimal antibiotic dosages in various ocular clinical conditions and surgical prophylaxis of the eye.

Table 14.1: Recommended non-toxic doses of anti-microbial infusion fluids for vitrectomy

Agent	*Dose (mg/ml)*
Aminoglyosides	
Gentamicin	0.008
Tobramycin	0.010
Amikacin	0.010
Penicillins	
Penicillin G	0.010
Methicillin	0.020
Oxacilin	0.010
Dicloxacillin	0.010
Clindamycin	0.009
Chloramphenicol	0.010
Lincomycin	0.010
Imipenem	0.010
Ciprofloxacin	0.010
Ofloxacin	0.010
Pefloxacin	0.010
Lomefloxacin	0.010
Sparfloxacin	0.010
Gatifloxacin	0.010
Moxifloxacin	0.010
Ceftazidine	0.040
Vancomycin	0.030

Table 14.2: Recommended doses of intravitreal antimicrobial agents

Agent	*Dose (mg/0.1ml)*
a. *Aminoglycosides*	
Gentamicin	0.10
Tobramycin	0.10
Amikacin	0.40
Netilmicin	0.10
Kanamycin	0.40
b. *Cephalosporins*	
Cefazolin	2.25
Cephalothin	2.0
Cephaloridine	0.25
c. *Penicillins*	
Methicillin	2.0
Oxacillin	0.50
Carbenicillin	2.0
Ampicillin	5.0
d. *Fluoroquinolones*	
Norfloxacin	0.10
Ciprofloxacin	0.10
Ofloxacin	0.10
Pefloxacin	0.10
Lomefloxacin	0.08
Sparfloxacin	0.08
Levofloxacin	0.10
Gatifloxacin	0.10
Moxifloxacin	0.10
Vancomycin	1.0
Clindamycin	0.45-1.0
Erythromycin	0.50
Roxithromycin	0.50
Clarithromycin	0.50
Chloramphenicol	2.0
Lincomycin	1.5
Imipenem	0.50

Table 14.3: Preparation of intravitreal antibiotic injections

Drug	*Vial size (Commercial)*	*Amount of initial diluent (ml)*	*Initial conc (per ml)*	*Aliquot (ml)*	*Vol Nos. (ml)*	*Final conc (per ml)*	*Final intravitreal dose in (0.1 ml)*
Amikacin	500 mg/2 ml	–	250 mg	0.1	6.15	4 mg	400 µg
Ampicillin	1 g	3.4	250 mg	0.3	1.2	50 mg	5 mg
Cefazolin	500 mg	2.0	225 mg	0.1	0.9	22.5 mg	2.25 mg
Chloram-phenicol	2 mg	1 g	100 mg	0.1	0.4	20 mg	2 mg
Clindamycin	300 mg/2 ml	–	150 mg	0.1	1.4	10 mg	1 mg
Gentamicin	80 mg/2 ml	–	40 mg	0.1	1.9	2 mg	200 ug
Kanamycin	500 mg/2 ml	–	250 mg	0.1	4.9	50 mg	5 mg
Vancomycin	500 mg	10.0	50 mg	0.2	0.8	10 mg	1 mg
Tobramycin	80 mg/2 ml	–	40 mg/ml	0.5 ml	0.5 ml	2 mg/ml	0.2 mg/ 0.1 ml

Table 14.4: Various topical antibiotic preparations (Fortified and commercial with dosages)

Antibiotic preparation	*Commercial drops*	*Fortified drops*	*Self life*	*Subconjunctival final doses*
Chloramphenicol	0.4-1.0%	5-10 mg/ml	15 days	100 mg
Penicillin	100000 units/ml	0.15-0.30 lac IU/ml	24 hours	1 million units/ml
Framycetin	0.5%	NE	NE	–
Gentamicin	0.3%	20 mg/ml	30 days (RT)	20-40 mg
Tobramycin	0.3%	20 mg/ml	30 days (RT)	20-40 mg
Amikacin	3%	10-20 mg/ml	30 days (RT)	25-50 mg
Sisomicin	0.3%	20 mg/ml	30 days (RT)	20-40 mg
Neomycin	0.17%	30-40 mg/ml	7 days ®	250-500 mg
Netilmycin	NE	15-20 mg/ml	7 days ®	–
Kanamycin	NE	10 mg/ml	7 days ®	–
Tetracycline	1	NE	NE	–
Polymixin B	0.5-1.0%	1-2 mg/ml	1 week ®	10000 units/ml
Bacitracin	NE	10000 units/ml	7 days ®	5000 units
Erythromycin	NE	5 mg/ml	14 days (RT)	100 mg/ml
Roxithromycin	NE	5 mg/ml	14 days (RT)	100 mg/ml
Clarithromycin	NE	5 mg/ml	14 days (RT)	100 mg/ml
Norfloxacin	0.3%	20 mg/ml	14 days ®	20-40 mg/ml
Ciprofloxacin	0.3%	20 mg/ml	14 days ®	20-40 mg/ml
Oxfloxacin	0.3%	20 mg/ml	14 days ®	20-40 mg/ml
Pefloxacin	0.3%	20 mg/ml	14 days ®	20-40 mg/ml
Lomefloxacin	0.3%	20 mg/ml	14 days ®	20-40 mg/ml
Sparfloxacin	0.3%	20 mg/ml	14 days ®	20-40 mg/ml
Levofloxacin	0.5%	20 mg/ml	14 days ®	20-40 mg/ml
Gatifloxacin	0.3%	20 mg/ml	14 days ®	20-40 mg/ml
Moxifloxacin	0.5%	20 mg/ml	14 days ®	20-40 mg/ml
Cephaloridine	NE	50 mg/ml	7 days ®	100 mg/ml
Cephamandole	NE	50 mg/ml	7 days ®	100 mg

Contd...

Contd...

Antibiotic preparation	*Commercial drops*	*Fortified drops*	*Self life*	*Sub conjunctival final doses*
Cephazolin	NE	50 mg/ml	7 days ®	100 mg
Cefoperazone	NE	40-50 mg/ml	7 days ®	100 mg
Cefadroxyl	NE	40-50 mg/ml	7 days ®	100 mg
Ceftriaxone	NE	130 mg/ml	10 days ®	100 mg
Ampicillin	NE	10 mg/ml	7 days ®	–
Penicillin G	NE	100000 units/ml	24 hours ®	1 million units ml
Methicillin	NE	4 mg/ml	7 days ®	–
Carbenicillin	NE	4 mg/ml	7 days ®	100 mg
Vancomycin	NA	20 mg/ml	1 week ®	25 mg
Clindamycin	NA	10 mg/ml	7 days ®	–
Ticarcillin	NA	6 mg/ml	7 days ®	–

For fortified drops use BSS or isotonic saline (For 5% fortified drops, 50 mg/ml, dissolve 500 mg of salt in 10 CC of BSS)

Table 14.5: Initial topical antibiotic therapy choice for external ocular infections based on Gram's stain findings

Bacteria type	*Drugs of choice (fortified)*	*Alternative drug (Fortified and Non-fortified)*
1. Gram-positive cocci	Cefazolin 100 mg/ml	Vancomycin 25 mg/ml Bacitracin 10000 units/ml Ciprofloxacin, Lomefloxacin } 20 mg/ml Gatifloxacin
2. Gram-positive bacilli	Penicillin G 100000 units/ml	Vancomycin—25-50 mg/ml Bacitracin—1000 units/ml
3. Gram-positive rods	Gentamicin 14 mg/ml	Tobramycin—14 mg/ml
4. Gram-negative cocci	Ceftriaxone 50 mg/ml	Ofloxacin, Lomefloxacin, Sparfloxacin, Moxifloxacin } 20 mg/ml Chloramphenicol—5 mg/ml
5. Gram-negative bacilli	Tobramycin 14 mg/ml Amikacin 10 mg/ml Ticarcillin 6 mg/ml	Gentamicin—14 mg/ml Polymixin B-50000 units/ml Ciprofloxacin, Ofloxacin, Gatifloxacin, Lomefloxacin } 20 mg/ml
6. Bacteria suspected (No organism seen)	Cefazolin 100 mg/ml and Tobramycin 14 mg/ml	Gentamicin—14 mg/ml or Amikacin—10 mg/ml plus Vancomycin—25 mg/ml or Lomefloxacin Sparfloxacin 20 mg/ml Moxifloxacin

Table 14.6: Topical antibiotic therapy for culture specific bacterial ulcers

Organism	*Topical (Fortified or non-fortified)*	*Subconjunctival*
1. *Pseudomonas*	Tobramycin 14 mg/ml or Amikacin—10 mg/ml Lomefloxacin, Sparfloxacin, Gatifloxacin }	Tobramycin 40 mg (1 ml) Amikacin 25 mg 20 mg/ml
2. *Staphylococcus*	Cefazolin 100 mg/ml Vancomycin 25-50 mg/ml or Bacitracin—10000 units/ml	Cefazolin —100 mg Vancomycin—25 mg Oxacillin—100 mg
3. *Proteus*	Gentamicin 14 mg/ml Tobramycin 14 mg/ml Amikacin 10 mg/ml Ceftriaxone 50 mg/ml	Gentamicin—20-40 mg Amikacin—25 mg Carbenicillin—100 mg
4. *Enterobacter* *E. coli* *Klebsiella* *Acinetobacter*	Tobramycin 14 mg/ml Amikacin 10 mg/ml Pefloxacin, Sparfloxacin, Lomefloxacin, Gatifloxacin } 20-40 mg	Tobramycin—40 mg Amikacin—25 mg Pefloxacin Sparfloxacin Lomefloxacin Moxifloxacin

Table 14.7: Specific antibiotics therapy for the treatment of bacterial endophthalmitis

Microorganisms	*Intravitreal injection*	*Systemic therapy*	*Topical/sub-conjunctival*
Staphylococcus	Vancomycin/Cefazolin	Cefazolin	Cefazolin/vancomycin
Streptococcus	Vancomycin/Cefazolin	Cefazolin and Ampicillin	Cefazolin/vancomycin
Haemophilus	Chloramphenicol	Ceftazidine/ Ciprofloxacin Gatifloxacin	Lomefloxacin/ Ciprofloxacin Moxifloxacin
Propioni-bacterium	Vancomycin	Penicillin/ Erythromycin Cloxithromycin	Vancomycin/ Penicillin Cefazolin
Coryne-bacterium	Vancomycin and Cefazolin	Cefazolin	Cefazolin
Bacillus	Clindamycin and Amikacin/ Vancomycin	Clindamycin and Gentamicin Ciprofloxacin Gatifloxacin	Clindamycin and Gentamicin/ Cipro/Sparfloxacin Moxifloxacin
Listeria	Ampicillin and Vancomycin	Ampicillin	Vancomycin

Contd...

Contd...

Microorganisms	*Intravitreal injection*	*Systemic therapy*	*Topical/sub-conjunctival*
Clostridium	Clindamycin/Penicillin	Clindamycin/ Penicillin	Clindamycin/ Penicillin
Nocardia	Amikacin	Cotrimoxazole	Amikacin
Pseudomonas	Amikacin/Ceftazidime	Moxifloxacin/ Ceftazidime	Gatifloxacilin/ Gentamicin/ Lomefloxacin
Enterobacter	Amikacin	Amikacin	Amikacin
Proteus	Sisomycin and Cefazolin	Cefazolin and Ofloxacin Moxifloxacin	Gentamicin Ofloxacin Gatifloxacin
Serratia	Amikacin	Gentamicin/ Lomefloxacin Gatifloxacin	Gentamicin/ Lomefloxacin Moxifloxacin
Klebsiella	Amikacin	Cefazolin/ Gentamicin	Cefazolin/ Gentamicin

BIBLIOGRAPHY

1. Agarwal Amar. Textbook of Ophthalmology, ed.1, New Delhi : Jaypee Medical Publishers, 2002.
2. Bartlett JD. Clinical Ocular Pharmacology, ed. 4. Boston: Butterworth-Heinemann, 2001.
3. Bartlett JD. Ophthalmic Drug facts. Lippincott – William and Wilkins, 2001.
4. Crick RP, Trimble RB. Textbook of Clinical Ophthalmology: Hodder and Stoughton, 1986.
5. Duane TD. Clinical Ophthalmology, ed. 4. Butterworth – Heinemann, 1999.
6. Duvall. Ophthalmic Medications and Pharmacology: Slack Inc, 1998.
7. Ellis PP. Ocular Therapeutics and Pharmacology, ed. 7. CV Mosby, 1985.
8. Fechner. Ocular Therapeutics. Slack Inc., 1998.
9. Fraunfelder. Current Ocular Therapy, ed. 5. WB Saunders, 2000.
10. Garg Ashok. Current Trends in Ophthalmology, ed. 1. New Delhi: Jaypee Medical Publishers, 1997.
11. Garg Ashok. Manual of Ocular Therapeutics, ed. 1, New Delhi: Jaypee Medical Publishers, 1996.
12. Garg Ashok. Ready Reckoner of Ocular Therapeutics, ed. 1. New Delhi: 2002.
13. Goodman LS, Gilman A. Pharmacological basis of Therapeutics, ed.7, New York: Macmillan, 1985.
14. Havener's, Ocular Pharmacology, ed. 6. CV Mosby, 1994.
15. Kanski, Clinical ophthalmology, ed. 4. Butterworth – Heineman, 1999.
16. Kershner. Ophthalmic Medications and Pharmacology: Slack. Inc., 1994.
17. Kucers A, Bennett NM. The use of Antibiotics, ed. 4. Philadelphia: JB Lippincott Company, 1987.
18. Olin BR et al. Drugs Facts and Comparisons: Facts and Comparisons, St. Louis, 1997.

19. Onofrey. The Ocular Therapeutics; Lippincott-William and Wilkins, 1997.
20. Rhee. The Wills Eye drug Guide: Lippincott – William and Wilkins, 1998.
21. Seal. Ocular infection management and treatment: Martin – Dunitz, 1998.
22. Steven Podos. Textbook of Ophthalmology. New Delhi: Jaypee Medical Publishers, 2001.
23. Zimmerman. Textbook of Ocular Pharmacology. Lippincott—William and Wilkins, 1997.

Chapter 15

Endophthalmitis Prevention Strategies

John D Sheppard (USA)

Perfected treatment strategies depend on a surgeon's preferences and individual patient needs.

Infectious complications following routine cataract surgery are the most feared of all ophthalmic infections, due to the high expectations for cataract operations in the 21st century. Endophthalmitis complicates approximately one in every 1,000 cataract operations. With clear corneal incisions, this rate may be rising. Risk factors cited in the peer-reviewed literature include extracapsular surgery, intracapsular surgery, clear corneal incisions, diabetes mellitus, prolonged surgical time, previous or concurrent trabeculectomy, repeated instrument entry and exit, chronic blepharitis, chronic conjunctivitis, keratitis sicca, ocular surface disease, capsular rupture, vitreous prolapse, and vitrectomy surgery. The potential for this risk may rise to one in every 100 cases with vitreous loss. Although rapid diagnosis and expeditious surgical intervention can preserve excellent visual function in many patients with endophthalmitis, preventive measures are the cornerstone of any surgical management strategy.

NEW CONCEPTS IN ENDOPHTHALMITIS TREATMENT

The landmark Endophthalmitis Vitrectomy Study (EVS), conceived by Dr Bernard Doft and completed in 1995, found that 70% of endophthalmitis cases were caused by coagulase-negative, gram-positive micrococci, overwhelmingly *Staphylococcus epidermidis*.[1] This study has revolutionized our treatment algorithm for postcataract surgery endophthalmitis, recognizing the essential aspects of vitreous-tap diagnosis and expeditious injection of intravitreal antibiotics, while surprisingly raising the threshold for pars plana vitrectomy for patients with light perception or worse-quality vision.

New data have extended our understanding of the pathogenesis and prevention of postoperative endophthalmitis since the completion of the EVS. Postcataract infections originate by one of three routes: (1) introduction through instrumentation at the time of surgery; (2) inoculation through the wound after cataract surgery and (3) (although extremely rarely) by endogenous spread from concurrently infected extraocular tissues, such as a tooth abscess or infected diverticulum. Material presented at the 2002 ARVO meeting in Fort Lauderdale, Florida, in particular offered insight into bacteriologic factors relevant to cataract surgery.

EXISTING LITERATURE

With experience and consideration of extensive laboratory data, most surgeons now believe that postcataract infections are introduced into the eye from the ocular surface. This belief brings into question the traditional use of topical perioperative aminoglycosides for cataract patients, especially when most endophthalmitides are gram-positive and aminoglycosides are so insoluble. In our analysis, gram-positive isolates from 163 patients with bacterial conjunctivitis were only 85% sensitive to tobramycin, while 97% were sensitive to levofloxacin, a third-generation fluoroquinolone, 83% to sulfasoxazole, 77% to ciprofloxacin, and only 75% to trimethoprim, commonly used in combination with the gram-negative agent, polymyxin B.[2]

Franco Recchia of Vanderbilt University and colleagues clearly showed that an increasingly higher percentage of postcataract infections are due to gram-positive organisms.[3] In a study of 493 consecutive patients with postcataract endophthalmitis, researchers cultured an organism from the vitreous in 318 cases (65%). During the last decade of the 20th century, gram-positive isolates increased from 92 to 97%. Furthermore, resistance rates to commonly used prophylactic antibiotics increased; resistance among all isolates to ciprofloxacin rose significantly (23 to 38%), while resistance to ciprofloxacin and cefazolin rose among coagulase-negative staphylococci (18 to 38%).

In his new study from Stanford University, Christopher Ta and associates compared the ability of 21 different antibiotics to cover coagulase-negative Staphylococcus organisms.[4] Researchers took preoperative conjunctival swabs from 66 patients prior to applying antibiotics or antiseptic. Their analysis concluded that, among the four fluoroquinolones tested, levofloxacin had the highest antistaphylococcal susceptibilty (91%) compared to norfloxacin (79%), ofloxacin (75%), and ciprofloxacin (73%). Conversely, resistance patterns also favored levofloxacin at only 5%, whereas norfloxacin was 18%, ciprofloxacin 20%, and ofloxacin 23%.

PRACTICAL CLINICAL PRACTICE

Revealing *in vivo* data from Frank Bucci, MD, in Wilkes-Barre, Pennsylvania, demonstrate that levofloxacin reaches therapeutic aqueous concentrations, therefore exceeding the MIC90 for both Staphylococcus and Streptococcus.[5] Dr Bucci found that 0.5% levofloxacin reached four- to seven-fold higher aqueous concentrations than 0.3% ciprofloxacin when administered according to identical preoperative regimens. The ciprofloxacin levels were below the established NCCLS MIC90 for both Staphylococcus and Streptococcus. Dr Bucci also noted that, higher intracameral levofloxacin concentrations could be achieved with a regimen of administering five drops every 10 minutes immediately prior to surgery, when compared to administering the drug four times per day for 2 days preoperatively. He achieved an additional 50% increase in aqueous levels by combining the two regimens.

Starr, Jensen and Fiscella[6] showed that, of 24 endophthalmitis cases in 9,079 patients, eyes receiving topical ofloxacin postoperatively developed endophthalmitis significantly less often than those receiving topical ciprofloxacin (P<.0009). According to these investigators, this difference in endophthalmitis rates may reflect differences in pharmacological and bioavailability properties that exist among fluoroquinolone antibiotics. Ciprofloxacin, the least soluble of available topical fluoroquinolones, achieves the lowest intraocular levels. Levofloxacin, with 3.3 times more active drug per drop than ofloxacin, might be the preferred choice at this time because of superior gram-positive coverage and solubility.

Even though some surgeons have popularized the use of antibiotic infusion through balanced saline-irrigating solutions during cataract surgery, a group of researchers in Arizona, led by Robert Snyder, MD, do not see the efficacy of this approach.[7] Dr Snyder and his colleagues noted that antibiotics chosen for infusion should be fast-acting, due to the limited time exposure to purported intracameral bacterial contaminants. The fluoroquinolones showed dose-dependent killing. On the other hand, vancomycin killing did not correlate with drug concentration relative to the MIC of Staphylococcus species tested. Fluoroquinolones may be more suitable for killing bacteria seeded into the anterior chamber than vancomycin. Because vancomycin concentration decreases rapidly in the anterior chamber following surgery completion, residual surviving organisms with exposure to this antibiotic of last resort could have a high likelihood of vancomycin resistance. Those who advocate aminoglycoside antibiotic infusion during routine surgery ignore both the severe potential retinal toxicity of this class, and waning gram-positive sensitivity.

MICROBIAL ANTIBIOTIC RESISTANCE

Careful clinical analysis customized to each prospective cataract patient by a knowledgeable, conscientious surgeon provides the best solution to endophthalmitis risk. There is no single agent capable of killing every microbe known to cause postoperative infections.[8] Even in this brief review of recent ARVO abstracts, epidemiologic patterns differ between hospitals, cities, and regions, a fact that renders each surgeon uniquely capable of understanding the peculiarities of their own bacteriologic environs. Although newer fourth-generation fluoroquinolones, such as moxifloxacin and gatifloxacin, may demonstrate increased potency for gram-positive bacteria over second- and third-generation drugs, the fourth-generations demonstrated no advantage for gram-negative coverage in a keratitis study conducted by Kowalski et al.[9] gram-negative resistance appears to cross all fluoroquinolone generations. Thus, miniscule but significant holes have appeared in the once-invincible fluoroquinolone family's gram-negative coverage spectrum. The best protection of all may be a thorough povidone-iodine preparation,[10] including the periorbital skin, lids, lashes, and conjunctival cul-de-sac.

Consistent routines, meticulous iodine preparation and reliable surgical technique, coupled with highly effective and penetrating topical antibiotics given frequently prior to surgery, provide our patients with the best defense against infection.

REFERENCES

1. Han DP, Wisniewski SR, Wilson LA, et al. Spectrum and susceptibilities of microbiologic isolates in the Endophthalmitis Vitrectomy Study. Am J Ophthalmol 1998;122:1-17.
2. Sheppard JD, Oefinger PE, Wegerhoff PE. Susceptibility patterns of conjunctival isolates to newer and established anti-infective agents. IOVS 2002 (abstr 1588) (suppl).
3. Recchia FM, Busbee BG, Pearlman RB, et al. Changing trends in the microbiologic aspects of post-cataract endophthalmitis. Arch Ophthalmol 2005;123:341-46.
4. Ta CN, Mino de Kaspar H, Chang RT, et al. Antibiotic susceptibility pattern of coagulase-negative staphylococci in patients undergoing intraocular surgery. IOVS 2002 (abstr 4444) (suppl).
5. Bucci FA. An *in vivo* comparison of the ocular absorption of levofloxacin versus ciprofloxacin prior to phacoemulsification. IOVS 2002 (abstr 1579) (suppl).
6. Starr MB, Jensen MK, Fiscella RG. A retrospective study of endophthalmitis rates comparing quinolone antibiotics, Am J Ophthalmol 2005:140;769-71.
7. Snyder RW, Krueger T, Nix DE. Kill curves for vancomycin versus 3rd generation quinolones. IOVS 2002 (abstr 4452) (suppl).
8. Benz MS, Scott IU, Flynn HW, et al. *In vitro* susceptibilities to antimicrobials of pathogens isolated from the vitreous cavity of patients with endophthalmitis. IOVS 2002 (abstr 4428) (suppl).
9. Kowalski RP, Karenchak LM, Romanowski EG, et al. An *in vitro* comparison of 2nd, 3rd, and 4th generation fluoroquinolones against bacterial keratitis isolates. IOVS 2002 (abstr 1585) (suppl).
10. Ciulla TA, Starr MB, Masket S. Bacterial endophthalmitis prophylaxis for cataract surgery: An evidence-based update. Ophthalmology 2002;109(1):13-24.

than tobramycin. This represents a significant reduction in dosing as compared to conventional drops that require anywhere from 3-8 doses per day.

The rate of ocular adverse events was 1.9% in the tobramycin comparison study. (Protzko,et al., 2006) The most frequently observed ocular adverse events in the overall study population were eye irritation (1.9%), conjunctival hyperemia (1.1%) and, worsening conjunctivitis (1.1%), which compares favorably with that of tobramycin and the topical fluoroquinolone, gatifloxacin (Zymar full prescribing information).

In a parallel study, participants were randomized to receive AzaSite or a vehicle that contained DuraSite and the preservative benzylkonium hydrochloride. The same 5 day treatment regimen was employed. The results demonstrated that microbiological and clinical outcomes were superior in participants who used AzaSite rather than vehicle. At the test-of-cure visit on day 6, treatment with AzaSite achieved clinical resolution in 63.1% (82/130) of participants compared to treatment with vehicle which achieved clinical resolution in 49.7% (74/149). The difference in resolution rate was 13.4% (95% CI:1.9 to 25%) and statistically significant (P=0.030) in favor of AzaSite.

Expanded Killing Profile

In vitro studies that supported the phase 3 clinical trials, indicated that clinical isolates that showed resistance to azithromycin *in vitro* were eradicated on the ocular surface by 1% solution of azithromycin in DuraSite. Clinical Laboratory and Standards Institute (CLSI) breakpoints were used to identify resistant bacteria. Most strains of Enterococcus faecalis and methicillin resistant staphylococci are resistant to azithromycin. Although strains of Hemophilus *influenzae* and *Streptococcus pneumoniae* with decreased susceptibility to azithromycin are rare, isolated reports have appeared in literature. (Cerquettu M, Cardines R Giufre M et al., 2004; Thornsberry C, Olgive PT, Holly HP et al., 1999). In the phase 3 studies, AzaSite eradicated 72.4% (21/29) of azithromycin-resistant *Staphylococcus* and *Streptococcus* strains isolated from the patient population. In addition, although the total number was small, AzaSite eradicated all of the oxacillin (methicillin) resistant strains (2/2) that were isolated from the patient population. (Abelson M et al., 2006). The efficacy of AzaSite against resistant organisms is almost certainly due to the extremely high tear film concentrations of azithromycin which were obtained.

CONCLUSION

Azithromycin is a semi-synthetic azalide derived from erythromycin. Favorable pharmacokinetics and bacterial spectrum make azithromycin an excellent candidate for the treatment of ocular surface infections. Significant milestones in formulation technology involving mucoadhesive polymers permitted the development of a stable eye drop with a high safety and tolerability profile and convenient once-a-day dosing. AzaSite is a significant improvement on the azithromycin molecule. The addition of the DuraSite drug delivery vehicle imparts stability and increased contact time with the ocular surface, which allows AzaSite to sustain high bactericidal tear film and conjunctival concentrations of azithromycin.

BIBLIOGRAPHY

1. Abelson M, Protzko EE, Shapiro AM, AzaSite. Clinical Study Group. A randomized trial assessing microbial eradication and clinical efficacy of AzaSite (1.0% azithromycin ophthalmic solution) vs. tobramycin in adult subjects with bacterial conjunctiv.
2. Bryskier A, Labro MT. Macrolides: New therapeutic prospects. Presse 1994;23(38):1762-66.
3. Cerquetti M, Cardines R, Giufre M, Mastrantonio P. HI Study Group. Antimicrobial susceptibility of Haemophilus influenzae strains isolated from invasive disease in Italy. J Antimicrob Chemo. 2004;54:1139-46.
4. Girard D, Bergeron JM, Millisen WB et al. Comparison of azithromycin, roxithromycin, and cephalexin penetration kinetics in early and mature abscesses. J Antimicrob Chemother 1993;Suppl E:17-28:1993.
5. Kuehne JJ, Yu AL, Holland GN et al. Corneal pharmacokinetics of topically applied azithromycin and clarithromycin. Am J Ophthalmol 2004;138:547-53.
6. Morrow GL, Abbott RL. Conjunctivitis. Am Family Physician 1998, 57 accessed at http://www.aafp.org/afp/980215ap/morrow.html, November 6, 2006.
7. Neu HC. Clinical microbiology of azithromycin. Am J Med 1991;91(3A):12S-18S.
8. Protzko E et al. A randomized trial assessing the safety and tolerability of 1.0% azithromycin ophthalmic solution vs. tobramycin in pediatric and adult subjects with bacterial conjunctivitis. Invest Ophthalmol Vis Sci. 2003. E-abstract@arvo.org. E-abstract 4958.
9. Retsema J, Girard A, Schelkly W, et al. Spectrum and mode of action of azithromycin (CP-62,993) , a new 15-membered-ring macrolide with improved potency against gram-negative organisms. Antimicrobial Agents and Chemo 1987;31:1939-47.
10. Rodvold KA, Piscitelli SC. 1993 New oral macrolide and fluoroquinolone antibiotics: An overview of pharmacokinetics, interactions and safety. Clin Infect Dis 1993;Suppl 1:S192-S199.
11. Thornsberry C, Olgive PT, Holly HP, Sahm DF. Survey of susceptibilities of Streptococcus pneumoniae, Haemophilus influenzae, and Moraxella catarrhalis isolates to 26 antimicrobial agents: a prospective U.S. study. Antimicrob Agents Chemother. 1999;43:2612-2623.
12. Williams JD, Sefton AM. Comparison of macrolide antibiotics. J Antimicrobi Chemother 1993;Suppl C:11-26.
13. Zymar [package insert]. Allergan, Inc; Irvine, Calif 2004.

Chapter 17

Tetracyclines for Ocular Surface Disease

Robert Latkany (USA)

The signs and symptoms of ocular rosacea, blepharitis, meibomian gland dysfunction, trachoma, recurrent corneal erosions, phlyctenular keratoconjunctivitis and ulcerative corneal thinning may all benefit from the use of an antibiotic from the tetracycline family (Fig. 17.1). The most common include tetracycline, doxycycline, and minocycline. Their benefit lies not so much in their ability to destroy bacteria but rather a plethora of mechanisms that prevent the degradation of the ocular surface.

For instance, tetracyclines block the production of matrix metalloproteinases (MMP-9), which are capable of destroying extracellular matrix proteins like collagen.[1] Its anti-collagenase activity may ultimately prove to be the reason why tetracyclines prevent further tissue degradation in corneal ulcers. This same action may also explain why the use of doxycycline has proven useful in the treatment and resolution of previously unresolved recurrent corneal erosions for up to 22 months.[2] Tetracyclines also block the production of lipases by Staphylococci[3] and alter the quality of meibum or meibomian gland secretions.[4] The enhanced functional quality of the meibum

Ocular rosacea
Blepharitis
Meibomian gland disease
Trachoma
Recurrent corneal erosions
Phlyctenular keratoconjunctivitis
Corneal ulcers
Dry eyes

Fig. 17.1: Diseases that can improve with tetracycline use

resulting from the reduction in free fatty acids and diglycerides remained 3 months after stopping a course of minocycline therapy.[4] Prolonged benefit may prove to be very useful as ongoing therapy may not be necessary and thereby limits potential side effects. The tetracycline family also works through immunomodulation[5] and by altering the ocular flora.[6] However, 3 months after stopping treatment the ocular lid flora returned almost back to baseline pretreatment levels.[6] More research is needed to determine which has greater therapeutic value, altering the quality of the meibum or reducing the ocular lid flora. Despite the obvious therapeutic value the question still remains how often and how long should a patient be prescribed a tetracycline?

There are a wide range of suggested dosages including doxycycline 100mg twice daily for up to 3 weeks then tapering down to 25 mg or 50 mg daily based on the therapeutic response[7] while others have had success with initial dosages of only 100 mg daily.[8] The recommended dosage of minocycline is 50 mg daily for 2 weeks and then increasing the dosage to 100 mg daily for up to 3 months.[6] The author prefers doxycycline 100 mg twice daily for 3 weeks and upon re-examination for therapeutic assessment will either stop treatment all together if there was no obvious improvement of clinical signs or symptoms or taper immediately down to 25 mg per day if there was an appreciable improvement for an additional month. Patients need to be made aware that dairy products can limit the absorption of tetracyclines. Tetracycline concerns, however, do not end there.

There are several side effects that warrant careful consideration as to when a patient should receive an antibiotic from the tetracycline family. Most notably, a recent article showed an increased likelihood of breast cancer with an increased number of days on systemic antibiotics.[9] Of equal importance, minocycline may induce autoimmune syndromes.[10] Other often reported side effects include scleral pigmentation and tooth discoloration.[11-13] Gastrointestinal side effects were noted in 12.5% of patients treated with 100 mg of doxycycline daily and 37.5% of patients treated with 1 gram of tetracycline daily.[14] So it is recommended to use doxycycline in patients with sensitive gastrointestinal issues.

The true anti-inflammatory benefit of the tetracycline family will need to be clarified with future studies. Conflicting studies only shed light on the fact that we are in the very early stages of understanding the exact mechanisms of action. In some areas where one could imagine a noticeable benefit with the use of tetracyclines none was found. Tetracycline did not show any reduction in corneal haze post-photorefractive keratectomy in a study involving 30 rabbits.[15] However, other areas show more promise such as chemical injuries where tetracyclines may inhibit the collagenolytic degradation of the cornea stroma.[16] The coverage can extend even further to involve all patients with dry eye disease secondary to meibomian gland disease and/or blepharitis as one study involving 39 ocular rosacea patients showed a significant improvement in tear break-up time from 5.7 seconds to 10.8 seconds after receiving 100 mg of doxycycline for 12 weeks.[8] These types of evaluations are necessary because we cannot rely on patients symptoms alone to judge efficacy because it is well known that signs do not often correlate with symptoms in ocular surface disease.

Even a lose dose of 20 mg of doxycycline twice a day proved effective in a study involving 300 eyes of patients with chronic meibomian gland dysfunction in improving tear break-up time, Schirmer's test, the number of symptoms reported and the degree of improved subjective symptoms.[17] This same study, interestingly enough, showed no statistical difference in improvement of any of the above between the groups of patients receiving the low dose of 20 mg of doxycycline twice a day and the high dose of 200 mg twice a day. So further comparative studies are necessary to assess what is the maximum dosage required to achieve a noticeable therapeutic benefit.

Other studies only highlight the early stages of our understanding of the use of tetracyclines with ocular surface disease. 16 patients received short-term minocycline therapy and showed an improvement of the turbidity of the meibomian gland secretions and microbial cultures; however, surprisingly, there was a decrease in aqueous tear volume and flow with increased evaporation.[18] Also equally disturbing was an *in vitro* study that showed doxycycline induced keratocyte cell death, and detachment of epithelial cells from their basement membrane.[19] It would be interesting to know if there is a therapeutic benefit with the use of a topical tetracycline cream or drop and if it shows any ocular surface toxicity. The use of a topical tetracycline may reduce systemic side effects but possibly increase surface related toxicity. And yet another concern lies in the open chronic use of this family of antibiotics and their possibility of developing resistance. Four of ten patients tested carried tetracycline resistant strains in a study involving 3 months of minocycline therapy.[6]

It is certain that there is a place for the anti-inflammatory properties of tetracyclines in a number of external diseases of the eye. However, it is also clear that more work is needed to clarify the exact mechanisms of action, the most effective dosage, the route of administration, and the total duration of therapy necessary with the use of these tetracyclines.

REFERENCES

1. Sadowski T, Steinmeyer J. Effects of tetracyclines on the production of matrix metalloproteinases and plasminogen activators as well as of their natural inhibitors, tissue inhibitor of metalloproteinases-1 and plasminogen activator inhibitor-1. Inflamm Res 2001;50:175-82.
2. Dursun D, Kim MC, Solomon A, et al. Treatment of recalcitrant corneal erosions with inhibitors of matrix metalloproteinases-9, doxycycline and corticosteroids. Am J Ophthalmol 2001;132(1):8-13.

3. Dougherty JM, McCulley JP, Silvany RE, Meyer DR. The role of tetracycline in chronic blepharitis. Inhibition of lipase production in staphylococci. Invest Ophthalmol Vis Sci 1991;32:2970-75.
4. Shine We, McCulley JP, Pandya AG. Minocycline effect on meibomian gland lipids in meibomianitism patients. Exp Eye Res 2003;76(4):417-20.
5. Thong YH. Immunomodulation by antimicrobial drugs. Med Hypotheses 1982;8:361-70.
6. Ta CN, Shine WE, McCulley JP, et al. Effects of minocycline on the ocular flora of patients with acne rosacea or seborrheic blepharitis. Cornea 2003;22:545-48.
7. Alvarenga LS, Mannis MJ. Ocular Rosacea. The Ocular Surface 2005;3(1):41-58.
8. Quarterman MJ, Johnson DW, Abele DC, et al. Ocular Rosacea. Signs, symptoms, and tear studies before and after treatment with doxycycline. Arch Dermatol 1997;133:49-54.
9. Velicer CM, Heckbert SR, Lampe JW, et al. Antibiotic use in relation to the risk of breast cancer. JAMA 2004;291:827-35.
10. Elkayam O, Yaron M, Caspi D. Minocycline-induced autoimmune syndromes: An overview. Semin Arthritis Rheum 1999;28:392-97.
11. Fraunfelder FT, Randall JA. Minocycline-induced scleral pigmentation. Ophthalmology 1997;104:936-38.
12. Bradfield YS, Robertson DM, Salomao DR, et al. Minocycline-induced ocular pigmentation.
13. Morrow GL, Abbott RL. Minocycline-induced scleral, dental, and dermal pigmentation. Am J Ophthalmol 1998;125:396-97
14. Frucht-Pery J, Sagi E, Hemo I, et al. Efficacy of doxycycline and tetracycline in ocular rosacea. Am J Ophthalmol 1993;116(1):88-92.
15. Corbett MC, O'Brart DP, Patmore AL, et al. Effect of collagenase inhibitors on corneal haze after PRK. Exp Eye Res 2001;72(3):253-59.
16. Ralph RA. Tetracyclines and the treatment of corneal stromal ulceration: A review. Cornea 2000;19(3):274-97.
17. Yoo Se, Lee DC, Chang MH. The effect of low-dose doxycycline therapy in chronic meibomian gland dysfunction. Korean J Ophthalmol 2005;19(4):258-63.
18. Aronowicz JD, Shine WE, Oral D, et al. Short-term oral minocycline treatment of meibomianitis. Br J Ophthalmol 2006;90(7):856-60.
19. Smith VA, Cook SD. Doxycycline—a role in ocular surface repair. Br J Ophthalmol 2004;88(5):619-25.

Chapter 18

Management of Endophthalmitis: Antibiotic Schedule and Dosages

Pei-Chang Wu, Hsi-Kung Kuo (Taiwan)

Endophthalmitis is defined by marked inflammation of intraocular fluids and tissues. When caused by micro-organisms, endophthalmitis often results in severe visual loss. The broad categories of endophthalmitis include postoperative (acute-onset, chronic or delayed onset, bleb-associated), posttraumatic, endogenous and miscellaneous, such as intravitreous triamcinolone associated endophthalmitis, microbial keratitis and suture removal (Table 18.1). These categories are important in predicting the causative organism and guiding therapeutic decisions before microbiological confirmation.

Table 18.1: Classification of endophthalmitis and most frequent organisms

1. Postoperative
   a. Acute-onset: coagulase (-) *staphylococci*(*Staph. epidermidis*), *Staphylococcus aureus*, *Enterococcus* species, *Streptococcus* species, gram-negative bacteria (*Pseudomonas*)
   b. Chronic: *P. acnes*, coagulase (-) *staphylococci*, fungi
   c. Bleb-associated: *Streptococcus* species, *Hemophilus influenza*, *Staphylococcus* species
2. Posttraumatic: *Bacillus* species, *Staphylococci*
3. Endogenous: *Candida* species, gram-negative bacteria (*Klebsiella pneumoniae*), *S. aureus*
4. Miscellaneous
   a. Corneal ulcer perforation: *Pseudomonas*, *Staphylococcus* species
   b. intravitreous triamcinolone associated
   c. suture removal associated

Acute postoperative endophthalmitis

Acute postoperative endophthalmitis is defined as the occurrence of intraocular infection within 6 weeks after surgery by the Endophthalmitis Vitrectomy Study (EVS).

Prophylaxis

In recent evidence-based literature, Cillua et al found preoperative irrigation with povidone-iodine (PI) to be a most strongly recommended technique based on the current clinical evidence (Table 18.2).[1] PI is a potent antiseptic with a wide spectrum of activity against both gram-positive and gram-negative bacteria, fungi and viruses. Antimicrobial activity contributes to the 1% free iodine released that occurs after contact with the skin for 30 seconds to 1 minute, and this effect will last for 1 hour.[2, 3] Iodine penetrates the cell wall and reacts with aminoacids and nucleotides, which ultimately disrupt the cell's protein synthesis. Despite the wide use of PI solutions as disinfectants in hospitals, these solution have been reported to be susceptible to contamination with *Pseudomonas cepacia*, which could be passed on to the patient.[4]

Preoperative preparation with 5% PI solution dropped into the conjunctival sac followed by a skin preparation of 10% PI solution has been recommended.[5] Our retrospective, case-controlled study found that patients who received 10% PI skin disinfection combined with 5% PI conjunctival disinfection had significantly less risk of developing post-cataract surgery endophthalmitis. However, a modified preparation method of 5% PI on both the skin and conjunctiva has been used in many institutes and for simple ocular surgery, such as intravitreous injection.[6, 7] Caution should be taken to avoid touching the lid margin and lashes when the needle is inserted into the eye.

Table 18.2: Prophylactic methods to prevent bacterial endophthalmitis after cataract surgery[1]

prophylactic intervention	*clinical recommendend*
Postoperative subconjunctival antibiotics	C
Preoperative lash trimming	C
Preoperative saline irrigation	C
Preoperative povidone-iodine antisepsis	B
Preoperative topical antibiotic therapy	C
Irrigating solutions containing antibiotics	C
Intraoperative heparin	C

Grade 'A' is considered very important or crucial to clinical outcome, grade 'B' as moderately important, and grade 'C' is of questionable use.

Intraocular Antibiotics

Intravitreal antibiotic therapy could reach far greater intraocular antibiotic concentration than any other method of administration. It is the main stay of treatment for infective endophthalmitis. In instances of instant and prompt treatment required in order to save the vision, inaccuracies of gram-staining results and unavailable culture results, broad-spectrum intravitreal antibiotics covering almost all the gram-positive and gram-negative bacteria are necessary. A few selected drugs are currently recommended, including vancomycin, ceftazidime and amikacin. In the EVS, the antimicrobial sensitivity profile of amikacin and ceftazidime was similar at 89% against gram-negative organism, and all gram-positive cocci were sensitive to vancomycin.[8]

Vancomycin

Vancomycin is the drug of choice for gram-positive bacteria in acute postoperative endophthalmitis. It is a bactericidal drug whose primary mode of action is inhibiting synthesis and assembly of the bacterial cell wall. It has a strong antimicrobial effect against gram-positive bacteria, especially *Staphylococcus aureus, Staphylcoccus epidermidis and Enterococcus,* including methicillin-resistant *Staphylococcus aureus.* In intraocular use, concentrations of up to 2 mg/0.1 mL have been demonstrated to be non-toxic to the retina.[9] The EVS recommended a dose of 1.0 mg/0.1 mL.[10] The half-life of the drug is reduced in inflamed eyes and prolonged in normal vitreous.[11] Even in inflamed eyes, therapeutic levels are still detected up to 72-84 hours after injection. Vancomycin is also cleared more rapidly in aphakic, vitrectomized eyes.[9, 11]

Ceftazidime

Ceftazidime is a third-generation cephalosporin that has a bactericidal effect by disrupting cell wall synthesis. Third-generation cephalosporins have strong antibacterial effects against gram-negative bacilli. They also have an added effect against *Streptococcus pneumonia, pyogenes* and other streptococci. Cephalosporins have little effect against *Staphylococcus aureus* but a strong effect against *Pseudomonas aeruginosa.* In contrast to the aminoglycosides, ceftazidime carries a lower risk of retinal toxicity and a broader therapeutic index. However, intravitreous ceftazidime was not evaluated in the EVS and it has been shown that in vitro ceftazidime precipitates in vitreous humor at body temperature, irrespective of the presence of vancomycin.[12] In clinical studies, ceftazidime has been demonstrated to precipitate in inflamed eyes resulting in possible subtherapeutic concentration. Reconstitution with normal saline as opposed to balanced salt solution produced less precipitation. Intravitreous ceftazidime is typically injected at a concentration of 2.25 mg/ 0.1 mL.[13] Like vancomycin, half-life is decreased in aphakic, vitrectomized and inflamed eyes.

Aminoglycosides

Aminoglycosides have a bactericidal effect through ionic interaction with the cell surface, energy dependent uptake phases and binding to ribosomes.

Amikacin has a strong bactericidal effect against aerobic and facultative gram-negative bacilli. It has a synergistic effect with vancomycin and other cell wall active antimicrobials (penicillins and cephalosporins). Aminoglycosides such as amikacin and gentamicin have been used for intravitreous injection. Gentamicin has been reported to cause macular toxicity.[14] Aminoglycoside-induced macular infarction is thought to result from an increased concentration by the gravity-induced accumulation of drugs on the macula in a supine patient. Although animal experiments[15] have shown that amikacin is safer than gentamicin, a potential for macular toxicity might still exist. Amikacin has been shown to cause macular infarction with loss of macular capillaries and pre-retinal hemorrhage.[16-18]

The standard intravitreous dose of amikacin is 0.4 mg/0.1 mL. This is the dose used in the EVS. Pharmacokinetic studies in animals were similar to vancomycin pharmacokinetics in the vitreous cavity. However, levels measured 24 hours after injection were equal to or less than the minimal inhibitory concentration (MIC) for most organisms sensitive to amikacin.[19] Lower concentrations in the vitreous may necessitate the need for repeat injections of amikacin if there is no response. No toxicity has been contributed to a single injection but repeated injections should be undertaken with caution due to the possible risk of macular infarction.[18, 19] Nasal side recumbency for about 30 minutes might be suggested after intravitreous injection of amikacin.

Repeated vitreous tapping and injection of antibiotics, together with pars plana vitrectomy, should be consider if there is no clinical improvement or if the condition deteriorates within 48 to 72 hours.[20]

Systemic Antibiotics

The systemic antibiotics that cross the blood retinal barrier include cefazolin, ceftazidime and ciprofloxacin.[21-23] In the EVS, intravenous ceftazidime and amikacin were evaluated, and it was concluded that these antibiotics did not alter final visual acuity or media clarity.[10] However, subsequent to the publication, this conclusion has come under question. First, these two drugs did not cover the most common micro-organisms of gram-positive bacteria in post-operative endophthalmitis. Second, intravenous amikacin has little intraocular penetration. The recommendation against intravenous antibiotic use was not warranted and might be based on inadequate data.

Intravenous vancomycin has been suggested as an alternative therapy to systemic ceftazidime and amikacin because of its superior gram-positive coverage. However, vancomycin penetrates poorly into the vitreous yielding an inadequate antibacterial effect.[24, 25]

Oral ciprofloxacin might be an effective drug against many common infecting organisms causing endophthalmitis.[26] However, older-generation fluoroquinolones (ciprofloxacin, ofloxacin and levofloxacin) are increasingly ineffective against some of the pathogens most commonly responsible for postoperative endophthalmitis. In contrast, the newer-generation fluoroquinolones (gatifloxacin and moxifloxacin) show promising results; they not only display effective activity against gram-negative bacteria, as do the older-generation fluoroquinolones, but also demonstrate enhanced potencies against gram-positive bacteria.[27] Orally administered gatifloxacin was able to penetrate into the non-inflamed human eye, and reach therapeutic levels in the aqueous and vitreous humors.[28] Gatifloxacin has a broad spectrum of coverage over the bacteria involved in endophthalmitis. It also has a low MIC of 90, good tolerability and excellent bioavailability after oral administration. Oral gatifloxacin has the ability to achieve rapid, effective levels in the aqueous and vitreous, with the notable exceptions of not achieving effective levels against *Enterococcus* or *Pseudomonas*. Gatifloxacin may thus represent a good adjunctive treatment for certain types of endophthalmitis.

Subconjunctival and Topical Antibiotic Therapy

Subconjunctival and topical antibiotics are often used to supplement intravitreal injections in attempt to increase the concentration of antibiotics within the anterior segment of the eye. Subconjunctival administration can reach therapeutic concentrations in the eye, especially in the aqueous humor. However, conflicting data regarding the intravitreal penetration after periocular antibiotic injection have been reported.[29] In addition, subconjunctival injection is more painful and could not be as frequently administrated as topical antibiotics. A risk of macular infarction when using gentamicin has also been reported.[14] Of the currently used antibiotics, the third-generation cephalosporins (ceftazidime and ceftriaxone) achieve the highest vitreous levels.

Topical application is associated with very poor vitreous penetration. However, significant intraocular levels of antibiotics can be achieved with frequent administration of highly concentrated solutions[30], especially if the corneal epithelium has been damaged. For acute-onset postoperative endophthalmitis, topical vancomycin (50 mg/mL) with amikacin (20 mg/mL) or ceftazidime (50 mg/mL) administered hourly is recommended. This regimen can then be adjusted for the specific organism after culture and sensitivity results are available.

Steroid Treatment

The early use of corticosteroids, in addition to antibiotics, reduces inflammation and subsequent retinal damage in endophthalmitis. Corticosteroid therapy may be administered topically, intravitreally or systemically. In the EVS, oral prednisone was used at a dose of 30 mg orally twice a day for 5 to 10 days.

Intravitreous dexamethasone has been increasingly employed as an alternative to systemic therapy. Dexamethasone sodium phosphate is typically used in an intravitreous concentration of 0.4 mg/0.1 mL. This is equivalent to 40 mg of oral prednisone. Experimental studies have shown that intravitreal dexamethasone has a large safety window and that it prolongs the half-life of intravitreal vancomycin.[31, 32] Triamcinolone acetonide (4 mg/0.1 mL) is more potent and equivalent to 50 mg of oral prednisone. Recently it has been reported that intravitreal triamcinolone combined with intravitreal antibiotics appear to have a safety profile similar to current modalities, with a favorable effect on visual recovery and function in acute postoperative endophthalmitis.[33]

Table 18.3: Recommended doses of initial management of infective postoperative endophthalmitis

Route	*Drug*	*Dose*
Intravitreal	Vancomycin	1 mg in 0.1mL
	Ceftazidime	2.25 mg in 0.1mL
	Amikacin	0.4 mg in 0.1mL
	Dexamethasone	0.4 mg in 0.1mL
Subconjunctival	Vancomycin	25 mg in 0.5mL
	Ceftazidime	100 mg in 0.5mL
Topical	Vancomycin	50 mg/mL drop q1h
	Amikacin	20 mg/mL drops q1h
Systemic	Fluoroquinolones (oral)	
	Gatifloxacin	400 mg bid

Vitrectomy

Vitrectomy debulks the vitreous cavity, reduces the load of bacteria and toxins, and makes space for intravitreous antibiotics. Only core vitrectomy is recommended, due to fear of causing retinal break as the vitrector is near to the fragile, inflamed retina in a cloudy vitreous. In addition, it is always combined with intravitreous antibiotic injection. The EVS concluded that immediate vitrectomy was not beneficial for patients with an initial visual acuity of hand movement or better.[10] Among patients with initial light-perception-only vision, it was three times more likely that a visual acuity of 20/40 or better would be achieved after vitrectomy. Complications of pars plana vitrectomy include infection, bleeding, cataract, glaucoma and retinal detachment.

In summary, the authors recommend the following for management of acute postoperative endophthalmitis. Noting the patient's unusual symptoms, carefully examining signs associated with infection and a highly alert mind in the physician are important in early intervention, especially for immunocompromised and diabetic patients. It is good to initiate topical antibiotics and cycloplegics immediately during close follow-up when there is suspicion of infection. The current choice of drugs is ciprofloxacin 0.3% or ofloxacin 0.3%. If infection is strongly suspected, the presenting vision is important in deciding between a vitreous tap and vitrectomy in conjunction with intraocular antibiotic injection. Culture of vitreous fluid from a vitreous tap or vitrectomy is essential for microbiology sensitivity patterns. The flow-chart for management of acute endophthalmitis is shown in Figure 18.1. For intravitreous antibiotic injection, we prefer intravitreal vancomycin (1 mg) and ceftazidime (2.25 mg) or amikacin (0.4 mg) combined with intravitreal dexamethasone (0.4 mg). The rationale and choice of systemic antibiotics is best left to the treating physician. Systemic fluoroquinolone is suggested.

Table 18.4: Antimicrobial agents: dosages for ophthalmic use

Drug	*Topical*	*Subconj. (in 0.5ml)*	*Intravitreal (in 0.1ml)*	*Intravenous dose*	*Oral dosage*
Aminoglycosides					
Gentamicin	14 mg/ml	20 mg	0.1 mg	1.4 mg/kg q 8-12hr	
Tobramycin	14 mg/ml	20 mg	0.1 mg	1.4 mg/kg IV, IV, q8-12hr	
Amikacin	20 mg/ml	25-50 mg	0.4 mg	7.5 mg/kg q12hr	
Cephalosporins					
Cefazolin	50 mg/ml	50 mg	2.0 mg	1 g q8h	
Cefotetan			3.0 mg	1 g q12h	
Ceftrizxone			2.0 mg	1-2 g q8h	
Ceftazidime	50 mg/ml	100 mg	2.25 mg	1-2 g q8h	
Penicillins					
Oxacillin	50 mg/ml		0.5 mg	2 g q4h	500 mg qid
Miscellaneous					
Clindamycin	20 mg/ml	15-40 mg	1 mg	600 mg q8h	150-450 mg qid
Ciprofloxacin	0.3%		0.1 mg	400 mg q12h	500-75 mg bid
Gatifloxacin					400 mg bid
Chloramphenicol	5 mg/ml	2 mg	750 mg q6h	250-750 mg qid	
Erythromycin	10 mg/ml		0.5 mg	500-1000 mg q6h	250-500mg qid
Vancomycin	50 mg/ml	25 mg	1-2 mg	1 g q12h	

Chronic Postoperative Endophthalmitis

There are two different types of chronic postoperative endophthalmitis, one is caused by *Propionibacterium acnes* and the other is caused by fungus. These micro-organisms should be considered especially when the initial culture result is negative. The culture plates should be investigated for at least 2 weeks. However, the culture rate is very low. Polymerase chain reaction (PCR) detection of bacterial DNA with specific primers from vitreous samples may prove a useful means of diagnosing delayed post-operative endophthalmitis.[34]

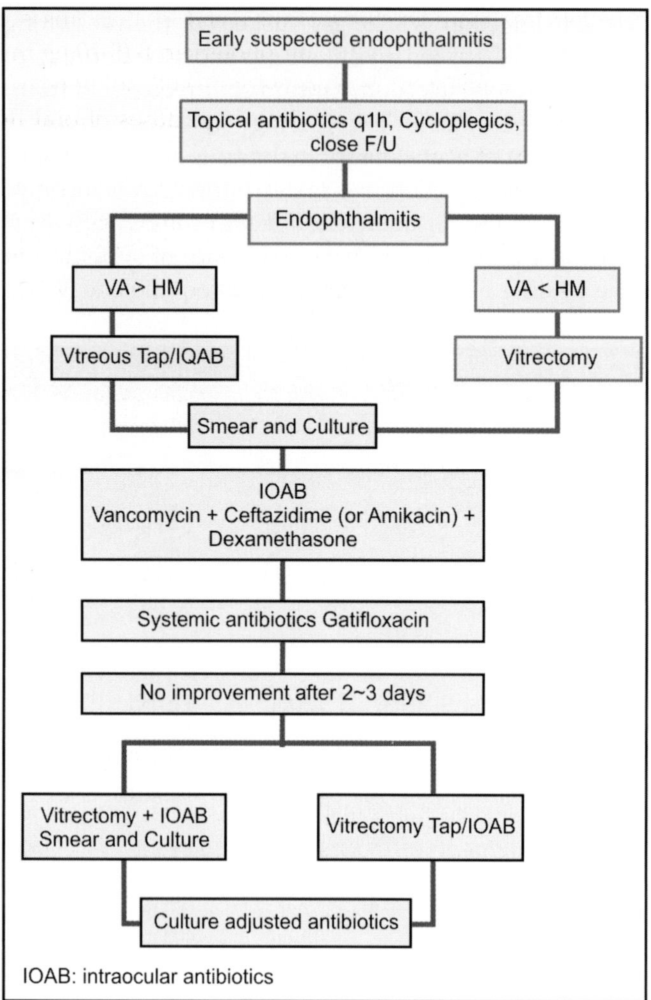

Fig 18.1: Flow-chart for the manage of acute postoperative endophthalmitis

There are two important retrospective studies by Aldave et al.[35] and Clark et al.[36] on *P. acnes* induced postoperative endophthalmitis. The choice for intravitreous antibiotic injection is vancomycin (1 mg in 0.1 mL). However, intravitreous injection of antibiotics alone is associated with a very high rate recurrence. Pars plana vitrectomy, partial capsulectomy and intravitreous antibiotic injection without intraocular lens (IOL) exchange are usually successful on long-term follow-up. For patients with recurrent intraocular inflammation, pars plana vitrectomy, total capsular bag removal, intravitreous antibiotic injection and IOL exchange or removal is a uniformly successful strategy.

Recommended treatment for chronic fungal endophthalmitis is pars plana vitrectomy and intravitreal injection of amphotericin B (5-10 μg in 0.1 mL).[37] Effective systemic amphotericin concentration is still unknown. In cases of yeast endophthalmitis (i.e. *Candida* species), high doses of oral fluconazole (400-600 mg/day) are recommended.[38]

Table 18.5: Antifungal dosages in ophthalmic use

Drug	*Topical*	*Subconj. (in 0.5ml)*	*Intravitreal (in 0.1ml)*	*Usual Intravenous dose*	*Oral dosage*
Polyenes					
Amphotericin B	2.5-10 mg/ml	300 μg	5-10 μg/ml	1mg/kg/day	
Natamycin	5%				
Nystatin	100,000 U/g ointment				
Imidazoles					
Fluconazole	2%				400 mg/day
Clotrimazole	1%	5-10 mg			60-150 mg/kg/day
Econazole	1%			30 mg/kg/day	200 mg tid
Ketoconazole	1-5%				200-400 mg/day
Miconazole	1%	5-10 mg	0.25 mg	25 mg/kg/day in 2-3 divided doses	
Thiabendazole	4%				25mg/kg/day
Pyrimidines					
Flucytosine	1%				50-150 mg/kg/day

Bleb-associated Endophthalmitis

It is important to distinguish between a localized bleb infection (blebitis) and true bleb-associated endophthalmitis. In cases of blebitis, topical antibiotics and subconjunctival antibiotics, such as vancomycin and ceftazidime, can usually be given in an out-patient setting.[39] Bleb-associated endophthalmitis is typically characterized by a delayed onset, more virulent pathogens and poor visual prognosis. Due to the more virulent microorganisms (*Streptococcus* species and *Hemophilus influenzae*) and resulting poor visual prognosis, immediate pars plana vitrectomy, and intravitreal injection of vancomycin and ceftazidime are recommended.[40] Topical and systemic antibiotics (vancomycin and ceftazidime) should be used.

Post-traumatic Endophthalmitis

Due to the initial injury, delay in primary wound repair and more virulent organisms (*Bacillus* or *Staphylococcus* species), post-traumatic endophthalmitis generally has a worse visual outcome than other categories. Endophthalmitis caused by *Bacillus* species is characterized by a rapidly progressive course, ring corneal infiltrates and, generally, a poor visual outcome, even with prompt therapy.[41] Prophylactic intravitreal broad spectrum antibiotic injection decreases the risk of post-traumatic endophthalmitis.[42] In addition, systemic antibiotics are usually administered.[43]

Endogenous Endophthalmitis

Endogenous endophthalmitis is more commonly diagnosed in immunocompromised and debilitated patients. Once the diagnosis of endophthalmitis is suspected, blood or urine cultures should be obtained and other organ involvement must be sought by consultation with an infectious disease specialist or internist. The use of systemic antibiotics is also usually undertaken.

Candida albicans is the most common organism causing endogenous fungal endophthalmitis and *Aspergillus* species is the second most common fungal cause.[44] The management of endogenous *Candida* endophthalmitis is generally tailored to the clinical situation. When chorioretinal infiltrates are present with no or minimal vitreous involvement, systemic therapy alone is recommended. With moderate or severe vitritis, or deterioration in spite of systemic therapy, vitrectomy and intraocular amphotericin B are recommended.

Endogenous bacterial endophthalmitis often is an initial finding leading to the diagnosis of bacterial endocarditis, sepsis and liver abscess in Asians. In patients with diabetes and liver abscess, endogenous *Klebsiella pneumoniae* endophthalmitis is endemic in the Chinese population.[45] It is a very fulminant infection and often results in poor visual outcome. Prompt diagnosis and vigorous treatment with intravitreous injections of vancomycin, amikacin and dexamethasone within 24 hours can save the patient's eyes and vision.[46] Systemic antibiotics and intraocular antibiotics are recommended. Early vitrectomy for endogenous *Klebsiella pneumoniae* endophthalmitis might be beneficial.[47] However, debilitation and confinement in bed because of the sickness in these patients often results in it being unlikely that anesthesia and surgery can be performed in the operating room.

Intravitreous Triamcinolone-associated Endophthalmitis

Triamcinolone injection has become popular for treating macula edema in many diseases. Although some patients appear to have an infectious endophthalmitis, many reports detail a "pseudoendophthalmitis" that resolves without invasive treatment, which might be caused by triamcinolone crystal in the anterior chamber or an inflammatory reaction to the solvent toxin.

Infectious endophthalmitis usually manifests acutely or subacutely with pain. It was concluded that in certain eyes injected with triamcinolone, the differential diagnosis should include a sterile, toxic endophthalmitis and it may be appropriate to observe the patient closely every 8 to 12 hours to determine if the inflammation is worsening or improving. However, if new symptoms develop more than several days after injection, infectious endophthalmitis should be presumed and treatment initiated immediately.[48]

CONCLUSION

Early recognition of endophthalmitis, together with appropriate and timely treatment, can often reduce visual loss.

REFERENCES

1. Ciulla TA, Starr MB, Masket S. Bacterial endophthalmitis prophylaxis for cataract surgery: an evidence-based update. Ophthalmology 2002;109(1):13-24.
2. Saggers BA, Stewart GT. Polyvinyl-Pyrrolidone-Iodine: An Assessment of Antibacterial Activity. J Hyg (Lond) 1964;62:509-18.
3. Connell JF, Jr., Rousselot LM. Povidone-Iodine. Extensive Surgical Evaluation of a New Antiseptic Agent. Am J Surg 1964;108:849-55.
4. Berkelman RL, Lewin S, Allen JR, et al. Pseudobacteremia attributed to contamination of povidone-iodine with Pseudomonas cepacia. Ann Intern Med 1981;95(1):32-6.
5. Johns KJ, Feder RS, Hamill MB, Miller-Meeks MJ. Surgery for Cataract. In: Johns KJ, Feder RS, Hamill MB, Miller-Meeks MJ (eds). Basic and Clinical Science Course Section 11: Lens and Cataract: American Academy of Ophthalmology, 2003-2004.
6. Ferguson AW, Scott JA, McGavigan J, et al. Comparison of 5% povidone-iodine solution against 1% povidone-iodine solution in preoperative cataract surgery antisepsis: a prospective randomised double blind study. Br J Ophthalmol 2003;87(2):163-7.
7. Ta CN. Minimizing the risk of endophthalmitis following intravitreous injections. Retina 2004;24(5):699-705.
8. Han DP, Wisniewski SR, Wilson LA, et al. Spectrum and susceptibilities of microbiologic isolates in the Endophthalmitis Vitrectomy Study. Am J Ophthalmol 1996;122(1):1-17.
9. Pflugfelder SC, Hernandez E, Fliesler SJ, et al. Intravitreal vancomycin. Retinal toxicity, clearance, and interaction with gentamicin. Arch Ophthalmol 1987;105(6):831-7.
10. Results of the Endophthalmitis Vitrectomy Study. A randomized trial of immediate vitrectomy and of intravenous antibiotics for the treatment of postoperative bacterial endophthalmitis. Endophthalmitis Vitrectomy Study Group. Arch Ophthalmol 1995;113(12):1479-96.
11. Coco RM, Lopez MI, Pastor JC, Nozal MJ. Pharmacokinetics of intravitreal vancomycin in normal and infected rabbit eyes. J Ocul Pharmacol Ther 1998;14(6):555-63.

12. Kwok AK, Hui M, Pang CP, et al. An in vitro study of ceftazidime and vancomycin concentrations in various fluid media: implications for use in treating endophthalmitis. Invest Ophthalmol Vis Sci 2002;43(4):1182-8.
13. Tanabe J, Kitano K, Suzuki T, et al. Nontoxic concentration of ceftazidime and flomoxef sodium for intravitreal use—evaluated by in-vitro ERG. Lens Eye Toxic Res 1990;7(3-4):677-83.
14. Campochiaro PA, Conway BP. Aminoglycoside toxicity—a survey of retinal specialists. Implications for ocular use. Arch Ophthalmol 1991;109(7):946-50.
15. D'Amico DJ, Caspers-Velu L, Libert J, et al. Comparative toxicity of intravitreal aminoglycoside antibiotics. Am J Ophthalmol 1985;100(2):264-75.
16. Campochiaro PA, Lim JI. Aminoglycoside toxicity in the treatment of endophthalmitis. The Aminoglycoside Toxicity Study Group. Arch Ophthalmol 1994;112(1):48-53.
17. Kumar A, Dada T. Preretinal haemorrhages: an unusual manifestation of intravitreal amikacin toxicity. Aust N Z J Ophthalmol 1999;27(6):435-6.
18. Seawright AA, Bourke RD, Cooling RJ. Macula toxicity after intravitreal amikacin. Aust N Z J Ophthalmol 1996;24(2):143-6.
19. Mandell BA, Meredith TA, Aguilar E, et al. Effects of inflammation and surgery on amikacin levels in the vitreous cavity. Am J Ophthalmol 1993;115(6):770-4.
20. Shaarawy A, Grand MG, Meredith TA, Ibanez HE. Persistent endophthalmitis after intravitreal antimicrobial therapy. Ophthalmology 1995;102(3):382-7.
21. Aguilar HE, Meredith TA, Shaarawy A, et al. Vitreous cavity penetration of ceftazidime after intravenous administration. Retina 1995;15(2):154-9.
22. Keren G, Alhalel A, Bartov E, et al. The intravitreal penetration of orally administered ciprofloxacin in humans. Invest Ophthalmol Vis Sci 1991;32(8):2388-92.
23. Martin DF, Ficker LA, Aguilar HA, et al. Vitreous cefazolin levels after intravenous injection. Effects of inflammation, repeated antibiotic doses, and surgery. Arch Ophthalmol 1990;108(3):411-4.
24. Ferencz JR, Assia EI, Diamantstein L, Rubinstein E. Vancomycin concentration in the vitreous after intravenous and intravitreal administration for postoperative endophthalmitis. Arch Ophthalmol 1999;117(8):1023-7.
25. Souli M, Kopsinis G, Kavouklis E, et al. Vancomycin levels in human aqueous humour after intravenous and subconjunctival administration. Int J Antimicrob Agents 2001;18(3):239-43.
26. Das T, Sharma S. Current management strategies of acute post-operative endophthalmitis. Semin Ophthalmol 2003;18(3):109-15.
27. Mather R, Karenchak LM, Romanowski EG, Kowalski RP. Fourth generation fluoroquinolones: new weapons in the arsenal of ophthalmic antibiotics. Am J Ophthalmol 2002;133(4):463-6.
28. Hariprasad SM, Mieler WF, Holz ER. Vitreous and aqueous penetration of orally administered gatifloxacin in humans. Arch Ophthalmol 2003;121(3):345-50.
29. Foster RE, Rubsamen PE, Joondeph BC, et al. Concurrent endophthalmitis and retinal detachment. Ophthalmology 1994;101(3):490-8.
30. Barza M. Antibacterial agents in the treatment of ocular infections. Infect Dis Clin North Am 1989;3(3):533-51.
31. Kwak HW, D'Amico DJ. Evaluation of the retinal toxicity and pharmacokinetics of dexamethasone after intravitreal injection. Arch Ophthalmol 1992;110(2):259-66.

32. Park SS, Vallar RV, Hong CH, et al. Intravitreal dexamethasone effect on intravitreal vancomycin elimination in endophthalmitis. Arch Ophthalmol 1999;117(8):1058-62.
33. Falk NS, Beer PM, Peters GB, 3rd. Role of intravitreal triamcinolone acetonide in the treatment of postoperative endophthalmitis. Retina 2006;26(5):545-8.
34. Hykin PG, Tobal K, McIntyre G, et al. The diagnosis of delayed post-operative endophthalmitis by polymerase chain reaction of bacterial DNA in vitreous samples. J Med Microbiol 1994;40(6):408-15.
35. Aldave AJ, Stein JD, Deramo VA, et al. Treatment strategies for postoperative Propionibacterium acnes endophthalmitis. Ophthalmology 1999;106(12):2395-401.
36. Clark WL, Kaiser PK, Flynn HW, Jr., et al. Treatment strategies and visual acuity outcomes in chronic postoperative Propionibacterium acnes endophthalmitis. Ophthalmology 1999;106(9):1665-70.
37. Ciulla TA. Update on acute and chronic endophthalmitis. Ophthalmology 1999;106(12):2237-8.
38. Luttrull JK, Wan WL, Kubak BM, et al. Treatment of ocular fungal infections with oral fluconazole. Am J Ophthalmol 1995;119(4):477-81.
39. Chen PP, Gedde SJ, Budenz DL, Parrish RK, 2nd. Outpatient treatment of bleb infection. Arch Ophthalmol 1997;115(9):1124-8.
40. Kangas TA, Greenfield DS, Flynn HW, Jr., et al. Delayed-onset endophthalmitis associated with conjunctival filtering blebs. Ophthalmology 1997;104(5):746-52.
41. Foster RE, Martinez JA, Murray TG, et al. Useful visual outcomes after treatment of Bacillus cereus endophthalmitis. Ophthalmology 1996;103(3):390-7.
42. Narang S, Gupta V, Gupta A, et al. Role of prophylactic intravitreal antibiotics in open globe injuries. Indian J Ophthalmol 2003;51(1):39-44.
43. Reynolds DS, Flynn HW, Jr. Endophthalmitis after penetrating ocular trauma. Curr Opin Ophthalmol 1997;8(3):32-8.
44. Weishaar PD, Flynn HW, Jr., Murray TG, et al. Endogenous Aspergillus endophthalmitis. Clinical features and treatment outcomes. Ophthalmology 1998;105(1):57-65.
45. Chen YJ, Kuo HK, Wu PC, et al. A 10-year comparison of endogenous endophthalmitis outcomes: an east Asian experience with Klebsiella pneumoniae infection. Retina 2004;24(3):383-90.
46. Chou FF, Kou HK. Endogenous endophthalmitis associated with pyogenic hepatic abscess. J Am Coll Surg 1996;182(1):33-6.
47. Yoon YH, Lee SU, Sohn JH, Lee SE. Result of early vitrectomy for endogenous Klebsiella pneumoniae endophthalmitis. Retina 2003;23(3):366-70.
48. Roth DB, Chieh J, Spirn MJ, et al. Noninfectious endophthalmitis associated with intravitreal triamcinolone injection. Arch Ophthalmol 2003;121(9):1279-82.

Chapter 19

Clinical Applications of Antimycotic Agents in the Eye

Niranjan Nayak (India)

INTRODUCTION

Fungal infections of the eye can give rise to severe ocular morbidity, often leading to blindness, if not treated early. In many tropical countries, including India, keratitis is the most frequently encountered fungal infection[1]. However, infections of the orbit, lids, lacrimal apparatus, sclera, conjunctiva and intra-ocular structures due to fungi are not uncommon. Early diagnosis followed by immediate therapeutic intervention may help in preventing many vision threatening complications. Thus, informations on the choice of appropriate antifungal agents and their clinical applications certainly help the ophthalmologist in the effective management of the cases. In the present review, discussion will mainly be focused on the therapeutic modalities for the most important clinical entities like keratomycosis, endophthalmitis, orbital cellulitis and dacryocystitis.

KERATOMYCOSIS

Keratomycosis or fungal infection of the cornea was described for the first time by Leber[2] in Germany in the year 1879. Since then it has been recognised as a major public health problem in the tropical parts of many developing countrie.[3-5] Corneal infection of fungal etiology may represent 40 to 50% of all cases of culture proven infectious keratitis.[3,6] If not treated early, this condition may lead to corneal blindness.

Treatment of Fungal Keratitis

If direct microscopic examinations of corneal scrapes or corneal biopsies yield definite results that are consistent with the clinical picture, treatment should be initiated immediately.[5] The antifugnal agents available today to combat fungal keratitis are not so well developed as those available against bacterial infections. Most of the available agents only inhibit the growth of the fungus necessitating the host defense mechanisms to eradicate the infection.[7]

The currently used antifungal agents belong to (1) Polyenes, (2) Azoles, including newer azoles (3) Pyrimidines, (4) other derivatives.

Polyenes

The polyene antibiotics bind to the ergosterol of fungal cell membrane, creating pores that disrupt the homeostatic mechanisms leading to cell death. *Nystatin* was the first polyene antifungal to be identified. It has been recommended for topical use (100,000 units). However, its only limitations are corneal toxicity and poor ocular penetration.[7]

Amongst all the polyenes, *Natamycin* is often the first drug of choice to be used for filamentous infections since it is commercially easily available. It is marketed as a 5% suspension for topical use. It has broad spectrum of acitivity against filamentous fungi. A 5% suspension in the eye is well tolerated. However, this drug may be ineffective in cases with deep stromal abscess because of poor corneal penetration.[7]

Amphotericin B has widely been used as a topical and systemic drug for ocular infections. Preparation of a 0.15% suspension of this drug , reconstituted from the 50 mg vial powder (for IV formulation) is universally adopted for topical use as the first line drug both for *Candida* keratitis as well as for keratitis due to other mycelial fungi.[8] After topical application, this drug can penetrate deep into the corneal stroma and 0.15% suspension is well tolerated, when instilled round the clock every 15 to 30 minutes.

Pyrimidines—5 Fluorocytosine is a synthetic pyrimidine analogue. This drug is available in the form of 1% suspension for topical use. It can be given orally (150 mg/kg) as well. It has synergistic effect if given in combination with amphotericin B in fungal keratitis. Its topical form is nontoxic to the eye. If given systemically, it may cause transient bone marrow depression and gastrointestinal upset. The main drawback of this drug is its limited spectrum of activity against filamentous fungi and rapid development of resistance by *Candida* species.[9,10]

Azoles—Azoles include the imidazoles and the structurally related N-substituted triazoles. These two share the same antifungal spectrum and similar mechanism of action. However, systemic triazoles have a longer half-life than imidazoles. The imidazoles include clotrimazole, miconazole and ketoconazole. The triazoles include fluconazole and itraconazole.

Clotrimazole is usually used topically for skin and genital *Candida* infections. It is marketed as a 1% lotion for fungal dermatitis and as 1% cream for Candida vaginitis. A 1% vaginal cream placed into an ophthalmic ointment container can be used for topical use in the eye for the treatment of keratomycosis.

Miconazole can be used as 1% eye drop, or through systemic infusion (20 mg/kg body weight)[1]. The 1% topical application is well tolerated and is reported to be quite successful in treating keratomycosis due to *Aspergillus* and *Candida* species.[12] A perspective series from India[13] found it to be effective in 64.7% of the cases when administered topically every 2 hours. It is usually reserved as a second-line drug in the management of fungal keratitis[2].

Ketoconazole is another imidazole with pharmacological properties similar to that of miconazole. However, it is less toxic and is easily absorbable from the gastrointestinal tract. It is available as oral preparation in the form of 200 mg tablets. It can also be administered topically as 2% eye drops. Studies on rabbit models[14,15] of keratitis showed effective intraocular penetration of ketoconazole after oral administration. This drug was also shown to be quite effective both as a prophylactic and a therapeutic agent after topical administration[16].

Fluconazole is a triazole compound, which can be administered both systemically (200-400 mg per day) and topically (0.2% eyedrops). After topical application, as 0.2% eyedrop it shows good penetration into the anterior chamber.[17] The preparation is also well tolerated in the eye.

Itraconazole is a newer triazole which has larger spectrum of activity than fluconazole against filamentous fungi.[2] However, its only drawback is its hydrophobicity, and hence tissue penetration is poor. A study from India reported an effectivity rate of 69% when topical or systemic itraconazole was used as the sole therapeutic agent for keratomycosis[18].

Coad et al,[19] on the basis of tube dilution minimal inhibitory concentration and minimal fungicidal concentration testing, determined that the imidazoles such as miconazole and ketoconazole consistently showed the lowest geometric mean titre for filamentus fungi. Thus, systemic azoles, in general have a good penetration and are frequently used for fungal keratitis. However, they have drug interactions and require monitoring of liver function tests.

Newer Azoles

Voriconazole is a new azole with broad spectrum efficacy for fungal keratitis and endophthalmitis. In a recent study,[20] *in vitro* susceptibility of various fungal isolates in infectious keratitis towards Voriconazole was 100%, towards ketoconazole 82.4%, amphotericin B 76.5%, itraconazole 67%, fluconazole 60% and 5-fluorocytocin 60%. Voriconazole MIC (90) was lowest for *Candida* species (0.016 mg/ml). They concluded that Voriconazole was a better alternative for the therapeutic management of *Candida* and *Aspergilus* ocular infections, as compared to other antifungals.

Testing of topical voriconazole in a rabbit model of *Paecilomyces* induced fungal keratitis, was quite encouraging.[21] It was observed that voriconazole therapy caused lesions to decrease within 8 days. Hyphal masses were present in the control infected eyes (not treated with the drug), but absent in the treated infected eyes (as observed after sacrificing the animals and examining the sections of the eyeball). It was therefore postulated that topical voriconazole was a good and effective alternative to topical amphotericin B, because *Paecilomyces* species were often resistant to amphotericin B. In yet another development, Ozbek et al,[22] emphasised the role of voriconazole in the management of *Alternaria* keratiits.

Other Derivatives

Echinocandins These drugs have recently emerged as valuable antifungal agents.These are cell wall acting agents unlike amphotericin B which acts on the cell membrane. These drugs inhibit β 1-3 glucan synthesis, and include Caspofungin and Micafungin . Recently, topical Caspofungin was tried in a rabbit model,[23] in which a 0.5% suspension of the drug was found to be as effective as 0.15% amphotericin B, in the treatment of keratitis caused by *Candida*.

Povidone-iodine (Betadine) and Polyhexamethyl Biguanide (PHMB) The effectiveness of Povodone-iodine (Betadine) and PHMB as topical antifungals was evaluated by a study group in India[24] in experimentally induced *Aspergillus fumigatus* keratitis in rabbits. Keratitis was induced by corneal intrastromal infection of spores of A fumigatus in four groups of six healthy rabbits each. Drugs used were 5% natamycin, 0.02% PHMB, 1% betadine and 0.5% hydroxypropyl methyl celllulose (HPMC) as control. The average healing time of ulcers were 21.5 ± 3.08 days for natamycin, 27.8 ± 2.28 days for PHMB, 36.4±2.57days for betadine and 38.2±4.7 for HPMC. While no corneal perforation occurred with Natamycin therapy, there was one perforation case with PHMB, three with betadine and 5 with HPMC. Thus, 1% betadine was not effective in fungal keratitis while 0.02%PHMB was moderately effective.

Silver sulfadiazine Another antifungal agent that has been used successfully in fungal keratitis is topical silver sulfadiazine, an ointment generally used for prophylactic purpose in patients with burns[2]. In a study of a series of 110 patients from India using the ointment 5 times a day, the drug was found to be effective in 76.3% of the cases caused by a variety of fungi, especially by *Fusarium* species[25]. A randomised clinical trial, conducted by the same workers[26], found silver sulfadiazine more effective than miconazole in a group of patients with keratomycosis (80% vs 55%). However, their view was that additional clinical trials were needed comparing silver sulfadiazine to polyenes in the treatment of mycotic keratitis.

Therefore, the overall view on the management of mycotic keratitis is that the condition responds slowly over a period of weeks to antifungal therapy. Thus, in order to evaluate the prognosis, clinical signs of improvement should carefully be noted which include diminution of pain, decrease in the size of the infiltrate, disappearance of satellite lesions, rounding of the feathery margins of the ulcer and hyperplastic masses or fibrous sheets in the region of healing fungal lesions.[3] Negative scrapings during treatment do not always indicate that fungal infection has been eradicated, since there may be active proliferation of the fungi deep in the stroma; hence therapy should be continued for at least 6 weeks, depending upon the antifungal agent selected (Table 19.1).

Table 19.1: Antifungal regime for keratomycosis

Yeasts First choice Amphotericin B 0.15% eyedrops Fluconazole (0.5% drops, 200 mg orally)	Alternatives Flucytocine (1% drops,150 mg/kg orally) Miconazole 1% drops,subcunjunctival/ injection Ketoconazole 1% drops Ketoconazole 200 mg bd orally
Filamentous fungi First choice Natamycin 5% drops	Alternatives Amphotericin B 0.15% drops + Flucytosine Itraconazole (1% cream + 200-400 mg orally)

Patients with deep stromal infections and those who have received corticosteroids appear to respond poorly to medical therapy.[27] Surgery may be necessary in such cases. Every attempt is made, however, to prolong medical therapy for as long as possible, since this renders the infecting fungus nonviable, thereby improving the outcome of surgery. At the same time surgery may help medical management by increasing drug penetration. For example, in small superficial corneal fungal infections, regular surgical debridement of the base of the ulcer helps elimination of fungi and necrotic material, facilitating the penetration of antifungal drugs into the corneal stroma[3].

ORBITAL CELLULITIS

Orbital cellulitis is an infection of the soft tissue surrounding the orbit. Orbital cellulitis of fungal origin is the most serious ocular infection with significant potential morbidity, including loss of vision, cavernous sinus thrombosis, intracranial spread of infection and occasionally death.[28,29] Therefore, it is essential that patients with periorbital infection need careful evaluation and treatment.

Treatment Modalities for Orbital Cellulitis

Systemic amphotericin B is the drug of choice. As has been emphasised earlier, the condition being acute and fatal, clinical diagnosis and positive smear report are quite suggestive of starting systemic amphotericin B therapy without waiting for the culture report which may take days. Conventional Amphotericin B being nephrotoxic, it is administered with gradually increasing dosage each day, starting with 0.25 mg/kg/day, increasing each day by 0.25 mg/kg/day till a dosage of 5 mg/kg/day is achieved.

The drug should be administered in the form of slow intravenous drip in 5% dextrose solution. During the course of therapy, constant monitoring of blood urea is recommended. In case of development of features of renal toxicity, systemic amphotericin B should be omited and in place of that oral itraconazole 200 mg twice daily for 4 to 6 weeks should be started. If there is no renal toxicity and the clinical condition of the patient improves after systemic administration of amphotericin B, then the patient is put on itraconazole therapy, amphotericin B being omited. Attempts have also been made to deliver amphotericin B directly to the infected orbital tissue, in the form of daily irrigation and packing.[30]

In addition to the aforementioned modalities, several novel formulations of amphotericin B have been tried clinically with excellent results, keeping in view the potent toxicity of the conventional drug. Such preparations include amphotericin B colloidal dispersion and liposomal amphotericin B.[30,31] However, controlled trials are needed to assess the efficacy of these lipid formulations and of the conventional Amphotericin B in the therapy of ophthalmic mycoses.

DACRYOCYSTITIS

Dacryocystitis is infection of the lacrimal sac. The primary lesion is the obstruction of nasolacrimal duct (NLD). As a result, there occurs obstruction to the normal flow of tears through the sac. This alongwith retained microbial contents give rise to inflammation of the sac.

Treatment of Dacryocystitis

Mycotic dacryocystitis responds well to topical administration of 5% natamycin. Somctimes, alongwith the topical application, local syringing of the sac with either amphotericin B (1.5 to 8 mg/ml) or Nystatin (100,000 units/ ml). solutions may be quite helpful.[32]

ENDOPHTHALMITIS

Endophthalmitis is an inflammatory reaction of intraocular fluid or tissues. Endophthalmitis can be infectious or non-infectious. Infectious endo-phthalmitis is one of the most serious and vision threatening complications of ophthalmic surgery. Infectious endophthalmitis may be postoperative, post-traumatic or endogenous.

Recommended Therapy for Endophthalmitis

Intravitreal Amphotericin B

The recommended dosage of intravitreal amphotericin B is 7.5 mg in 0.1 ml (prepared from a 50 mg vial by serial dilution). Table 19. 2 illustrates the details of the steps for preparation of intravitreal formulation of amphotericin B.

Table 19.2: Amphotericin B (AmB) for intraocular injection (7.5 μg/ml)
a. Inject 10 ml water into the bottle with 50 mg dry AmB. Shake until transparent (50 mg Am B)
b. Take 1 ml of this into a 10-ml syringe (5 mg Am B)
c. Dilute with water to 10 ml, shake well
d. 1 ml of the above (500 μg Am B) is diluted with water to 6.7 ml and must be shaken (74.62 μg/ml Am B)
e. Take 0.1 ml of this with an insulin syringe (7.4 μg Am B)

Systemic

Ketoconazole 200 mg tid orally is also advocated. However, intravenous amphotericin B is quite effective. This is administered by IV infusion in 5 % dextrose solution, starting with 0.25 mg/kg on the 1st day, increasing by 0.25 mg/kg/day till a total dosage of 0.6 mg/kg is achieved.

Influence of Fungal Species on Therapeutic Outcome of Infection

The therapeutic implications of the above clinical entities are often influenced by the various fungal species causing the infections. For example the situation is quite alarming in cases of endophthalmitis caused by species of *Candida* other than C *albicans.* These *Candida* species are reportedly showing in vitro resistance to fluconazole. In addition, *C. tropicalis* is intrinsically resistant to many azole compounds. Thus, newer azoles like voriconazole and posaconazole are worth trying.[22]

Similarly, considering about mycotic keratitis one would surely appreciate that the most common fungi like *Fusarium* species produce very severe infection with rapid onset of perforation of the cornea. Vision may be completely lost if timely therapeutic intervention is not initiated.[33,34] The same is true for keratitis due to *Aspergillus flavus* and *Pseudallescheria boydii.* Keratis. In all the above situations the organisms give rise to severe form of keratitis with very poor clinical improvement, in spite of all possible medical therapy and may thus require surgical intervention.[35,36]

Considering the aforementioned clinical situations,therapy of such cases always remains a challenge before the treating ophthalmologist[22] and thus, testing for antifungal drug susceptibility seems to be a suitable solution to this.[28,36]

Some progress has been made in this field during the past decade with the standardisation of various parameters of antifungal sensitivity testing.The methods currently recommended by CLSI (Clinical and Laboratory standard Institute) have been adopted by many laboratories for the standardisation of the techniques both for filamentous fungi and yeasts and reproducibilities of the results have been claimed.[37-40]

A recent study,based upon such testing, documented the superiority of voriconazole over itraconazole towards fluconazole resistant *Candida* isolates. Thus, antifungal drug sensitivity testing in a routine laboratory could help the clinician in prescribing drugs which are effective against a particular clinical isolate, rather than putting the patient on empirical therapy without knowing whether the patient is going to respond to the prescribed treatment or not. In this context, the results of a recent study [41] are noteworthy. While studying on the risk factors and treatment outcome in fungal keratitis the authors highlighted the importance of selecting the appropriate antifungal agent particularly for patients who were refractory to the primary therapy [41]. In addition to this there are scanty reports of inadequetly treated fungal keratitis (becuause the sensitivity pattern was not known) leading to serious complications like endophthalmitis.[42] All the above mentioned observations only point towards one thing that antifungal susceptibility testing is a prerequisite in the management of all problematic clinical situations mentioned above.

Of all the clinical conditions mentioned above, orbital cellulitis is the one the clinical outcome of which which is invariably fatal unless appropriate and timely therapeutic measures are undertaken. This is especially so if there is intracranial spread, which is not unusual in an immuno-compromised patient. More importantly, *Mucor* and *Rhizopus* can give rise to a fulminant and acutely fatal disease when the patient is ketoacidotic. In such cases, the prognosis is very poor.[43,44]

Although the best available therapeutic modality in such cases is intravenous amphotericin B, problem sometimes arises in managing the cases. This is owing to the fact that fungal isolates from deep seated infections like this often show higher MICs for amphotericin B. Thus the patient might have to be put on a high dose regime, i.e. 5 mg/kg/day of the drug, with a constant watch on blood urea and creatinine levels. In case of blood chemistry abnormality, the drug should be replaced with oral pasaconazole.[44]

Mycotic dacryocystitis, though uncommon invariably responds satisfactorily to topical antifungals mentioned above. However, if medical management fails, surgery is advocated.

In spite of the above mentioned effective antifungal regime , the clinical outcome of fungal dacryocystitis, especially those due to *Aspergilli* or *Candida* is not quite encouraging. About 40% of the cases managed by medical treatment alone do recur, whereas around 80% of those who undergo surgery alongwith medical treatment get cured.[32,45]

REFERENCES

1. Srinivasan R, Kanungo R, Goyal JL. Spectrum of oculomycosis in South India. Acta Ophthalmol 1991;69:744-9.
2. Abad JC, Foster CS. Fungal keratitis. Intl Ophthalmol Clinic 1996 ; 36 : 1-15.
3. Agarwal V, Biswas J, Madhavan HN, et al. Current perspectives in infectious keratitis. Indian J Ophthalmol 1994;42:171-92.
4. Sharma S,Srinivasn M,George C. The current status of Fusarium species in mycotic keratitis in South India. Indian J Med Microbiol 1993;11:140-7.
5. Thomas PA. Fungal infections of the cornea. Eye 2003;17:852-2.
6. Vajpayee RB, Ray M, Panda A, Sharma N, Taylor HR, Murthy GV, Satpathy G, Pandey RM. Risk factors of pediatric presumed microbial keratitis. Ann Ophthalmol 2002;34:204-310.
7. Walsh TJ, Pizzo A. Treatment of systemic fungal infections: recent progress and current problems. Eur Clin Microbiol Infect Dis 1988;1:460-75.
8. Tanure MA, Cohen EJ, Grewal S, Rapuano CJ, Laibson PR. Spectrum of fungal keratitis at Wills Eye Hospital, Philadelphia, Pennsylvania. Cornea 2000;19: 307-12.
9. Beggs WH. Mechanism of synergistic interaction between amphotericin B and flucytosine. J Antimirob Chemother 1986;17:403-4.
10. Viviani MA. Flucytosine-what is its future? J Antimicrob Chemother 1995 ; 35 : 241-4.
11. Pflugfelder SC, Flynn HW, Zwickey TA, et al. Exogenous fugnal endophthalmitis. Ophthalmology 1988;95:19-30.
12. Fitzsimons R, Peters AI. Miconazole and ketoconazole as satisfactory first-line treatment for keratomycosis. Am J Ophthalmol 1986;101:605-8.
13. Mohan M, Panda A, Gupta SK. Management of human keratomycosis with miconazole. Aust N Z J Ophthalmol 1989;17:295-7.
14. Komadina TG, Wilkes TD, Shock JP. et al Treatment of *Aspergillus fumigatus* keratitis in rabbits with oral and topical ketoconazole. Am J Ophthalmol 1985;99: 476-9.
15. Hemady RK, Foster CS. Intra-ocular penetration of ketoconazole in rabbits. Cornea 1992;11:329-33.
16. Oji EO. Ketoconazole: a new imidazole agent has both prophylactic potential and therapeutic efficacy in keratomycosis in rabbits. Int Ophthalmol 1982;5: 163-7.
17. Behrens-Baumann W, Klinge R, Richel R. Topical flucanazole for experimental *Candida* keratitis in rabbits. Br J Ophthalmol 1990;74:40-2.
18. Rajasekaran J, Thomas PA, Kalavathy CM, Joseph PC, Abraham DJ. Itraconazole therapy for fungal keratitis. Indian J Ophthalmol 1987;35:157-60.
19. Coad CT, RobinsonNM, Weilhelmus KR. Antifungal sensitivity testing for equine keratomycosis. Am J Vet Res 1985;46:676-8.

20. Marangon FB, Miller D, Giacore JA, Alfonso EC. Invitro investigation of voriconazole susceptibility for keratitis and endophthalmitis fungal pathogens. Am J Ophthalmolol 2004;137:820-5.
21. Sponset W, Chen N, Dang D, Paris G, Graybill J, Najvar LK, Zhou L, Lam KW, Glickman R, Scribbick F. Topical voriconazole as a novel treatment for fungal keratitis Antimicrob Agents Chemother 2006;50:262-8.
22. Ozbek Z, Kang S, Sivalingam J, Rapuano CJ, Cohen EJ, Hammersmith KM. Voriconazole in the management of *Alternaria* keratitis. Cornea 2006;25:242-4.
23. Goldblum D, Fruch BE, Sarra GM, Katsoulis K, Zimmerli S. Topical caspofungin for treatment of keratitis caused by *Candida abicans* in a rabbit model. Antimicrob Agetns Chemother 2005;49:1359-63.
24. Panda A, Ahuja R, Biswas NR, Satpathy G, Khokhar S. Role of .02% polyhexamethyl biguanide and 1% puvidone iodine in experimental *Aspergillus* keratitis. Cornea 2003;22:138-41.
25. Mohan M, Gupta SK, Kalra VK, Vajpayee RB, Sachdev MS. Silver sulphadiazene in the treatment of mycotic keratitis. Indian J Med Res 1987;85:572-5.
26. Mohan M, Gupta SK, Kalra VK, Vajpayee RB, Sachdev MS. Topial silver sulphadiazine—a new drug for ocular kratomycosis. Br J Ophthalmol 1988;72: 192-5.
27. Wilhelmus KR, Jones DB. *Curvularia* keratitis. Trans Am Ophthalmol Soc 2001; 99:111-32.
28. Israele V, Nelson JD. Periorbital and orbital cellulitis. Pediatr Infect Dis J 1987; 6: 404-10.
29. Jackson K, Barker SR. Clinical implications of orbital cellulitis. Laryngoscope 1986;96:568-74.
30. Khoo SH, Band J, Denning DW. Administering amphotericin B—a practical approach. J Antimicrob Chemother 1994;33:203-13.
31. Walker S, Tailor SAN, Lee M, et al. Amphotericin B in lipid emulsions : stability, compatibility and in vitro antifungal acitiviy. Antimicrob Agents Chemother 1998; 42:762-6.
32. Ghose S, Mahajan VM. Microbiology of congenital dacryocystitis:its clinical significance. J Ocul Ther Surg 1985;4:54-7.
33. Jones BR. Principles in the management of oculomycosis. Am J Ophthalmol 1975; 79:719-51.
34. Vemuganti GK, Garg P, Gopinathan U, et al. Evaluation of agent and host factors in progression of mycotic keratitis : a histologic and microbiologic study of 167 corneal buttons. Ophthalmology 2002;109:1538-46.
35. Bloom PA, Laidlaw DA, Easty DL, Warnock DW. Treatment failure in case of fungal keratitis caused by *Pseudallescheria boydii*. Br J Ophthalmol 1992 ; 76 : 367-8.
36. Ozkurt Y, Oral Y, Kuleckei Z, Benzonana N, Ustaoglu R, Dogan OK. Pseudallescheria boydii keratitis. J Paed Ophthalmol Strabismus 2006;43:114-5.
37. Pujol I, Guarro J, Sala J and Riba MD. Effects of incubation temperative, inoculum size, and time of reading on broth microdilution susceptibility test results for Amphotericin B against Fusarium. Antimicrob Agents and Chemother 1997;41: 808-11.
38. Espinel-Ingroff A, Barchiese F, Cuenca – Estrella M, et al. International and multicenter comparison of EUCAST and CLSI M27-a2 broth microdilution methods for testing susceptibility of candida species to flucanazole, itraconazole, posaconazole and voriconazole. J Clin Microbiol 2005;43:3884-9.

39. Roma, Kaushal Anju, Roy P and Singh H. Antifungal susceptibility patern of non-albicans *Candida* species and distribution of species isolated form candidaemia cases over a 5 year period. Indian J Med Res 1996;106:171-6.
40. Nguyen MH, and Yu CY. Influence of incubation time, inodulum size, and glucose concentration on spetrophotometric endpoint : determinants of Amphotericin B, fluconazole and itraconazole. J Clin Microbol 1999;37:141-5.
41. Lalitha P, Prajna NV, Kabra A, Mahadevan K, Srinivasan M. Risk factors and Rx outcome in fungal keratitis. Ophthalmology 2006;113:526-30.
42. Rosenberg KD, Flynn HW Jr., Alfonse EC, Miller D. *Fusarium* endophthalmitis following keratitis associated with contact lens. Oph Surg Laser Imaging 2006; 37:310-3.
43. Lessner A, Stern GA. Preseptal and orbital cellulitis. Infect Dis Clin of North America 1972;6:933-52.
44. Rutor T, Cockerham KP. Periorbital zygomycosois (Mucormycosis) trated with posaconazole. Am J Ophthalmol 2006;142:187-8.
45. Ghose S, Jha RK, Nayak N, Satpathy G, Bajaj MS, Pushker N, Balasubramaniam ST, Prasad R. Current microbial correlates of the eye and nose in dacryocystitis-their clinical significance. Proceedings of All India Ophthalmological Society Conference 2005;437-9.

Chapter 20

Ocular Drug Toxicity (Complications)

Ashok Garg (India)

Ocular tissue undesired side effects have been seen by every ophthalmologists in their practice involving various drugs used topically and systemically for the treatment of various ocular problems. An adverse drug reaction (ADR) is an undesirable response to a drug occurring during or following a course of therapy. The types of adverse effects of drugs on the eye may be mild and transient like temporary decrease in vision, abnormal pupillary responses, Accommodation impairment, color vision disturbance, abnormal eye movements to serious side effects like cataract, glaucoma and retinal damage which may seriously disrupt in ocular functions.

It is essential for every ophthalmologist to have complete insight to recognize and prevent vision threatening complications from adverse effects of drug reactions. It is essential for the ophthalmologist to obtain a careful history with special attention to particular medication used. The clinicians shall be fully aware of certain oculotoxic drugs and their side effects to detect the drug related ocular disorder.

Before going into details of complications of various topical ocular formulations, let me remind you that for certain drugs with potential ocular toxicity a careful pre-treatment examination should be performed before the drug is administered specially if:

a. The drug shall be used for a long period of time.
b. If it is known to have established severe toxic effects.

Patients taking such drugs should undergo frequent monitoring examinations so that if the symptoms do arise, the drugs can be withdrawn immediately.

Often reversible effect are observed while the patient is off the drug and later after resolution of the effects, the drug regimen may be restarted at a lower dose. The pre-treatment examination should include following parameters:

I. **Visual acuity:** Check visual acuity for near and distance vision with and without pin-hole testing and spectacles (if required).
II. **Pupillary responses:** Check pupil size, briskness of reactions (direct and consensual) to light and convergence reflex.
III. **Ocular motility examination:** Check complete motility in all field directions of gaze with ductions, versions and convergence.
IV. **Intraocular pressure monitoring:** Periodic tonometry should be done as intraocular pressure rise is sensitive adverse effect of certain topical formulations.
V. **Slit-lamp examination** is essential as certain drugs affect the conjunctiva, cornea and lens.
VI. **Ophthalmoscopy:** Perform ophthalmoscopy (Direct and indirect) with dilation as certain drugs may produce changes in the retina, macula and the optic nerve.
VII. **Specific retinal function examinations:** These examinations include:
- Electroretinography (ERG)
- Fundus photography
- Visual field analysis
- Color vision tests
- Visual evoked potential (VEP)
- Fluorescein angiography

Generalized ocular manifestations of drug toxicity
- Reduced visual acuity due to transient changes in refractive errors, anterior and posterior segment toxicity.
- Blurring of vision may be caused by mydriasis and cycloplegia as well as anterior and posterior segment toxic changes.
- Color vision disturbances that may include hallucination, altered perception and diminished sensitivity.
- Ocular movement abnormalities include neuromuscular myesthenic block, paralytic strabismus, diplopia and oculogyric crisis.
- Severe conjunctival inflammation and corneal opacification.
- Glaucoma.
- Cataract development.
- Optic nerve pathology (optic neuritis).
- Exophthalmos, retinal hemorrhage, vasculopathy, retinal pigment epitheliopathy and macular edema.

Ocular adverse drug reactions (OADR) may be predictable and unpredictable. In 80-90% of cases OADR caused by drugs can lead to complete loss of vision also. The causes of adverse drug reactions are summarised as follows:
- Exaggeration of intended pharmacological effects.
- Concomitant administration of drugs with synergistic effects.
- Immunological mechanism

- Idiosyncratic reactions
- Cytotoxic reactions
- Genetically determined enzymatic defects.
- Error in self administration of the drugs.

Here in this chapter I shall discuss the main systemic and local complications due to the use of various topical ocular formulations and ocular surgery adjuncts prescribed by ophthalmologists in their day to day practice. In modern high tech scenario it is important to have complete insight into the complications of prescribing ophthalmic formulations.

COMPLICATIONS OF TOPICAL ANTIMICROBIAL AGENTS

Topical antimicrobial drugs—antibiotics, antifungals, antivirals and anti-parasitics are the most common drugs prescribed by ophthalmologists. These drugs used to treat a wide variety of infectious diseases ranging from mild conditions to vision threatening infections such as corneal ulceration and endophthalmitis. Topical antimicrobial agents are often used in postocular surgical phase for the prophylaxis of infections. Although these drugs are effective, however, in some cases complications may arise from their use. In this chapter, I review the common and serious complications of the use of topical antimicrobial drugs.

Systemic Complications

A major advantage of the topical use of drugs is that high local drug level can be achieved with minimal systemic absorption, However, idiosyncratic and immunological reactions can occur with exposure to minute quantities of drugs. Two such reactions that may occur related to the use of topical anti-microbial drugs are aplastic anemia and Stevens-Johnson syndrome.

Aplastic Anemia

It is a well know, potentially fatal complication of the ingestion of drugs. Chloramphenicol a commonly used topical ophthalmic antibiotic is the most common cause of drug related aplastic anemia. Bacterial breakdown product of chloramphenicol may be responsible for this complication in susceptible individuals.

Chloramphenicol has two known effects on the bone morrow.

1. Dose related reversible suppression of the bone marrow affecting mainly the red blood cell line.
2. Progressive marrow aplasia.

Stevens-Johnson Syndrome

It is an acute dermatitis with severe mucous membrane involvement that most commonly occurs in association with *Mycoplasma pneumoniae* infection or as a reaction to variety of drugs. In the milder from of disease there is symmetrical involvement with skin lesions affecting mainly the extremities. Mucous membrane involvement is mild and generally limited to one surface. The disease generally resolves in 1 to 4 weeks without important sequelae.

In major form cutaneous eruptions are more variable in morphological features, area of extent of involvement.

Lesions may become confluent, bullar may form and there may be toxic epidermal necrolysis.

Drug induced cases of STS generally occur after 7-14 days of drug therapy but may occur within hours if patients had previous exposure to the drug. Sulfonamides are the drugs most commonly complicated as causes of SJS followed by penicillins.

Phenylbutazone and barbiturates. Patients should be questioned about previous exosure to sulfonamides and especially about any reaction to these drugs before ophthalmic sulphonamide preparations are prescribed.

Local Complications

Most of the complications of topical antimicrobial drugs affect only local structure. They may be immunological or allergic in origin, related to toxicity of the drug or refect a lack of specificity of effect against the organism being treated. Local side effects may be caused by preservatives which are combined in commercially available antimicrobials.

Non Specific Local Complications

1. *Contact dermatoconjunctivitis:* It is a cell mediated reaction and most commonly related to the use of topical ophthalmic medications. Patients are usually sensitized to previous exposure to the drug. Because of popularity of topical neomycin - polymixin B – bacitracin combination, many individuals are sensitized to neomycin, a common cause of this condition. This disease begins 24-72 hours following repeated instillation of the drug.

The patient complains of itching. Chronic changes include thickening of skin and hyperpigmentation and sometimes mild ectropion may occur.

Initially findings will be more apparent in the lower conjunctiva and eyelid but eventually the entire eye and upper lid are involved in the process.

Conjunctival involvement takes the form of papillary conjunctivitis.

The diagnosis of contact dermatoconjunctivitis is generally made on the basis of clinical appearance of the patient. In patients taking several topical ophthalmic drugs, the specific offender can be identified by cutaneous patch testing.

In addition to neomycin other drugs that may cause CDC are topical gentamicin, tobramycin, idoxiuridine trifluridine, natamycin, atropine and commonly used preservatives like thiomersal and EDTA. The treatment of CDC requires identification and discontinuation of the offending agent.

Chronic Follicular Conjunctivitis

CFC may occur as a complication of the long-term topical use of the drug. Affected patients complain of chronic redness and mild discharge. In general follicular reaction involves both the the upper and lower palpebral conjunctiva but it is most apparent in the lower fornix.

Drug related CFC is a diagnosis of exclusion.

Idoxiuridine is the most common cause of CFC among the anti-microbial drugs. Sulfonamids are also another cause for CFC. The conjunctivitis resolve in 6 weeks after discontinuation of offending drug.

Punctate Marginal Keratitis

It occurs either during the acute stages of infectious conjunctivitis or as a hypersensitivity reaction to topical drugs. The most common topical antimicrobial drug implicated is gentamicin but several other drugs like atropine, mydriatics and epinephrine may also cause.

PKM treatment involves the discontinuation of the offending agent. In addition topical steroids may be useful.

Keratitis Medicamentosa

It refers to corneal epitheliopathy related to the use of certain topical medications. In milder form KM may affect only the lower cornea. In more severe forms, the entire corneal epithelium may become involved. The epithelium may slough and superficial stromal edema and necrosis may lead to corneal scarring and vascularization. KM must be suspected in any patient with epithelial keratitis of any degree. The antivirals appear to be most common cause of medication induced epithelial keratitis. A 2 week course of idoxuridine or trifluridine will nearly always cause KM. Among the antibiotics the aminoglycoside, neomycin, gentamicin and tobramycin appears to be drugs that may cause KM. Preservative Benzalkonium commonly used in prep of topical antibiotics may also cause desquamation of the outer two layers of the corneal epithelium.

The treatment of KM is discontinuation of all topical medications. Early recognization of the problem is essential since advanced disease may take 2-3 months to clear. The use of non-preserved artificial tears may ameliorate symptoms. In extreme causes, use of bandage soft contact lenses may relieve pain until the epithelium begin to heal. Patient should understand the nature of disease as prolonged time may be required for disease resolution.

Inhibition of Epithelial Wound Healing

Antimicrobial drugs exert their effects by one of two broadly defined mechanisms of action – (i) Disruption of cell wall (ii) Inhibition of intracellular metabolic process.

To heal an epithelial defect, the bordering epithelium must replicate and slide to fill the defect. In addition epithelial defects may persist following any type of corneal infection and antibiotics, antifungals or antivirals may be used beyond the period that is needed to eradicate the infecting organisms. Antimicrobial drugs that inhibit intracellular metabolic processes may have a deleterious effect on healing of corneal epithelium.

Although topical antimicrobials may not have an appreciable effect on the healing of healthy epithelium following a mechanical injury but these agents may have a markedly deleterious effect on the healing of persistent epithelial defects that occur in neurotrophic, post-surgical and post-infections corneas and in corneas that have suffered chemical injuries.

The first step in treating such cases is to assess the patients topical medications and to eliminate or reduce to lowest possible level of all those might interfere with epithelial healing.

Specific Local Complications

Sulfonamides

Calcific band shaped keratopathy has been reported with use of topical sulfonamides. This was most likely complication caused by the preservative since band keratopathy is known to be caused by chronic exposure to organic mercurials.

Amphotericin B

Salmon colored subconjunctival nodules have been seen following S/C injection of amphotericin B in doses greater than 5 mg. Histological exam of nodules revealed numerous histiocytes in an area of fibrosis in addition to lymphocytes and plasma cells. The lesions eventually resolved but permanent yellowing of conjunctiva remains.

Idoxiuridine

IDU has been reported to cause punctal or canalicular stenosis. It has been attributed to cicatrical changes occurring in patients who have had a CFC related to the drug.

Propamidine

Propamidine isoethionate is a nonspecific conjunctivitis remedy. It can cause intraepithelial microcystic lesions related to the use of topical preparation. The lesions are asymptomatic and resolved without sequelae following discontinuation of the drug.

COMPLICATIONS OF STEROIDS

Corticosteroids are important therapeutic agents that are used to treat ocular inflammation commonly.

Complications of steroids are related to dose and duration of therapy. The clinician must consider all the possible complications when counseling and treating patients with vision threatening disease.

Corticosteroids

Few adverse effects of steroids occur with short-term therapy. Most problems occur with long-term therapy. However long-term and short-term adverse effects are grouped together. In general, the lower the maintenance dose, lesser the side effects. These adverse effects are produced both by topical and systemic steroid therapy.

Topical Steroids

Dermatitis

Periocular dermatitis resulting from long-term use of fluorinated steroid drops or ointment have been reported. This dermatitis is similar to perioral dermatitis and should not be confused with allergic contact dermatitis.

Infection and Ulceration

Inappropriate use of topical steroids by patient and registered medical practitioners lead to infectious keratitis especially herpetic keratitis. Reactivation of herpes simplex virus in patients who have undergone penetrating keratoplasty is especially common in patients who were previously treated with steroid antibiotic combination (Figs 20.1 to 20.4).

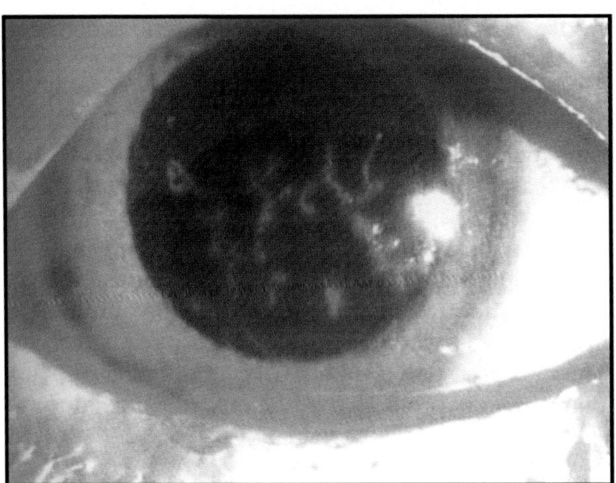

Fig. 20.1: Fluorescein stain of dendritic ulcer with numerous branches made worse by the use of topical steroid eyedrops

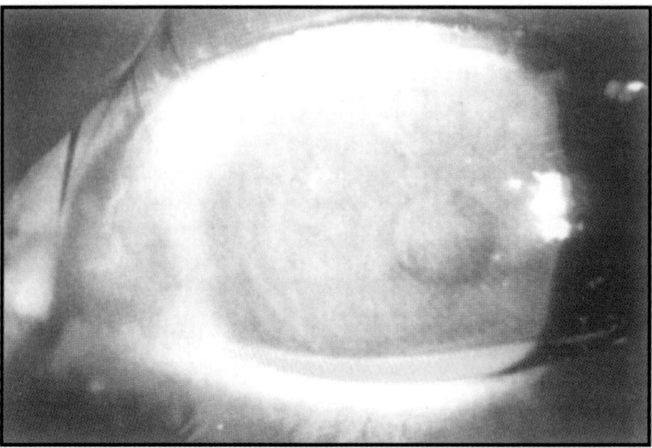

Fig. 20.2: Steroid-induced dendritic keratitis. Fluoresein stain of dendritic ulcer

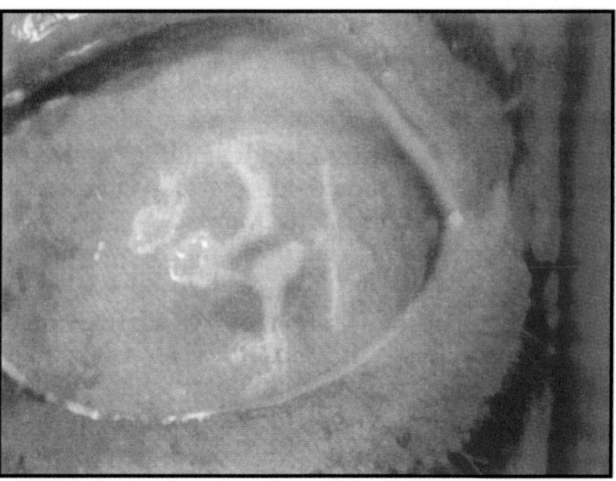

Fig. 20.3: Steroid-induced dendritic keratitis. dendritic ulcer under magnification with fluorescein stain (Courtesy: Kanski Clinical Ophthalmology, Butterworth International Edition)

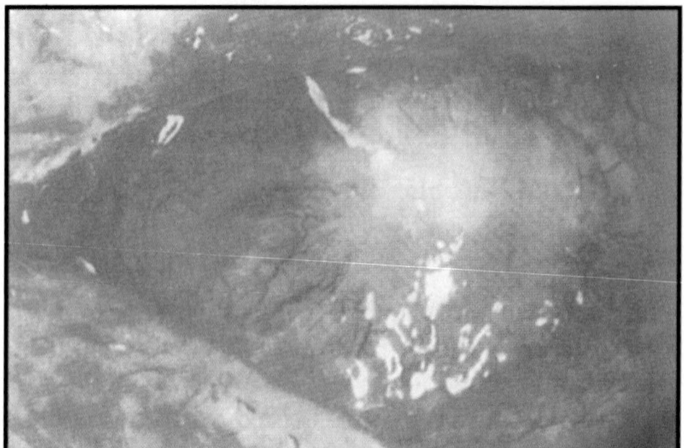

Fig. 20.4: Steroid-induced fungal keratitis (Courtesy: Kanski Clinical Ophthalmology, Butterworth International Edition)

Delayed Wound Healing

Corneal wound healing may be inhibited by proliferation of fibroblasts and new vessels. Ocular surgery may be carried out but the surgeon may use interrupted suture techniques and delay suture removal for few weeks.

Cataracts

Cataract development especially posterior subcapsular type has shown to occur after prolonged treatment with steroid drops and ointments. With the stoppage of the steroids, some of these changes are either partially or totally reversible. Visual impairement is variable. Once visual impairement has taken place, complete resolution of lenticular opacification cannot be expected. The pathophysiology of steroid induced cataract formation is by mechanism affecting water transport by increasing cation influx. This leads to excess water in cells. Causing intumescence of the cell and a disparity of refractive index from the surrounding medium (Figs 20.5 and 20.6).

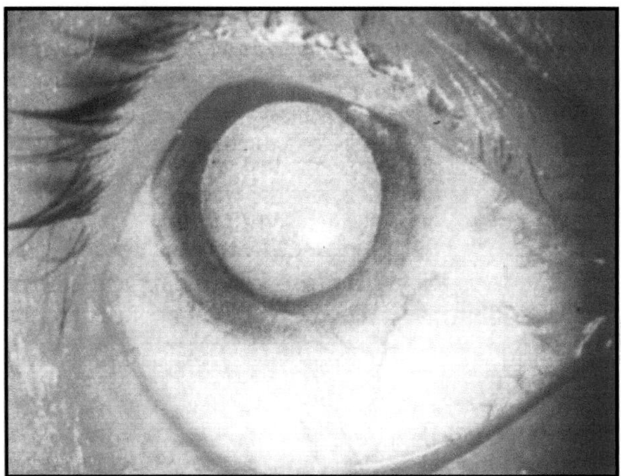

Fig. 20.5: Steroid-induced cataract (Mature type)

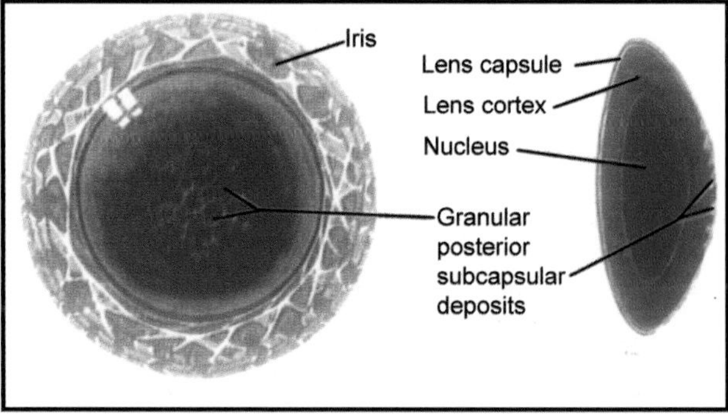

Fig. 20.6: Steroid-induced cataract (posterior subcapsular type)

The steroids also bind to specific amino acids groups with in the lens cell fibers. These combined factors are responsible for the lost in transparency.

Elevated IOP (Steroid Induced Glaucoma)

Prolonged use of corticosteroids may cause an elevation of intraocular pressure, leading to optic nerves damage and visual field. Changes synonymous with chronic open angle glaucoma.

As ophthalmologists we are familiar with abuse of long-term steroids use for minor inflammation by patient himself. So, ophthalmologists should monitor all patients on steroids, no matter what preparation or initial IOP to watch for any increase in IOP. The elevation of IOP can occur with in days of starting therapy or it can occur months later on. Patients with myopia greater than 5 diopters or a history of glaucoma are more susceptible to this complication. Raised IOP by steroids is related to cytoplasmic and nuclear receptors for steroids that have been shown in trabecular meshwork.

Steroid-induced elevations in IOP appear to be secondary to decreased facility of aqueous outflow. The mechanisms include accumulation of glycosaminoglycans or an increase in debris in the trabecular meshwork due to inhibition of phagocytosis.

The frequency and severity of IOP rise is greater with topical application than with systemic administration.

The patient is usually asymptomatic unless the intraocular pressure increases enough to cause corneal edema (Decreased vision, halos, photophobia or pain). Clinical signs of prolonged elevation of IOP include optic nerve cupping and visual field defects (Figs 20.7 to 20.11).

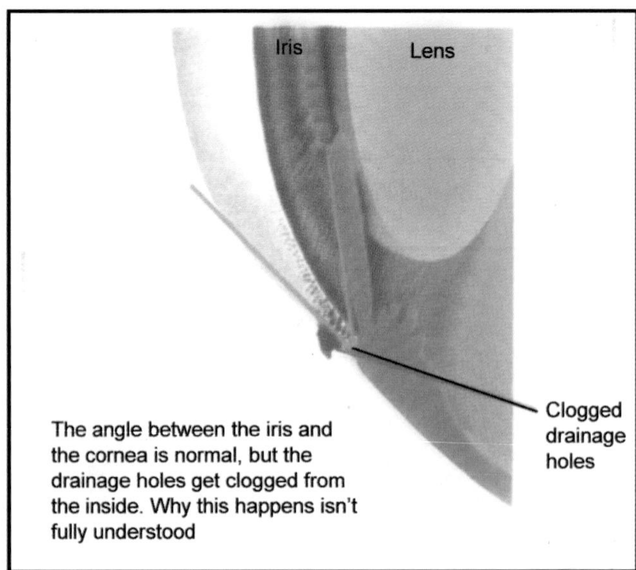

Fig. 20.7: Steroid-induced glaucoma (chronic open angle type) (Courtesy: Allergan India Limited)

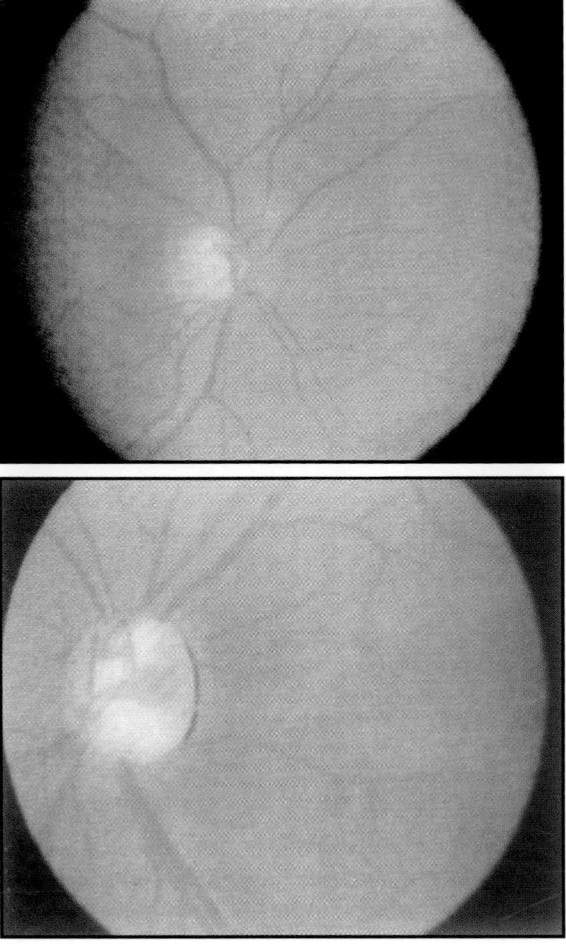

Fig. 20.8: Steroid-induced glaucoma (large terminal glaucomatous cup with C/D ratio 1.0 and optic atrophy)

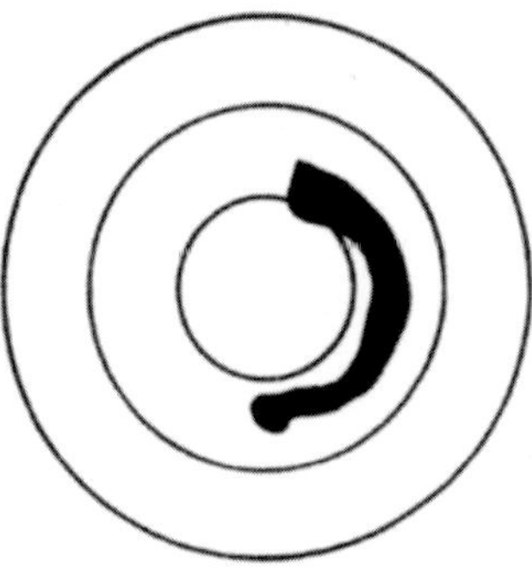

Fig. 20.9: Steroid-induced glaucoma visual field loss (arcuate scotoma in early glaucoma)

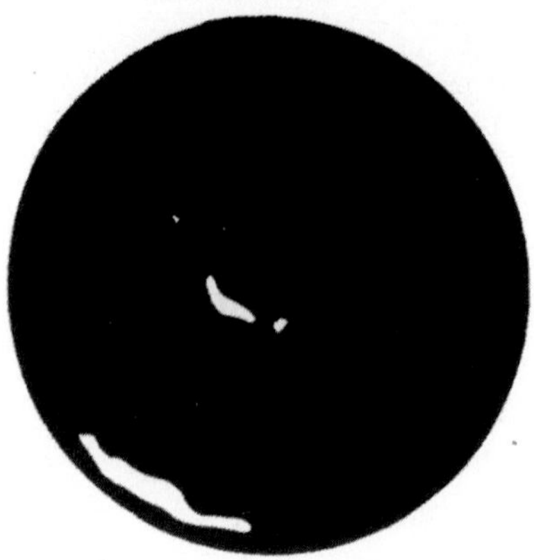

Fig. 20.10: Steroid-induced glaucoma, severe visual field loss in advanced glaucoma

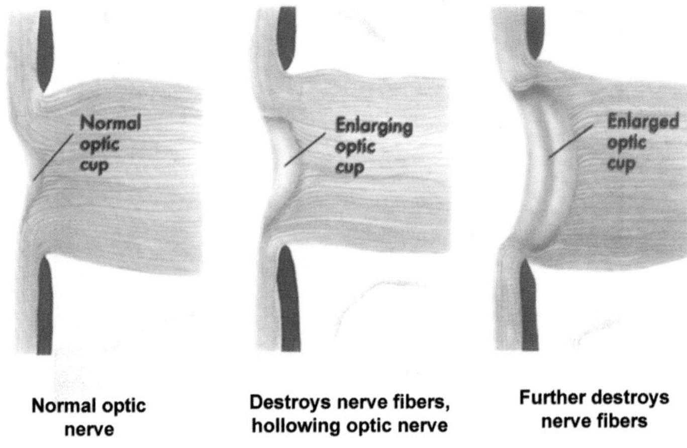

Fig. 20.11: Progression of glaucoma (steroid-induced)

Steroid-induced IOP elevations almost always respond with in days to weeks of stopping the steroids. It is not always possible to abruptly stop steroids because of underlying ocular condition being treated.

It is important to note that although most patients will respond to hypotensive agents, the hypertensive effect can occur in susceptible individuals who are already on hypotensive agents when steroids are added for either ocular or systemic diseases.

In those patients in whom hypotensive agents are unable to control IOP in steroid induced glaucoma Argon laser trabeculoplasty and glaucoma filtering surgery are necessary treatment modalities.

Periocular Steroids

One of the rare but most dangerous complications of injections behind Tenon's capsule is penetration of globe and accidental intraocular injection, substantial retinal damage has also been reported when the vehicles in which steroids are commonly packed react. The preservatives and the osmolality of the vehicle can cause retinal degeneration, preretinal membrane formation, cataract formation. Other complications of injection itself includes retrobulbar hemorrhage, proptosis of globe and fibrosis of extraocular muscles.

Increased IOP may also occur with depot injections of long acting steroids. Injections of long acting steroids are not indicated in patients with episcleritis and scleritis.

Systemic Steroids

Systemic steroids affect patients in many ways. A number of side effects seem to occur early on, in the treatment. The classical clinical triad that contributes to the moon-face appearance of some patients using systemic steroids comprises ptosis, chemosis and swelling of the periorbital tissues.

Various Adverse Effects

1. *Abnormalities of the hypothalmic—pituitary adrenal axis:* Soon after start of steroid therapy abormalities of hypothalamic-pituitary gland adrenal axis including decreased cortisol, adrenal axis response to ACTH and blunted response to insulin induced hypoglycemia can occur. Long-term therapy may blunt this effect.

However, low does maintenance and alternate day therapy will minimize this effect.

Steroids should be withdrawn slowly as quick tapering often result in flare up of ophthalmic disease and can leave the patients with adrenal suppression. Too rapid a decrease in steroids can also result in pseudorheumatism. Systemic steroids can also cause retardation of growth in children and secondary amenorrhea in females.

2. *Mood changes:* Steroids induce euphoria depression, headache, hallucination and psychosis. Suicidal tendencies may also increase. Previous history of psychiatric problems is not believed to increase the tendency for patients to manifest such behavioral disturbances during therapy.

3. *Increased intracranial pressure:* Steroids may cause benign increase in intracranial pressure. Pseudotumor cerebri is most commonly indicated by headache while the patient is taking steroids.

4. *Ophthalmic changes:* Studies have shown the presence of exophthalmos induced by exogenous steroids. Other ocular effects are:

- Ocular palsy due to extraocular muscles myopathy.
- Thining and thickening of sclera.

- Refractive changes due to electrolyte and water shifts.
- Posterior subcapsular cataracts.
- Elevation of IOP.
- Papilledema, visual fields changes like scotoma, constriction and glaucoma field defects.
- Ptosis, subconjunctival hemorrhage.
- Visual hallucinations, mydriasis, ciliary body epithelial microcysts.
- Color vision defects, myopia, diplopia.
- Myasthenic block and toxic amblyopia.
- Central serous retinopathy.
- Herpes keratitis activation.
- Retinal hemorrhages, edema, abnormal ERG and VEP.
- Pseudotumor cerebri.

5. *Diabeties:* Systemic steroids induce glucose intolerance owing to increased hepatic gluconeogenesis and decreased peripheral utilization.

Previously healthy non-diabetic patients can develop hyperosmolar, hyperglycemic non-ketotic coma.

Such patients may be treated with diet restriction, weight loss, oral hypoglycemic agents and if necessary by insulin. By halting the steroids, induced diabetes will resolve, however, it may take several months.

6. *Infections:* Steroids make patients more susceptible to infections. These include bacterial, viral, fungal and parasitic infections.

7. *Alternations in lipid metabolism:* Steroids have two effects on lipid metabolism

   1. Marked redistribution of body fat resulting in classic cushingoid appearance of a patient with moon face, buffalo hump and wasting of the extremities.
   2. Facilitation of lipolysis of the triglycerides of adipose tissue.

8. *Coronary risk factors:* Hypertension is commonly found in patients treated with systemic steroids with an increased incidence in patients with underlying impaired renal function. The exact mechanism that causes hypertension is not clear. Researchers believe that an increased in plasma serum volume, glomerular filtration and decrease in plasma renin concentration and increase in renal vascular resistance may cause hypertension.

9. *Dermatological effects:* Hirsutism and acne occur in about 10% of patients on long-term systemic steroid therapy.

10. *GIT disorders:* Superficial punctate gastric erosions with hemorrhage may occur and are reversible with cessation of steroid therapy. So patients are advised to use antacid cover when taking oral steroids. Steroids used for more than 30 days or short-term use of large doses may cause peptic ulcers. The incidence of peptic ulcers is 1.8% . This risk is also dependent on the patients underlying disease state, age, nutritional status and concomitant drug use and past history of ulcers.

Other GIT effects are:
- Visceral perforation
- Pancreatits
- Nausea
- Increased appetite.

11. *Osteoporosis:* Patients on prolonged therapeutic regimes of steroids often develop osteoporosis. Post-menopausal women, elderly people and immbolised patients are more susceptible to this complication osteoblastic activity is inhibited and bone resorption increases leading to the loss of trabecular bone especially in spine, rib and distal radii. Steroids may cause increased urinary calcium loss and decreased enteric absorption which may lead to secondary hyperparathryoidism and bone resorption. Aseptic necrosis of femoral head can be devastating.

12. *Myopathy:* Muscle weakness with wasting of proximal limb and girdle occurs more readily with fluorinated steroids than with other steroids. Most patients improve with the cessation of the medication but recovery may be slow and incomplete.

13. *Leukocytic and platelet aberrations:* Use of steroids tends to be accompanied by an increase in the no of circulating WBC which is due to increased rate of entrance of polymorphonuclear leukocytes into the blood from the bone marrow.

Thrombocytosis and thrombocytopenia have also been reported to increase.

14. *Hematological changes:*
- Ecchymosis
- Purpura
- Easy bruising.

These are common in elderly patients and are believed to be caused by diminished phagocytosis and alterations of connective tissue.

Subconjunctival and retinal hemorrhage may also be seen in patients who develop purpura and ecchymosis.

15. *Anaphylaxis:* A rare but serious complication of IV steroids is an anaphylactoid reaction in asthmatics. CNS manifestations associated with IV steroids include headache, lethargy, confusion, seizures, hemiplegia and loss of vision.

16. *Renal effects:* These are:
   - Sodium retention, potassium loss
   - Hypokalemic alkalosis
   - Fluid retention

17. *General effects:*
   - Increased sweating
   - Subcutaneous tissue atrophy.

BIBLIOGRAPHY

1. Agarwal Amar. Textbook of Ophthalmology, ed.1. New Delhi: Jaypee Medical Publishers, 2002.
2. Bartlett JD. Clinical Ocular Pharmacology, ed.4. Boston: Butterworth-Heinemann, 2001.
3. Bartlett JD. Ophthalmic Drug facts. Lippincott – William and Wilkins, 2001.
4. Crick RP, Trimble RB. Text book of Clinical Ophthalmology: Hodder and Stoughton, 1986.
5. Duane TD. Clinical ophthalmology, ed. 4. Butterworth – Heinemann, 1999.
6. Duvall. Ophthalmic Medications and Pharmacology. Slack Inc, 1998.
7. Ellis PP. Ocular Therapeutics and Pharmacology, ed. 7. CV Mosby, 1985.
8. Fechner. Ocular Therapeutics. Slack Inc., 1998.
9. Flach AJ. Non Steroidal Anti-inflammatory drugs in Ophthalmology : Int Ophthalmol Clinic 1993;33:1.
10. Franzie JP. Steroids: Int Ophthalmol Clinic 1993;33:9.
11. Fraunfelder. Current Ocular Therapy, ed. 5. WB Saunders, 2000.
12. Garg Ashok. Current Trends in Ophthalmology, ed. 1. New Delhi: Jaypee Medical Publishers, 1997.
13. Garg Ashok. Manual of Ocular Therapeutics, ed. 1. New Delhi: Jaypee Medical Publishers, 1996.
14. Garg Ashok. Ready Reckoner of Ocular Therapeutics, ed.1. New Delhi: 2002.
15. Goodman. LS, Gilman. A. Pharmacological basis of Therapeutics, ed.7. New York: Macmillan, 1985.
16. Havener's. Ocular Pharmacology, ed 6. CV Mosby, 1994.
17. Kanski. Clinical Ophthalmology, ed. 4. Butterworth – Heineman, 1999.
18. Kershner. Ophthalmic Medications and Pharmacology. Slack. Inc., 1994.
19. Leibowitz HM. Anti-inflammatory Medications. Int Ophthalmol Clinic, 1980; 20: 117.
20. Olin BR et al. Drugs Facts and Comparisons. Facts and Comparisons, St. Louis, 1997.
21. Onofrey. The Ocular Therapeutics. Lippincott-William and Wilkins, 1997.
22. Rhee. The Wills Eye drug Guide. Lippincott – William and Wilkins, 1998.
23 Steven Podos. Textbook of Ophthalmology. New Delhi: Jaypee Medical Publishers, 2001.
24 Zimmerman. Textbook of Ocular Pharmacology. Lippincott and William and Wilkins, 1997.

SECTION THREE

Classification of Anti-inflammatory Drugs and Their Clinical and Surgical Applications in Ophthalmology

Chapter 21

Update on Anti-inflammatory Drugs in Ophthalmology

Ashok Garg (India)

Various anti-inflammatory drugs developed so far have been directed against various cellular and chemical mediators of inflammation, e.g. mast cells, lymphocytes, leukocytes, complement histamine, plasma kinins, proteolytic enzymes and various derivates of arachidonic acid anti-inflammatory drugs can broadly be classified as:

1. Corticosteroids
2. Non-steroidal anti-inflammatory drugs (NSAIDs)
3. Immunosuppressive agents.

CORTICOSTEROID

Since their introduction into ocular therapy, corticosteroids have been useful in control of inflammatory and immunological diseases of the eye. The anti-inflammatory effects of corticosteroids are non-specific and they inhibit inflammation without regard to cause. Topical corticosteroids exert an anti-inflammatory action. Aspects of the inflammatory process such as Hypremia, cellular infiltration, vascularization and fibroblastic proliferation are suppressed. Steroids cause inhibition of inflammatory reponse to inciting agents of mechanical, chemical or immunological nature. Topical corticosteroids are effective in acute inflammatory conditions of conjunctiva, sclera, cornea, lids, iris, ciliary body and anterior segment of the globe. They are effective in ocular allergic conditions. In the treatment of ocular diseases, the route depends on the site and extent of the disorder.

The mechanism of the anti-inflammatory action is shown to be potentiation of epinephrine vasoconstriction, stabilization of lysosomal membranes, retardation of macrophage movement prevention of Kinin release, inhibition of lymphocyte and neutrophil function, inhibition of prostaglandin synthesis and in prolonged use decrease of antibody production. By inhibition fibroblastic proliferation, Symblepharon formation in chemical and thermal burns may be prevented. Decreased scarring with clearer corneas following topical corticosteroid therapy is the result of inhibiting fibroblastic proliferation and vascularization. The use of corticosteroids in ocular diseases remains largely empirical but some general principles should be kept in mind.

1. Type and location of inflammation determines which route of administration is appropriate.
2. Dosage is largely determined by clinical experience and should be reassessed at frequent intervals during the course of therapy.
3. Therapy should be reduced gradually, not discontinued abruptly.
4. The minimum effective dose should be used for the shortest time necessary.
5. Individualize dosage.
6. Maintain close follow-up to assess the effects of therapy on the disease and possible adverse effects to the patient.
7. Patient compliance watch with the drug regimen is important in resolution of the inflammation.

Clinical use experience indicate that corticosteroids differ in their ability to suppress inflammation.

They fall into three categories.

1. Glucocorticoids
2. Mineralocorticoids
3. Sex hormones
4. Only the glucocorticoids are of importance in ophthalmic field.

They have powerful anti-inflammatory action and it is this property that has made them such an important agent in the treatment of many ocular diseases. However they have a number of adverse effects.

Steroids may be administered locally in the form of eye drops, ointments, injections (Sub-conjunctival, sub-Tenon, retroequatorial, retrobulbar, intracameral, intravitreal and intralesional) and systemically in form of tablets or injections.

Indications

Topical corticosteroids are used for the treatment of steroid responsive inflammatory conditions of the palpebral and bulbar conjunctiva, lid, cornea and anterior segment of the globe. Indications for topical use include various allergic and hypersensitivity conditions of the eye like.

- Postoperative phase of Excimer Laser and LASIK surgery.
- Iatrogenic inflammation of the eye.
- Contact dermatitis of eye lids.
- Pseudophakic inflammation and after phacoemulsification.
- Non-specific superficial keratitis.
- Allergic conjunctivits and Blepharitis
- Vernal conjunctivitis

- Phlyctenular keratoconjunctivitis.
- Herpes zoster keratitis
- Disciform and Interstital keratitis.
- Corneal graft reactions.
- Anterior and Panuveititis.
- Episcleritis and Scleritis
- Chlazion, iritis, cyclitis
- Hemangioma
- Post keratoplasty phase.
- Superficial punctate keratitis.
- Traumatic inflammation of eye.
- Corneal injury from chemical, radiation or thermal burns.

Use higher strengths for moderate to severe inflammations. In difficult cases of anterior segment eye diseases, systemic therapy may also be required in addition.

Contraindications

Topical corticosteroids should not be used in acute superficial herpes simplex keratitis, fungal diseases of ocular structures, vaccinia, varicella and other viral diseases of cornea and conjunctiva, ocular tuberculosis, hypersensitivity and after uncomplicated removal of superficial corneal foreign body.

Topical steroids are not effective in Sjögrens keratoconjunctivitis. Acute Purulent untreated eye infections may be masked or activity enhanced by topical steroids.

Stromal herpes simplex keratitis treatment with steroid medication require great caution.

Usage of topical steroids in pregnancy and lactation. Safety of intensive or protracted use is not fully substantiated. Use with caution, when clearly needed and when potential benefits outweigh potential hazards.

Administration and Dosage

Topical steroid treated duration varies with the type of lesion and may extend from few days to several weeks depending on therapeutic response. Replase may occur if therapy reduced too rapidly.

Taper over several days. Relapse more common in chronic active lesions usually respond to retreatment.

TOPICAL SOLUTIONS

Instil 1-2 drops into the conjunctival sac every hour during the day and every 2 hours during the night in acute inflammatory conditions of the eye in Mild to moderate inflammation use dosage of 1 drops every 4-6 hours.

OINTMENTS

Apply a thin coating in lower conjunctival sac 3-4 times a day in severe inflammation. In mild to moderate one application at bed time may be suffice to control symptoms. Ointments are specially convenient when eye pad is used and may be preparation of choice when prolonged contact of drug with ocular tissues is needed.

Various topical steroidal agents used in ophthalmology are

Dosage and duration of steroids is disease specific.

A. **HYDROCORTISONE:**
   1. Acetate suspension - 0.5 to 2.5%
   2. Acetate solution – 0.2%
   3. Acetate ointment – 1.5%

B. **PREDNISOLONE:**
   1. Acetate suspension – 0.12%, 0.25% and 1.0%
   2. Sodium phosphate solution – 0.12%, 0.5% and 1.0%
   3. Phosphate solution – 0.5%
   4. Phosphate ointment – 0.25%

C. **DEXAMETHASONE:**
   1. Sodium phosphate solution - 0.1%, 0.05%, 0.01%
   2. Suspension – 0.1%
   3. Sodium phosphate ointment – 0.05%

D. **BETAMETHASONE:**
   1. Sodium phosphate solution 0.1%
   2. Sodium phosphate ointment – 0.1%

E. Triamcinolone acetonide in form of suspension and ointment – 0.1%

F. **PROGESTERONE LIKE AGENTS:**
   1. Medrysone suspension – 1%
   2. Fluorometholone suspension – 0.1% (FML), 0.25% (FML Forte) and ointment (0.1%)
   3. Fluorometholone acetate suspension 0.1%

G. **RIMEXOLONE OPHTHALMIC SUSPENSION 1%**

H. **LOTEPREDNOL ETABONATE OPHTHALMIC SOLUTION 1%**

Some group of the steroidal drops have better intraocular penetration than others. Dexamethasone and Betamethasone have better intraocular penetration than Triamcinolone and hydrocortisone. New generation steroids like Rimexolone, Fluorometholone are powerful corticosteroids with very low risk of IOP spikes.

Medrysone (Hydroxy methyl progesterone) have poor intraocular penetration.

Full strength topical Corticosteroids are indicated in severe allergic or immunological responses, severe uveitis with hypopyon but without corneal epithelial break and microbial infective element, iatrogenic and pseudophakic inflammation and in post excimer PRK laser and LASIK surgery phases.

In severe forms of anterior uveitis or iatrogenic inflammation, topical steroid therapy may require supplementation with periocular injection or systemic steroids.

Medysone is usually recommended for minor reaction involving lids and conjunctiva. Its efficacy has not been demonstrated in iritis or uveitis.

In certain ophthalmic inflammatory diseases where full strength topical steroids are not indicated diluted steroid regime should be used Topical Dexamethasone phosphate (0.01 diluted soln) is commonly prescribed by the ophthalmologists. The diluted corticosteroids (1:10) have clear advantages in the therapy of ophthalmic disorders. These are:

1. Enhance resistance to infection.
2. Possess effective anti-inflammatory response even in 1:20 dilutions.
3. Do not enhance microbial fungal flora of their lesions.
4. Do not produce ocular hypertension.
5. Do not delay healing when used in 1:10 dilution.
6. Do not enhance collagenase release.
7. Effective control of allergic conditions of conjunctiva.
8. Stabilize the corneal endothelial function.
9. Do not produce keratopathy.
10. Does not cause dry eye.

Thus advantages of diluted corticosteroids are non-promotion of organismal growth, non-interference in healing processes without compromising their therapeutic effects strict, precaution should be taken that topical steroid are never stopped suddenly to avoid high chances of recurrence of disease and adverse effects owing to tissue addiction. The therapy must be tapered gradually in dose and frequency over a period of time. The diluted corticosteroid regime should be continued for a period of one week after the clinical cure.

Since the advent of new generation topical corticosteroid like Rimexolone and Fluorometholone topical steroid therapy has revolutionized. Unlike topical Dexamethasone, Betamethasone, Prednisolone and Hydrocortisone ophthalmic solutions, these new generation steroids have low incidence of adverse effect specially rise of IOP spikes leading to steroid induced Glaucoma. Let me discuss these new generation topical steroids here.

Rimexolone

Rimexolone (Vexol) 1% ophthalmic suspension is first new ocular steroid with classic steroid power in 20 years. With this unique new design rimexolone displays a strong effinity for human glucocorticoid receptor and high *in vitro* activity. It has powerful anti-inflammatory effect like other steroids but significantly with low risk of IOP spikes similar to FML (0.1% solution).

Its mechanism of action is similar to topical FML.

Indications

Topical Rimexolone (1%) is

- Highly effective in reducing postoperative inflammation of eye. (Intraocular surgery) In post-surgery inflammation following Excimer Laser PRK and LASIK surgery.
- In pseudophakic inflammation of the eye.
- Highly effective in treating anterior uveitis
- Treating allergic conjunctivitis, Keratoconjunctivitis.

Contraindication

It should not be used in

- Dendritic keratitis
- Vaccinia varicella
- Mycobacterial infection of the eye.
- Fungal disease of the eye.
- Acute purulent untreated infections which may be masked or enhanced by the presence of steroid
- Persons with hypersensitivity to any component.
- Pregnancy, Lactating mothers and in children.

Dosage

1% ophthalmic sterile multi dose suspension (5 and 10 ml vials). Patient is advised to put one drop in the affected eye 3-4 times a day. Dosage can be safely increased depending upon severity of the condition. Rimexolone provides well tolerated, comfortable, ease to use therapy.

Adverse Reactions

In addition to standard adverse effects of topical steroids being discussed separately in details, Topical Rimexolone can cause.

Blurred vision, discharge, discomfort, ocular pain, foreign body sensation, Hyperemia, increased fibrin, dry eye, conjunctival edema, corneal staining, photophobia, non-ocular adverse effect although very low can be headache, hypotension, rhinitis, taste perversion and Pharyngitis.

Fluorometholone (FML)

FML is new generation topical corticosteroid being prescribed maximally by ophthalmologists world wide. It is powerful anti-inflammatory agent of steroidal group. Chemically it is 9-Fluor 11B, 17-dihydroxy-6-x- Methyl pregna – 1,4 – diene 3, 20 dione.

In topical suspension (0.1 and 0.25% FML forte) it is available with liquid film (polyvinyl alcohol). It is well tolerated in ocular tissues and is distributed throughout the ocular tissues rapidly.

Mechanism of Action

Topical Fluorometholone acts by inhibiting the inflammatory response to a variety of inciting agents. They inhibit the edema, fibrin Deposition, Capillary dilation, Leukocyte migration, phagocytic activity. Capillary proliferation, fibro blast proliferation, Deposition of collagan and scar formation associated with inflammation. It inhibits the synthesis of histamine within mast cells. FML also decreases prostaglandin synthesis and retard epithelial regeneration. The special character of topical FML is that it has powerful anti-inflammatory property similar to topical Dexamethasone, Betamethasone and Prednisolone (diluted and undiluted) but has a significant lower propensity to increase intraocular pressure which leads to steroid induced Glaucoma.

Indications

For steroid responsive inflammation of the palpebral and bulbar conjunctiva, Cornea and anterior segment of the globe.

- In iatrogenic inflammation specially after Excimer Laser PRK and LASIK Surgery, Pseudophakic inflammation.
- In phacoemulsification (Postsurgical inflammation).
- Disciform and interstitial keratitis
- Panuvictis
- Scleritis and episcleritis
- Traumatic inflammation of the eye.

Contraindications

Contraindications are similar to standard topical therapy already mentioned in the chapter.

Precaution should be taken while prescribing topical FML medication for herpes simplex keratitis involving stroma as it requires greater and frequent slit-lamp microscopy for adverse effects.

Topical FML should not be used for injection.

Dosage and Administration

FML is available as sterile suspension in 5 ml vials in strength of 0.1% and 0.25% (FML forte). Besides it, FML is also available as ophthalmic ointment (0.1%) and as acetate suspension (0.1%).

Patients should be advised to instil one drop of topical FML into conjunctival sac 2-4 times daily. During the initial 24-48 hours the dosage may be safely increased to 2 drops every hour depending upon severity of the condition.

Care should be taken not to discontinue therapy prematurely and abruptly. Unique features of Topical FML suspension are:

- It efficacy on ocular surface well established all over the world.

- It is safer than currently available low dose preparations which are upto 10 times diluted.
- It is microfine suspension which ensures uniform particle distribution, longer residence time and rapid absorption.
- Its liquifilm advantage soothes, cools, enhances patient confort and microfine suspension minimizes mechanical irritation.
- Has least risk to raise IOP spikes established worldwide through clinical trials.

Due to these special features Topical FML suspension is most widely and frequently prescribed by ophthalmologists worldwide specially to control iatrogenic inflammation in Modern High tech ophthalmic surgery of PRK, LASIK and Phacoemulsification.

Loteprednol Etabonate

Loteprednol etabonate (0.5% Ophthalmic solution) is latest topical corticosteroid on the anvil.

It is a novel, site reactive Corticosteroid with powerful anti-inflammatory activity similar to Dexamethasone and FML with marked low propensity to increase IOP spike.

Loteprednol etabonate (0.5%) is structurally similar to other corticosteroids and is a soft drug. Soft drug is a biologically active compound with predictable inactivation to nontoxic moieties after achieving its therapeutic role. The design of this drug incorporates a "Soft spot" into the structure that undergoes a predictable metabolic inactivation leading to lower toxicity and more specific action on target organ.

It has high lipophilicity with good intraocular penetration and its predictable degradation is depicted to provide an improved safety profile. That is the reason it causes less increase in intraocular pressure than Dexamethasone.

Predictable intraocular conversion of the drug to an inactive compound reduces the amount of active corticosteroid in the trabecular meshwork. Loteprednol etabonate (0.5%) is indicated in steroid responsible inflammatory condition of the eye, iatrogenic and pseudophakic inflammation of the eye and in anterior uveitis whereas Loteprednol 0.2% has been approved for seasonal allergic conjunctivitis.

It is available as 0.2 and 0.5% ophthalmic suspension in 2.5, 5 and 10 ml vials.

The relatively low incidence, transient nature and reversibility of ocular pressure increase reported with Loteprednol indicate that it can provide an additional treatment choice for ocular inflammatory conditions.

In Post PRK and LASIK surgery inflammation its specific role is being clinically tried with initial encouraging results. The advent of new anti-inflammatory drugs with fewer side effects is the need of the hour and is a welcome step. Several new drugs have been developed and clinical trials show promising results. New drugs such as Loteprednol etabonate may be an important addition to the therapeutic armamentarium of the practicing ophthalmologist in near future.

Corticosteroids drops are used either in solo or in combination of topical antibiotics to produce synergistic effect.

Topical Steroid Antibiotic Combinations

Various topical steroid – antibiotic combinations used in ophthalmic field are.

1. Dexamethasone (0.1%) with neomycin (0.5%) in solution form.
2. Dexamethasone (0.1%) with neomycin (0.35%) and Polymixin B (10000 units/ml) suspension or ointment.
3. Dexamethasone (0.1%) with chloramphenicol (0.5 to 1%) Solution.
4. Dexamethasone (0.1%) with framycetin (0.3%) suspension.
5. Dexamethasone (0.1%) and tobramycin (0.3%) suspension.
6. Dexamethasone (0.1%) with chloramphenicol (1%) and Polymixin B 5000 I.U. solution and oint.
7. Dexamethasone (0.1%) with gentamyecin (0.3%) – solution.
8. Dexamethasone (0.1%) with ciprofloxacilin (0.3%)
9. Dexamethasone (0.1%) with ofloxacilin (0.3%)
10. Dexamethasone (0.1%) with lomefloxacilin (0.3%)
11. Dexamethasone (0.1%) with sparfloxacilin (0.3%)
12. Dexamethasone (0.1%) with gatifloxacilin (0.3%)
13. Dexamethasone (0.1%) with moxifloxacilin (0.5%)
14. Betamethasone (0.1%) with neomycin (0.5%) – solution
15. Betamethasone (0.1%) with chloramphenicol (0.5%) in solution and ointment form.
16. Betamethasone (0.1%) with gentamicin (0.3%) in solution
17. Hydrocortisone (0.5%) with chloramphenicol (0.5%) Solution.
18. Hydrocortisone (0.5%) with neomycin (0.5%) oint and Solution.
19. Hydrocortisone (1.5%) and neomycin (0.5%) ointment.
20. Hydrocortisone 10 mg/gm, polymixin B 0.5 mg/gm, bacitracin 400 units/gm and neomycin 5 mg/gm ointment.
21. Hydrocortisone (1%) with gentamicin (0.3%) – suspension.
22. Hydrocortisone (0.5%) with chloramphenicol (1%) – ointment.
23. Prednisolone (0.5%), neomycin 0.35% and Polymixin B 10000 units/ml suspension.
24. Prednisolone (1%) with gentamicin (0.3%) suspension.
25. Prednisolone (0.2) with sulphacetamide (10%) and phenylephrine (0.12%) – solution.
26. Fluorometholone (0.1%) with neomycin (0.35%) in solution.
27. Fluorometholone (0.1%) with Gentamicin (0.9%) in solution.
28. Fluorometholone (0.1%) with tobramycin (0.3%) in solution.
29. Ofloxacin (0.3%) with prednisolone (0.5%) in solution.

Topical Antibiotic Steroid Combinations are Indicated In

- In treatment of anterior segment inflammatory disorders which may be threatened with or complicated by bacteria sensitive to antibiotics.
- In pre and postoperative phase of intraocular surgery where the possibility of infection with susceptible organisms exists.
- In chronic anterior uveitis and corneal injury from chemical, radiation or thermal burns.

Contraindications

- In acute untreated purulent ocular infections caused by microc organisms not sensitive to antibiotics in steroid combination.
- Acute superficial herpes simplex (dendritic keratitis).
- Vaccinia varicella and other viral diseases of the conjunctiva and cornea.
- Fungal diseases
- Ocular tuberculosis
- Hypersensitivity of drug.
- In diseases due to micro-organisms resistant to associated antibiotic with concerned steroid combination, infection may be masked enhanced or activated by the steroid.
- Prolonged use may result in overgrowth of non-susceptible organisms.

Topical steroid-antibiotic combination advantage is that when decision is taken to administer such drugs combination, there is greater patient compliance and convenience with the added assurance that the appropriate dosage of both the drugs is administered. When both the drugs are in the same formulation compatibility of ingradients is assured and the correct volume of drug is delivered and retained. In antibiotic steroid topical combination, steroids provided powerful anti-inflammatory effect while associated antibiotic provide broad spectrum bactericidal effect. Even pus, exudates and bacteria growth products cannot inactivate the antibiotics in such combinations.

Dosage and Administration

Patient is advised to put 1-2 drops in the conjunctival sac 2-4 times daily. Care should be taken not to discontinue the treatment prematurely and abruptly.

Adverse Reactions

In addition to topical steroid complications already mentioned in this chapter, the most frequent reactions reported are ocular discomfort, irritation upon instillation of the medication and punctate keratitis. These reactions resolve with the discontinuation of the medication.

In present day ophthalmic practice Topical Fluorometholone neomycin (FML-neo), Dexamethasone – Tobramycin and Dexamethasone – neomycin – Polymixin B combinations are commonly prescribed as effective treatment when infection and inflammation or injection and allergy co-exists.

Systemic Corticosteroids

Systemic steroids are the mainstay of treatment of inflammation of the posterior segment and orbit. They are used as supplement to topical steroids in severe inflammation of the anterior segment of the eye.

Anti-inflammatory effect of Dexamethasone is 30-50 times more than that of cortisone, prednisolone is 5 times more potent than cortisone as an anti-inflammatory agent.

INDICATIONS FOR SYSTEMIC STEROIDS

- Posterior uveitis.
- Sympathetic ophthalmia
- Papillitis and retrobulbar neuritis
- Anterior ischemic optic neuropathy.
- Scleritis
- Severe anterior uveitis
- Malignant exophthalmos
- Orbital pseudotumor
- Herpes Zoster ophthalmicus
- IOL implantation
- Refractive keratotomy
- Vogt – Koyanagi – Harada syndrome

Dosage, duration and type of systemic steroids use depends upon the severity and type of ocular diseases in which it is required.

Complications

Complications of topical steroids are due to their intraocular penetration, collagenolytic and immuno-susppressive properties.

Topical steroids must be used with caution in herpetic keratitis and never stops steroid therapy abruptly.

COMPLICATIONS OF TOPICAL STEROIDS

- Reduced resistance of viral, bacterial and fungal infections.
- Cataract (Posterior subcapsular cataract type)
- Raised intraocular pressure in susceptible patients (Glaucoma open angle type) with optic nerve damage defects in visual field and acuity.
- Secondary ocular infections from fungi and viruses liberated from ocular tissues.
- Delayed wound healing

- Dry eye
- Ptosis
- Mydriasis
- Perforation of globe when used in conditions where there is thinning of cornea and sclera
- Systemic corticosteroids produce several ocular side effects on extensive use. There are -

1. Posterior subcapsular cataract
2. Activation of infections
3. Glaucoma, exophthalmos, papilledema CRV.

Detailed adverse effects of topical and systemic steroids are being discussed in a separate chapter in this book.

The undesirable effects of steroids led to the development of non-steroidal anti-inflammatory agents which are relatively free of serious side effects.

NON-STEROIDAL ANTI-INFLAMMATORY DRUGS (NSAIDs)

Classification and Structure of NSAIDs (Fig. 21.1)

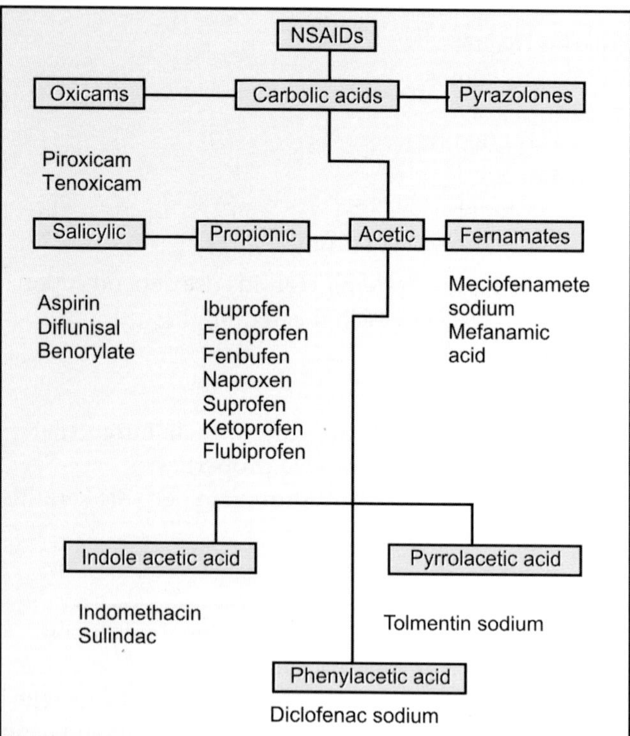

Fig. 21.1: Classification of nonsteroidal anti-inflammatory drugs (NSAIDs)

NSAIDs are chemically hetrogenous group that can be grouped into seven major classes.

- Salicylates
- Fenamates
- Indoles
- Phenylalkanoic acids
- Pyrazolones
- Phenylacetates
- Pyrazolones
- Phenylactates
- Paraminophenols

The chemical feature shared by all these classes is the absence of cholesterol derived steroid nucleus hence the term non-steroidal (Fig. 21.2). The pharmaceutical emphasis has been on the indoles, phenylacetates and phenylalkanoic acids because of instability in solution and hence high ocular toxicity of salicylates. Fenamates and phyrazolone derivatives. Specific drugs belonging to each class are listed in (Tables 21.1 and 21.2).

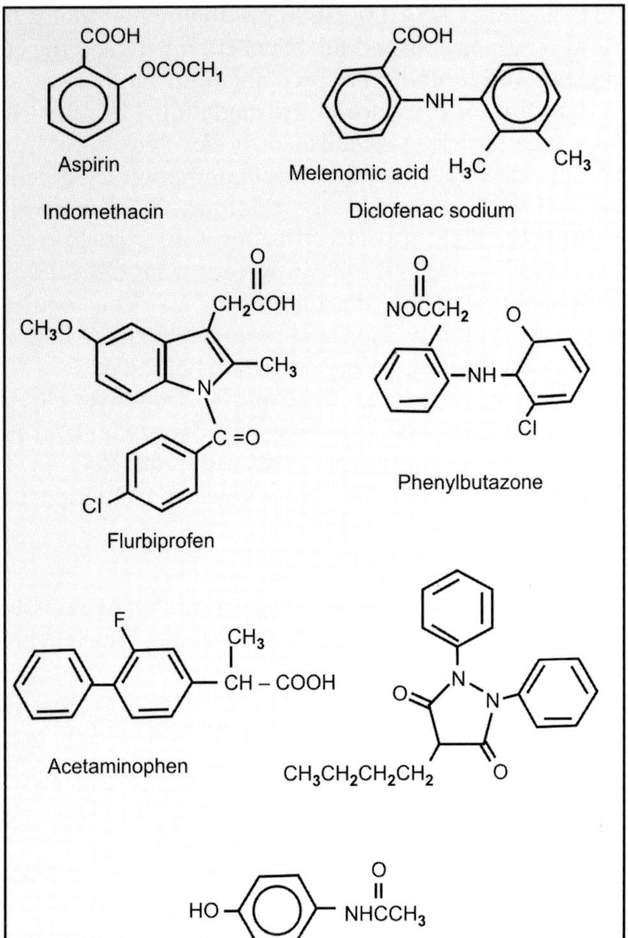

Fig. 21.2: Chemical structures of various NSAIDs

Mechanism of Action

NSAIDs act mainly as anti-inflammatory agents by inhibiting cyclo-oxygenase and Lipoxygenase enzymes which lead to inhibition of products like prostaglandins, thromboxane and leukotriens which induce inflammation (as shown in Fig. 21.3). Ocular actions of prostaglandins cause miosis, increased vascular permeability, break down of blood-aqueous barrier, conjunctival hyperemia and changes in intraocular pressure. Lipoxygenase products which are generated from.

In the treatment of ocular inflammation need of non-steroidal anti-inflammatory drugs was felt due to severe complications associated with more established corticosteroid therapy. Although a overlap between the mechanisms of action of both NSAIDs and steroids exists, yet the use of NSAIDs in ophthalmology is safer than the use of cortecostiroids as NSAIDs are relatively free of potential adverse effects of steroids.

The history of role of NSAIDs use in ophthalmology dates back to 1971 when Vane and Smith established the connection between the clinical effect of acetylsalicylates and inhibition of prostaglandin synthesis.

Since the detection of presence of prostaglandins in rabbit iris tissue in 1955, this substance has been established in elevated levels in the anterior chamber that have been associated with inflammation triggered by trauma, uveitis, cataract, IOL surgery and laser iridotomy. It is now well know that NSAIDS produce their clinical effect by inhibiting cyclo-oxygenase and subsequent prostaglandin synthesis. In Recent time topical NSAIDS have become commercially available throughout the world as ocular eye drops thus gaining due acceptability in ophthalmology which are now widely used in iatrogenic and other inflammatory conditions of the eye.

Arachidonic acid include leukotriene and hydroperoxy eicosate traenoic acid (HPETES). These products like prostaglandins also cause an inflammatory response following tissue injury and have a potent effect on the immune responses. Prostaglandins have also been implicated in allergic reactions also.

Inhibition of Prostaglandin Synthesis

Synthesis of cyclo-oxygenase products can be inhibited by non-steroidal anti-inflammatory drugs (NSAIDs). Depending on step at which action is exerted they have been categorized in two types.

1. **Type I inhibitors:** Type I inhibitors inhibit cyclo-oxygenase therefore the cyclic endperoxide O_2 and H_2 are not formed, thus the whole range of PG_3 thromboxane A_2 and PGI_2 cannot be synthesized. Examples of type I inhibitors include salicylates, the fenamates, propionic acid derivatives and indomethacin.
2. **Type II inhibitors:** Type II inhibitor inhibit isomerases and reductases i.e. the step from cyclic endperoxide to PGE_2, PGF_2 etc. e.g. pyrazolones.

NSAIDs have free radical scavenging activity during inflammation and thus help in the prevention of tissue damage.

Table 21.1: Systemic non-steroidal anti-inflammatory agents

Drug class	*Drug name*	*How supplied (mg) (Commercially)*	*Typical adult daily dose (mg)*
Salicylates	Aspirin	325-925	650-975 mg q4h
	Diflunisal	250,500	250 qid
	Choline magnesium trisalicylate	250,500	1000-1500 mg bid
	Sodium salicylate	325-650	325-650 mg q3-4h
Fenamates	Mefenamate	250	250 qid
	Meclofenamate	50,100	50-100 qid
Indoles	Indomethacin	25,50,75 (slow release)	25,50 tid-qid,75 bid
	Sulindac	150,200	150-200 bid
	Tolmetin	200,400,600	400 tid
Phenyl acetic acids	Diclofenac	25,50,75	50-75 bid
	Nepafenac	25, 50	25-50 bid
Phenyl alkanoic acids	Fenoprofen	200,300,600	300-600 tid
	Ketoprofen	25,50,75	75 tid-50 qid
	Piroxicam	10,20	10 bid, 20 daily
	Flurbiprofen	50,100	100 tid
	Ketorolac	10	10 qid
	Naproxen	250, 375, 500	250-500 bid
	Naproxen Na	275,550	275-550 bid
	Ibuprofen	200,300,400,600,800	400-800 tid
	Nabumetone	250,300	1 g q night
Pyrazolones	Phenyebutazone	100	100 tid-qid
	Oxyphenyl butazole	100	100 tid-qid
Paraaminophenols	Acitaminophen	80,325,500,650	650 q 4h

Table 21.2: Topical non-steroidal anti-inflammatory agents

Drug name	*How supplied commercially*	*Typical dose*
1. Flurbiprofen	0.03% solution	1 drop every 30 minutes, 2 hours pre-operatively (total dose-4 drops)
2. Suprofen	1.0 % solution	2 drops at 1,2 and 3 hours pre-operatively or every 4 hours while awake on the day of surgery
3. Diclofenac	0.1 % solution	-qid
4. Nepafenac	0.1% suspension	-qid
5. Ketorolac	0.4% and 0.5% solution	-tid
6. Indomethacin	(a) 0.5-1.0% suspension (b) 0.1% ophthalmic solution	-qid
	Freshly prepared Topical NSAIDs	
1. Asprin	1.0 % solution	-qid
2. Acetyl Salicylic acid	0.03% solution	-qid
3. Diflunisol	0.03% solution	-qid
	OINTMENTS	
1. Oxyphenbutazole	10% ointment	HS-bid
2. Pheylbutazone	10% ointment	HS-bid

Arachidonic Acid (AA) Metabolites and Inflammation

A variety of phenomena in the inflammatory response are mediated by three interrelated plasma derived factors the complement, kinin and Clotting system (As shown in Figure 21.4).

The products derived from metabolism of AA affect a variety of biological processes including inflammation and hemostasis. AA metabolism proceeds along one of two major pathways.

Lipoxygenase or cyclo-oxygenase. The cyclo-oxygenase (Cox) enzymes exists in two forms Cox 1- and Cox-2. Cox1 is found in mast cells. It is thought that the prostanoids it produces are involved in normal hemostasis. Cox-2 is induced inflammatory cells by an inflammatory stimulus. Thus has relevance for the mechanisms of action of present and future NSAIDs.

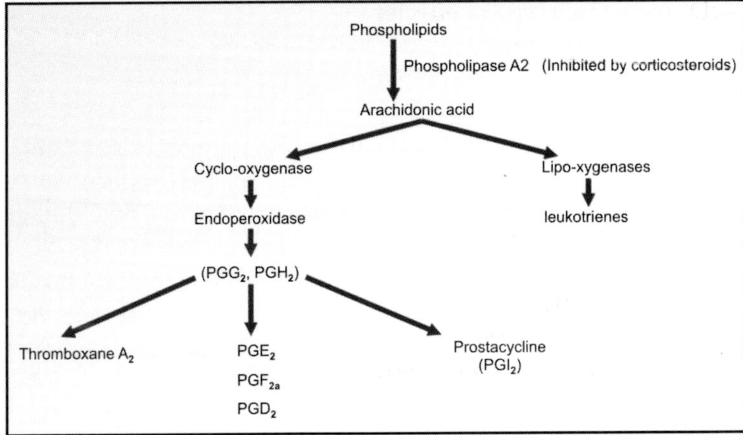

Fig. 21.3: Mechanism of action of NSAIDs

Pharmacokinetics

NSAIDs are well absorbed after oral administration and have measurable ocular penetration. NSAIDs are 90 to 99% protein bound and therefore are easily recovered from ocular tissues. However topical NSAIDs appear to penetrate the eye better than oral administration. Topical instillation of these drugs provides adequate levels of agents in ocular tissue and aqueous humour for inhibition of Prostaglandin synthesis. However topical NSAIDs can gain access to the systemic circulation via mucosal absorption. Therefore even local administration of NSAIDs can be accompanied by systemic toxicity if nasolacrimal occlusion and eyelid closure are not employed following eye drop instillation.

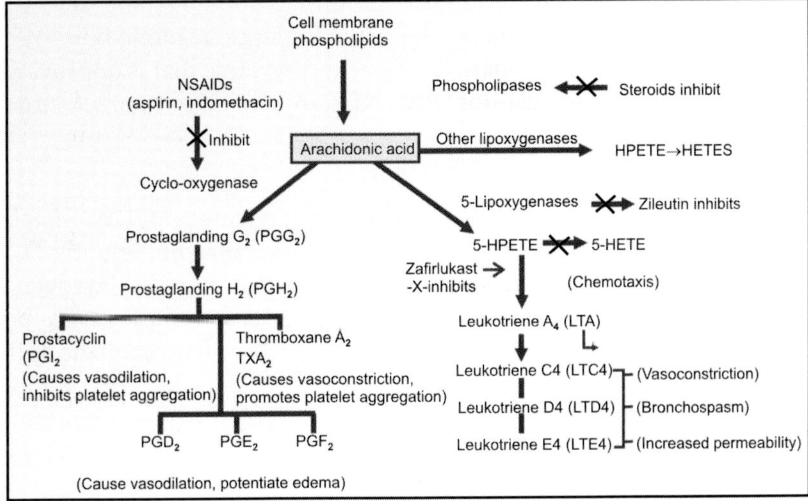

Fig. 21.4:Arachidonic acid metabolites and their role in inflammation

NSAIDs have three type of effects:

- Anti-inflammatory effect
- Analgesic effect
- Anti-pyretic effect

In ophthalmology these drugs are used primarily for their anti-inflammatory effects and when required for the analgesic effect.

NSAIDs are inhibitors of both isoenzymes Cox-1 and Cox-2 though they vary in degree of inhibition of each.

The anti-inflammatory action is mediated by their inhibition of Cox-1. Drugs with selective action on Cox-2 could bring in a major advancement. The anti-inflammatory effect of NSAIDs varies. Drug such as indomethacin and piroxicam are strongly anti-inflammatory some such as naproxan, ibuprofen and nambumetone are moderately anti-inflammatory while drugs like paracetamol have essentially no anti-inflammatory activity.

In ophthalmic topical preparations Flurbiprofen 0.03% DICLOFENAC (0.1%), ketorolac (0.5%), indomethacin (1%) and suprofen (1%) are commonly used.

Topical NSAIDs when used stabilize the blood-ocular barriers and are as effective in reducing iatrogenic inflammation as topical corticosteroids. NSAIDs like steroids are also used systemically specially when their action needs to be combined with anti-inflammatory effects or when higher intra-ocular levels are desirable such as in CME or diffuse retinitis.

Topical NSAIDs like indomethacin (Indole derivative) is commercially available as 1% aqueous suspension. A 0.1% indomethacin ophthalmic solution has recently been commercially launched. The phenyl alkanoic acids are water soluble and are formulated as ophthalmic solutions. Flurbiprofen (0.03%) and suprofen (1%) are approved by FDA (USA) for intra-operative use to inhibit miosis during cataract surgery. Ketorolac tromethamine (0.5%) has been approved for the treatment of seasonal allergic conjunctivitis While Topical Diclofenac (1%) is a phenylacetic acid derivative that is approved by FDA for use to minimize post-operative inflammation after cataract surgery.

Ocular Indications for Use of NSAIDs

1. **Maintenance of Intra-operative Mydriasis:** Adequate pupillary dilatation specially its maintenance during intra-ocular surgery undergoing ECCE and in posterior segment procedures (Vitreo-retinal surgery). Endogenous factors other than prostaglandins and surgical techniques have been responsible for this condition. NSAIDs use can cause pharmacological effect on the pupil lessening intra operative miosis. NSAIDs that are commonly used for this purpose include Topical Flurbiprofen 0.3%. Suprofen 1% and Indomethacin 1% Suspension. Clinical datas have shown that topical Indomethacin 1% suspension or 0.1% ophthalmic solution maintain pupillary dilatation in statistically significant higher number of patients

undergoing cataract surgery. Topical Flurbiprofen and Suprofen solutions are commonly used by ophthalmologists to inhibit intraoperative miosis. This pharmacological activity of NSAIDS is of potential clinical benefit because decreasing pupil size is a well established risk factors for vitreous loss and zonular breaks during ECCE with IOL implantation.

2. **Reduction of Postoperative Inflammation:** Topical NSAIDs drops are potentially useful in managing postoperative inflammation following intra- ocular surgery. Fluorophotometric analysis offers a quantitative means of studying anterior chamber inflammation.

Several clinical studies have shown the efficacy of NSAIDs specially Indomethacin 1%, Flurbiprofen 0.03%, Ketorolac 0.5% and Diclofenac 0.1%. On postoperative inflammation NSAIDs positive effect has been reported both in intracapsular and extra capsularcataract surgery. Flurophotometry study have shown that topical NSAIDs achieve better inflammation control than the corticosteroids in Double masked randomized studies. Topical Diclofenac 0.1% and Indomethacin 1% suspension or 0.1 ophthalmic solution have been proved to be better in controlling inflammation after cataract surgery. Latest studies have strongly advocated the use of topical diclofenac 0.1% four times daily starting 24 hours after cataract surgery to control post- operative inflammation. It is possible practically to prescribe a topical NSAIDs for a topical corticosteroid to control iatrogenic inflammation specially in eyes with significant steroid responsive glaucoma.

3. **Prevention and Treatment of Aphakic and Pseudophakic Cystoid Macular Edema:** Cystoid macular edema (CME) is the most common cuase of visual decline following cataract surgery. Angiographically proven CME after cataract surgery occurs in 50 to 70% of patients undergoing ICCE and in 20-30% patients who undergo ECCE. The common denominator of all the CME is believed to be mainly prostaglandin mediated breach of blood-retina barrier clinical studies have shown that oral and Topical NSAIDs are effective in the prophylaxis of angiographic pseudophakic and aphakic CME.

Topical NSAIDs specially topical Indomethacin 1% and Flurbiprofen 0.03% when prescribed to patients postoperatively undergoing cataract surgery resulted in improved Snellan visual acuity and decrease in the incidence of post surgical angiographic CME.

In summary:

a. Topical NSAIDs are effective in preventing post surgical angiographic CME when topical or sub-tenon corticosteroid is given concurrently.
b. Prophylactic treatment with topical NSAIDs has a beneficial effect on visual function.

c. Topical NSAIDs are also effective in the treatment of angiographically documented subclinical CME and this can turn into improved visical function.

d. Topical NSAIDs are also effective in treating Chronic symptomatic established CME (of 6 months or greater duration) 1% Topical Fenoprofen and oral indomethacin has been shown to be quite effective in such condition. In the treatment of CME, standard recommendation is to use combination of a topical corticosteroid and topical NSAIDs and then tapering of corticosteroid as the clinical situation improves.

4. **Uveitis:** In contrast to postsurgical inflammation, many forms of uveitis require prolonged steroid therapy to control inflammation. Of course, the risk of iatrogenic glaucoma and cataract becomes substantial in these situations. Therefore, NSAIDs are gaining a more secure position in the treatment of certain uveitis.

Systemic NSAIDs have shown to prevent attacks of juvenile rheumatoid arthritis associated iridocyclitis, acute non-granulomatous anterior uveitis and chronic iridocylitis.

In cases of posterior uveitis and secondary vasculitis, oral NSAIDs are shown to be effective in eliminating macular edema and preventing recurrence. Standard recommend regime is combination of topical corticosteroid and an oral NSAIDS (specially Diclofenac 75 mg bd daily) as initial therapy.

5. **Scleritis and Episcleritis:** Systemic NSAIDs are agents of choice in the treatment of non necrotizing, simple diffuse and nodular scleritis. Furthermore when a steroid is needed, the duration and dose of the steroid may be reduced with the adjunctive use of an NSAIDs.

6. **Allergic and Giant Papillary Conjunctivitis:** Vernal Keratoconjunctivitis most commonly occurs in children and young adults. It shares with contact lens – associated giant papillary conjunctivitis (GPC) the common finding of giant papillae. Ketorolac 0.5% ophthalmic solution is effective in reducing eye itching often associated with allergic conjunctivitis. It can also be useful in cases of steroid induced open angle Glaucoma and also to prevent cataract formation. 1% Topical suprofen has been shown to effective in the treatment of contact lens related GPC.

Recent studies have shown that 1%. Acetyl salicylate and 1% piroxicam solutions are effective in treating seasonal allergic conjunctivitis.

7. **Reduction of Discomfort After Refractive Surgery:** Topical Keortolac 0.5% has been reported to be effective in the management of certain corneal conditions. Well known analgesic effect of topical ketorolac has been shown to reduce corneal pain following Excimer Laser PRK surgery.

Combination of Topical Diclofenac 1% and topical steroid (FML) has been shown to be statistically superior to corticosteroid alone in controlling post PRK myopic regression.

Topical NSAID have been used to lessen pain and inflammation after Nd Yag and photocoagulating lasers.

The use of topical Indomethacin 1% has been found to be effective to treat symptoms associated with corneal scars, edema, infiltrates and erosions.

Various Topical NSAIDs used Commonly in Ophthalmic Practice Worldwide are

PHENYLALKANOIC ACIDS

Flurbiprofen

It is one of the most potent NSAIDs of this group which is found to be very effective in various ocular conditions. Topical Flurbiprofen is available as 0.03% in ophthalmic solution (5 ml pack). It is indicated for the inhibition of intra-operative miosis. It is also indicated for treatment of post-operative (iatrogenic) and post laser trabeculoplasty, inflammation of anterior segment of the eye. It has no significant effect on IOP.

Dosage

For inhibition of intraoperative miosis, a total of four drops of topical Flurbiprofen should be administered in the eye by instilling one drop every half hour beginning two hours befor surgery.

One drop should be instilled into the conjunctival sac every four hours for one week following laser trabeculoplasty or 2-3 weeks after other surgical procedures.

Topical Flurbiprofen is contraindicated in Dendritic Keratitis and in individuals who are hypersensitive to the drug. Precaution should be taken as there exists the potential for cross-senstivity to acetylsalicyclic acid and other NSAIDs a histidine drug.

Use of Flurbiprofen sodium with an anti-infective drug in the presence of ocular infections should be monitored closely.

Adverse Reactions

The most frequent adverse reactions reported with the use of Topical Flurbiprofen solution are transient burning and stinging upon instillation and other minor symptoms of ocular irritation.

It may cause an increased bleeding tendency of ocular tissues in conjunction with surgery.

Ketorolac Tromethamine

It is recently introduced topical NSAIDs.

It is a new alpha substituted aryl acetic acid. It has both analgesic and anti-inflammatory properties. It is highly soluble in water.

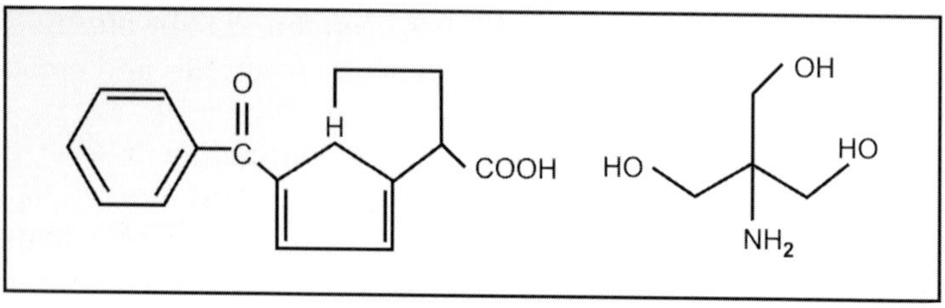

Fig. 21.5: Chemical structure of ketorolac tromethamine

As it is non-narcotic, non-steroidal agent, its mechanism of action is by its ability to inhibit prostaglandin biosynthesis (Fig. 21.5). Ocular administration of Ketorolac reduces prostaglandin E_2 levels in aqueous humour clinical studies have shown that the mean concentration of PGE_2 was 80 pg/ ml in aqueous humour prior to start of Topical Ketorolac treatment which was reduced drastically to 28 pg/ml in the eye receiving Ketorolac ophthalmic solution. It has no significant effect upon Intraocular pressure.

Ketorolac ophthalmic solution has following salient features.

- It can be safely administered in conjunction with other ophthalmic medications such as antibiotics, beta blockers, carbonic anhydrase inhibitors, cycloplegic and mydriatics.
- Inhibit Leukocyte accumulation even better than Dexamethasone.
- Microfine suspension helps in uniform distribution and rapid absorption.
- Lesser propensity to raise IOP than Low dose and comparable dose Dexamethasone.
- Proven safety in children.

Indications and Usage

- Indicated for relief of ocular itching due to seasonal allergic conjunctivitis. It significantly reduces conjunctival inflammation, lid edema, foreign body sensation and photophobia.
- Post Excimer PRK Surgery pain management.
- Chronic conjunctivitis.
- Iatrogenic inflammation of the eye.
- Treating Aphakic and Pseudophakic CME.
- For treating episcleritis, patients with corneal edema or erosions.
- For prophylaxis associated with retinal detachment surgery.

Dosage and Presentation

- Topical Ketorolac tromethamine ophthalmic solution is available in strength of 0.4 and 0.5%. The recommended dose is one drop four times a day in seasonal allergic. Conjunctivitis, Post PRK pain management and in iatrogenic inflammation of the eye. On topical use it is distributed throughout ocular tissues.

- Systemic 10 mg tablets (one tablet 3-4 times daily depending upon the severity of pain.
- Injection 1 ml ampoule containing 4.35 mg of Ketorolac.
- Precautions should be taken regarding its potential for cross-sensitivity to acetylsalicylic acid, Phenylacetic acid derivatives and other NSAIDs.
- There is report that it may cause increased bleeding of ocular tissues including hyphema in conjunction with ocular surgery as it has potential for increased bleeding time due to interference with thrombocyte aggregation.

Adverse Reactions

On topical use Ketorolac is well tolerated except for transient stinging and burning sensation on instillation. Other ocular adverse effects reported are ocular irritation, allergic reactions, superficial ocular infections and superficial Keratitis. On systemic use it can cause GIT disturbances like Nausea, vomiting, constipation, Anorexia, Pain and Ulceration. Dermatological and Hypersensitivity reactions, CNS effects like Headache, Dizziness, Depressions, Confusion and Insomnia.

Suprofen

It is available as 1% topical ophthalmic solution. Following topical application it achieves significant intraocular levels and inhibit the release of prostaglandin E_2 and F_{2x} and thromboxane B_2 from the inflammed cornea more effective.

It is good NSAIDs in treating Giant papillary conjunctivitis, Iatrogenic inflammation of eye and in preventing intraoperative miosis.

Dosage

It is available as 5 ml pack in 1% conc. Patient is advised to put 2 drops at 1,2,3 hours pre-operatively and four times a day postoperatively and in other ocular inflammatory conditions. Besides these NSAIDs, the other Phenylalkanoic acid derivative used in topical form are:

- Fenoprofen (0.3%)
- Ibuprofen (0.5%)
- Ketoprofen (1.0%)
- Naproxen (0.5%)
- Piroxicam (1%)

INDOLES

Indomethacin

Topical Indomethacin is used in the form of 1% aqueous suspension and recently introduced 0.1% ophthalmic solution.

- It is an excellent NSAIDs to treat aphakic and pseudophakic CME following Cataract Surgery and retinal detachment surgery.
- It has an excellent anti-inflammatory property in treating iatrogenic inflammation, Episcleritis and patients of corneal edema and erosions. It has good intraocular penetration.

Its mechanism of action and adverse reactions are similar to other NSAIDs mentioned earlier in this chapter.

In other indole NSAIDs used topically are:

1. Tolmetin (5% ophthalmic solution)
2. Surindac (1%)

PHENYLLACTIN ACID

Diclofenac

Diclofenac sodium is a potent non-steroidal anti-inflammatory drug with analgesic activity which inhibites prostaglandin synthesis. Sodium salt of diclofenac is commercially used. It is one of the most widely prescribed NSAID (Either topical or systemic) in ophthalmology. It is most commonly used for its marked anti-inflammatory and analgesic activities in ophthalmology (Fig. 21.6).

Indications

1. In topical form it is most commonly prescribed in iatrogenic inflammation, Pseudophakic inflammation of the eye following cataract and IOL Surgery.
2. In aphakic, pseudophakic CME following intra-ocular surgery.
3. In reduction of post excimer Laser PRK surgery pain in the patients.
4. Inhibition of surgically induced miosis during intraocular surgery.

Dosage and Administration

- In topical form it is used as ophthalmic solution in strength varying from 0.1 to 1%. It has good intraocular penetration. Patient is advised to put

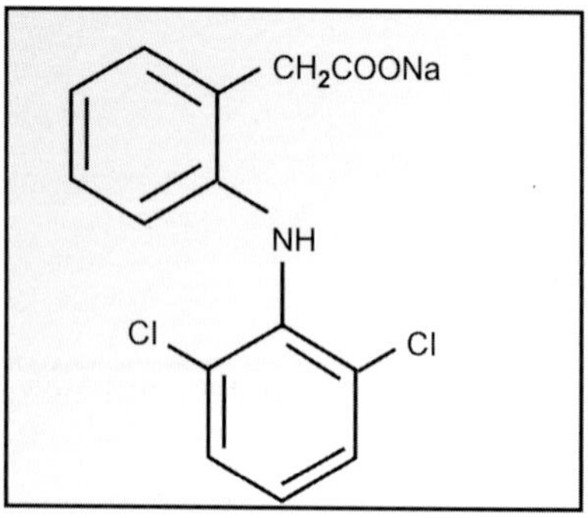

Fig. 21.6: Chemical structure of diclofenac

one drop 4 times a day post operatively till the complete clinical cure is achieved. For pre-operative use 1 drop of topical diclofenac 0.1% solution may be instilled in the affected eye 5 times during 3 hours (prior to surgery).

- In systemic form. It is available as tablet in the strength of 25, 50 and 75 mg. Patient is given oral dose in certain ocular condition where systemic administration is warranted in addition to Topical use.
- It is also available in injection form as 75 mg/3 ml ampoule.

In certain cases of severe postoperative pain 1-2 Deep intramasscular injection is indicated following cataract surgery for analgesic effect.

Topical diclofenac does not cause rise in intraocular pressure. It is contraindicated in patients allergic or senstive to asprin or other NSAIDS. Patients with blurred vision should not drive or operate machinery and soft contact lenses should not be worn during the treatment period.

Place of Ocular Diclofenac in Therapy

As the world population ages, cataract becomes an even more common problem facing clinicians and surgeons.

Indentification of effective pharmacological method of treating or preventing acute inflammatory processes associated with Surgical extraction of cataract constitute an important goal of pre and postoperative management.

NSAIDs have more recently become a focal point in the search for an alternative anti-inflammatory adjunct to cataract surgery. The activity of this class of drugs is by inhibiting prostaglandin synthesis.

Topical Diclofenac a potent NSAIDs has shown equivalent efficacy (when formulated as 0.1% solution) to dexamethasone 0.1% solution in attenuating signs of ocular inflammation. The drug is similar to indomethacin 0.1% in preventing elevation of IOP following cataract surgery. The occurrence and severity of cystoid macular edema is lessened with prophylactic instillation of topical diclofenac and drugs appears to prevent surgically induced miosis to greater degree.

Adverse Reactions

Topical diclofenac solution is well tolerated except for a transient localized burning and tingling sensation as reported by some patients.

On systemic use GIT disturbances, Headache, dizziness, rash, pruritis, peripheral edema, GI bleeding and peptic ulcer etc.

Nepafenac

Nepafenac is recently introduced a very potent non-steroidal antiinflammatory drug (NSAID) with analgesic activity which inhibits prostaglandin synthesis.

Nepafenac ophthlamic suspension is the first and only prodrug ocular NSAID which delivers highly effective therapy to the sites. It has target specific action and activates in key ocular tissues for excellent pain and inflammation control with no burning or stinging sensation.

Because of Nepafenac pro drug structure, its suspension penetrates the cornea rapidly and becomes an active metabolite in vascular tissue. Activation is greatest in the retina and choroid the most vascular ocular tissue so it has highest activation in the target tissues where CME occurs.

Its prodrug structure is well tolerated with little to no irritation, has an excellent safety profile and penetrates the eye well in its native form. It can be activated to provide an effective concentration of amfenac at target tissues which reduces intraocular inflammation.

This novel pro drug rapidly penetrates ocular tissues and is converted intraocularly from nepafenac to amfenac NSAID a potent commercially.

Nepafenac is available as Topical ophthalmic suspension 0.1%. It has an excellent intraocular penetration. It is also available in systemic form in tablet form in strength of 500 mg.

Indications

a. In topical form it is most commonly prescribed in iatrogenic inflammation of the eye following cataract surgery, Phaco surgery.
b. For cataract prophylaxis.
c. CME treatment and prophylaxis.
d. Refractive surgery prophylaxis and treatment.

Topical Nepafenac does not cause rise in intraocular pressure.

Adverse Effects

Topcial Nepafenac is quite safe. However ocular side effects reported are decreased visual acuity, Foreign body sensation, sticky sensation and capsular opacity etc.

Contraindications

Nepafenac ophthalmic suspension should not be administered while wearing contact lenses. It is contraindicated in patients with previously demonstrated hypersensitivity to any of the ingradients in the formulation or the NSAIDs. Concomitant use of topical Nepafenac and Topical steroids may increase the potential for healing problems.

General Local and Systemic Toxicity of NSAIDs

The most common adverse reactions after topical instillation as already described in individual NSAIDs pharmacokinetics are transient blurring, stinging and hyperemia of the conjunctiva.

Manufacturers have used various new formulation methods to minimize this potential discomfort.

Indomethacin solution in sesame seed oil was abandoned in favor of aqueous suspension or ophthalmic solution. Suprofen is prepared with 1% caffeine because it is less irritating in this form. Ketorolac is formulated as tromethamine salt as its moeity enhances the aqueous solubility and results in solution which is less irritating to the eye.

In addition allergic and hypersenstive reactions have been reported with topical NSAIDs. Systemic administration of NSAIDs can be accompanied by serious side effects such as gastrointestinal, central nervous system, hematological, renal, liver, dermatological and metabolic changes. It appears though these effects are largely avoided by topical administration.

Therefore, NSAID use much be carefully monitored for adverse events as it is good practice with any new drug treatment.

BIBLIOGRAPHY

1. Agarwal Amar. Text book of ophthalmology, ed.1, New Delhi : Jaypee Medical Publishers, 2002.
2. Bartlett. JD Clinical Ocular Pharmacology, ed.4, Boston : Butterworth-Heinemann,2001
3. Bartlett. JD, Ophthalmic Drug facts : Lippincott – William and Wilkins, 2001.
4. Crick. RP, Trimble RB. Text book of clinical ophthalmology : Hodder and Stoughton, 1986.
5. Duane. TD. Clinical ophthalmology, ed. 4 : Butterworth – Heinemann, 1999.
6. Duvall. Ophthalmic Medications and Pharmacology : Slack Inc, 1998.
7. Ellis. PP. Ocular Therapeutics and Pharmacology, ed. 7 : C.V. Mosby, 1985.
8. Fechner, Ocular Therapeutics : Slack Inc., 1998.
9. Flach. AJ, Non steroidal Anti-inflammatory drugs in Ophthalmology : Int. ophthalmol. Clinic, 1993; 33 : 1.
10. Franzie JP. Steroids : Int. Ophthalmol. Clinic, 1993; 33 : 9.
11. Fraunfelder. Current Ocular Therapy, ed. 5 : W.B. Saunders, 2000.
12 Garg Ashok. Current Trends in ophthalmology, ed. 1, New Delhi : Jaypee Medical Publishers, 1997.
13. Garg Ashok. Manual of Ocular Therapeutics, ed. 1, New Delhi : Jaypee Medical Publishers, 1996.
14. Garg Ashok. Ready Reckoner of Ocular Therapeutics, ed.1, New Delhi : 2002.
15. Goodman. LS, Gilman. A. Pharmacological basis of Therapeutics, ed.7, New York: Macmillan, 1985.
16. Havener's. Ocular Pharmacology, ed. 6: C.V. Mosby, 1994.
17. Kanski, Clinical ophthalmology, ed. 4: Butterworth – Heineman, 1999.
18. Kershner. ophthalmic Medications and Pharmacology: Slack. Inc., 1994.
19. Leibowitz HM. Anti-inflammatory Medications: Int. Ophthalmol. Clinic, 1980; 20: 117.
20. Olin BR et.al. Drugs Facts and Comparisons. Facts and Comparisons, St. Louis, 1997.
21. Onofrey. The Ocular Therapeutics; Lippincott-William and Wilkins, 1997.
22. Rhee. The Wills Eye drug Guide: Lippincott – William and Wilkins, 1998.
23. Steven Podos. Text book of ophthalmology, New Delhi: Jaypee Medical Publishers, 2001.
24. Zimmerman. Text book of Ocular Pharmacology : Lippincott and William and Wilkins, 1997.

Chapter 22

Management of Iatrogenic Inflammation of the Eye

NR Biswas, GK Das, Viney Gupta (India)

For the treatment of any type of inflammation including iatrogenic, both the asteroids and non-steroidal anti-inflammatory drugs may be used.

The corticosteroids are essential drugs in ophthalmological diseases. It is a boon to the patients when it is used with proper indications. It is a two-edged sword, however and can cause serious complications and side effects if it is used unwisely. Are we using corticosteroids judiciously? This question must always be kept in mind and answered before instituting this therapy. Before planning the corticosteroid therapy, we must keep in mind its ocular hazards. In clinical practice corticosteroids are often used as shotgun therapy or as a placebo when all is not going well. This practice must be discouraged.

TOPICAL APPLICATION

The route of administration of corticosteroids depends primarily on the site of involvement. Topical therapy is effective in anterior segment diseases, including disorders of lids, conjunctiva, cornea, iris and ciliary body. Ease of application, relatively low cost, and absence of systemic complications strongly favour local routes whenever they are effective.

The course of posterior segment disease (chorioretinitis, optic neuritis, and posterior scleritis) is not appreciably affected by topical corticosteroids and requires systemic therapy.

a. **Are diluted corticosteroid drops effective in controlling intraocular inflammation?**

   It was demonstrated that diluted corticosteroids have therapeutic anti-inflammatory effect in strengths of 0.01 and 0.005 percent.

b. **Corticosteroids in infective corneal diseases:** Local installation of corticosteroids in frank suppurative conditions are generally considered as contraindications to their use. In experimental studies the available 0.1 percent dexamethasone further diluted as 1:10 or 1:20 dilution had no virus or fungal replications enhancing effect when instilled 10 times a day, while

1:5 dilution or undiluted available dexamethasone drops (0.1%) enhanced virus and fungal growth. Moreover, adequately diluted corticosteroid does not increase the risk of enhancing the collagenase effect.

c. **Corticosteroid therapy in vernal conjunctivitis and allergic disorders:** The use off corticosteroids locally has a beneficial effect in vernal conjunctivitis. But prolonged use is attended by unwanted side effects like cataracts, glaucoma and secondary keratoconus.
d. **Use of corticosteroids in alkali burns of cornea and conjunctiva:** The use of corticosteroids in alkali burns is obligatory and seems beneficial.
e. **Use of corticosteroids in pseudophakic bullous keratopathy (PBK):** The effects of 5% hypertonic sodium chloride drop and deturgescent drops, prepared by mixing betamethasone eyedrops (0.1%) 1 ml; glycerin, 1 ml and artificial tear drops 8 ml, achieving 10% glycerin and 1:0 betamethasone eye drops (0.1%), were compared in a controlled clinical trial in 50 cases of PBK. These were instilled 10 times a day. The deturgescent drops were significantly superior in subjective as well as objective parameters like discomfort, foreign body sensation, corneal clarity and improvement in vision, etc. as compared to 5% hypertonic saline.
f. **Ocular hypertensive effect of corticosteroids:** Surgical trauma causes inflammation which demands the use of corticosteroids to prevent the trabecular meshwork, corneal endothelium and other inner structures of the eye from damage by inflammatory response as well as its debris. But, ocular hypertension inducing effects restrict their wide usage. In this regard, 1:10 or 1:20 diluted steroid did not have any ocular hypertensive effect.

The use of 1:10 or 1:20 dexamethasone (0.1%) for specified periods is safe to be used in glaucoma patients after intraocular surgery or when there is an associate uveitis, as there should be negligible risk of producing hypertension.

Systemic Therapy

Prednisone has become a corticosteroid of choice because it is inexpensive, short acting, and relatively free from sodium retention. It may be used in divided doses, a single daily dose, or a single alternate day dose.

Single daily dose For long term low-dosage maintenance (as for chronic uveitis), a single, morning, daily dose of prednisone may be optimal.

Alternate day therapy The undesirable side effects of systemic corticosteroid therapy can be substantially reduced by using alternate day therapy rather than divided dosage. Briefly stated, the entire total dose of corticosteroid that would have been given during a 2-day period is administered as a single dose every other morning.

Repository Injection

The ophthalmologist who wishes to administer corticosteroids by "subconjunctival" injection should consider use of the repository form of methyl-prednosolone acetate (Depo-Medrol). Thus suspension form of prednisolone provides a constant source of corticosteroid that lasts for 2 to 4 weeks.

Intravitreal Injection

Intravitreal 0.1 ml (Dose 50 mg/ml) is injected to prevent proliferation of fibroblast. It seems helpful to combat proliferative vitreoretinopathy.

Controlled Release Vehicles

Ocusert devices delivering 10mg of hydrocortisone acetate/hr were used to treat allergic conjunctivitis.

Pulse Therapy

Slow intravenous infusion of 100 mg Prednisolone daily for consecutive three days shows good response in Harada's disease. If needed, repeat dose can be given after 14 days.

Indications

In general, corticosteroid therapy may be helpful for all allergic ocular diseases, for most non-pyogenic inflammations (episcleritis, scleritis, uveitis, interstitial keratitis, optic neuritis and the like), and for the reduction of immunologic responses.

Use in Ocular Surgery

1. Cataract
2. Corneal graft rejection
3. Glaucoma surgery
4. Retinal detachment
5. Vitreous surgery
6. Strabismus
7. Intraocular foreign body

Contraindications and Complications

Systemic Complications

- Peptic ulceration
- Osteoporosis
- Femoral head ischemia necrosis

- Pseudotumor cerebri
- Exophthalmos.

Local Contraindication and Complications

- Superinfection
- Activation of tuberculosis
- Uveitis
- Glaucoma
- Corticosteroid mydriasis
- Corticosteroid induced cataract

The severe scleritis associated with rheumatoid arthritis, an example of immunological disorder does respond to corticosteroid treatment but the patient may suffer structural loss of sclera upto more severe scleromalacia as a result of treatment.

Sympathetic ophthalmia is a classic example of a disease responsive to corticosteroid therapy, but requires prolonged therapy.

Nonspecific iridocyclitis and chorioretinitis, as well as herpetic keratitis do seem to benefit from corticosteroid therapy.

Posterior ocular effects require systemic administration or retrobulbar injection.

Responsive Diseases

Boeck's Sarcoid Uveitis

The response of Boeck's sarcoid uveitis to corticosteroid therapy may be very gratifying. Topical use of corticosteroids and mydriatics is often insufficient to arrest the disease. Addition of systemic corticosteroid therapy has frequently given prompt subjective relief, followed within a few weeks by considerable objective improvement. Up to 200 mg daily was used and produced a consistently favourable symptomatic effect.

Orbital Myositis

Acute inflammation of one or more extraocular muscles may be a sequel to upper respiratory infections. These painful restrictions of movement may respond promptly to corticosteroid therapy.

Ocular Pemphigoid

Although pemphigoid is characteristically a slowly progressive chronic subepithelial scarring process, episodes of acute inflammation may occur. These typically are nonresponsive to topical corticosteroid therapy. Systemic corticosteroids in dosage of 60 to 100 mg/day have caused remission of the disease.

Herpes-zoster

In a small series of 11 patients with herpes-zoster, very favorable results were reported from the systemic administration of cortisone or ACTH.

Neoplasms

Hemangiomas, intracranial plasmacytoma, medulloblastoma, Ewing's tumors respond well to corticosteroid therapy.

Tolosa-Hunt Syndrome

Recurrent unilateral, painful, acute ophthalmoplegia responds dramatically to corticosteroid therapy within 2 to 3 days. A daily dosage of 60 mg prednisone was used.

Anterior Segment Ischemia

Prednisolone 1% was used four times daily, with gradual clearing of the corneal edema and anterior chamber cellular reaction.

Pseudotumor Cerebri

Dexamethasone 0.5 mg is prescribed three doses daily for 3 weeks.

Toxoplasmosis

It can be treated with high corticosteroid doses (up to 100 mg prednisone per day for a prolonged period with specific antitoxoplasmic therapy).

Other Indications

Corticosteroid is found to be useful in cysticercosis.

Use of Nonsteroidal Anti-inflammatory Drugs in Inflammation

In the treatment of ocular inflammation, the appeal of nonsteroidal anti-inflammatory drugs (NSAIDs) hinges on the complications associated with the more established therapy for ocular inflammation, i.e. corticosteroids. Although an overlap exists between the mechanisms of action of both, the use of NSAIDs may be safer than the use of corticosteroids, as the latter may produce adverse effects such as glaucoma, opportunistic infections, and posterior subcapsular cataracts. In sharp contrast, topical NSAIDs are known to cause only minor adverse effects such as burning, stinging and hyperemia of the conjunctiva.

Ocular Inflammation

A simple definition of ocular inflammation would be inflammation of any part of the eye. Intraocular inflammation can be subdivided into inflammation of the anterior and posterior segments of the eye. The cardinal signs of ocular inflammation are hyperemia, increased vascular permeability, edema, and cellular (leukocytes, mast cell, platelets, etc) infiltration into ocular fluids and tissues. In experimental anterior uveitis, miosis and a rise in intraocular pressure which is usually due to the breakdown of the blood-aqueous barrier with subsequent release of protein and fibrin into the aqueous humor, but not of cellular infiltration, is observed. Inflammation after paracentesis usually disappears within 2 to 3 hr.

To understand the history of NSAID use in ophthalmology, one must appreciate the relevance of prostaglandins in the eye. In 1971, Vane and Smith established the connection between the clinical effect of acetylsalicylate and inhibition of prostaglandin systesis.[1,2] It is now well-known that aspirin and other NSAIDs produce their clinical efficacy by inhibiting cyclooxygenase and thus inhibiting prostaglandin synthesis (Fig. 22.1). Specific drugs belonging to each class are listed in Tables 22.1 and 22.2.

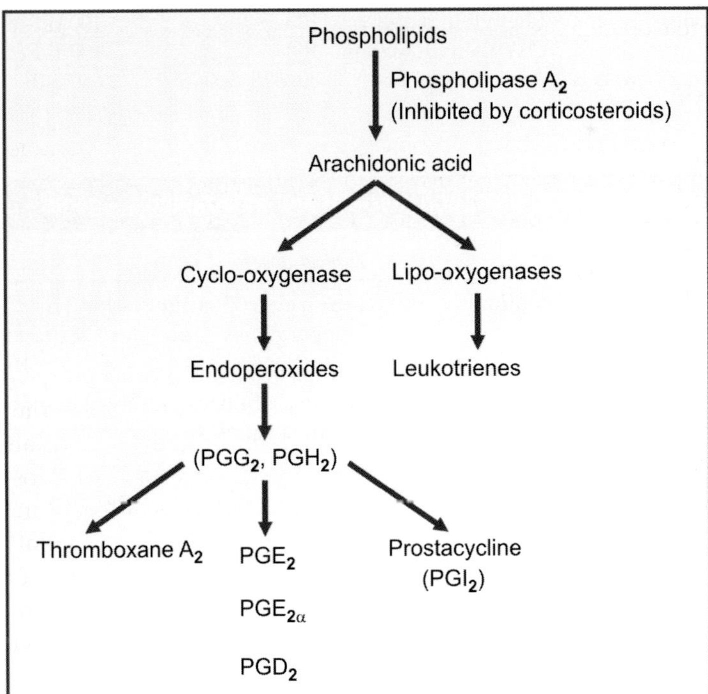

Fig. 22.1: Mechanism by which nonsteroidal anti-inflammatory drugs produce their clinical effect

Table 22.1: Systemic nonsteroidal anti-inflammatory agents

Drug	*Drug name*	*How supplied (mg)*	*Typical adult daily dose (mg)*
Salicylates	Aspirin	325-925	650 q4h
	Diflunisal	250, 500	250-500 bid
Fenamates	Mefenamate	250	250 qid
	Meclofenamate	50, 100	50-100 qid
Indoles	Indomethacin	25, 50, 75 (slow release)	25-50 tid-quid, 75 bid
	Sulindac	150, 200	150-200 bid
	Tolmetin	200, 400, 600	400 tid
Phenylacetic acids	Diclofenac	35, 50, 75	35-75 bid
Pheynylalkanoic acids	Fenoprofen	200, 300, 600	300-600 tid
	Ketoprofen	25, 50, 75	75 tid - 50 quid
	Piroxicam	10, 20	10 bid, 20 daily
	Flurbiprofen	50, 100	100 tid
	Ketorolac	10	10 qid
	Naproxen	250, 375, 500	250-500 bid
		275-550	275-550 bid
		200, 300, 400	
	Ibuprofen	600, 800	400-800 tid
Pyrazolones	Phenylbutazone	100	100 tid-qid
	Oxyphenybutazone	100	100 tid-qid
Paraaminophenols	Acetaminophen	80, 325, 500, 650	650 q4h

Table 22.2: Topical nonsteroidal anti-inflammatory agents

Name	*Strength*	*Typical doses*
Flurbiprofen	0.03% solution	1 drop every 30 minutes for 2 hr Preoperatively (Total dose: 4 drops)
Suprofen	1.0% solution	2 drops at 1.2 and 3 hours preoperatively or every 4 hours while awake on the day of surgery
Diclofenac	0.1% solution	qid
Ketorolac	0.5% solution	tid
Indomethacin	0.5%-1.0% suspension	qid

Mechanism of Action

NSAIDs act mainly as anti-inflammatory agents by inhibiting cyclooxygense and lipo-oxygenase enzymes which lead to inhibition of products like prostaglandins, thromboxane and leukotrienes which induce inflammation. Ocular actions of prostaglandins include an increase in vascular permeability, breakdown of the blood-aqueous barrier and induction of miosis.[3]

Cystoid Macular Edema (CME)

Topical NSAIDs are effective in preventing postsurgical angiographic CME when topical or subTenon's corticosteroid injections are given concurrently. Only one study (involving 50 patients) has demonstrated similar effect with a topical NSAID in the absence of concurrent corticosteroid therapy.[4] Several studies have demonstrated that prophylactic treatment with a topical NSAID has a beneficial effect on visual function. In one study, this effect was shown even in the absence of concurrent corticosteroid therapy. Topical NSAIDs also are effective in the treatment of angiographically documented subclinical CME, and this can translate into improved visual function. Oral NSAIDs have also been shown to be effective in both the prevention and treatment of CME after cataract surgery. However, a study demonstrating a positive effect on visual function with oral promote one NSAIDs still is lacking. There is no strong evidence to promote one NSAID over another.

Postoperative Inflammation

Fluorophotometric analysis has made available a quantitative means of studying anterior chamber inflammation. With this tool, it has been possible to evaluate, in a reproducible fashion, the effect of NSAIDs on postoperative inflammation. By using both slit lamp and fluorophotometric analysis as a part of randomized double-masked placebo-controlled studies, several topical NSAIDs like indomethacin 1.0%[5], flurbiprofen 0.03%[6], ketorolac 0.5%[7,8] and diclofenac 0.1%[9] have been shown to reduce postoperative inflammation. The positive effect of NSAIDs was seen in both intracapsular and extracapsular cataract surgery. It is important to note that whereas in most of the studies, corticosteroids were given concurrently, two of these studies were conducted without concurrent corticosteroid therapy.[7,8] In these studies, topical ketorolac 0.05% proved to be better than placebo in controlling inflammation after cataract surgery.

In the treatment of postsurgical inflammation, the superiority of NSAID over placebo has led to a comparison of NSAIDs with corticosteroid. Ketorolac 0.5%[10] and diclofenac[11] were compared to dexamethasone and prednisolone, respectively. In both studies, there was no significant difference in the reduction of postoperative inflammation by slit-lamp examination between patients on NSAIDs and those on corticosteroid topical therapy. However, it should be noted that in the ketorolac study, a subTenon injection of corticosteroid was given to all the patients and this may have contributed to the lack of difference between the two treatment groups. Concurrent corticosteroid therapy was not a factor in the study comparing diclofenac with prednisolone. When fluorophotometry was used in both comparative studies, it was found that control of inflammation in the topical NSAID treatment group was better achieved than in the corticosteroid groups.

Regardless of the preceding findings, it is a common practice to use topical corticosteroid alone to control post cataract surgery inflammation. Nevertheless, the U.S. food and Drug Administration (FDA) has approved the use of the diclofenac 0.1% four times daily, starting 24 hours after cataract surgery for this purpose. Thus, it is possible to substitute a topical NSAID for a topical corticosteroid to control postoperative inflammation, especially in eyes with significant steroid responsive glaucoma.

Uveitis

In contrast to postsurgical inflammation, many forms of uveitis require prolonged steroid therapy to control inflammation. At times, the therapeutic effort must be escalated to the use of subtenon injections or oral administration of corticosteroid. Of course, the risk of iatrogenic glaucoma and cataract becomes substantial I these situations. Therefore, NSAIDs are gaining a more secure position in the treatment of certain forms of uveitis.

Scleritis and Episcleritis

Topical NSAIDs have no proven efficacy in the treatment of episcleritis. In fact, they appear to be less effective than topical corticosteroids in reducing episcleral injection and pain associated with episcleritis.[12] In contrast, systemic NSAIDs are the agents of choice in the treatment of nonnecrotizing simple, diffuse, and nodular scleritis.[13] One may have to proceed sequentially through several different NSAIDs until one find the one that works. Furthermore, when a steroid is needed, the duration and dose of the steroidal may be reduced with the adjunctive use of an NSAID.

Allergic and Giant Papillary Conjunctivitis

Vernal keratoconjunctivitis most commonly occurs children and young adults. It shares with contact lens-associated giant papillary conjunctivitis (GPC). The common finding of giant papillary conjunctivitis on the upper palpebral conjunctiva. The standard treatment for both is topical steroids until a topical mast cell stabilizer takes effect.

Side Effects of NSAIDs

Common adverse effects following instillation of topical NSAIDs include burning, stinging, and hyperemia of conjunctiva. Allergic and hypertensive reactions are also reported following use of topical NSAIDs. Systemic side effects following use of NSAIDs mainly include gastritis, but are unlikely to occur with topical administration.

CONCLUSION

NSAIDs have wide potential for use in various ocular disorders, though the effects vary from one individual to another and the effect is unpredictable. More research is required to develop newer NSAIDs which can be used for various inflammatory disorders of the eye with more effective action with minimal ocular toxicities.

Currently corticosteroids are still the drugs of choice in the treatment of ocular inflammation. However, because their prolonged use may result in severe ocular side effects, it would be therapeutically beneficial to develop nonsteroidal anti-inflammatory drugs that have similar or greater efficacy than steroids but not their ocular side effects.

REFERENCES

1. Flck AJ. Cyclo-oxygense inhibitors in Ophthalmology. Surv Ophthalmol 1992;36:259-84.
2. Gilman AG, Rall TC, Nies AS, Taylor P. The pharmacologic basis of therapeutics. Elmsford: Pergamon 1990;638-81.
3. Abramson SB, Weisman G. The mechanism of nonsteroidal anti-inflammatory drugs. Arthritis Rheum 1989;32:1-9.
4. Flach AJ, Jampol LM, Weinberg D, et al. Improvement in visual acuity in chronic aphakic and pseudophakic cystoid macular edema after treatment with topical 0.5% ketorolac tromethamine. Am J Ophthalmol 1991;112:514-19.
5. Sanders DR, Kraff ML. Steroidal and nonsteroidal anti-inflammatory agents. Effects on postsurgical inflammation and blood-aqueous barrier breakdown. Arch. Ophthalmol 1984;102:1453-6.
6. Sabiston MB, Tessler D, Summersk H, et al. Reduction of inflammation following cataract surgery by flurbiprofen. Ophthalmic Surg 1987;18:873-7.
7. Flach AJ, Graham J, Kruger LP, et al. Quantitative assessment of postsurgical breakdown of the blood-aqueous barrier following administration of ketorolack tomethmine solution. A double-masked, paired comparison with vehicle-placebo solution study. Arch Ophthalmol 1988;106:344-7.
8. Flach AJ, Lavelle CJ, Olander KW, et al. The effect of ketorolac 0.5% solution in reducing postsurgical inflammation following ECCE with IOL. Double masked, parallel comparison with vehicle. Ophthalmology 1988;95:1277-84.
9. Vickers FF, McGuigan LJB, Ford C, et al. The effect of diclofenac sodium ophthalmic drops on the treatment of postoperative inflammation. Invest Ophthalmol Vis Sci (ARVO suppl) 1991;32:793.
10. Flach AJ, Kraff MC, Sanders DR, et al. The quantitative effect of 0.5% ketorolac tromethamine solution and 0.1% dexamethasone sodium phosphate solution on postsurgical blood aqueous barrier. Arch Ophthalmol 1988;106:480-83.
11. Kraff MC, Sanders DR, McGuigan L, et al. Inhibition of blood aqueous humour barrier breakdown with diclofenac. A fluorophotometric study. Arch Ophthalmol 1990;108:380-3.
12. Lyons CH, Hakin KN, Watson PG. Topical flurbiprofen: An effective treatment for epoiscleritis? Eye 1990;4:521-25.
13. Vitale A, Foster CS. Nonsteroidal anti-inflammatory drugs. In. Zimmerman TJ, (Ed): Textbook of Ocular Pharmacology. New York: Lippincott-Raven, 1995.

Chapter 23

Management of Post-Refractive Keratitis

Eric D Donnenfeld (USA)

Laser in situ keratomileusis (LASIK) is the most commonly performed surgical procedure to correct refractive errors and is the most common elective procedure performed in the United States. LASIK offers many benefits over photorefractive keratectomy, including increased visual rehabilitation, decreased stromal scarring, less postoperative pain, less irregular astigmatism, minimal regression, and the ability to treat a greater range of refractive disorders.[1,2] Compared to other refractive procedures, LASIK preserves the integrity of Bowman's membrane and the overlying epithelium, thus decreasing the risk of microbial keratitis. However, microbial keratitis following LASIK has become an increasingly recognized, sight-threatening complication of refractive surgery.[3-10]

The incidence of infectious keratitis following LASIK is unknown and can vary widely depending on the study. One large, retrospective study investigating the complications associated with LASIK surgery found an incidence of two infections in 1,062 eyes,[7] and another similar study found an incidence of one infection in 1,019 eyes.[8] A more recent case series of LASIK-associated infections encountered at a single institution quotes an estimated incidence between 1:1000 and 1:5000.[9] Based on a comprehensive review and analysis of the published literature on infections following LASIK, Chang and colleagues[5] also noted that the incidence of infection after LASIK can vary widely (0-1.5%). The American Society of Cataract and Refractive Surgery (ASCRS) Cornea Clinical Committee developed a post-LASIK infectious keratitis survey and conducted a survey of the organization's members in 2001 and again in 2004.[10] In the 2001 survey, there was an incidence of 1 infection for every 2919 procedures performed by physicians returning the questionnaire (116 post-LASIK infections were reported by 56 LASIK surgeons who had performed an estimated 338,550 procedures). These results are contrasted to 1 infection for every 2131 procedures performed by physicians returning the questionnaire in 2004. The increase in incidence of infections is presumably due to an increase in gram-positive resistant organisms, most likely due to methicillin resistant *Staphylococcus aureus*. Culture results revealed opportunistic infections and gram-positive bacteria as the most common organisms in 2001 (Fig. 23.1A). In contrast, as noted above, in 2004 gram-positive bacteria have increased in incidence while opportunistic infections, specifically atypical mycobacteria, have seen a marked reduction (Fig. 23.1B).

In 2004, the epidemic of atypical mycobacteria that was seen in 2001 (Fig. 23.1B) ended. Cases from atypical mycobacteria decreased from 48% to 5%. This decrease is presumably due to the use of fourth-generation fluoro-

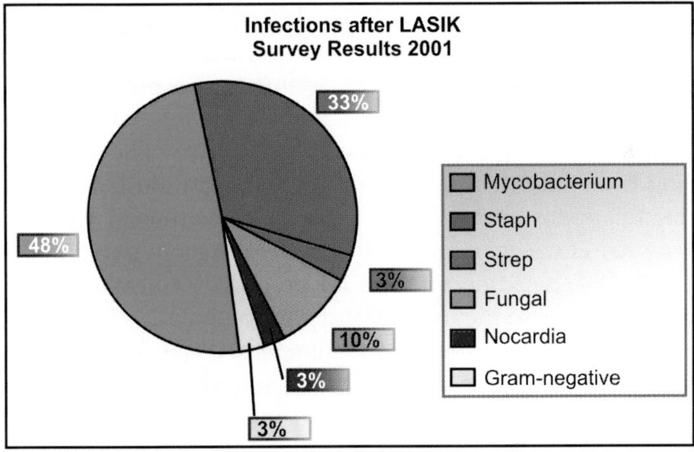

Fig. 23.1A: ASCRS 2001 culture results of post-LASIK infectious keratitis

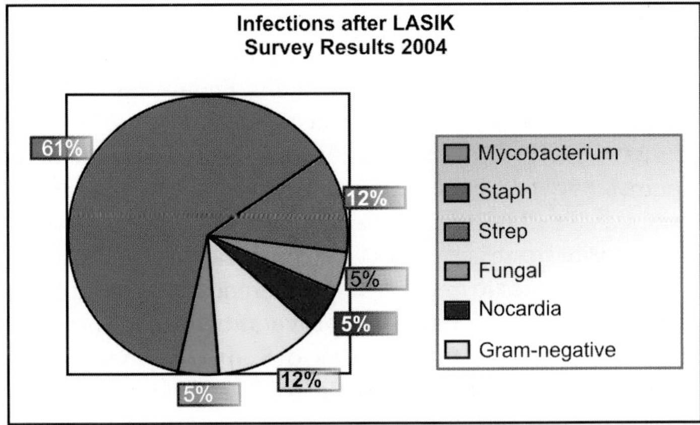

Fig. 23.1B: ASCRS 2004 culture results of post-LASIK infectious keratitis

quinolones and improved sterile technique. It was interesting to note that no patient who received a 4th generation fluoroquinolone as prophylaxis developed an atypical mycobacteria infectious keratitis in the 2004 survey. However, the overall incidence of infectious keratitis increased in 2004 from 2001.

The results of these surveys and an analysis of the trends seen in the data can help to guide prophylaxis and treatment of infections keratitis following LASIK. Infectious keratitis is a potentially devastating complication of LASIK. A high degree of suspicion coupled with a rapid diagnosis and appropriate therapy can result in visual recovery. For prophylaxis against a post-LASIK infectious keratitis there are several steps which can be implemented. Preoperatively, all patients considering refractive surgery should have a thorough examination of their eyelids and lacrimal apparatus. Treatment of infectious lid disease prior to LASIK with hot compresses and a topical antibiotic ointment applied three times daily to the lid margin may decrease the risk of a bacterial keratitis. A small minority of clinicians recommend performing monocular surgery or the use of separate instruments when performing bilateral surgery.[11] Some clinicians recommend the use of sterile drapes, gowns, gloves and masks by the treating physician and assisting technician. A 10% betadine solution lid prep prior to cataract surgery has been shown to decrease the incidence of endophthalmitis following cataract surgery and is recommend by many clinicians when performing LASIK.[12] Proper sterilization techniques can prevent the use of contaminated instruments. As several epidemics of atypical mycobacteria have been associated with the use of non-sterile water to clean instruments or the use of ice during LASIK surgery, all fluids applied to the eye before, during and after LASIK should be sterile.[13]

Antibiotic prophylaxis for LASIK should emphasize the need to provide broad-based spectrum coverage with gram-positive emphasis. The antibiotic should be non-toxic to promote epithelial healing and should provide coverage against atypical mycobacteria which is the most common opportunistic organism responsible for post-LASIK infections. Finally, the antibiotic should penetrate effectively into the cornea and achieve therapeutic levels in the mid stroma. Fourth generation fluoroquinolones (gatifloxacin 0.3% and moxifloxacin 0.5%) for antibiotic prophylaxis of LASIK and PRK are recommended as they best meet the criteria listed above.[13] We begin topical therapy 1 hour prior to surgery and at the conclusion of LASIK we dehydrate the cornea for 1-2 minutes to improve flap adherence and then apply antibiotic directly on the dehydrated flap to improve antibiotic absorption into the cornea. With PRK, we place the antibiotic directly onto the stromal bed and soak the bandage contact lens in antibiotic for 30 seconds prior to placing the contact lens on the eye. Postoperatively, patients receive a fourth generation fluoroquinolone four times a day for 5 days with LASIK and for one day after the epithelial defect has closed with PRK.

We divide infectious keratitis following LASIK into rapid onset within the first two weeks of surgery and late onset which can occur from 2 weeks to 3 months following surgery.[13] The organisms seen in early onset infectious keratitis within the first two weeks are common bacterial pathogens such as staphylococcal and streptococcal species. Gram-negative organisms are rare. The organisms seen in late onset infectious keratitis after two weeks are usually opportunistic such as fungi, *Nocardia* and atypical mycobacteria. The published literature review of LASIK-associated infections by Chang and colleagues supports this classification of infection.[5] Based on their study, gram positive organisms were more likely to present within 7 days of surgery ($p = 0.001$) while mycobacterial infections were more likely to present 10 or more days after surgery ($p < 0.001$).[5]

Since the organisms responsible for infectious keratitis following LASIK often will not respond to empiric therapy, as with the results from the previous survey, we recommend lifting the flap, scraping, and culturing all suspicious cases, and selecting appropriate culture media including blood agar, chocolate agar, Sabouraud's agar and thioglycolate broth.[13] For infectious keratitis after two weeks, we recommend a growth media for atypical mycobacteria such as Lowenstein-Jensen or Middlebrook 7H-9 media in addition to the previous culture media. If these special media are unavailable, we recommend using blood agar as atypical mycobacteria grow quite well on these plates. At the time of culture we also recommend scraping the infiltrate and performing a Gram stain, Gomori-methenamine silver stain, and Ziehl-Neelsen stain to rule out unusual pathogens such as nocardia, atypical mycobacteria, and fungi. In cases in which cultures are negative and the infection continues to a corneal biopsy or PCR should be considered.

For the treatment of both rapid-onset and delayed-onset infectious keratitis, it is recommended to elevate the flap and culture. Irrigation of the flap interface with an appropriate antibiotic solution (fortified vancomycin 50 mg/ml for rapid-onset keratitis and fortified amikacin 20 mg/ml for delayed-onset keratitis) may be helpful. For rapid-onset keratitis, we recommend a fourth-generation topical fluoroquinolone such as gatifloxacin 0.3% or moxifloxacin 0.5% be given in a loading dose every 5 minutes for 3 doses and then every 30 minutes alternating with an antimicrobial which is rapidly bacteriocidal and has increased activity against gram-positive organisms, such as cefazolin 50 mg/ml every 30 minutes.[13] In patients who work in a hospital environment or have been exposed to a hospital surgical setting or healthcare environment, there is an added risk of methicillin-resistant *staphylococcus aureus* (Solomon R, Donnenfeld E, Perry H, et al. Methicillin Resistant *Staphylococcus aureus* Infectious Keratitis Following Refractive Surgery. Presented as a paper at the American Society of Cataract and Refractive Surgery Symposium on Cataract, IOL, and Refractive Surgery, San Diego, Calif, 2004). In those patients who work in a hospital environment or have had exposure to a healthcare environment, we recommend the substitution of vancomycin 50 mg/ml every

30 minutes instead of cefazolin to provide more effective therapy against MRSA. In addition, we advocate the use of oral doxycycline 100 mg twice daily (to inhibit collagenase production) and also recommend discontinuing corticosteroids.

For delayed-onset keratitis, which is commonly due to atypical mycobacteria, *Nocardia* and fungi, we recommend beginning therapy with amikacin 35 mg/ml every 30 minutes alternating with vancomycin 50 mg/ml every 30 minutes, starting oral doxycycline 100 mg BID, and discontinuing corticosteroids. Alternative therapy for delayed-onset keratitis, which would cover atypical *Mycobacteria*, includes clarithromycin and fourth-generation fluoroquinolones. This treatment will not cover fungal infections, and therefore, treatment for all cases of infectious keratitis should be modified based on culture and scraping results and response to therapy.

Infectious keratitis after LASIK frequently presents with inflammation in the corneal interface, which can mimic diffuse lamellar keratitis (DLK). DLK usually occurs within the first few days following LASIK, unless there is postoperative ocular trauma.[14] The appearance of an interface inflammation more that one week following LASIK should be presumed to be infectious unless proven otherwise. Since DLK usually presents with a diffuse appearance while infectious keratitis has focal area of infiltration, any focal infiltrate surrounded by inflammation following LASIK should be considered infectious until proven otherwise.

In conclusion, infectious keratitis is a potentially devastating complication following LASIK. Culture results reveal gram-positive bacteria as the most common organisms. Infectious keratitis may present as late as months following LASIK, and its frequent misdiagnosis at initial presentation may result in significant vision loss. Antibiotic prophylaxis for LASIK should emphasize the need to provide broad-based spectrum coverage with gram-positive emphasis. For treatment, we do not recommend empiric therapy as most organisms are opportunistic and do not respond to conventional therapy. A high degree of suspicion with flap elevation and culturing should be performed on all eyes suspected of infectious keratitis following LASIK.

REFERENCES

1. Hersh PS, Brint SF, Maloney RK, et al. Photorefractive keratectomy versus laser in situ keratomileusis for moderate to high myopia: a randomized prospective study. Ophthalmology 1998;105:1512-23.
2. Azar DT, Farah SG. Laser in situ keratomileusis versus photorefractive keratectomy: an update on indications and safety. Ophthalmology 1998;105: 1357-8.
3. Garg P, Bansal AK, Sharma S, Vemuganti GK. Bilateral infectious keratitis after laser in situ keratomileusis: a case report and review of the literature. Ophthalmology 2001;108:121-5.
4. Solomon A, Karp, CL, Miller D, et al. Mycobacterium interface keratitis after laser in situ keratomileusis. Ophthalmology 2001;108:2201-8.

5. Perry HD, Doshi SJ, Donnenfeld ED, et al. Herpes simplex reactivation following laser in situ keratomileusis and subsequent corneal perforation. CLAO J 2002;28:69-71.
6. Chang MA, Jain S, Azar DT. Infections following laser in situ keratomileusis: an integration of the published literature. Surv Ophthalmol 2004;49:269-80. after laser in situ keratomileusis. J Cataract Refract Surg 2002;28:898-9.
7. Stulting RD, Carr JD, Thompson KP, et al. Complications of laser in situ keratomileusis for the correction of myopia. Ophthalmology 1999;106:13-20.
8. Lin RT, Maloney RK. Flap complications associated with lamellar refractive surgery. Am J Ophthalmol 1999;127:129-36.
9. Karp CL, Tuli SS, Yoo SH, et al. Infectious keratitis after LASIK. Ophthalmology 2003;110:503-10.
10. Solomon R, Donnenfeld ED, Azar DT, Holland EJ, Palmon FR, Pflugfelder SC, Rubenstein JB. Infectious keratitis after laser in situ keratomileusis: results of an ASCRS survey. J Cataract Refract Surg 2003;29:2001-6.
11. Kohnen T. Infections after corneal refractive surgery: can we do better? (editorial). J Cataract Refract Surg 2002;28:569-70.
12. Speaker MG, Menikoff JA. Prophylaxis of endophthalmitis with topical povidone-iodine. Ophthalmology 1991;98:1769-75.
13. Donnenfeld ED, Kim T, Holland E, et al. Management of infectious keratitis following laser in situ keratomileusis. J Cataract Refract Surg 2005;31:2008-11.
14. Stulting RD, Randleman JB, Couser JM, Thompson KP. The epidemiology of diffuse lamellar keratitis. Cornea 2004;23:680-8.

Chapter 24

Conjunctival Allergen Challenge for Evaluating Anti-inflammatory Therapy

Mitchell H Friedlaender, Daphne Breshears (USA)

ABSTRACT

Background: Ocular allergic reactions are typically evaluated subjectively for erythema, edema, and itching. Objective measurements may have greater accuracy and reproducibility than subjective methods.

Objective: To apply objective measurements of erythema, edema, and ocular surface sensation (the EES Method) to ocular allergic reactions induced by conjunctival allergen challenge (CAC).

Methods: Twenty allergic subjects were evaluated 5 minutes before and 5 minutes after CAC for objective and subjective signs of conjunctival erythema, edema, and sensation. Objective evaluations were determined by spectroradiometry (erythema), a fractional millimeter reticule in a slit lamp microscope eyepiece (edema), and aesthesiometry (ocular surface sensation). Subjective evaluations were performed by observation (erythema and chemosis), and questioning the subject (itching). Repeat measurements were made after instillation of a vasoconstrictor/antihistamine eyedrop.

Results: Objective measurements of erythema and eyelid edema increased significantly after CAC ($p < 0.001$). Subjective measurements of erythema, chemosis, and itching also increased significantly after CAC ($p < 0.001$). The objective measurement of sensation decreased after CAC, but the change was not statistically significant. After treatment with a vasoconstrictor/antihistamine eyedrop, a significant decrease in erythema (but, not edema or sensation) could be measured objectively and subjectively ($p < 0.001$). There was a correlation between objective and subjective measurements of erythema and edema following CAC ($r_s = 0.838$ and 0.893, respectively), and for the reduction of erythema after treatment with a vasoconstrictor/antihistamine eyedrop ($r_s = 0.822$).

Conclusion: Ocular allergic reactions and the effects of antiallergic treatment can be measured objectively by the EES (erythema, edema, sensation) Method, and subjectively, by observation and questioning.

INTRODUCTION

Conjunctival allergen challenge (CAC) has been used for over one hundred years to confirm the diagnosis of systemic allergy,[1] study the ocular features of the allergic reaction,[2-5] and evaluate antiallergic therapy.[6-9] Conjunctival reactions are typically graded subjectively on the basis of severity. Conjunctival erythema and conjunctival edema, or chemosis, are usually graded by observation on a 0 to 4 scale. Itching is graded on a 0 to 4 scale by questioning the subject. While subjective methods are useful for documenting large differences in allergic signs and symptoms, they are less useful for documenting small differences. In addition, a reaction may be graded differently when viewed by multiple examiners, and even a single examiner may grade two identical reactions differently.

Attempts have been made previously to evaluate ocular allergic reactions objectively by measuring ocular surface temperature,[2] chemical mediators in the tear film,[2,5,10-14] and cellular responses after CAC.[4,13,14] Such objective measurements are, for the most part, cumbersome, time consuming, expensive, and imprecise. For objective measurements to be useful in studies with multiple evaluations of large numbers of allergic patients, they must be quick, accurate, and easy to record.

Recently, we have found that allergic and toxic conjunctival reactions can be evaluated objectively with simple, accurate, and reproducible methods. Conjunctival erythema can be measured with a spectroradiometer, a device for measuring the color of reflected light.[15] Eyelid edema can be measured using a fractional millimeter reticule in the eyepiece of a slit lamp microscope. Ocular surface sensation can be measured with aesthesiometry.

The purpose of this study is to determine if conjunctival erythema, edema, and ocular surface sensation can be measured before and after allergen challenge, and after administration of vasoconstrictor-antihistamine eye drops. We also sought to determine whether there is a correlation between erythema, edema, and sensation when measured objectively and subjectively.

Methods

Conjunctival Allergen Challenge

Twenty subjects with allergy to either cat dander, grass, or ragweed were recruited. All subjects had participated in previous CAC studies, and all had positive skin and conjunctival tests to specific allergens when previously tested. The study was approved by the Scripps Clinic Human Subjects Committee, and all subjects signed approved consent forms. Thirty microliters of allergen were instilled in the inferior conjunctival cul-de-sac of both eyes beginning with a low dose (Table 24.1). If necessary, medium and high doses of allergen were instilled at 5-minute intervals until a moderate, subjective allergic reaction (itching = 2, and redness = 2) was achieved.

Table 24.1: Allergen concentrations used for conjunctival allergen challenge

	Low	*Medium*	*High*
Cat dander	2,500 AU/ml	5,000 AU/ml	10,000 AU/ml
Grass	10,000 PNU/ml	20,000 PNU/ml	40,000 PNU/ml
Ragweed	10,000 PNU/ml	20,000 PNU/ml	40,000 PNU/ml

Objective Measurements

Erythema Conjunctival erythema was measured using a PR-650 Spectrascan spectroradiometer (Photo Research Inc., Chatsworth, CA), 5 minutes before and 5 minutes after CAC. Using consistent room illumination and subject positioning, the spectroradiometer was placed on an adjustable tripod 18 inches from the subject's eye. With the subject looking up, a 5 mm focusing spot was positioned on the inferior bulbar conjunctiva. Using the u′ measurement of the 1976 Commission Internationale d'Eclairage (CIE), a mean of three consecutive readings was calculated.

Edema Anterior to posterior width of the lower eyelid margin was measured using a fractional millimeter reticule in the eyepiece of a slit-lamp microscope (Haag-Streit, Bern, Switzerland). The measurement was made posteriorly from the gray line (the junction of the skin and conjunctiva at the lid margin) to the posterior most central eyelash.

Sensation Ocular surface sensation was measured using the aesthesiometer of Cochet and Bonnet (Luneau, Chartres, France). This device has an adjustable nylon filament which can be extended from 0 to 6 cm. With the filament fully extended, sensation was tested on the conjunctival side of the 6 o'clock limbus (the junction of the cornea and conjunctiva), one millimeter from the cornea. The filament was shortened by 0.5 cm increments until the subject perceived the sensation of touch. The shorter the filament, the more force is delivered to the eye, and the easier it is for the subject to perceive the sensation of touch. The filament length which first produced a threshold sensation of touch was recorded.

Subjective Measurements

Conjunctival erythema, chemosis, and itching were graded 5 minutes before and 5 minutes after CAC by observation at the slit lamp microscope, using a 0 to 4 scale (Table 24.2).

Instillation of Vasoconstrictor/Antihistamine Eyedrops

Fifteen minutes after CAC, eyes were randomized so that one eye of each subject received one drop containing 30 microliters of a solution of naphazoline hydrochloride 0.025% and pheniramine maleate 0.3%, and the fellow eye received 30 microliters of normal saline.

Table 24.2: Subjective grading of erythema, chemosis, and itching

0	None
1	Mild
2	Moderate
3	Moderately severe
4	Severe

Repeat Measurements

All objective and subjective measurements were repeated 5 minutes before, and 5 minutes after instillation of eyedrops.

Statistical Analysis

Data were analyzed using a paired sample t-test. A probability value of 0.05 was considered statistically significant, and data are presented as means ± the standard deviation. Spearman rank-correlation coefficients were calculated to determine if there was a correlation between objective and subjective measurements.

RESULTS

Conjunctival Allergen Challenge

All 40 eyes had an onset of conjunctival allergic reactions within 5 minutes of allergen challenge, and all reactions achieved at least moderate intensity (redness = 2, itching = 2). Ten subjects required low dose allergen (6 cat dander, 3 grass, 1 ragweed), and 10 subjects required medium dose allergen (5 cat dander, 3 grass, and 2 ragweed). Both eyes of each subject required the same allergen dose in all cases, and reactions of the two eyes were of similar intensity.

Objective Measurements

Erythema

Conjunctival erythema increased after CAC (Fig. 24.1). The mean u′ value for erythema before CAC was 0.280 ± 0.01, and the mean u′ value 5 minutes after CAC was 0.293 ± 0.01 ($p < 0.001$).

Edema

Mean lower lid edema increased after CAC (Fig. 24.2). Mean lid edema before CAC was 1.10 mm ± 0.08 mm, and 1.31 mm ± 0.04 mm after CAC ($p < 0.001$).

Sensation

Ocular surface sensation decreased after CAC (Fig. 24.3). Mean ocular surface sensation before CAC was 3.2 ± 2.2 mm, and 3.1 ± 1.8 mm after CAC. This difference was not statistically significant ($p = 0.72$).

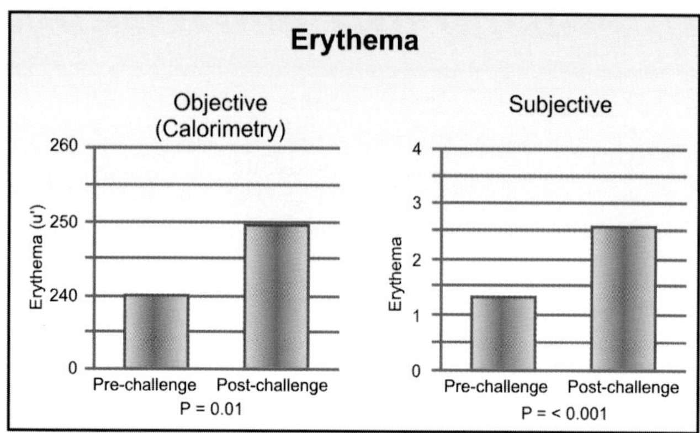

Fig. 24.1: Objective and subjective measurements of conjunctival erythema before and after conjunctival allergen challenge

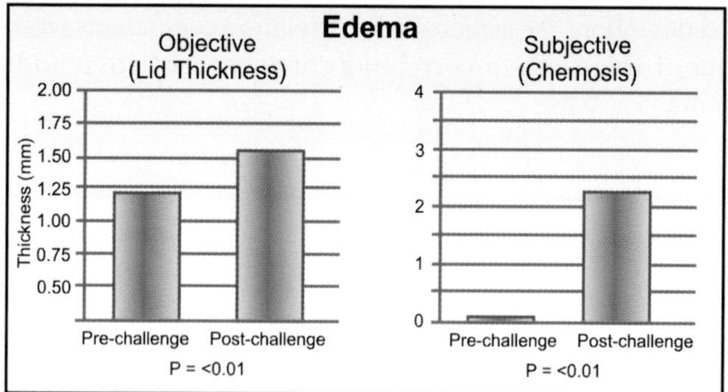

Fig. 24.2: Objective measurement of lower eyelid edema and subjective measurement of chemosis before and after conjunctival allergen challenge

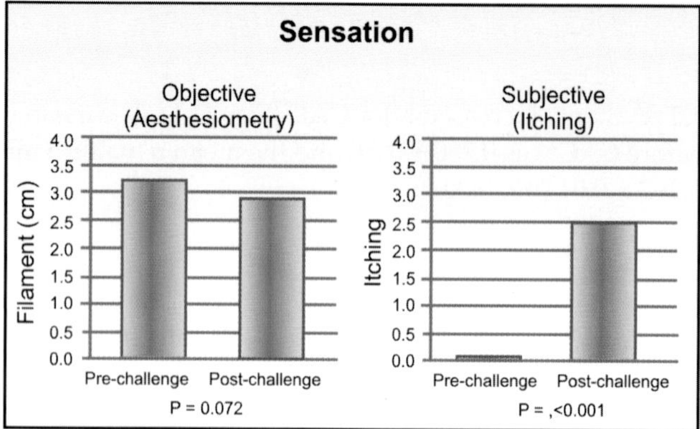

Fig. 24.3: Objective measurement of ocular surface sensation and subjective measurement of itching before and after conjunctival allergen challenge

Subjective Measurements

Erythema

Erythema increased significantly after CAC (Fig. 24.1). Mean erythema before CAC was 0, and 2.0 ± 0.39 after CAC ($p < 0.001$).

Edema

Chemosis increased after CAC (Fig. 24.2). Mean chemosis was 0 before CAC, and 2.0 ± 0.42 after CAC ($p<0.001$).

Itching

Itching increased after CAC (Fig. 24.3). Mean itching before CAC was 0, and 2.0 ± 1.2 after CAC ($p<0.001$).

Statistical Analysis

Following CAC, Spearman rank-correlation analysis showed a correlation between objective and subjective measurements of conjunctival erythema ($r_s = 0.838$), and between lower lid edema and chemosis ($r_s = 0.893$).

SUMMARY

The results of objective and subjective testing are summarized in Table 24.3.

Repeat Measurements after Instillation of Vasoconstrictor/Antihistamine Eyedrops

In eyes receiving naphazoline/pheniramine eyedrops, objective erythema diminished from a mean u′ value of 0.290 ± 0.02 to 0.278 ± 0.02 ($p < 0.001$)

Table 24.3: Comparison of objective and subjective measurements of ocular allergic reactions before and after conjunctival allergen challenge indicating significant (S), or not significant changes (NS), and correlation (C) between objective and subjective methods

Objective
Erythema, S, C
Eyelid edema, S, C
Sensation, NS
Subjective
Erythema, S, C
Chemosis, S, C
Itching, S

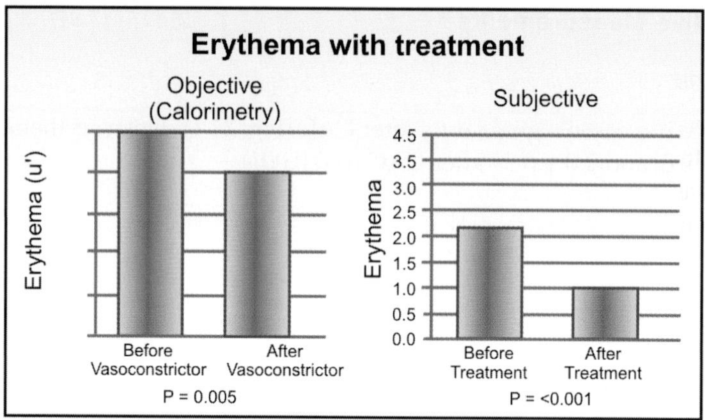

Fig. 24.4: Objective and subjective measurements of conjunctival erythema before and after treatment of ocular allergic reactions with one drop of a vasoconstrictor/antihistamine eyedrop

(Fig. 24.4). Objective evaluation of eyelid edema and ocular surface sensation did not change significantly. Subjective erythema decreased from 1.8 ± 0.02 to 0.08 ± 0.02 ($p < 0.001$), but itching, and chemosis, did not change significantly. There was a correlation between objective and subjective measurements of conjunctival erythema ($r_s = 0.822$).

In eyes receiving saline eyedrops, objective and subjective measurements of erythema, edema, itching, and ocular surface sensation did not change significantly.

DISCUSSION

Objective measurements have the advantage of being highly reproducible, and free of subjective influences.[16,17] If objective measurements can be made quickly and accurately, they should be useful in CAC. Objective measurements would not be expected to vary from one study to another, or from one examiner to another. Erythema and edema measurements should be graded consistently on any given day by any given examiner.

Attempts have been made in the past to objectively quantify ocular inflammation after CAC.[2,11,12] These attempts have been cumbersome, variable, and sometimes expensive. Mediator studies are usually difficult to perform, and require highly precise collection techniques.[11] These studies involve lengthy and costly techniques which must be performed in a laboratory setting.

Ideally, objective measurements of ocular inflammation should be rapid and easy to perform. They should be standardized and adaptable from one center to another. Spectroradiometry, fractional millimeter measurements, and aesthesiometry, the EES (erythema, edema, sensation) method seem to fulfill the criteria for desirable objective measurements of ocular inflammation.

Spectroradiometry measures the color coordinates that describe any color in the visible spectrum. Color can be measured in several ways. We have chosen the u′ coordinate of the 1976 Commission Internationale d'Eclairage. This measurement is easily obtainable, since it can be read directly from the display of the colorimeter, and it increases proportionally with increasing intensity of conjunctival erythema.

Eyelid edema can be easily measured with a fractional millimeter reticule in the eyepiece of a slit lamp microscope. Increased lid edema most likely reflects edema of the palpebral conjunctiva in response to mast cell degranulation following allergen challenge. We have chosen to measure the width of the lower eyelid centrally from the gray line posteriorly to the posterior most central eyelash. This direct measurement of lid thickness is straightforward and reproducible.

Aesthesiometry is a technique for measuring corneal sensation.[18-20] The aesthesiometer of Cochet and Bonnet is commercially available and easy to use. Our impression is that ocular surface sensation is slightly reduced after CAC, and the amount of reduction may be proportional to the intensity of inflammation. Although this study showed a mild reduction of ocular surface sensation following CAC, the reduction of ocular surface sensation from baseline levels was not statistically significant. We anticipate that further studies with larger numbers of subjects will help clarify the relationship of ocular surface sensation to the ocular allergic reaction.

These studies demonstrate that objective measurements of erythema, but not edema or ocular surface sensation, can be documented following treatment with a vasoconstrictor/antihistamine eyedrop. A similar reduction in conjunctival erythema was reported following the use of vasoconstrictor/antihistamine eye drops in normal subjects.[21] This is not surprising, since these eye drops are known to be highly effective in reducing conjunctival erythema. These drops are less effective in reversing edema and altering ocular surface sensation.

It remains unclear whether objective measurements are superior to subjective measurements for evaluating ocular allergic reactions. Subjective measurements showed greater differences in erythema, conjunctival edema, and itching from baseline evaluation to post challenge evaluations. On the other hand, the small standard deviation of objective measurements suggests a certain precision and repeatability of objective measurements.

We believe objective measurements of the ocular allergic reaction provide new ways in which allergic reactions can be quantified. We believe that further study and refinement of objective measurements of ocular allergic reactions will improve our ability to measure these reactions with less variability and greater objectivity.

REFERENCES

1. Blackley CH. Experimental researches on the cause and nature of catarrhous acativas. In: Hay Fever or Hay Asthma. London: Bailliere, Tindal, Cox, Ltd., 1873.
2. Friedlaender MH. Conjunctival provocation tests: A model of human ocular allergy. Trans Am Ophthalmol Soc 1989;87:577-97.
3. Allansmith MR, Baird RS, Greiner JV, Bloch KJ. Late-phase reactions in ocular anaphylaxis in the rat. J Allergy Clin Immunol 1984;76:49-55.
4. Leonardi A, Secchi AG, Briggs R, Allansmith MR. Conjunctival mast cells and the allergic late phase reaction. Ophthalmic Res 1992;24:234-42.
5. Leonardi A, Borghesan F, Faggian D, et al. Tear and serum soluble leukocyte activation markers in conjunctival allergic diseases. Am J Ophthalmol 2000;129:151-8.
6. Friedlaender MH, Harris J, LaVallee N, et al. Evaluation of the onset and duration of effect of azelastine eye drops (0.05%) versus placebo in patients with allergic conjunctivitis using an allergen challenge model. Ophthalmology 2000;107: 2152-7.
7. Abelson MB, Allansmith MR, Friedlaender MH. Effects of topically applied ocular decongestant and antihistamine. Am J Ophthalmol 1980;90:254-7.
8. Ciprandi G, Cerqueti P, Sacca S, et al. Levocabastine versus cromolyn sodium in the treatment of pollen-induced conjunctivitis. Ann Allergy 1990;65:156-8.
9. Emmi L, Rossi O. A new H1-blocking antihistamine. Critical review of pharmacological and clinical studies [Italian]. Minerva Medica 2002;79:219-27.
10. Kari O, Salo OP, Halmepuro L, Suvilehto K. Tear histamine during allergic conjunctivitis challenge. Graefes Arch Clin Exp Ophthalmol 1985;223:60-2.
11. Proud D, Sweet J, Stein P, et al. Inflammatory mediator release on conjunctival provocation of allergic subjects with allergen. J Allergy Clin Immunol 1990;85: 896-905.
12. Margrini L, Bonini S, Centofanti M, et al. Tear tryptase levels and allergic conjunctivitis. Allergy 1996;51:577-81.
13. Abelson M, Chambers WA, Smith LM. Conjunctival allergen challenge. A clinical approach to studying allergic conjunctivitis. Arch Ophthalmol 1990;108:84-8.
14. Bonini S, Magrini L, Rotiroti G, et al. The eosinophil and the eye. Allergy 1997;52:44-7.
15. Simpson T, Chan A, Fonn D. Measuring ocular redness: First and second order (luminance and chromaticity) measurements proved more informative than second order (spatial structure) measurements. Optom Vis Sci 1998;75 (Suppl):125.
16. Fieguth P, Simpson T. Automated measurement of bulbar redness. Invest Ophthalmol Vis Sci 2002;43:340-7.
17. Efron N, Morgan PB, Katsara SS. Validation of grading scales for contact lens complications. Ophthalmic Physiol Opt 2001;21:17-29.
18. Beuerman RW, McCulley JP. Comparative clinical assessment of corneal sensation with a new aesthesiometer. Am J Ophthalmol 1978;85:812-5.
19. Lawrenson JG, Corbett MC, O'Brart DPS, Marshall J. Effect of beam variables on corneal sensitivity after excimer laser photorefractive keratectomy. Br J Ophthalmol 1997; 81:686-90.
20. Barequet IS, Soriano ES, Green WR, O'Brien TP. Provision of anesthesia with single application of lidocaine 2% gel. J Cataract Refract Surg 1999;25:626-31.
21. Simpson TL, Sin T. The effect of topical vasoconstriction on bulbar redness measured objectively. ARVO Abstract, May 8, 2002.

Chapter 25

Steroid Therapy for Allergic Ocular Disease

John D Sheppard (USA)

New Concepts in Topical Steroid Therapy

Ophthalmic use of steroids has been a balancing act for many years. Therapeutically the clinician must balance the benefits of steroids against the risks. Nevertheless, by avoiding steroids in the past, patients may not have received the optimal treatment for certain diseases. As a result, patients with ocular surface and corneal diseases can develop unnecessary pain, surface damage, and internal ocular cicatrization. As a student of ophthalmology, the astute clinician follows the lessons and embraces the ideas of respected mentors. But as the science has grown and changed, therapeutic options change as well. Now with more experience utilizing newer steroid molecules and more aggressive approaches to ocular inflammatory diseases including allergy, ophthalmology and optometry see a clear picture of appropriate steroid use, acknowledging the low incidence of side effects and embracing the potent therapeutic effects.

Treatment wisdom dictates that it is far better to utilize a potent agent infrequently as opposed to prescribing a weaker agent frequently. The more potent agent can be used as infrequently as once per day, thus improving compliance, reducing costs to the patient, and also reducing exposure of the ocular surface to preservatives found in most topical ocular anti-inflammatory agents. Steroids certainly fulfill this billet.

The True Risk to Benefit Profile for Allergic and Ocular Surface Disease

Years ago, instructors told soon-to-be-ophthalmologists that steroids were not a first-choice treatment because they carried serious risks.

Considerations include cataracts, 'steroid dependence,' IOP response, delayed wound healing and opportunistic infections made us fear corticosteroids. This fear was rooted in the strong corticosteroid molecules such as prednisolone acetate, which had serious potential side effects, particularly with chronic use. These agents controlled inflammation, but they were stronger than they typically needed to be, unlike modulated designer corticosteroids we can use today. Previously clinicians either avoided steroids completely except for severe blinding diseases, or discontinued treatment before it was effective or reduced the concentration to an ineffective level. Only by treating hundreds of external disease patients does the corneal external disease specialist as well as the comprehensive ophthalmologist learn that a little tincture of steroid is one of the most effective ways to control many types of ocular surface disease, including chronic dry eye, allergy and blepharitis. These 3 conditions represent the bulk of external diseases, and a significant percentage of emergency presentations to the eye care practitioner.

Another lingering idea is so-called steroid dependence. 'Steroid dependence' is not really a dependence. Certainly, we haven't seen addiction or classic withdrawal reactions from steroids. There is clearly a rebound in inflammation, however, when steroids are withdrawn too rapidly or without any weaning or tapering process whatsoever. There are two likely reasons for this misconception. First, some patients need steroids to manage chronic diseases where the blood-aqueous barrier has broken down. And second, patients might appear to need more steroids because they have not received enough steroids. They seem to rebound or develop new problems, but it's really a return of an inadequately treated condition.

Some patients develop chronic irreversible breakdown of the blood aqueous barrier due to severe disease, inadequately treated disease, misdiagnosed inflammatory disease, or poor compliance. It can be virtually impossible to control uveitis or eliminate flare in these patients. Similarly, chronic ocular surface inflammation due to atopic conditions can produce irreversible vascular changes in the lids and conjunctiva that remain perpetually inflamed or red despite massive regular doses of seemingly appropriate topical anti-inflammatory medications.

Insufficient Steroid Treatment: Adversely Impacts/Outcomes

Early intervention with corticosteroids can help save a patient's vision, although clinicians don't always seize this opportunity. One of the biggest problems in corneal external disease referral practices is under-utilization of topical steroids by referring physicians. By sparing the steroids early, they may be creating far worse outcomes for patients down the road. The sequelae to inflammation may be irreversible damage to the ocular surface, or even the retina and the eye itself. In the case of allergy, ocular surface scarring can occur in a number of locations, including the bulbar and tarsal conjunctiva, the lacrimal ductules, the cornea, and even the lids and adnexae. We can prevent this irreversible damage, and corticosteroids are usually the answer. Nervously withholding steroids will hurt patients in many ways. Witholding topical steroids in severe ocular surface disease or allergy is not beneficial in either the short-term or long-term for patient care. This decision to prescribe steroids hinges on a clinician's basic understanding of their role in treating inflammatory disease. Although it is compassionate to give a corticosteroid to control inflammation and make patients feel better, the most important goal is to interrupt the inflammatory and subsequent cicatricial process. If we see a reversible process, we can intervene early with corticosteroids and control the inflammation enough to return the patient's anatomy to normal. Topical steroids work wonders when begun early.

The Nature of Allergic Disease

Molecular Biology Allows Better Understanding of Ocular Allergic Diseases

Recent decades have seen an explosion of knowledge about the nature of allergic ocular disease. No longer accepted as part of aging or a necessary evil for the unfortunate, the disease is recognized as inflammatory in nature — and controllable. Remarkably, the basic mechanism of inflammatory ocular surface tissue damage is highly similar in patients with a wide variety of disease processes, including dry eye, allergy and blepharitis. Thus, adequate therapy for one disease may assist in control of concomitant disease. Similarly, the correct treatment for the wrong diagnosis may still produce patient satisfaction.

Reversible Inflammation

The inflammatory, reversible nature of allergic ocular surface disease is widely accepted today. If a patient has herpes and significant stromal inflammation, we prescribe steroids to prevent irreversible scarring and avoid a corneal transplant. Ocular allergy is the same type disease, and early anti-inflammatory therapy can achieve the same beneficial result. The target tissue here is generally the tarsal and bulbar conjunctiva, where severe protracted cases can produce subconjunctival scarring, eyelid deformity, trichiasis and entropion, and progressive gradual obliteration of the lacrimal ductules leading to dry eye.

Experience also has taught that ocular allergy sometimes has a systemic trigger. There is no doubt that ocular allergy is a biphasic inflammatory disorder, with early phase histamine release and mast cell degranulation, followed by late phase reactants, vasodilation, leukocyte diapedesis, and long term vascular permeability alterations. These changes can eventually lead to scarring, particularly with the onset of eosinophil major basic protein release, a highly toxic degratory protein responsible for the rapid corneal tissue loss seen in vernal ulcers among other processes. Systemic allergy, such as an exacerbation of rhinitis, sinusitis, eczema or asthma can trigger ocular allergy flares. Similarly, Stern and colleagues showed that dry eye also a true inflammatory disease, and in many patients, inflammation gradually progresses and tear production decreases. But some patients have a history of an acute episode of a systemic, sometimes infectious, disease followed quickly by an acute episode of severe dry eye. This is a systemic autoimmune phenomenon.

Thus patients with inflammatory insult, from acute allergic conjunctivitis, to chronic vernal, to epidemic keratoconjunctivitis may develop cicatricial changes leading to lid disease or dry eye. These patients become contact lens intolerant and highly symptomatic around classic dry eye stimuli. The inflammatory stimulus triggers a mechanism that goes beyond the disease process and damages the entire ocular surface unit, from corneal nerves, to conjunctiva, to lids to lacrimal gland.

The cardinal aspect of ocular surface disease is that the underling etiology is many times driven by some sort of T-cell malfunction and therefore immunomodulation may be required. As cornea specialists, many clinicians have certainly realized that even a small dose of topical steroids does wonders for patients that have dry eye. As a rule, steroids reduce ocular surface inflammation and further normalize goblet cell numbers, for example, and reduce surface T-cell surface markers just as topical cyclosporine might. A number of companies are working on a lower dose, even lower yet than the concentrations that you might see in loteprednol as Lotemax 0.5% or Alrex 0.2% (Bausch and Lomb), Pred Forte (prednisolone acetate 1%), or FML (fluorometholone 0.1%, both Allergan), or a topical steroid that would reduce ocular surface inflammation as a primary treatment for the underlying etiology of the dry eye. Rimexolone (Alcon) in very low concentrations may be a useful agent for this strategy, and is currently in Phase III clinical trials.

Combined Surface Diseases: Present Diagnostic Challenges

Rapid Diagnosis of Dry Eye, Blepharitis and Allergy

Classic allergic disease is readily diagnosed, particularly when itching or systemic manifestations are obvious. Concomitant ocular disease is another story. A multifaceted phenomenon, dry eye disease can present as an amalgamation of different processes. Simultaneously, these conditions may include any combination of keratitis sicca, allergy, blepharitis, eyelid deformity, neurotrophic keratitis, nutritional deficiencies and previous eye surgery.

One of the most difficult aspects of managing dry eye is diagnosing it. First, patients don't always recognize their symptoms, describe them inaccurately or offer insufficient detail. Blepharitis or environmental changes can cloud the diagnosis as well. But once a clinician suspects dry eye disease, proper testing—in particular, supravital staining with flurorescein, lissamine and Rose Bengal — can clarify the diagnosis quickly. Once blepharitis is suspected, eversion of the superior tarsus similarly reveals the greatest amount of potentially diagnostic information.

Clarify Concomitant Ocular Surface Disease

Dry eye patient questionnaires include important questions like: Do your eyes feel dry? Itchy? Does it feel like you have something in your eye? When do your eyes bother you? What other medical conditions do you have? Thus it is possible to quantify not only the signs but also the symptoms of dry eye — redness, burning, itch, foreign body sensation. Although only some patients complain about these, others are stoic and don't mention them. It is very important to know what to look for and how to look. Patients often don't volunteer their history, especially if they've had a problem for years and see it as a normal part of getting older or common to everyone in their own age group. If we can train our staff to obtain a good history, we can diagnose patients early. Patients present with various combinations of dry eye signs and symptoms. Some patients feel bad and look good, and other patients look bad and feel good. Patients who look bad may have a neurotropic component so they just don't feel what they should, and neurotropic ocular surface disease can be extremely serious in its advanced stages.

It is important to caution against diagnosing allergy alone, advising further dry eye testing or tarsal eversion to rule out concomitant disease. Many corneal experts note that ocular allergies are over-diagnosed, and dry eye is very under-diagnosed, True itching is a symptom of allergic eye disease, along with burning, discomfort and other complaints, but the term 'itching' frequently sends us off on the wrong course. Patients often use 'itching' to describe foreign body sensation. Then we start looking for allergic eye disease and may prescribe anti-allergy medications to manage what's really dry eye. Conversely, patients treated with lubricants alone for dry eye will fare far better when treated for allergy utilizing a standard, aggressive anti-allergy regimen.

Tear Film and Schirmer's Testing

If symptoms indicate dry eye disease, the next step is to administer standard tests. Measure the volume of the tear meniscus, look for debris and possibly check tear film break-up time using fluorescein. The gold standard in ophthalmology has been Schirmer's testing with and without anesthesia. The Schirmer test is important in diagnosing Sjögren syndrome. A score of 0 — no wetting whatsoever — is a diagnosis of true Sjögren syndrome. Such a patient likely suffers from a systemic autoimmune disease and faces a risk of epithelial erosion or stromal melt, and should be observed and treated aggressively. Rose bengal or lissamine green will show significant abnormal tear film disruption that fluorescein won't show, and are especially useful for delineating the degree of conjunctival surface diseases. These supravital stains are essential to ocular surface disease evaluations. Thus, with highly depressed Schirmers tests or severe staining patterns, begin anti-inflammatory therapy that very day and send every such patient for a collagen vascular work-up to look for systemic disease. With fluorescein alone, we can detect dry eye only in its advanced stage. Rose Bengal or lissamine green will show significant abnormal tear film disruption that fluorescein won't show. By using either of these stains, we can detect conjunctival pathology in the interpalpebral area that we'd certainly miss with fluorescein. Lissamine green staining is a key factor in diagnosing dry eye. Thus with supravital staining, physicians can better recognize dry eye disease. Improved understanding of the disease, combined with better treatment regimens, put reversal of this inflammatory disease within easy reach. The astute clinician understands and addresses the interaction of dry eye, allergy, blepharitis, environmental factors, and systemic disease when treating ocular surface inflammation.

Sjogren's Syndrome Can Accompany Allergic Disease

Dry eye disease encompasses aqueous tear deficiency, mucin deficiency, lipid layer abnormalities and exposure due to eyelid abnormalities. In terms of aqueous tear deficiency, clinicians often differentiate between patients with Sjögren syndrome, which damages the lacrimal glands, and non-Sjögren patients.

This differentiation is intellectually important, however, the treatment for the two types of patients is the same today. Sjögren patients have more severe dry eye and are at risk for stromal inflammation and necrosis. In the past, we classified Sjögren patients as actively inflamed, in contradistinction to age related acquired tear deficiency. Now, with awareness that all dry eye patients have inflammation in the conjunctiva and the lacrimal gland, our concept of the disease spectrum has changed our approach. Instead of using anti-inflammatories to treat only Sjögren syndrome, we use them to treat all aqueous deficient patients: it's just a matter of degree. The histopathology is identical for Sjögren and non-Sjögren dry eye. The FDA clinical studies of cyclosporine ophthalmic emulsion 0.05% (Restasis) showed the conjunctival biopsy proven histopathogenesis of ocular surface disease was the same among Sjögren and non-Sjögren patients, but the former had systemic problems that warranted action.

Sjögren-related uveitis, scleritis, keratitis or vasculitis may be the first presentation of extrasynovial inflammatory disease. Early intervention is essential, before systemic problems develop, and referral to primary physicians or a rheumatologist may interrupt an otherwise devastating systemic illness.

Innovative Strategies for Ocular Surface Diseases

Dry Eye and Ocular Allergy have Overlapping Therapeutic Profiles

Clinicians have finally started to think that other eye diseases might contribute to allergy. For instance, posterior blepharitis is one major disease category that clearly occurs concomitantly with dry eye and allergy.

As a result, clinicians would apply blepharitis treatments like topical steroids, oral doxycycline and warm compresses to dry eye, and the dry eye would improve as the lid disease improved. Similarly, allergy affects the entire conjunctival surface. With a chronically inflamed tarsus, the patient bathes the corneal epithelium with inflammatory cells and cytokines. Thus, allergy patients may have seasonal or environmental exacerbations of dry eye symptoms and vice versa.

Now that we understand that inflammation is the key component of dry eye as well as allergy, we've entered a new era of formulating concomitant therapy for the condition. The intention is to simplify the regimen while reducing toxicity from topical medications. Substituting an aqueous replacement simply washes the problem away temporarily. What's really needed is better endogenous tear production, both in quality and quantity.

At the first encounter with a moderate to severe dry eye patient, an anti-inflammatory agent prescription is clearly indicated instead of punctal occlusion. The prescription form of cyclosporine ophthalmic 0.05% emulsion (Restasis) in low concentration, with high bioavailability and a specially formulated micelle lipid base, gives us an agent that replaces the aqueous component and lipid component of tears. By replacing the essential oil and mucin tear layers while providing an ideal delivery strategy for the cyclosporine the 0.05% topical cyclosporine emulsion is biochemically designed and formulated to control ocular surface inflammation. Restasis compared to much higher but less bioavailable concentrations of cyclosporine that were used in the past clearly has less better tissue penetration with lower toxicity. Restasis has been effectively utilized for patients with concomitant allergy and dry eye, as well as vernal and atopic disease.

Newer agents are under investigation to eliminate safely the tear film deficiency and surface inflammation of dry eye disease. These include FK-506 or tacrolimus (Sucampo), pimecrolimus (Novartis), Ecabet sodium (Ista), and the P2Y2 agonist diquafasol tetrasodium (Prolacria, Inspire), a secretagogue. Pimecrolimus (Elidel cream dermatologic) and Tacrolimus (Protopic ointment dermatologic) have been tainted by recent reports of a potential link with cancer. Topical ocular investigations of tacrolimus have as a result been terminated.

Clinicians have also begun to link dry eye with systemic medications, such as antihistamines, antidepressants, diuretics and such HMG Co-A reductase inhibitors as Mevacor, Zocor and Lipitor. But no one until recently realized the importance of inflammation to the condition. Thus a strong common link to allergic ocular surface disease.

In the past, a diagnosis of dry eye prompted a therapy regimen that usually included: treatment of aggravating factors, such as blepharitis; tear supplementation; lid hygiene; and finally, punctal occlusion. Many patients were not well served. Tear substitutes are still address aggravating factors, but inflammation control is still central to improvement.

Punctal Occlusion: Past and Present

Prior to modern punctual plug technology, dry eye patients received punctual occlusion through cautery or pre-cut cat-gut or collagen dissolving temporary plugs. Prior to the advent our understanding of inflammation as the underlying etiology of dry eye, punctual occlusion was a primary therapeutic intervention. This approach has changed drastically as both the literature and clinical experience revealed problems with early punctal occlusion. Now the paradigm has really changed because we know plugs can trap 'bad tears.' Pflugfelder and colleagues have shown that punctal occlusion can worsen a Schirmer's test score, and premature occlusion can harm the biofeedback loop to the ocular surface enervation. In the old paradigm, we gave dry eye patients some artificial tears and occluded their puncta. The eyes looked moist, but they were still red and painful. The patient had more tears and maybe even a better Schirmer's test, but often was not content. Using a bathtub analogy to describe the situation, one would obviously drain the dirty water and refill it before the next bath. The same applies to punctal plugs: in an eye with inflammatory mediators like cytokines, interleukin and neutrophils, punctual plugs trap these inflammatory cells on the ocular surface. With the new anti-inflammatory approach, treatment improves not only the quantity of tears, but also the quality of the tear film on the ocular surface.

In this approach, physicians start by improving the quality of the tear film, eliminating the cytokines, down-regulating the T-cell activation on the ocular surface and improving goblet cell production and the mucin layer of the tear film by reducing ocular surface inflammation. If anti-inflammatory therapy doesn't work or it doesn't work completely — and that often happens in moderate and severe cases — then follow with punctal occlusion 4 to 6 weeks after starting anti-inflammatory therapy. The occlusion therapy can be trialed with properly sized collagen plugs, then after a month of no epiphora, a silicone plug inserted.

By prescribing an anti-inflammatory first, physicians have greater success with punctal occlusion. The anti-inflammatory makes a big difference because we mitigate pro-inflammatory mediators of the pain seen in allergy and dry eye. If a new patient already has punctal plugs, anti-inflammatory therapy is still recommended, although not the preferred order.

Therapy for Every Allergy Level

The first line of treatment for ocular allergy depends on the degree of disease severity. Many patients already are using some type of over-the-counter artificial tears or vasoconstrictor. If a patient presents with mild allergy, it is best to continue with a tear replacement, with preference to preservative-free or vanishing preservative preparations, such as Refresh (Allergan), Systane (Alcon) or GenTeal (Novartis). These generally produce a less toxic effect on the ocular surface.

Physicians also must consider patients' other medications or practices that may exacerbate pre-existing allergic and dry eye disease and interfere with therapy. Many of these patients need better contact lens-wearing regimens, or they should stop wearing their contact lenses, particularly if there is concomitant dry eye and allergy. Patients with superior tarsal disease are also prone to more severe contact lens intolerance. Some can also taken off oral diuretics because they were taking them unnecessarily for underlying hypertension or resolved fluid retention. It is incumbent upon clinicians to help patients identify and control environmental situations that aggravate their dry eye and allergic disease. Patients might stay up late at night and not use their artificial tears, or sleep upon dust mite infested or down pillows. They might have terrible humidity control in the winter, or an adverse work environment laden.

Nutrition is also an important topic for discussion. Some patients have a soda-and-potato-chips diet, which robs their mucous membranes of essential dietary components, including essential fatty acids like gamma linoleic acid (GLA) and omega-3 fatty acids, which are very good for dry eye as well as allergy. Similarly, poor diets are laden with pro-inflammatory omega-6 fatty acids, saturated fats, and trans fats, all of which up-regulate inflammatory pathways that worsen allergic disease.

Basic education about dry eye disease, allergic environmental factors, and proper contact lens care are an essential element of early therapy. Patients often arrive in our offices dissatisfied because they haven't had anti-inflammatory treatment, and they demand a cure. Allergy, dry eye and blepharitis are not curable. This is a lifelong process, and the disease can progress with age or repeated insult.

Treating Moderate to Severe Disease

Moderate to severe allergic disease is easy to detect. Severe itching, redness, papillary tarsal conjunctivitis, discharge, limbal hyperemia, and even chronic follicles betray the underlying allergic etiology. On the other hand, patients with moderate to severe dry eye can be challenging to detect. Regardless, early diagnosis is essential for their ocular health.

We need to examine high-risk dry eye patients carefully. This group includes people who take medications that dry their eyes, have collagen vascular disease, are postmenopausal, abuse contact lenses or work in a very dry environment. They may have severe, rapid disease progression without even feeling the symptoms.

Once diagnosed with moderate to severe dry eye, anti-inflammatory therapy should be started immediately. When patients are using transiently preserved tears but are still breaking through on this therapy and showing dry eye signs and symptoms, they always need anti-inflammatory therapy. Signs may be minimal with subtle fluorescein, lissamine green or Rose Bengal staining, and minimal depression of the tear meniscus. Many of the most severely affected patients receive two medications, cyclosporine ophthalmic emulsion 0.05% (Restasis) b.i.d. and loteprednol etabonate ophthalmic suspension (Lotemax or Alrex) b.i.d. The loteprednol induces an initial rapid response with increased comfort; and the cyclosporine provides preservative-free immunomodulation in the long-term. Patients can use the loteprednol during the day and the cyclosporine before and after sleeping. Those who have stinging trouble with cyclosporine may go on q.i.d. loteprednol. Those who do not tolerate loteprednol can use chilled cyclosporine t.i.d. to start.

Dosages can be titrated to individual needs. For example, increase the dosage and frequency of loteprednol with the severity of dry eye disease — low for mild to moderate patients, higher for severe patients and highest for patients with concomitant ocular surface disease. One might prefer the lower concentration of loteprednol found in Alrex for mild cases.

Combining agents produces many favorable results. Not only do patients have a better experience with this approach, but they also have better outcomes with this combination. The loteprednol and the cyclosporine both have anti-inflammatory effects, but they use different mechanisms of action on different stages of the inflammatory process. Together, the dual-action mechanism and the synergy between the two drops deliver better outcomes faster. It is desirable to bring the ocular surface to homeostasis at about 4 to 6 months, and then see patients less frequently — enough to pick up any changes.

Tapering and Titration

In severe or chronic cases, better judgment warns against tapering steroids early, even when patients feel better. Instead, strive to eliminate every last cell in a uveitic patient, every last papillae in an allergic patient, and every last punctuate corneal stain in a dry eye patient. If absolute control is not established, then as dosage of steroids is decreased, the patient will show a rejuvenated response and have an increased risk of developing terrible consequences, such as chronic inflammation, cicatrization, chronic cystoid macular edema with cystic edema, and even epiretinal membrane formation in severe atopic patients or complex post-operative cases. Patients with advanced uveitic disease, for example, may develop hypotony as the ciliary body shuts down. Similarly, we don't want to allow permanent structural changes in the lacrimal gland, limbal stem cells or conjunctival mucosa. Allergic patients can exhibit prolonged post-cataract cystoid macular edema, presumably because the choroid, and not the conjunctiva, contains the highest concentration of mast cells in the body.

Regardless of the etiology of ocular surface inflammation, begin tapering anti-inflammatory medications for patients who are feeling well at about the 6-month mark. However, they still need to use the medications to treat any acute episodes that arise. Patients will have episodes of discomfort, so they must use loteprednol 0.5% one to four times a day on those days. There is no standard for tapering loteprednol in dry eye patients because the disease is so individual. It is necessary to titrate the medication to the disease. Patients with concomitant ocular surface disease — perhaps blepharitis or severe peri-ocular cutaneous allergy, vernal or tarsal conjunctival changes or concomitant rosacea — receive a higher initial dose and maintenance dose of loteprednol or other steroid. Exacerbations may be more frequent and require pulse-dosing at a higher frequency and intensity. With loteprednol it is possible to titrate to the patient, the disease and the response. In the long run, it enables minimization of the cumulative dose. Loteprednol's markedly reduced risk of glaucoma and cataract enables this facility.

Perspective on Risks

Because ketone steroids, loteprednol and cyclosporine work so differently and cyclosporine performs well as a constant b.i.d. medication, it is not usually necessary to taper cyclosporine in patients on both drugs. In the Ilyas study, patients on loteprednol 0.2% for years had insignificant risks for glaucoma. Part of the individualized approach to tapering anti-inflammatory medications is thus to lower the dosage. The 0.2% (Alrex) dose is lower, and the safety profile is even better than that of loteprednol 0.5% (Lotemax).

Far from ignoring the possibility of steroid-related risks, clinicians should choose to put them in perspective. Although steroids are less risky with close observation and newer formulations, we still have to remember the risks and the benefits. We can fix cataracts, but we can't fix permanent cicatrization of the ocular surface, obliteration of the lacrimal ductules or changes in corneal clarity. Corneal ectasia and opacification are irreversible changes, often necessitating a $25,000 corneal transplant. Many severe corneal problems, including severe scarring from vernal corneal ulceration, can be eliminated or controlled rapidly with topical steroids.

Environmental Control

In addition to sophisticated topical anti-inflammatory medications, environmental control is key to the control of ocular surface diseases. For the allergy patient, even on aggressive topical therapy, simple removal of antigens through intelligent management of the sleep and work space can provide tremendous relief and thereby a reduction in required medications. For the dry eye patient, removal of convection currents from fans and open window or convertible automobiles can make a huge difference. For both diseases, hand washing and avoidance of eye rubbing behavior is important to reduce mast cell degranulation and itching, and to avoid secondary bacterial infections and lash deformities associated with excessive lid manipulation.

One of the worst challenges is air travel where the relative humidity is below 20%. Thus, always forewarning patients prior to airline travel is judicious. Occasionally patients with known pre-existing dry eye return from dry climates with corneal ulcers because of the unfamiliar low humidity in that environment. Such an environmental change warrants patient education and increased lubrication. Many seaside locations on the other hand are blessed with year-round natural humidification.

Blepharitis Exacerbates Dry Eyes and Allergy

Cornea specialists see a great deal of blepharitis or chronic meibomian gland dysfunction. These patients experience significant discomfort and often take time to receive a diagnosis. As with dry eye disease, clinical findings for blepharitis point to inflammation as the basis of pain and discomfort. Fortunately, with accurate diagnosis and proper treatment, these patients can get much-needed relief.

Blepharitis Diagnosis

Blepharitis, also called meibomianitis or meibomitis for posterior lamellar lid disease, is caused by inspisation of the meibomian glands. Normal lipid secretions do not melt at body temperature, so they become saturated fats effectively cloggin the meibomian gland orifices. Bacteria grow in these lipids and secrete degratory enzymes such as lipases and collagenases, sequentially leading to lid ocular surface inflammation. Ocular surface stability breaks down because the lipids degrade into soaps and fatty acids. The tear film becomes inflammatory, which is a good reason not to put plugs in these eyes as a first line treatment. Plugs actually trap unhealthy tears on the ocular surface, exacerbating symptoms. This situation is often unrecognized clinically.

Tear film break-up time in these patients is generally shortened. The tear film has lost its lipid layer over the surface, so the diagnosis is readily apparent. When bubbly tiny soap suds appear in the meniscus and along the lower lid margin, normal lipid is breaking down into soaps and fatty acids: classic meibomian gland dysfunction.

Schirmer's test results may be normal or even high for these patients because this blepharitis causes an evaporative dry eye. Blepharitis can have serious long-term effects, so fast diagnosis and effective treatment are important. Chronic inflammation can cause corneal scarring, so these patients are at high risk for eventual costly corneal transplantation. Whenever corneal neovascularization (KNV) and corneal scarring are findings, aggressive therapy is indicated. Patients with blepharitis also may have no corneal symptoms, but their conjunctiva may be minimally injected. One characteristic of all blepharitis patients is discomfort, whether it's pain, burning, ache, or photophobia.

Patients with blepharitis frequently have rosacea, regardless of their race, so secondary infections are common. Treatment with both systemic and topical medications, as well as lid scrubs and dietary changes is indicated.

Topical Ointments: Bacitracin and Erythromycin

Meibomian gland dysfunction often results in secondary infections. The most likely culprit is *Staphylococcus*, so a rotation between erythromycin and bacitracin provides good gram-positive coverage. After a short-term trial with bacitracin ointment for a month or two, a switch to erythromycin helps because prolonged use of a single antibiotic will create resistance. Many staphylococcal organisms are already resistant, particularly to erythromycin, but much higher levels can be obtained with surface application than with systemic drugs, the standard upon which MIC data are based. Thus the surface concentration afforded by drops and ointments may sufficiently surpass standard MIC levels utilized in all microbiology laboratories.

Systemic Therapy

Blepharitis is a chronic disease, so patients require continuous treatment. The centerpiece is anti-inflammatory therapy. Blepharitis patients are at risk for KNV, which can progress to opacification, so aggressive first-line therapy wtih oral doxycycline, hot compresses and dietary supplements containing flaxseed and fish oils is recommended. Among the tetracyclines, doxycycline has a greater anti-inflammatory, anti-collagenolytic effect than tetracycline or minocycline. For patients with gastrointestinal intolerance, minocycline may be preferred.

With blepharitis, it is important to start the patient on a preservative free topical solution, and then when they're comfortable, one can have the luxury of switching to a transiently preserved artificial tear solution. Topical steroids are also very helpful in the initial and long-term strategic picture. Above all, however, the oral agents have proven efficacious, particularly for posterior lamellar disease. Patients can start with doxycycline, 50 mg four times a day, or 100 mg bid, always with food. High-dose tetracycline is less effective and far less well tolerated: only 50% of patients can continue high doses because of gastrointestinal side effects and photosensitivity. A lower 20 mg doxycycline preparation (Periostat) given bid is also acceptable anti-inflammatory, anti-lipid drug therapy.

Many patients, especially those with rosacea, may need to take doxycycline for a prolonged period. There is generally little difficulty in prescribing male patients with nearly continuous doxycycline therapy when indicated, giving perhaps a 1 month hiatus every summer when the sun is highest. Some have been successfully treated with low dose doxycycline for decades. After 2 to 4 months of treatment, patients can initially stop the medication if they get better. If symptoms come right back, they must necessarily resume therapy. A significant number of patients take doxycycline for 3 or 4 months, stop it for a few months, and then go back. Some patients can learn to titrate their own medication.

Tetracyclines have been in use for a long time for meibomitis, a very comfortable method of treatment. However, a February 2004 issue of The Journal of the American Medical Association looked at antibiotic risk and antibiotic use in relation to the risk of breast cancer. The investigators found that with the tetracyclines, those women who cumulatively were on tetracycline for longer than seven weeks doubled their risk of getting breast cancer and doubled their risk of dying from breast cancer. The effect was related specifically to cumulative dose. Currently there is a one in eight risk that a women will get breast cancer anyway: therefore with chronic tetracyclines we are potentially doubling that risk to one in four. This is a major clinical, psychological and medicolegal concern.

As a result of that keynote publication, therapeutic recommendations have to be altered for women who might require chronic oral doxycycline therapy. For patients with mild to moderate meibomitis or posterior blepharitis on omega-3 supplementation alone, oral antibiotic therapy is not necessary. Those severe blepharitis sufferers with severe disease can be kept on low-dose doxycycline, 20 mg or 50 mg a day, along with omega-3 supplementation, with informed consent regarding the breast cancer risk of course. In more severe patients, simply stop the doxycycline at four weeks and then maintain on omega-3 supplementation alone. Unfortunately, no alternative regimen exists for these severely affected female patients. On the horizon is a topical doxycycline preparation (Alacrity) which may revolutionize the treatment of ocular rosacea, but will not benefit patients with facial cutaneous disease.

Loteprednol, Metranidozol, Topical Doxycycline, and Cyclosporine

For particularly challenging patients with significant conjunctival injection and corneal findings, long-term topical anti-inflammatory therapy becomes mandatory. Newer agents such as loteprednol 0.5% (Lotemax) are indicated. Loteprednol has a well documented dual safety and efficacy profile resulting from its retro-metabolic engineered ester biochemistry. This allows for break down of all free steroid molecules into bio-inactive compounds if not initially bound to the glucocorticoid receptor. Other topical ketone steroids such as prednisolone acetate, dexamethasone or rimexolone can be prescribed, but with closer attention to the potential for secondary steroid induced glaucoma. Many of these patients are truly members of the "steroid for life club," which includes severe blepharitis, severe chronic dry eye, ocular cicatricial pemphigoid, post chemical burn, Stevens-Johnson, severe Vernal, atopic keratoconjunctivitis, corneal allograft patients, and uveitis sufferers.

Patients respond quickly to topical steroids like loteprednol 0.5%. Some patients have chronic pain without corneal pathology. They utilize lid hygiene with preferred products such as Ocusoft (Cynacon) or Eye Scrub (Novartis) and take doxycycline, yet the eye remains uncomfortable. For these topical steroids provide rapid relief. A starting dose of four times a day with subsequent taper, either to intermittent use or twice a day long-term to control inflammation and discomfort.

Several other topical and systemic compounds have useful secondary anti-inflammatory effects. These include metronidazole, which is available in oral or topical form from a compounding pharmacy. Some patients with rosacea find it helpful to use the ointment on their eyelids. Many with concomitant oculo-facial disease respond to topical therapy to the skin on the nose, cheeks, or chin. This is accomplished with metronidazole 1% gel (Galderma) or metronidazole 0.75% lotion or cream.

Steroids also can work well in combination with cyclosporine ophthalmic emulsion 0.05% (Restasis). Cyclosporine is helpful for chronic blepharitis. Steroids control the inflammation better than cyclosporine, but there is a synergy between the two. The cyclosporine in effect becomes a steroid sparing agent, similar in philosophy to the use of multiple chemotherapeutic agents to arrest cancer. Together, steroids and cyclosporine alter the deleterious milieu of an inflamed ocular surface by improving tear quality and quantity, increasing goblet cell density, and producing more and better mucin. In addition, steroids combined with cyclosporine also treat lid disease, reducing inflammation and creating a better lipid layer on the tear film surface. Thus, combination anti-inflammatory therapy treats and improves every component of the tear film. The 0.05% cyclosporine preparation from Allergan is also preservative free, further enhancing the integrity of the inflamed ocular surface on chronic therapy.

Off-label studies of cyclosporine reveal that it works well for allergic eye diseases, such as vernal keratoconjunctivitis and giant papillary conjunctivitis. Milder forms of allergic eye disease, such as seasonal allergic conjunctivitis, also may benefit. But these milder forms tend to be more transient and not necessarily matched to cyclosporine as a first-line therapy. On the other hand, if a patient has allergy and dry eye, concomitant chronic use of cyclosporine significantly attenuates the seasonal exacerbation of eye disease.

It is also necessary to work with patients' internists, allergists, oncologists, hematologists or rheumatologists to prescribe the simplest, most cost-effective repertoire of medications. By juggling the patients' systemic medications, we can significantly improve, simplify and reduce the cost of therapy.

Nutrition for Blepharitis and Ocular Allergy

Dietary changes may help resolve meibomian gland dysfunction and reduce the time patients need to use doxycycline. Nutritional supplementation with omega-3 fatty acids clearly has a salutary effect for all forms of ocular surface disease. A therapeutic dose of supplements includes iso-pentanoic acid, eicosapentaenoic acid, cod liver oil, other fish oils, flaxseed oil, and black currant seed oil, an excellent source of gamma linoleic acid (GLA). These oral supplemental agents taken commensurate with doxycycline and minocycline help limit the time patients need to take the prescription component of their regimen, thus reducing side effects. This multi-faceted approach focuses on the root problem of inflammation and the effects of meibomian gland dysfunction, ocular surface cytokine and T cell activiation, and mast cell degranulation.

The currently available commercial sources of omega fatty acids now available to ophthalmologists in the United States are flaxseed oil, which is predominantly omega-3, Hydroeye (ScienceBased Health, Corte Madera, Calif.), which is a mixture of omega-3 and omega-6, and BioTears (Biosyntryx, Lexington, S.C.), which is very similar. There are a few additives to these formulations, but they are basically a combination of omega-6 and omega-3. The Science Based Health formulation is continuously updated to most accurately reflect current nutritional research, and contains only fresh natural ingredients. TheraTears Nutrition (Advanced Vision Research, Woburn, Mass.), is more predominantly omega-3s. Tears Again Hydrate (Cynacon) contains primarily flaxseed oil with evening primrose oil as a source of GLA.

These are five choices among others, or one may recommend a simple trip to the health food store for the flaxseed oil, Omega-3, or black currant seed oil alone or in combination. Hydroeye and BioTears are a combination of black currant seed oil and cod liver oil, so there is a plant source of omega fatty acid and a fish source of omega fatty acid, again combining omega-6 and omega-3. Although a combination of omega-3 and beneficial omega-6s is preferred, it is better to have the patient use the flaxseed oil instead of nothing. The omega-3 in flaxseed oil is generally less bioavailable than that of fish oil, but some patients also have a seafood allergy precluding the most common supplemental source of omega-3.

Steroids for Contact Lens Wearers and Refractive Surgery Patients

Awareness of Ocular Surface Disease

Another point to be aware of is the constellation of ocular surface disease that creates discontent with contact lenses in the younger LASIK population, including allergy and blepharitis. There are many perturbations of overlapping presentations, including the itch that you see in dry eye that may be partially allergy, and the tear film break-up time acceleration you might see with concomitant blepharitis. This all comes into play with a therapeutic approach. There is overlap in the dry eye success story of the therapy of omega-3s with blepharitis, and certainly Restasis (Allergan, Irvine, Calif.) and topical steroids are effective against allergy as well.

Steroids can be effectively utilized for both difficult contact lens patients and those with upcoming refractive surgery. The same therapeutic tenets apply: close observation, titration of dosage to the individual patient's needs, and maximum utilization of all therapeutic options available.

In a landmark Wisconsin retrospective study of 360 myopic lasik patients by Boorstein in 2003, pre-emptive treatment with an oral antihistamine in an allergic patient population reduced the risk of developing DLK. Atopy is therefore a patient-specific risk factor for the development of DLK after primary bilateral LASIK for either myopia or myopic astigmatism. Atopic individuals benefited from preoperative treatment to minimize the incidence of DLK and the potential for visual loss. The lessons of the study can be furthered by evaluation of topical rather than drying systemic anti-histamines to reduce potential DLK in allergic patients, as well as prophylactic topical steroids prior to Lasik in allergic individuals. Thus, with the entire ocular surface milieu in mind, preventive therapy is essential. Surgeons must consider not just the etiology of dry eye or the tarsal surface changes seen in chronic allergy, since these conditions are clearly interrelated, but also medication use, both topically and systemically.

Challenging Refractive Patients and Informed Consent

In clinical practice, every surgeon sees problem patients — the ones whose dry eye and allergy are unidentified, ignored, or become dry following refractive surgery. Many troubled patients travel from doctor to doctor, disgruntled with their primary surgeon, and they're the last patient you want to see on a busy day because they complain, they have other psychosomatic problems, they're extremely disgruntled with the other doctor whose lawyer you're trying to bypass altogether if humanly possible, and they eat up a lot of chair time with really minimal problems, and minimal findings, and maximal symptoms. Thus, we know that dry eye and allergy, which predispose to poor outcomes and unpredictable refractive surgery results, are so important to the informed consent process. These shattered hopes are often a result of falsely high expectations for elective surgery.

The most highly effective way to minimize the deleterious effects that allergy and dry eye can have on LASIK outcomes is to take proactive preventive steps. Placing patients into a routine that manages allergy or any existing irritation due to dry eye is invaluable.

With a dry eye prior to LASIK, the primary goal leading up to surgery is to achieve a healthy ocular surface. More frequent artificial tears will help and can be continued postoperatively. Familiarizing patients with this rigorous schedule as early as possible before surgery is helpful not only in preparing the ocular surface for LASIK, but in developing the discipline to use the drops with enough frequency to avoid complications.

The best approach for ocular allergic LASIK candidates is the same as that for all ocular allergic patients: topical therapy. New generation anti-allergic agents prevent the release of histamine, cytokines and other pro-inflammatory and proliferative mediators such as those involved in corneal trauma and healing, including IL-8, ICAM-1. Generally these patients are better treated with topical anti-allergic agents such as mast-cell stabilizer/antihistaminic solutions that won't compromise, and may even enhance, corneal wound healing. For example, agents such as olopatadine have been shown to decrease the release of tryptase from mast cells in vitro. In human clinical study, these agents stabilize the conjunctival mast cells.

Parallel to the routine of artificial tears for dry eye, a regular regimen of anti-allergy eyedrops before LASIK can get patients out of the habit of rubbing their eyes, decreasing the risk of their continuing to do so after LASIK and dislocating their flaps.

Careful diagnosis of allergy and dry eye is naturally an important step in optimizing the success of LASIK. A specific medication history concerning the use of oral antihistamines, over-the-counter ocular allergy drops, nasal sprays, diuretics, anti-depressants and other drying agents or anti-pruritic agents is essential for identifying allergy. Also, the anatomic location and severity of allergic symptoms should be identified, including sinusitis, rhinitis, pharyngitis, dermatitis, eczema, asthma, food intolerance, and of course conjunctivitis.

Accurate assessment of tear-film status may also be predictive of postop dry eye symptoms. Since allergy and dry eye can sometimes be confused with one another, tear film quantification would allow for a precise differential diagnosis in ambiguous cases. You can optimize ocular surface health by discontinuing oral antihistamines in the pre-operative period and begin supplementing a typical LASIK medication regimen with potent topical anti-allergy therapy or preservative free artificial tears.

Recognition of allergy and dry eye as risk factors for LASIK complications is something that takes little time or effort, but may have profound effects upon the surgical outcome. Recognition allows for the identification of a patient category that may benefit from pre-operative prophylactic therapy and closer postoperative observation. It is always better to treat the eye than to not treat it and run the risk of complications.

Certainly, the astute clinician can offer an allergic or dry eye patient PRK where the risk is lower, and now there is a conglomerate of other alternative procedures, including clear lens extraction, phakic IOLs, the Crystalens (Eyeonics, Aliso Viejo, Calif.), and the recently approved ReSTOR lens (Alcon) and ReZoom lens (AMO). So the informed consent process becomes even more complex when presented with an ocular surface disease patient, when they really need to know about these alternative therapies. LASIK patients complain bitterly when they have not effectively anticipated going from being healthy to past the reserve and into a dry eye. Likely their biggest complaint is fluctuating, or decreased vision, often ahead of symptoms of irritation. Visual disturbance postoperative LASIK secondary to manifestations of dry eyes and severe ocular allergies are common yet avoidable. Nevertheless, all potential refractive patients should be made aware of the potential for interference by ocular surface diseases and the need for continued vigilance, particularly during the peri-operative period.

BIBLIOGRAPHY

1. Armaly MF. Statistical attributes of the steroid hypertensive response in the clinically normal eye. I. The demonstration of three levels of response. Invest Ophthalmol 1965;4:187-97.
2. Asano-Kato N, Toda I, Hori-Komai Y, Tsubota K. Allergic conjunctivitis as a risk factor for laser in situ keratomileusis. J Cataract Refract Surg 2001;27:1469-72.
3. Bartlett JD, Woollery TW, Adams, CM. Identification of high intraocular pressure responders to topical ophthalmic corticosteroids. J Ocul Pharmacol 1993;9:35-45.
4. Bartlett JD, Horwitz B, Leibovitz R, et al. Intraocular pressure response to loteprednol etabonate in known steroid responders. J Ocul Pharmacol 1993;9:157-65.
5. Biswas J, Ganeshbabu TM, Raghavendran SR, et al. Efficacy and safety of 1% rimexolone versus 1% prednisolone acetate in the treatment of anterior uveitis – a randomized triple masked study. Int Ophthalmol 2004;25:147-53.
6. Boorstein SM, Henk HJ, Elner VM. Atopy: a patient specific risk factor for diffuse lamellar keratitis. Ophthalmology 2003;110:131-7.
7. Brown NA, Bron A, Hardin JJ, Dewar HM. Nutrition supplements and the eye. Eye. 1998;12(Pt. 1):127-133. Review.
8. Ilyas H, Slonim CB, Braswell GR, et al. Long-term safety of loteprednol etabonate 0.2% in the treatment of seasonal and perennial allergic conjunctivitis. Eye Contact Lens 2004;30:10-3.
9. Leibowitz HW, Bartlett JD, Rich D, et al. Intraocular pressure-raising potential of 1.0% rimexolone in patients responding to corticosteroids. Arch Ophthalmol 1996;114:933-7.
10. Leibowitz HM, Kupferman A. Antiinflammatory Medications. In Clinical Pharmacology of the Anterior Segment. Holly FJ, ed. Int Ophthalmol Clinics 1980;20(3):117-34.
11. The loteprednol etabonate US uveitis study group. Controlled evaluation of loteprednol and prednisolone acetate in the treatment of uveitis. Am J Ophthalmol 1999;127:537-44.
12. McCluskey P, Powell RJ. The eye in systemic inflammatory diseases. Lancet. 2004;364:2125-33.
13. Pflugfelder SC, Solomon A, Dursun D, Li DQ. Dry eye and delayed tear clearance: A call to arms. Adv Exp Med Biol 2002;506(Pt B):739-43. Review.

14. Pflugfelder SC. Antiinflammatory therapy for dry eye. Am J Ophthalmol 2004;137:337-42.
15. Pflugfelder SC, Maskin SL, Anderson B, et al. A randomized, double-masked, placebo-controlled, multicenter comparison of loteprednol etabonate ophthalmic suspension, 0.5%, and placebo for treatment of keratoconjunctivitis sicca in patients with delayed tear clearance. Am J Ophthalmol 2004;138:444-57.
16. Ramamurthy NS, Rifkin BR, Greenwald RA, et al. Inhibition of matrix metalloproteinase-mediated periodontal bone loss in rats: A comparison of 6 chemically modified tetracyclines. J Periodontol 2002;73:726-34.
17. Restasis package insert.
18. Sheppard J, Alison N, Martin D, et al. Diquafosol tetrasodium is effective in a broad spectrum of patients with dry eye. Poster presented at The Association for Research in Vision and Ophthalmology (ARVO) 2004 Annual Meeting. 2004 April 25-29; Fort Lauderdale, Florida, USA.
19. Stern ME, Beuerman RW, Fox RI, et al. The pathology of dry eye: The interaction between the ocular surface and lacrimal glands. Cornea 1998;17:584-589.
20. Stern ME, Beuerman RW, Fox RI, et al. A unified theory of the role of the ocular surface in dry eye. Adv Exp Med Biol 1998;438:643-51.
21. Christine M. Velicer, PhD; Susan R. Heckbert, MD, PhD; Johanna W. Lampe, PhD, RD; John D. Potter, MD, PhD; Carol A. Robertson, RPh; Stephen H. Taplin, MD, MPH: Antibiotic Use in Relation to the Risk of Breast Cancer; JAMA 2004;291:827-35.
22. Yang H-Y, Fujishima H, Toda I, et al. Allergic conjunctivitis as a risk factor for regression and haze after photorefractive keratectomy. Am J Ophthalmol 1998;125:54-8.
23. Yolton DP. Use of Topical Steroids for the Treatment Of Anterior Segment Ocular Disease, Pacific University College of Optometry, 2006.

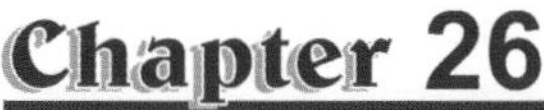

Chapter 26

Anterior Uveitis

Jorge L Alio, Mohammed Ahmed (Spain)

DEFINITION AND DEMOGRAPHY

Anterior uveitis (AU) is an inflammatory process that affects the tissue structures of the anterior uvea, that is the iris and the ciliary body. The terms iritis and iridocyclitis are more or less equivalent although some ophthalmologists use the term iritis to refer to mild AU whereas others consider iridocyclitis a more severe form of AU.

According to the studied geographical area, it was found to constitute between 30 and 73 percent of all cases of uveitis. In Spain anterior uveitis represents 70 percent of all uveitis cases, while in studies done in Belgium showed anterior uveitis to represent 51 percent of all cases. It is evident that the epidemiology of anterior uveitis differs to a certain extent from one studied area to another.[1-4]

CLINICAL MANIFESTATIONS

Symptoms

Pain

Pain due to anterior uveitis occurs with significantly variable intensity and a radiation pattern along the area of the ophthalmic branch of the trigeminal nerve. It is caused by spasm of the ciliary muscle and sphincter pupillae as well as irritation of the ciliary nerves caused by the inflammatory mediators. It is usually aggravated by accommodation, ocular movement and finger touch.

Photophobia

Presence of cells and plasmoid aqueous in the anterior chamber causes light scattering and photophobia which may be severe enough to hinder ocular examination.

Decreased Vision

In the first episode, it is usually caused by miosis and the diminished transparency of the plasmoid aqueous. In recurrent cases it may be caused by the former reasons or rather by complications such as cataract and glaucoma.

Tearing

A reflex irritation causes an increase in tear production via the lacrimal gland stimulation by the parasympathetic supply.

Signs

Ciliary Injection

It is marked perilimbally. It is characterized by injection of the deep episcleral arterioles. The conjunctiva can be moved freely over these arterioles and they cannot be affected by topical vasoconstrictive agents.

Reactive Miosis

The spastic constriction and pinpoint pupil is due to ciliary body spasm and tonic contraction of the sphincter pupillae. Edema of the iris stroma and paresis of dilator pupillae may also contribute to the extreme miosis.

Plasmoid Aqueous

Plasmoid aqueous occurs due to the exudation that occurs from iris vessels due to the disruption of the blood-aqueous barrier. It is composed of inflammatory cells, proteins (responsible for the Tyndall phenomenon). In severe cases, fibrin causes what is termed as plastic iritis. The Tyndall phenomenon is the optical effect caused by the foreign particles suspended in the aqueous when viewing the contents of the anterior chamber by the slit lamp. Distinction should be made between the presence of flare and that of cells in the anterior chamber (Fig. 26.1). Cells are larger than protein conglomerates, round and bright. The presence of cells is a necessity to diagnose "active" iritis. It is cells that cause the hypopyon when they gravitate in the anterior chamber (Fig. 26.2). On the other hand flare is caused by fibrin and not by cells.

Keratic Precipitates (KPs)

Keratic precipitates are macrophages and neutrophils that have been exudated from the iris vessels as a part of the chemotactic process of intraocular inflammation. As a result of convection currents in the anterior chamber, they become deposited on the back surface of the cornea. They gravitate and tend

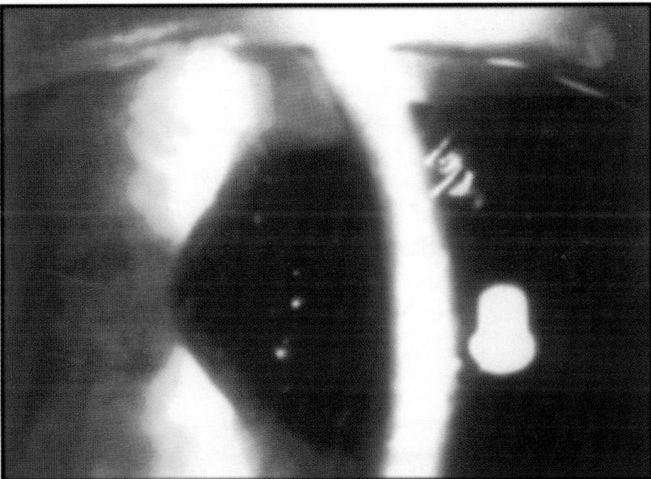

Fig. 26.1: Cells and flare in the anterior chamber. Note that cells are large nonpigmented while flare is formed of protein conglomerates which are smaller and pigmented

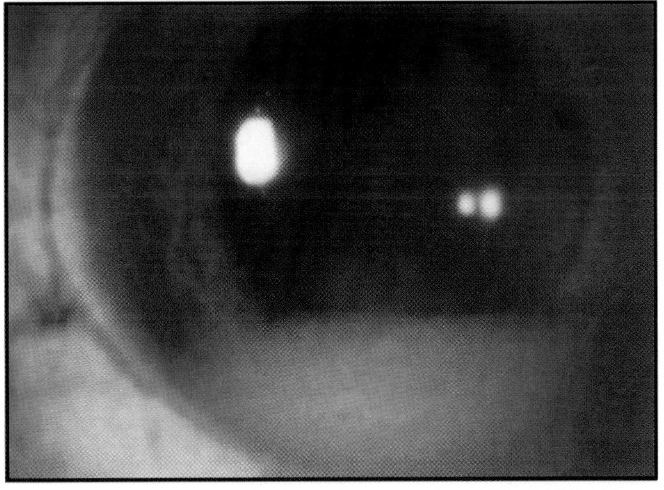

Fig. 26.2: Formation of hypopyon due to the presence of a large number of inflammatory cells in the anterior chamber

to form a triangular shape with an inferior base. The distribution, pattern and color of the KPs give very valuable clues in the diagnosis of the cause of iridocyclitis

- Large, white KPs or what is termed "Mutton fat" deposits are usually associated with granulomatous iridocyclitis (Fig. 26.3)
- Fine, dust-like KPs scattered all over the posterior surface of the cornea are characteristic of herpetic uveitis and Fuch's heterochromic iridocyclitis (Fig. 26.4)

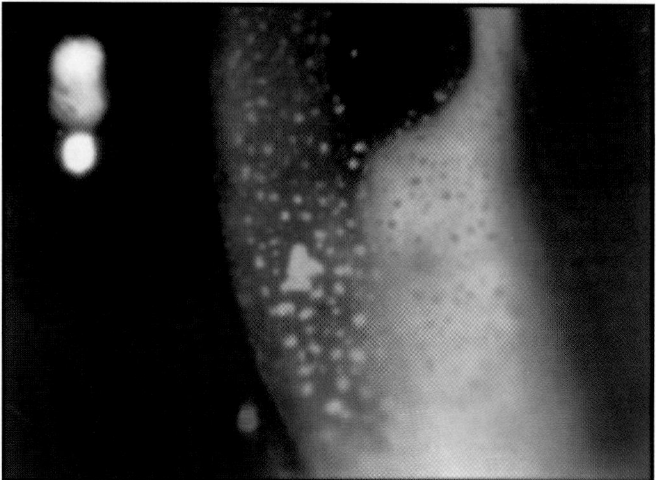

Fig. 26.3: Large KPs "mutton fat" in a case of acute AU in a patient with ankylosing spondylitis

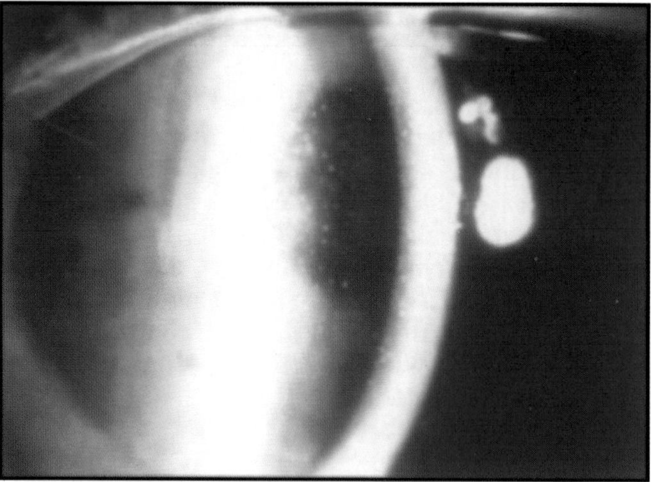

Fig. 26.4: Fine dust-like KPs in a case of herpetic uveitis

- Brown pigmented KPs are usually old standing as the iris pigmented epithelial cells participate in their formation, while light colored KPs suggest a recent affection (Fig. 26.5).

Synechiae

Synechiae occur due to the organization of fibrin laid down from fibroblasts that adhere the iris to the anterior surface of the lens—posterior synechiae (Fig. 26.6) which may induce a progressive lenticular changes or those that

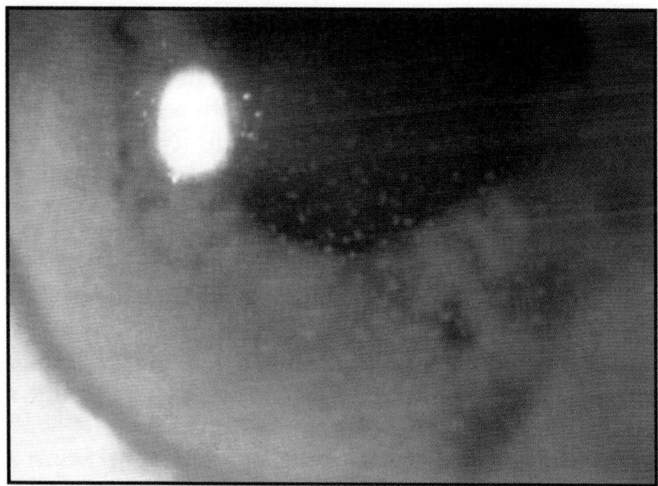

Fig. 26.5: Brown-pigmented KPs in a case of chronic AU

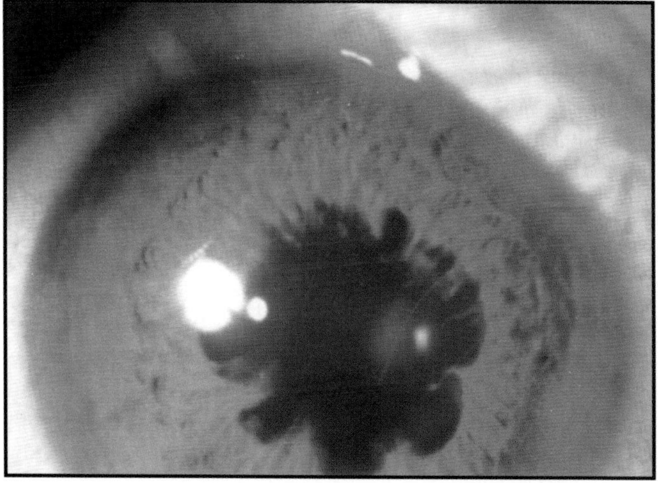

Fig. 26.6: Posterior synechiae and irregular pupil in a case of chronic indolent AU

cause adherence of the peripheral iris to the corneal endothelial surface, covering the angle structures (peripheral anterior synechiae) and may induce a chronic angle-closure glaucoma.

Nodules

Nodules are characteristic of granulomatous iritis, they are aggregates of epithelioid cells and lymphocytes in the iris stroma either on the pupillary border (Koeppe's nodules), or the larger peripheral ones near the iris root—Bussaca's nodules (Fig. 26.7).

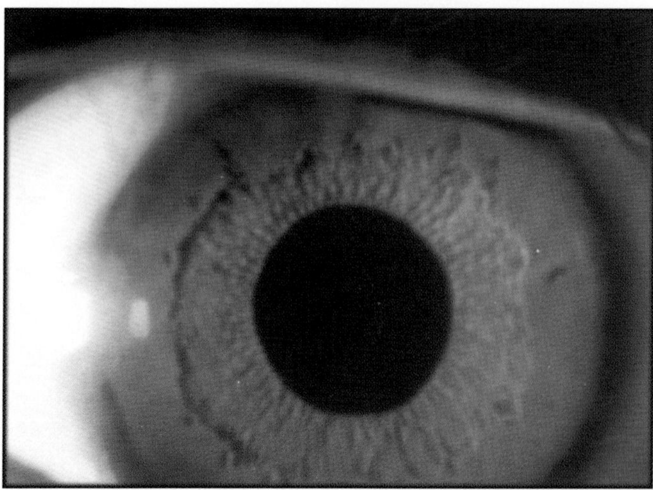

Fig. 26.7: Iris nodules (*Bussaca*) in a suspected case of sarcoidosis

The Lens

The lens may remain clear except for some fibrinous deposits in the pupillary area during the acute phase. Opacification may occur later on due to the inflammatory process or the use of corticosteroids.

Increased Intraocular Pressure

This usually occurs due to the associated trabeculitis and the increased viscosity of the plasmoid aqueous.[5] Other mechanisms involved will be discussed in detail in the section of complications. Goldmann tonometry should be performed without fluorescein or at the end of biomicroscopy as fluorescein may obscure flare and cells assessment.

Many classifications of the severity of anterior uveitis have been proposed as the classification proposed by Hogan *et al*.[6] In our opinion, the most practical scoring system is the one introduced by Ben Ezra *et al*.[7] This classifies the severity of anterior uveitis according to the two "active and rapidly changing signs", i.e. the number of cells and flare intensity using the widest slit lamp beam at 1.00 mm height with maximum luminance of Haag-Streit (or equivalent) slit lamp. Uveitic scoring system (USS) is based on grading the two previously mentioned signs (Table 26.1).

INSTRUMENTAL EXAMINATION

Recently, attempts were made to quantitate the above findings using the laser flare meter (kowa 1000), the Laser cell meter (kowa 500) and the fluorophotometry (Flourotron, Master), but their advantages for routine use by the ophthalmologist has to be further evaluated.[8]

Table 26.1: Uveitic scoring system (USS)

Clinical sign	*Grade*	*Description*
Flare intensity	0	Nil to trace
	1	Mild noticeable
	2	Moderate without plastic aqueous
	3	Marked with plastic aqueous
	4	Severe with fibrin deposits and/or clots
Cell count	0	< 5 cells/field
	1	5-10 cells/field
	2	11-20 cells/field
	3	21-50 cells/field
	4	> 50 cells/ field
	5	Hypopyon formation

Anterior chamber flare intensity
Grade 0 = nil to trace flare, Grade 1 = mild noticeable, Grade 2 = moderate without plastic aqueous, Grade 3 = marked with plastic aqueous, Grade 4 = severe with fibrin deposits and/ or clots (iris details hazy).

Anterior chamber cells count
Grade 0 = nil: <5 cells/field, Grade 1 = mild: 5-10 cells/field, Grade 2 = moderate: 11-20 cells/ field, Grade 3 = marked: 21-50 cells/field, Grade 4 = severe: >50 cells/field, Grade 5 = Hypopyon formation.

DIFFERENTIAL DIAGNOSIS

The differential diagnosis of acute AU is with all causes of the acute red eye. The presence of discharge indicates the presence of conjunctivitis; the presence of a corneal lesion with sharp pain readily relieved by one drop of local anesthesia indicates the presence of keratitis; the high tension with sudden marked loss of vision, mid-dilated pupil and edematous cornea suggests an acute angle-closure glaucoma and the presence of localized area of ciliary injection without having constricted pupil or posterior synechiae indicates anterior episcleritis/scleritis.

One particular case should be differentiated from AU is the acute anterior ischemic syndrome. The etiology of this condition is either atherosclerotic changes, carotid artery disease, peripheral vascular insufficiency or extensive extraocular muscle surgery. In the anterior segment, signs include perilimbal vascular congestion, corneal edema, cells and flare in the anterior chamber, rubeosis iridis and frequently severe orbital pain (ocular angina). In cases with associated posterior segment affection, the patient also experiences amaurosis fugax.

The other group that should be differentiated from anterior uveitis is the so-called Masquerade syndromes, these are namely most of the intraocular malignancies, the complex retinal detachments and some cases of microhyphemas. Intraocular malignancies are: the famous retinoblastoma which occurs in the young, mostly diagnosed before the age of three. It presents with a variety of signs the most common of which is leukocoria. Apart from complex genetic tests and tumor marker detection such as alpha-fetoprotein (AFP) and CEA, the most practical investigation to detect retinoblastoma in children is the search for calcification by CT or radiographs. Melanoma is also well differentiated by clinical picture, ultrasound, radioactive P uptake, MRI, CT, and radio investigations such as positron emission tomography (PET). Metastasis can be detected by monitoring the primary sites and by radioactive P uptake, while reticulum cell sarcoma can be detected through a vitreous sample. Complex retinal detachments with opacities in the media can be diagnosed by ultrasonography.

ANCILLARY TESTS FOR THE ETIOLOGICAL DIAGNOSIS OF ANTERIOR UVEITIS

These fall into one of the following groups:
- HLA phenotyping
- Immunological tests
- Anterior chamber puncture
- Specific tests for each syndrome.

HLA Phenotyping

The value of HLA typing is the early diagnosis of the cause of uveitis before the onset of systemic signs and the etiological diagnosis in cases of atypical mixed clinical picture.

HLA typing for some important specific ocular inflammatory states include:
- Acute anterior uveitis—HLA-B27, HLA-B8
- Ankylosing spondylitis—HLA- B27, HLA-B7
- Juvenile rheumatoid arthritis—HLA-DR4
- Vogt-Koyanagi-Harada disease—MT-3.

Immunological Tests

Tests of connective tissue disorders: The most valuable of these tests are those detecting autoantibodies since they not only differentiate various types of collagen diseases but also can imply the expected prognosis, for example, it is well known that patients with antinuclear antibodies (ANA) carry a much worse prognosis than those with no ANA in juvenile rheumatoid arthritis (JRA).[9]

Aqueous Sampling by Anterior Chamber Puncture

Technique

Aqueous sampling is a rather easy procedure. After local anesthesia and immobilization of the globe, a puncture is made with a 27G needle which is introduced as tangentially as possible to the limbus. This allows for sampling of 150 U of aqueous. A 5 ml blood sample is also obtained, centrifuged and both samples are divided into equal parts for further testing of cytology and local production of antibodies.[10]

Interpretation of Results for Immunoglobulin Detection

Three tests are run on the obtained samples, namely the C Quotient (Goldman Witmer), C′ Quotient, and the level of IgG production.

The C quotient compares the antibody/protein ratio of a specific single antibody in both the aqueous and the serum. If found to be more in aqueous than in serum, this is an indirect evidence of the responsibility of this specific antigen. The C′ quotient compares the value of several antibodies at the same time to detect the prevalence of one of them. It has been agreed that when several viral antibodies are found, the C′ quotient should be used, while if only one exists, the C quotient test is used.

The third test that evaluates the nonspecific IgG production by calculating the IgG/albumin in the aqueous (R2) and the same ratio in the serum (R1). Normally the R2/R1 is less than 1. If increased, it denotes an immunological intraocular inflammation.

Specific Tests for each Syndrome

- *Chest radiographs for TB and sarcoidosis*: The four radiological patterns found in sarcoidosis is either hilar lymphadenopathy alone, hilar lymphadenopathy with parenchymal reticular affection, parenchymal affection alone or progressive interstitial fibrosis.
- Bamboo-shaped spine sign in sacroiliac region in ankylosing spondylitis.
- Angiotensin converting enzyme (ACE) levels, bronchial lavage, serum calcium and radioactive gallium-67 uptake for sarcoidosis.
- Viral studies including monoclonal antibody detection, viral cultures from infected cells and vesicle aspirations for herpetic cases.
- HIV test.

COMPLICATIONS OF ANTERIOR UVEITIS

The complications that can appear in the course of anterior uveitis are as follows.

Complicated Cataract

The lens opacity can occur as a complication of the inflammatory process (complicated cataract) or due to the prolonged use of corticosteroids (iatrogenic). In the former group, anterior subcapsular opacities may occur due to lens epithelial cell necrosis and fibrous metaplasia with the production of subcapsular collagen deposition sandwiched between epithelial cells

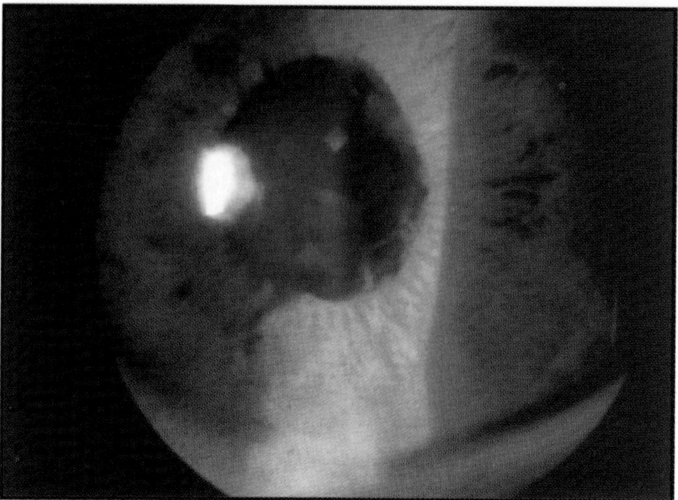

Fig. 26.8: Constricted pupil and nonresponding pupil with accompanying lenticular changes in a case of chronic indolent AU

(duplication cataract).This usually occurs in the presence of posterior synechiae (Fig. 26.8). In the latter group, as well as in cases with associated posterior chamber inflammation, migration of the equatorial subcapsular epithelium to the posterior pole producing colored interference patterns or the polychromatic luster.

It should be noted that these cataracts cause a significant loss of visual function due to their posterior location in the lens near to the nodal point of the eye, and due to the accompanying small pupil. Surgery also differs from that of usual cataracts since these small pupils should be stitched wide to allow safe capsulorhexis and phacoemulsification. It is in our belief that phacoemulsification is the safest technique when performed on selected cases as extracapsular cataract extraction (ECCE) is usually not preferred in these eyes with borderline endothelial cell function and in the presence of an experienced surgeon, a decision of phacoemulsification is always wise.

Glaucoma

The main mechanisms that cause increased IOP in cases of anterior uveitis are either inflammatory trabeculitis causing a decrease in size of the spaces of Fontana, blockage of the trabeculum with inflammatory cells, the consequential formation of peripheral anterior synechiae, the associated pupillary block caused by a seclused pupil, the difficulty in drainage of the viscous plasmoid aqueous, the associated episcleral congestion or the prolonged use of topical corticosteroids.

Iris Atrophy

Iris atrophy is often apparent either as a diffuse loss of iris stromal tissue or as localized patches. These changes have no evident influence on function. However, these atrophic areas of the iris are more permeable to the aqueous humor. Therefore, in their presence, an acute glaucomatous attack is extremely rare.

Synechiae (Either Posterior or Peripheral Anterior Synechiae)

The latter type usually develops if the anterior chamber shallows. In the presence of fibrin within the aqueous humor, adhesions between the iris and the endothelial surface of the cornea are created. These are more prone to occur in the periphery, where the distance between these two structures is narrowest.

Cyclitic Membrane

A cyclitic membrane covering the pupillary area may develop and is usually associated with recurrent acute inflammatory attacks. It is another bad prognostic sign, as it is usually accompanied by new vessel growth. These vessels are fragile and may bleed spontaneously (Fig. 26.9).

Band Keratopathy

Band keratopathy occurs due to the deposition of calcium in the subepithelial level. This spares the spots where there are corneal nerves and so presents clinically as a honeycomb deposition in the interpalpebral fissure. It occurs

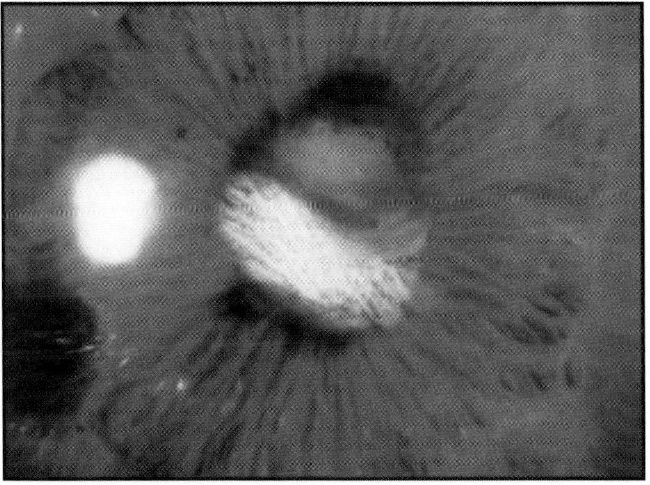

Fig. 26.9: A thick cyclitic membrane in a case of chronic AU

most frequently with juvenile rheumatoid arthritis (JRA). Treatment is carried out either by chelation which is the application of ethylenediaminetetraacetic acid (EDTA) with a concentration of 1 to 2 percent or the much expensive sodium versenate. If chelation does not do the trick then superficial keratectomy should be carried out. Excimer laser surgery (phototherapeutic keratectomy) is an excellent alternative for the surgical technique.

Corneal Endothelial Decompensation

Corneal endothelial decompensation is mostly observed during attacks of acute glaucoma. Mild localized decompensation may be detected. These are, however, of a transient nature in most cases and are due to an immune reaction directed specifically against the corneal endothelial cells.

Hypotony and Phthisis Bulbi

Hypotony may occur due to hyposecretion of aqueous humor caused by inflammation of the ciliary body or the formation of a cyclitic membrane and its subsequent contraction causing ciliary body detachment and the excessive drainage of aqueous through the uveoscleral route. If the condition does not reverse either spontaneously or by surgical removal of the membrane, Phthisis may occur with internal disorganization of the globe with scleral thickening and osseous metaplasia in the uveal tract.

SPECIFIC CLINICAL ENTITIES OF ANTERIOR UVEITIS

Iridocyclitis associated with HLA-B27
A-without systemic disorders
B-with systemic disorders:
Spondyloarthropathies:
1. Ankylosing spondylitis
2. Reiter's syndrome
3. Psoriatic arthritis
4. Chronic inflammatory bowel disease
5. Juvenile chronic arthritis.

Infectious anterior uveitis
- Herpetic iridocyclitis
- Bacterial and fungal iridocyclitis
- Associated with systemic infectious disorders: tuberculosis syphilis, Lyme's disease and leprosy

Fuch's heterochromic syndrome

Glaucomatocyclitic crisis

Idiopathic anterior uveitis

Traumatic iridocyclitis

Phacoantigenic anterior uveitis.

Iridocyclitis associated with HLA-B27

HLA-B27 denotes a genotype located on the short arm of chromosome 6 present between 1.4 percent and 8 percent of general population. 50 to 60 percent of acute AU may be HLA-B27 related either with or without associated systemic disorders.[11] The group of systemic disorders often associated with HLA-B27 is called *spondyloarthropathy* which accounts for 40 percent of all cases of AU and is a seronegative for the rheumatoid factor, this group includes:

Ankylosing Spondylitis

Ankylosing spondylitis is a common idiopathic chronic inflammatory arthritis affecting the axial skeleton. More common in males than females.[12]

Presentation is usually in the second or third decade with chronic backache. The course in men is usually more severe than in women.

Characteristic highly suggestive findings

- Radiographs for the lower back may show a bamboo-shaped spine before the patient has any skeletal complaints that is why spine radiograph should be carried out for all young males with acute unilateral iridocyclitis.

Ocular features These are usually in the form of unilateral, acute nongranulomatous AU, both eyes may be affected but show these features at different times. It should be noted that ocular features occur in 30 percent of patients with AS. Conversely 30 percent of males with acute iritis will eventually have AS.

Reiter's Syndrome

The classic triad of Reiter's syndrome is: urethritis, conjunctivitis and seronegative arthritis.

Urethritis is usually nonspecific and usually accompanied by an attack of dysentery. It occurs usually as a primary presentation before any other feature.

The last feature to present itself is acute arthritis which affects the knees and ankles. Other features include the periarticular features including plantar fascitis, Achilles tendonitis and calcaneal periostitis.

Moderately specific findings include extraarticular features including mouth ulcers, genital ulcers and circinate balanitis which confuses this disease with Behcet's syndrome, keratoderma blennorhagica which are skin lesions which confuses it with psoriasis.

Ocular features These usually present after urethritis but before arthritis. Mucopurulent conjunctivitis, acute iritis and keratitis are the main features. They occur in 20 percent of the patients.[13]

Psoriatic Arthritis

Seven percent of the patients suffering from psoriasis develop ocular features.

Highly specific findings include: Symmetrical arthritis during the fourth or fifth decade occurs along with psoriatic nail affection and sausage-shaped deformity of the digits.

Ocular features include conjunctivitis that occurs in 20 percent of the cases. Acute iritis occurs but is less common than in AS or Reiter's syndrome. Keratitis and secondary Sjögren syndrome may also occur.[14]

Juvenile Rheumatoid Arthritis

Juvenile rheumatoid arthritis (JRA) was defined as an idiopathic arthritis that persists at least for three months in a patient under the age of 16 years. Females are affected more, one of three presentations may occur.[15]

Systemic JRA or as previously called "Still's disease". It constitutes 20 percent of all types of JRA. It presents with maculopapular rash, fever, serositis, lymphadenopathy and hepatosplenomegaly. The development of arthritis and arthralgia is uncommon in this group. Ocular affection is rare.

Polyarticular JRA accounts for a further 20 percent of JRA cases. Arthritis involves five or more joints, most commonly the knees followed by the ankles and wrists. Systemic features are usually absent. Uveitis is uncommon.

Pauciarticular JRA accounts for 60 percent of JRA cases. Less than five joints are affected, most commonly the knee. Some of these group remain pauciarticular while the rest develop polyarthritis. The possibility of uveitis is high.

High-risk factors for development of uveitis in JRA are early onset, positive for antinuclear antibodies (ANA) and HLA-DW5 and HLA-DPw2.[16]

It has been postulated that the ophthalmic follow-up regimen for these patients would be: annual for systemic onset, every 9 months for polyarticular, every 6 months for polyarticular + ANA, every 4 months for pauciarticular and every 3 months for pauciarticular + ANA.

Ocular features

Bilateral chronic anterior uveitis occurs in 70 percent of cases. The course is usually asymptomatic and the eye is quiet (white uveitis). The severity and duration of intraocular inflammation varies widely between patients and 25 percent of cases show persistent uveal inflammation for several years, in this subgroup band keratopathy occurs in 40 percent, cataract in 30 percent and secondary glaucoma in 15 percent.[17]

Uveitis caused by JRA is one of the potentially damaging syndromes that may necessitate the usage of cytotoxic agents in its treatment.

Chronic Inflammatory Bowel Disease (Crohn's Disease and Ulcerative Colitis)

The general features of this syndrome include arthritis, erythema nodosum, hepatitis, sclerosing cholangitis and pyoderma gangrenosum. It is weakly associated with HLA-b27. Ocular features include conjunctivitis, keratoconjunctivitis sicca, episcleritis and scleritis. Chronic anterior uveitis occurs in 70 percent of cases with ocular involvement.

Infectious Anterior Uveitis

Herpetic Iridocyclitis

Herpetic iridocyclitis may result from either herpes zoster or herpes simplex infection. It presents as an acute or chronic anterior uveitis in the presence or absence of corneal involvement.[18]

Herpes simplex: This is usually associated with disciform keratitis but may occur without corneal affection. In the presence of keratitis, a bacterial corneal infection should be ruled out since it also presents with a corneal lesion together with signs of anterior chamber reaction. In some cases, the virus can be isolated from the anterior chamber. It is not clear if the anterior chamber reaction represents an active viral replication or a hypersensitivity to the viral antigen as occurs in the case of disciform keratitis. Treatment of this type of iridocyclitis should always include the use of an umbrella of antiviral drugs such as acycloguanosine 3 percent ointment under which topical steroids can be used with caution since it can activate the viral infection.

Herpes zoster: This causes an anterior uveitis in 50 percent of cases.The characteristic features include the presence of patchy or sectoreal iris atrophy associated with other signs of nongranulomatous iridocyclitis. The main pathological process is an obliterative vasculitis caused by the virus particles. The finding of a hemorrhagic hypopyon is suggestive enough of the herpetic etiology of the iritis. Although the finding of serum antibodies does not provide a definite diagnosis since they appear positive in the majority of adults, the clues to diagnose zoster uveitis include

- Associated diminished corneal sensitivity
- Presence of corneal nummular lesions
- Transillumination iris defects
- Postherpetic scarring and pigmentation which may be found on the patient's scalp.

The treatment is based on the administration of topical cycloplegics and corticosteroids under an umbrella of topical and systemic antiviral drugs unless there is an active epithelial infection. The drug of choice is acyclovir in the dose of 500 mg, 5 times/day for 10 days.

Specific tests for herpes infections include aspirations from affected vesicles, viral cultures, monoclonal antibody detection and viral DNA replication and detection using polymerase chain reaction (PCR) and DNA hybridation techniques.

A special mention should be done on the acute retinal necrosis (ARN) syndrome, although a primary posterior segment disease, this bimodal disease which is caused by herpes simplex in the young and herpes zoster in the elderly has significant anterior segment signs such as lid edema, conjunctivitis, scleritis and nongranulomatous iridocyclitis.

In addition to laser photocoagulation and vitreoretinal surgery for the posterior segment affection, the treatment of iridocyclitis caused by ARN is the same as that of herpetic iridocyclitis.

Bacterial and Fungal Iridocyclitis

Bacterial and fungal corneal ulcers often produce anterior uveitis, the most common risk factors include corneal trauma and contact lens use. A Gram stain with cultures and sensitivity aid in diagnosis and treatment and are indicated for all patients with severe or centrally located ulcers. Despite the presence of uveitis, corticosteroids should be avoided until the infection is well-controlled.

Associated with Systemic Infectious Disorders

Systemic infections account for less than 10 percent of all cases of AU but can cause significant morbidity and even death if unrecognized or treated inappropriately. Two systemic infections in particular, syphilis and tuberculosis are prevalent enough in patients with uveitis to warrant consideration.

Syphilis

Syphilis causes uveitis in 1 percent of the cases. Although syphilitic infection has decreased markedly during the past decades, it has recently shown a surge due to the worldwide AIDS epidemic.

Syphilis has always kept up with its reputation in being " the great mimicker", it can simulate any form of uveitis. Although the main signs of syphilitic uveitis occur in the posterior segment, anterior uveitis occurs in 4 percent of patients with secondary and tertiary syphilis. The anterior uveitis may be granulomatous or nongranulomatous and usually develops into a chronic iridocyclitis. The condition becomes bilateral in 50 percent of the cases. Early in the course of the iritis, dilated iris capillaries form the very famous 'roseolae' which change later into the larger yellow iris papules. Although one of the manifestations of tertiary syphilis, the presence of iris gummata is extremely rare.

Posterior segment affection results in unifocal or multifocal chorioretinitis, neuroretinitis and optic neuritis. Other ocular features include Argyll Robertson pupils and ocular motor palsies.

The management of ocular syphilis is the same as neurosyphilis. It consists of 12 to 24 megaunits of aqueous penicillin IV for 10 days followed by IM 2.4 MU for 3 weeks. Patients with sensitivity can be treated by erythromycin.

Tuberculosis

As in syphilitic uveitis, iridocyclitis occurs in 1 percent of cases of TB. The diagnosis of tuberculous iridocyclitis is always presumptive and based on indirect evidence although it can be partly confirmed by the famous tuberculin test, isoniazid test or a positive chest radiograph.

The iridocyclitis is usually granulomatous and usually associated with choroiditis and retinal vasculitis.[19] Treatment usually follows one of the well known antituberculous protocols and should be carried out together with the internist.[19]

Fuch's Heterochromic Iridocyclitis

Although conventionally named like that, Fuch's syndrome is no longer considered a uveitis and nowadays many ocular pathologists believe that it is a degenerative disease in spite of the increased level of serum IL-2R. Fuch's syndrome is often misdiagnosed and maltreated more than any other uveitis syndrome. It represents 2 percent of all cases of uveitis.

Presentation is as mild chronic unilateral and in 10 percent of cases is bilateral, with diminished visual acuity either due to vitreous floaters or due to the development of complicated cataract. Examination shows the presence of KPs which are characteristically small, round, nonpigmented and scattered throughout the corneal endothelium. A universal finding is the absence of posterior synechiae. Iris stromal atrophy and rubeosis iridis occur along with Koeppe nodules.[20]

Heterochromia occurs in the form of hypochromic discoloration of the affected iris. In less frequent cases, the affected iris aquires a much darker color (paradoxical Fuch's). In general a dark iris becomes more dark and a light colored iris becomes lighter in color.

Complications include: cataract which has good prognosis with cataract extraction,[21] except for the possibility of bleeding from rubeosis if intraocular pressure (IOP) is lowered rapidly or by paracentesis (Amsler's sign) and glaucoma which is a chronic open-angle glaucoma caused by trabecular sclerosis, rubeosis or fine peripheral anterior synechiae. Treatment with corticosteroids or cycloplegics has no objective importance, follow-up examination is recommended for early detection of glaucoma.

Glaucomatocyclitic Crisis

Glaucomatocyclitic crisis or Posner-Schlossman's syndrome is characterized by attacks of unilateral marked elevation of IOP associated with signs of anterior uveitis. It presents in middle-aged adults with a predilection for patients with HLA-DW54. Many theories for the pathogenesis of this condition have been suggested, including a possible viral etiology, but none was definitely proven.[22]

Clinically IOP elevation of up to 60 mm Hg can occur with an accompanying haloes, blurred vision and pupillary dilatation.

In spite of the presence of anterior chamber and vitreous reaction, posterior synechiae do not occur and optic nerve cupping and field changes do not occur.

Treatment is with topical nonsteroidal antiinflammatory drugs (NSAIDs), corticosteroids and antiglaucoma measures. No effective measure could be done to avoid a recurrent attack.

Idiopathic Anterior Uveitis

In spite of the breakthrough in the laboratory diagnosis of the etiology of anterior uveitis syndromes, 40 percent remain classified as idiopathic, they lack both systemic disorder and HLA-B27 associations.

Although these patients are classified as having idiopathic anterior uveitis on the basis of negative laboratory tests it should be repeated after six months to detect any seroconversion.

The good thing about pure idiopathic anterior uveitis is that it responds very well to the standard treatment of iridocyclitis in the form of topical steroids and cycloplegics.

Traumatic Iridocyclitis

Traumatic iridocyclitis may be induced by exogenous trauma or iatrogenic following surgery, when it becomes chronic, an indolent infectious origin for the continuing inflammatory reaction has to be looked for.

Phacolytic Iridocyclitis

Nowadays, this is a rare cause of AU. It is induced by leakage of lens protein into the anterior chamber causing for start low-grade granulomatous reaction followed by an intense inflammatory reaction which can be accompanied by a sudden rise of IOP.

Kawasaki Disease

Also called mucocutaneous lymph node syndrome, it is characterized by fever, polymorphous exanthem, oral mucous membrane erythema, bilateral conjunctival congestion and asymmetric nonsuppurative cervical adenopathy. Systemic vasculitis may lead to coronary arteritis and sudden death.[23] Ocular features include bulbar conjunctival congestion and transient acute AU which is mild, bilateral and resolves without treatment.

DECISION MAKING IN ANTERIOR UVEITIS IN AN ALGORITHMIC APPROACH[24] (FIG. 26.10)

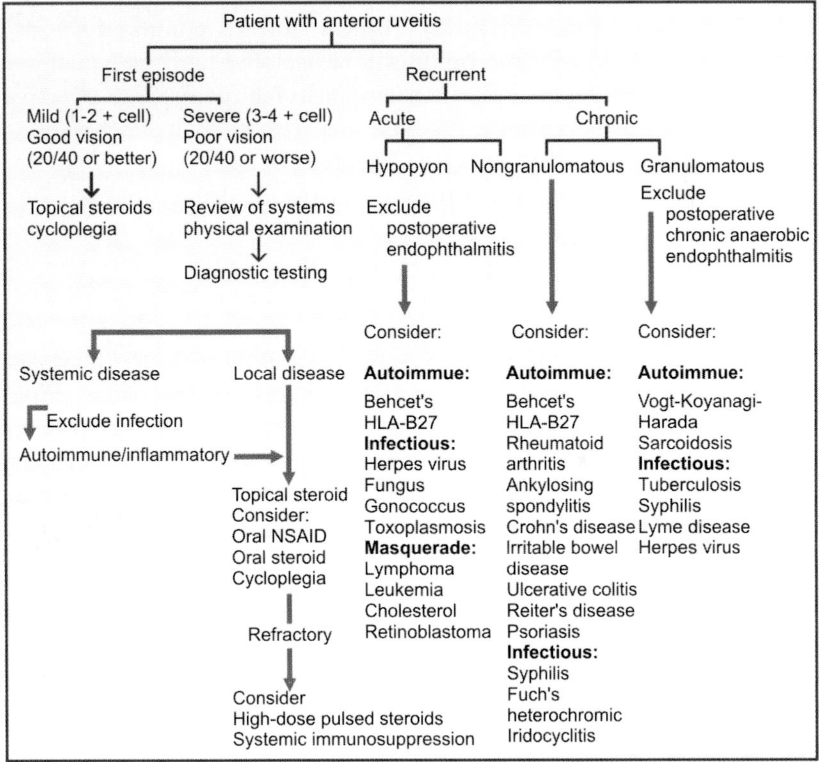

Fig. 26.10: Algorithmic approach to decision making in patient with anterior uveitis

MANAGEMENT

Treatment of Anterior Uveitis

Treatment should be classified as immediate treatment of the acute attack, treatment for recurrent cases, treatment to prevent recurrence and special lines of management.

Treatment of the Acute Attack

Essentially, treatment of AU should be confined to the use of drugs delivered locally. This recommendation is to be strictly followed in cases with unilateral ocular involvement and in most of bilateral cases. In few cases of bilateral involvement with severe inflammation and an imminent danger of irreversible affection of vision, systemic treatment of corticosteroids with low mineralo-corticoidal effect may be considered. Also when AU is associated with systemic disease, treatment of the associated systemic disorder should be integrated with the local treatment.[25-29]

Local treatment consists of antiinflammatory drugs combined with cycloplegics. The most efficient local antiinflammatory drugs are the corticosteroid preparations (drops, ointments or depot of steroids injected subconjunctivally, or periorbitally). Topical steroids commonly used are dexamethasone 0.1 percent and prednisolone acetate 1 percent. Nonsteroidal antiinflammatory drugs as indomethacin and voltaren are less effective in treatment of AU, also cyclosporin A eyedrops are equally ineffective because of poor intraocular penetration of this lipophilic drug.[30]

The frequency of instillation of corticosteroid drops depends on the intensity of the intraocular inflammation and on the sensitivity of the patient. Despite their high efficacy, corticosteroid drops may often induce secondary glaucoma, cataract and opportunistic infections. Therefore, their delivery has to be limited to minimal needs.

Cycloplegics are also used to prevent the formation of posterior synechiae and relaxes the ciliary muscle spasm. The type and frequency of cycloplegic eyedrops to be used depend mainly on whether there are developments of posterior synechiae and whether ciliary muscle spasm contributes to the ocular pain. When aches are a major symptom, atropine sulfate 1 percent eyedrops should be used. During the acute attack and especially if a shallowing of the anterior chamber is observed, a combination of scopolamine 0.3 percent and neosynephrine 10 percent may be used until the posterior synechiae are broken, a wick of cotton soaked in a solution of 1/1000 epinephrine can be inserted in the lower fornix, or 0.05 percent ml of this solution can be injected subconjunctivally around the limbal areas facing the most tenacious synechiae.[31] To prevent recurrence of the synechiae, cyclopentolate 1 percent can be used for maintenance of a dilated pupil. If the formation of posterior synechiae is not a major feature, a more short-acting solution like tropicamide 0.5 percent may be prescribed. The use of short-acting preparations can allow normal near-task activities without marked interference and affection of fixation for reading and writing.

Treatment of Recurrent Cases

This implies the use of the previously described measures along with the use of systemic steroids. The most commonly used drug is prednisone 1 mg/kg/ day with a maximum of 60 to 80 mg/day. The whole dose is usually given in the early morning to maintain the circadian rhythm for corticosteroids. Unless the drug is given for more than three weeks, neither tapering of the dose nor ACTH injection will be needed.

Treatment to Prevent Recurrences

This depends upon the specific treatment of each individual syndrome. A note worth mentioning is the indications of cytotoxic drugs in the treatment of anterior uveitis. These include uveitis caused by juvenile chronic arthritis, Behcet's disease and Vogt-Koyanagi-Harada syndrome. The most popular drugs are chlorambucil, cyclophosphamide and cyclosporin A. The latter is a T-cell suppressor which does not cause bone marrow suppression. It can be combined with steroids to speed remission. The dose of cyclosporin A is 3 mg/kg/day. Most cases of recurrent endogenous uveitis can be fully controlled by the above regimen.

The new horizon in the treatment of uveitis lies in the use of the promising new drugs such as the agent FK 506 which is a new immunosuppressor with fewer side effects, the use of monoclonal antibodies against specific lymphocytes and the new trend of using antioxidants such as vitamin C. The value of these modes of treatment in the long-term control of uveitis is still to be investigated.

REFERENCES

1. Dernonchamps JP. Epidemiology of uveitis in Belgium—a preliminary study. Proceedings of the Third International Symposium of Uveitis Kluger: New York 1993;157-9.
2. Sugita M, Enomoto Y, NaLaura S, et al. Epidemiological study on endogenous uveitis in Japan. Proceedings of the Third International Symposium of Uveitis Kluger: New York 1993;161-3.
3. Couto C, Merlo JL. Epidemiological study of patients with uveitis in Buenos Aires, Argentina. Proceedings of the Third International Symposium of Uveitis Kluger: New York 1993;171-4.
4. Weiner A, BenEzra D. Clinical patterns and associated conditions in chronic uveitis. Am J Ophthalmol 1991;111:151-8.
5. BenEzra D, Wysenheek YS, Cohen E. Increased intraocular pressure during treatment for chronic uveitis. Graefe's Arch Clin Exp Ophthalmol 1997;235:200-3.
6. Hogan MD, Kimura SJ, Thygeson P. Signs and symptoms of uveitis I—anterior uveitis. Am J Ophthalmol 1959;47:155-60.
7. BenEzra D, Forrester JV, Nussenblatt RB, et al. Uveitis Scoring System, Springer-Verlag: Berlin 1991;1-16.
8. Alió JL, Sayans JA, Chipont E. Flare-cell meter measurement of inflammation after uneventful cataract surgery with intraocular lens implantation. J Cataract Refract Surg 1997;23:935-9.
9. Roberton DM, Cabral DA, Malleson PN, et al. Juvenile psoriatic arthritis—follow up and evaluation of diagnostic criteria. J Rheumatol 1995;23:166-70.
10. Nussenblatt RB, Scott M, Palestine AG. Diagnostic testing of uveitis. Uveitis Fundamentals and Clinical Practice 1996;(2nd ed):79-90.
11. Tay Kearney ML, Schwam BL, Lowder C, et al. Clinical features and associated systemic diseases of HLA-B27 uveitis. Am J Ophthalmol 1996;121:47-56.
12. Brewerton DA, Caffrey M, Hart FD, et al. Ankylosing spondylitis and HLA-B27. Lancet 1973;1:904-7.

13. Lee DA, BarLer SM, Su WPD, et al. The clinical diagnosis of Reiter's syndrome. Ophthalmology 1986;93:355-56.
14. Roberton DM, Cabral DA, Malleson PN, et al. Juvenile psoriatic arthritis—follow up and evaluation of diagnostic criteria. J Rheumatol 1995;23:166-70.
15. Cassidy JT, Levinson JE, Bass JC, et al. A study of classification criteria for diagnosis of juvenile rheumatoid arthritis. Arthritis Rheum 1986;29:274-81.
16. Wolf MD, Lichter PR, Ragsdale CG. Prognostic factors in the uveitis of juvenile rheumatoid arthritis. Ophthalmology 1987;94:1242-8.
17. Chylack LT, Bientang DC, Bellows AR, et al. Ocular manifestations of juvenile rheumatoid arthritis. Am J Ophthalmol 1975;79:1026-33.
18. Womack LW, Liesegang TJ. Complications of herpes ophthalmicus. Arch Ophthalmol 1983;101:42-45.
19. BenEzra D. Diseases of the choroid and anterior uvea. Michaelsorz's Textbook of the Fundus of the Eye (3rd ed): Livingstone: Edinburgh 1980;667-712.
20. BenEzra D: Fuchs' heterochromic cyclitis. Ocular Inflammation Basic and Clinical Concepts (1st ed): 1999;305-12.
21. Nicholas PJ. Cataract surgery using heparin surface-modified intraocular lenses in Fuchs' heterochromic uveitis. Ophthalmic Surg 1995;26:49-52.
22. Posner A, Schlossman A. Syndrome of unilateral recurrent attacks of glaucoma with cyclitis symptoms. Arch Ophthalmol 1948;39:517-28.
23. Bligand CA. Kawasaki disease and its diagnosis. Pediatr Dermatol 1987;4:75-84.
24. Scales DK. Anterior uveitis. Decision Making in Ophthalmology (2nd ed) 2000;350-1.
25. BenEzra D, Nussen Blatt RB, Timonen P. Optimal Use of Sandimmun in Endogenous Uveitis Heidelberg: Springer-Verlag: Berlin 1988;1-22.
26. Dick AD, Azim M, Forrester JV. Immunosuppressive therapy for chronic uveitis—optimising therapy with steroids and cyclosporin A. Br J Ophthalmol 1997;81:1107-12.
27. Whitcup SM, Nussenblatt RB. Immunologic mechanisms of uveitis. Arch Ophthalmol 1997;115:520-5.
28. BenEzra D. Immunosuppressive treatment of uveitis. Int Ophthalmol Clin 1990;30:309-13.
29. BenEzra D. Treatment aspects in ocular Behçet's. Asia Pacific J Ophthalmol 1991;3:15-19.
30. BenEzra D. The role of cyclosporine eye drops in ocular inflammatory diseases. Ocul Immunol Inflam 1993;1:159-62.
31. Alió JL, Hosny M. Anterior uveitis. Ocular Inflammation Basics and Clinical Concepts (2nd ed) 1999;213-26.

Chapter 27

Uveitis Treatment Strategies

Jean Deschênes, LI Gisêle (Canada)

INTRODUCTION

Advances in the fields of immunology and pharmacology have expanded the therapeutic options for autoimmune diseases.

Two important discoveries in the field of ocular immunology have enabled progress in the treatment of uveitis: firstly, the characterization of the cytokine and interleukin profile during ocular inflammation, and secondly, the development of an animal model for uveitis induced by specific antigens have permitted the testing of new medications.

Progress in pharmacology, in particular, the ability to selectively target the immune system and the development of new preparations for systemic and local treatment, has paved the way for new treatment modalities.

CURRENT THERAPIES

Despite their known side effects, corticosteroids remain the principal agents used in the treatment of acute episodes of uveitis and are, unfortunately, sometimes necessary as adjuvants in maintenance therapy of chronic uveitis.

The main anti-inflammatory effects of corticosteroids are an attenuation of hypersensitivity reactions, an inhibition of cytokine and eicosanoid production and a sequestration of lymphocytes in the spleen, bone marrow and lymph nodes and out of the intravascular circulation. Their mechanism of action involves stabilization of the blood-ocular barrier and an inhibition of cellular migration during acute ocular inflammation.[1] Topical steroids are indicated in the treatment of anterior uveitis. The frequency of administration depends on the severity of the inflammation. A severe inflammatory reaction in the anterior chamber with presence of fibrin may necessitate a loading dose of one drop of 1 percent prednisolone acetate or of 0.1 percent dexamethasone given each minute during the first five minutes of each hour.[2,3] Conversely, less severe inflammation may be treated with fluorometholone. Betamethasone did not produce a good response in a group of patients under observation, including those with mild, non-serious forms of uveitis.

Cystoid macular edema (CME) a complication of anterior and intermediate uveitis, can be treated with sub-Tenon injections of 40 mg of triamcinolone acetonide. Before opting for this form of treatment prior episodes of steroid-induced elevations in intraocular pressure (IOP) must be ruled out.[4] When the inflammation threatens bilateral vision, treament with oral prednisone (1-2 mg/kg/day) may be used.[4]

When steroids are part of maintenance therapy in chronic uveitis, the addition of an aminobiphosphonate, such as alendronate (inhibitor of osteoclastic activity and promoter of osteoblastic activity) must be considered to mitigate steroid-induced osteoporosis.

In uveitis patients resistant to oral prednisone or intolerant of another immunosuppressive agent, intravenous therapy with methylprednisolone (1-2 g/day for 2-3 days) may be a valuable therapeutic approach in controlling sight threatening inflammation.[4]

Nonsteroidal anti-inflammatory drugs (NSAIDs) represent another group of well-known medications particularly useful in the therapy of chronic uveitis. NSAIDs inhibit cyclooxygenase, the enzyme necessary for the production of prostaglandins which are powerful mediators of inflammation. The principal characteristic of NSAIDs is their reduction of complications, notably CME[5,6] by preventing prostaglandin-mediated vasodilation and vascular leakage.[7] NSAIDs may also be used to control postoperative inflammation. Ketorolac tromethamine and diclofenac sodium were demonstrated to be as effective as prednisolone acetate in controlling inflammation following cataract extraction.[8,9]

There are two types of cyclooxygenase enzymes: COX-1 and COX-2. The first is a constitutive enzyme which produces a constant secretion of prostaglandins responsible for various physiologic functions. The second is an inducible enzyme regulated by diverse cytokines. Metabolities of COX-2 induce vasodilatation, chemotaxis and chronic breakdown of the blood-ocular barrier.[10]

A therapeutic regime involving selective NSAIDs targeting COX-1 or COX-2 may be useful in the stabilization of chronic non-granulomatous uveitis. Selective inhibitors of the COX-2 enzyme are better tolerated, thus larger doses may be administered. Numerous COX-2 inhibitors are presently in clinical trials and some are commercially available. An attractive feature of COX-2 inhibitors is the absence of the gastrointestinal side effects and of the inhibition of platelet aggregation associated with non-selective NSAIDs. Among the COX-2 inhibitors, celecoxib, known commercially as Celebrex,[11] has shown promise in the treatment of rheumatoid arthritis.

Immunosuppressive agents are indicated in the therapy of sight-threatening forms of uveitis resistant to corticosteroids and affecting patients who require long-term systemic corticosteroids.

Methotrexate, cyclophosphamide, leukeron, imuran and cyclosporin are mainly used in the treatment of severe uveitis.[4] Methotrexate is the first line immunosuppressive agent used in uveitis resistant to corticosteroids because of its demonstrated efficacy in the treatment of rheumatoid arthritis,[12] the reversibility of its side effects and minimal toxicity.

Methotrexate works by inhibiting the enzyme dihydrofolate reductase (DHFR) thereby preventing the production of tetrahydrofolate, a metabolite necessary for the production of nucleotides. Consequently, methotrexate prevents RNA and DNA synthesis and non-selectively inhibits T and B cell proliferation. The recommended dose is 7.5 mg per week with the addition of folic acid, 1 mg three to five days per week, to prevent adverse side effects. Folic acid should not be started until the 24 hours for methotrexate absorption have elapsed. During the first two months of methotrexate treatment, hepatic and hematologic profile monitoring should be performed every second week, then occurs regularly every two to four months.

Micophenolate mofetyl (MMP) is a new immunosuppressive agent which has been useful in the prevention of organ rejection in renal transplant patients.[13] The selective and non-competitive inhibition of inosine monophosphate dehydrogenase by MMP leads to a *de novo* inhibition of guanosine-derived nucleotides. These mechanisms act on the cellular and humoral immune responses and upregulate adhesion molecules during an inflammatory episode. MMP may be used in conjunction with cyclosporin or corticosteroids.[14] The recommended dose is 1 g/day, and its administration demands regular monitoring of the hematologic profile in order to prevent severe neutropenia.

Tacrolimus (FK506), macrolide antibiotic, has potent immunosuppressive properties. It inhibits signal transduction pathways which promote T-cell activation and recruitment. The molecular mechanism of action is mediated by an inhibition of the phosphorylase activity of calcineurin[15] resulting in a failure to activate genes, such as IL-2, necessary for T-cell proliferation.[16] Small scale clinical trials, mostly involving patients with Behcet's disease, have shown Tacrolimus to be beneficial in patients with sight-threatening inflammation[17,18] refractory to cyclosporin. Tacrolimus is effective at therapeutic doses of approximately 100 times less than that of cyclosporin.[19] A daily dosage of 0.10 to 0.15 mg/kg body weight/day has been suggested as an appropriate dosage.[20] Side effects of Tacrolimus are similar to those of cyclosporin. In studies of Tacrolimus-based immunosuppression for rejection prophylaxis after cardiac transplantation, Tacrolimus was associated with less hypertension and hyperlipidemia and no difference in renal function, hyperglycemia or infection incidence when compared to cyclosporin-based immunosuppression.[21]

FUTURE TREATMENTS

Although the previously described medications have efficacious immunosuppressive activity, their non-selective action results in systemic complications such as opportunistic infections and renal or hepatic toxicity. Such diverse clinical problems demand a broad range of therapeutic approaches. One therapeutic option is local treatment. The efficacy of ganciclovir administered via an intravitreal continuous release device in treating AIDS associated cytomegalovirus (CMV) retinitis has stimulated the development of similar devices for other medications. Intravitreal devices releasing cyclosporin and leflunomide have been shown to suppress ocular inflammation in animal models.[22] New local delivery systems for dexamethasone are also being developed. An anterior chamber implant releasing dexamethasone has shown to have similar efficacy to dexamethasone eyedrops in reducing postcataract surgery inflammation.[23]

Another approach involves specific regulation of the immune response using immunomodulatory agents. This approach represents a relatively new route in the treatment of autoimmune diseases. The immunomodulatory agents aim to selectively reduce CD4 cell differentiation, proliferation and production of Th1 type cytokines. Th1 cells are a subgroup of helper T cells associated with the cytokines IL-2 and IFN-γ. The other subgroup consists of Th2 cells which have a different cytokine profile. The Th1-type cytokine profile is associated with initiation of disease and the delayed hypersensitivity response whereas the Th2-type profile is linked to disease suppression.[20] The delayed hypersensitivity response plays a key role in the pathogenesis of most cases of uveitis. Downregulating the production and activity of Th1 cytokines will dampen this response in favor of a less vigorous type of immune response.

Although few immunomodulatory agents are currently being used to treat uveitis, a number of these agents have undergone clinical trials and the results are on the verge of appearing.

Interferon gamma (IFN-γ) is a chemotactic factor of type-1 T helper cells (Th1). Th1 type cytokines increase delayed hypersensitivity reactions. IFNγ activity may be downregulated by IFN-alpha-2. Systemic recombinant IFN-alpha-2a has been shown to be efficacious in the treatment of severe forms of vasculitis, an example being Behcet's disease.[24-26] The main inconveniences are its administration as intramuscular injections (three million IUs) three times per week and the associated flu-like symptoms.

Leflunomide is a new agent which inhibits lymphocyte proliferation and prevents the cycle of adhesion molecules. Its main active metabolite is A77 1726, a malononitriloamide, which prevents the proliferation of lymphocytes by inhibiting the *de novo* synthesis of pyrimidines, cytokines and tyrosine kinase growth receptors. In a phase II clinical trial, leflunomide revealed high tolerability and efficacy in patients with advanced rheumatoid arthritis.[27] A randomized clinical trial comparing leflunomide (20 mg/d), methotrexate (7.5-15 mg/wk) and placebo as treatments for rheumatoid arthritis showed superior clinical responses in patients receiving leflunomide. Common adverse reactions included gastrointestinal complaints, skin rash, reversible alopecia and asymptomatic transaminase elevations.[28] Combination therapy of low dose leflunomide and methotrexate, thereby preventing the respective drug-related side effects, may be the optimal treatment strategy. The biochemical mechanisms underlying their therapeutic efficacy are quite different.[29]

Meanwhile, leflunomide has shown *in vitro* activity against CMV including multidrug-resistant strains. Leflunomide is hypothesized to inhibit protein kinase-mediated phosphorylation of CMV proteins. This activity may potentially enable leflunomide to simultaneously mitigate a common complication of immunosuppression, CMV disease.[30]

Etanercept has been demonstrated to diminish the activity of rheumatoid arthritis in patients already receiving methotrexate treatment. Etanercept, a soluble recombinant tumor necrosis factor receptor, binds and inactivates TNF, an important mediator of inflammation. The medication must be administered subcutaneously (25 mg twice a week) as an adjuvant to methotrexate. The combination of etanercept and methotrexate is safe and well tolerated making this combination therapy a promising treatment.[31,32]

The agent daclizumab (zenapax), a monoclonal antibody directed against the IL-2 receptor, has demonstrated the ability to reduce acute rejection of renal allografts when used with cyclosporine or with corticosteroids.[33] Monoclonal antibody against the IL-2 receptor selectively dampens IL-2-mediated proliferation of T helper cells. The antibodies target the CD25 antigen, which functions as the IL-2 receptor, thereby preventing the receptor's internalization and signal transduction in T helper lymphocytes.

In a phase I/II clinical trial, daclizumab was administered to patients instead of their standard immunosuppressive therapy. Monoclonal antibody therapy appeared to prevent the expression of severe sight-threatening intraocular inflammatory disease over a 12-month period and was associated with improvements in visual acuity. The medication was tolerated without requiring dose reduction.[34] The main foreseeable drawbacks of daclizumab are its intravenous administration at 4 week intervals.

Somatic gene therapy appears to be a feasible therapeutics approach. The use of viral or other types of vectors to deliver specific genes to ocular tissues and replace defective genes has been accomplished. However, certain conditions remain to be achieved: efficient uptake of genetic vectors into target cells, high frequency vector integration into host cell chromosomes and low vector immunogenicity. Gene therapy enables the delivery of therapeutic genes to target cells and the appropriate localization of gene products. Using this approach, immunosuppressive cytokines and anti-inflammatory factors can be produced by vectors injected into cells of the retinal pigment epithelium (RPE) and in other ocular tissues.[35]

The expression of transcription factors, once encoded by vectors, may even upregulate or downregulate specific genes capable of producing or decreasing production of certain molecules.[36]

These various approaches to the treatment of uveitis are based on modifying the type of hypersensitivity reaction involved in ocular inflammation. Their common objective is an attenuation of Th1-type cytokine expression in favor of a Th2-type cytokine profile as the latter is associated with disease suppression. This goal would be best achieved by a combination of modalities encompassing immunosuppression, immunomodulation and (or) genetic therapy applied to the treatment of intraocular inflammation.

REFERENCES

1. Leibowitz HM, Kupferman A. Anti-inflammatory medications. Ophthalmol Clin 1980;20:117-34.
2. Nussenblatt RB, Palestine AG. Uveitis: Fundamentals and Clinical Practice. Year Book Medical Publishers: Chicago 1989;104-44.
3. Lightman S. Use of steroids and immunosuppressive drugs in the management of posterior uveitis. Eye 1991;5:294-98.
4. Nussenblatt RB, Witcup
5. Jampol LM, Sanders DR, Kraff MC. Prophylaxis and therapy of aphakic cystoid macular edema. Surv Ophthalmol 1984;28(Suppl):535-39.
6. Kraff MC, Sanders DR, Jampol LM et al. Prophylaxis of pseudophakic cystoid macular edema with topical indomethacin. Ophthalmology 1982;89:885-90.
7. Jampol LM. Pharmacologic therapy of aphakic cystoid macular edema—a review. Ophthalmology 1982;89(8):891-97.
8. Heier J, Cheetham JK, Degryse R et al. Ketorolac tromethamine 0.5% ophthalmic solution in the treatment of moderate to severe ocular inflammation after cataract surgery—a randomized, vehicle-controlled clinical trial. Am J Ophthalmol 1999;127(3):253-59.
9. El-Harazi SM, Ruiz RS, Feldman RM et al. A randomized double-masked trial comparing ketorolac tromethamine 0.5%, diclofenac sodium 0.1%, and prednisolone acetate 1% in reducing post-phacoemulsification flare and cells. Ophthalmic Surgery and Lasers 1998;29(7):539-44.
10. De Witt DL. Cox-2 selective inhibitors—the new super aspirins. Mol Pharrmacol 1999;55(4):625-31.
11. Gierse JK, Kabolt CM, Walker MC et al. Kinetic basis for selective inhibition of cyclooxygenases. Biochem J 1999;339(Pt3):607-14.
12. Verhoeven AC, Boers M, Tugwell P. Combination therapy in reumathoid arthritis—updated sytematic review. Br J Rheum 1998;37:612-19.
13. The Tricontinental Mycophenolate Mofetil Renal Transplantation Study Group Transplantation. A blinded, randomized clinical trial of mycophenolate mofetil for the prevention of acute rejection cadaveric renal transplantation 1996;61(7):1029-37.
14. Vanrenterghem YF. Impact of new immunosuppressive agents on late graft outcome. Kidney Int Suppl 1997;63:S81-83.
15. Jacobson P, Uberti J, Davis W et al. Tacrolimus—a new agent for the prevention of graft-versus-host disease in hematopoietic stem cell transplantation, Bone Marrow Transplantation 1998;22(3):217-25.
16. Ho S Clipstone N, Timmerman L, Northrop J et al. The mechanisms of action of cyclosporine A and FK 506. Clinical Immunology and Immunopathology 1996;80(3 Pt 2):S40-45.

17. Mochizuki M, Masuda K, Sakane T et al: A clinical trial of FK506 in refractory uveitis. Am J Ophthalmol 1993;115:763-69.
18. Sloper CM, Powell RJ, Dua HS. Tacrolimus (FK506) in the treatment of posterior uveitis refractory to cyclosporine. Ophthalmology 1999;106(4):723-28.
19. Tocci MJ, Matkovich DA, Collier KA et al. The immunosuppressant FK506 selectively inhibits expression of early T cell activation genes. J Immunol 1989;143:718-26.
20. Nussenblatt RB, Whitcup S, Palestine AG. Uveitis. Fundamentals and Clinical Practice. 2nd ed Mosby-Year Book: St. Louis, 1996.
21. Taylor DO, Barr ML, Radovancevic B et al. A randomized, multicenter comparison of tacrolimus and cyclosporine immunosuppressive regimens in cardiac transplantation—decreased hyperlipidemia and hypertension with tacrolimus. Journal of Heart and Lung Transplantation. 1999;18(4):336-45.
22. Jaffe GJ, Chang-Sue Yang Xiao-Chun Wang, Cousins WS, et al. Intravitreal sustained release cyclosporine in the treatment of experimental uveitis.
23. Tan DT, Chee SP, Lim L, Lim AS. Randomized clinical trial of a new dexamethasone delivery system (Surodex) for treatment of post-cataract surgery inflammation. Ophthalmology 1999;106(2):223-31.
24. Pivetti-Pezzi P, Accorinti M, Pirraglia MP et al. Interferon alpha for ocular Behcet's disease. Acta Ophthalmologica Scandinavica 1997;75(6):720-22.
25. Georgiou S, Monastirli A, Pasmatzi E et al. Efficacy and safety of systemic recombinant interferon-alpha in Behcet disease. Journal of Internal Medicine 1998;243(5):367-72.
26. Kotter I, Eckstein AK, Stubiger N et al. Treatment of ocular symptoms of Behcet's disease with interferon alpha 2a: a pilot study. British Journal of Ophthalmology 1998;82(5):488-94.
27. Tedesco Silva H. Jr, Morris RE. Leflunomide and malononitriloamides. Expert Opinion on Investigational Drugs 1997;6:51-64.
28. Strand V, Cohen S, Schiff M et al. Treatment of active rheumatoid arthritis with leflunomide compared with placebo and methotrexate. Leflunomide Rheumatoid Arthritis Investigators Group. Arch Internal Med 1999;159(21):2542-50.
29. Kremer JM. Methotrexate and leflunomide—a biochemical basis for combination therapy in the treatment of rheumatoid arthritis. Semin Arthritis and Rheuma 1999;29(1):14-26.
30. Waldman WJ, Knight DA, Lurain NS et al. Novel mechanism of inhibition of cytomegalovirus by the experimental immunosuppressive agent leflunomide. Transplantation 1999;68(6):814-25.
31. Weinblatt et al. A trial of Etanercept, a recombinant tumor necrosis factor receptor: Fc Fusion protein, in patients with reumathoid arthritis receiving methotrexate. N Engl J Med 1999;340:253-59.
32. O'Dell JR. Anticytokine therapy—a new era in the treatment of reumathoid arthritis? N Engl J Med 1999;340:310-12.
33. The Daclizumab double therapy study group. Reduction of acute renal allograft rejection by Daclizumab Transplantation 1999;67:110-15.
34. Nussenblatt RB, Fortin E, Schiffman R, et al. Treatment of noninfectious intermediate and posterior uveitis with the humanized anti-Tac mAb: a phase I/ II clinical trial. Proceedings of the National Academy of Sciences of the United States of America 1999;96(13):7462-66.
35. Nussenblatt R, Csaky K. Perspectives on gene therapy in the treatment of ocular inflammation. Eye 1997;11:217-21.
36. Wright FA. Gene therapy for the eye. BJ Ophthalmol 1997;81:620-23.

Chapter 28

Optimizing Visual Outcomes with NSAIDs Therapy in Cataract and Refractive Surgery

Eric D Donnenfeld, Henry D Perry (USA)

Ophthalmic nonsteroidal anti-inflammatory drugs (NSAIDs) are becoming a cornerstone for the management of ocular pain and inflammation. Their well-characterized anti-inflammatory activity, analgesic property, and established safety record have also made NSAIDs an important tool to optimize surgical outcomes. Ophthalmic NSAIDs currently play four principle roles in ophthalmic surgery including the prevention of intraoperative miosis during cataract surgery, management of post-operative inflammation, the reduction of pain and discomfort following cataract and refractive surgery, and the prevention and treatment of cystoid macular edema following cataract surgery.

Ocular inflammation is characterized by redness, swelling, and/or pain associated with irritation or trauma to the eye. Common triggers of ocular inflammation include allergies, meibomian gland dysfunction, ocular diseases (traumatic iritis, peripheral corneal inflammatory keratitis, episcleritis, and unilateral nongranulomatous idiopathic iritis), and most importantly ophthalmic surgical procedures.

The strict regulation of inflammatory reactions within the eye is vital in maintaining both anatomical integrity and visual function. Left unregulated, inflammation within the eye may lead to extensive ocular damage, resulting in impaired vision.

Ocular inflammatory pathways commence with the triggering of the arachidonic acid cascade. The cascade is triggered either by mechanical stimuli (such as the case of surgically-inflicted trauma) or by chemical stimuli (such as foreign substances or allergens). Prostaglandins are generated in most tissues by activation of the arachidonic acid pathway. Phospholipids in the cell membrane are the substrate for the enzyme phospholipase A to cause generation of arachidonic acid and, in turn, the enzymes cyclo-oxygenases and lipoxygenases act on arachidonic acid to produce a family of chemically distinct prostaglandins, and leukotrienes (McColgin). Clinical symptoms of prostaglandin production include hyperemi, miosis, poor vision, pain, and cystoid macular edema (CME).

It is well accepted that inhibition of prostaglandin synthesis and release reduces the inflammatory response induced by surgery and allergies, thereby reducing the clinical symptoms of prostaglandin production (McColgin). Prostaglandin synthesis can be suppressed by inhibiting phospholipase A2, which inhibits the release of arachidonic acid from the intracellular stores, or by inhibiting the conversion of arachidonic acid to prostaglandin via the cyclo-oxygenase pathway. Multiple portions of this pathway can be blocked and different classes of anti-inflammatory medications have differing effects on this pathway. For example, corticosteroids interfere with the activity of phospholipase A2, thereby inhibiting the release of arachidonic acid and the production of all arachidonic acid metabolites including prostaglandins (Polansky and Weinreb, 1984).

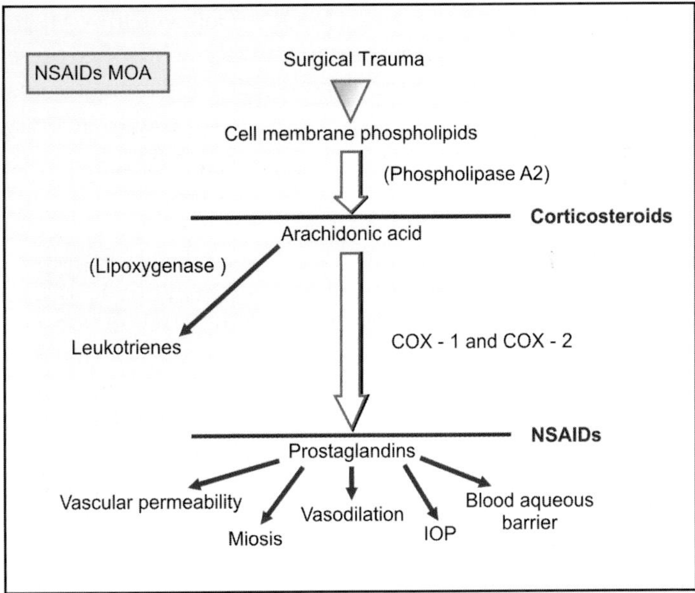

Fig. 28.1: Prostaglandin synthesis

In contrast, the nonsteroidal anti-inflammatory drugs (NSAIDs) specifically and irreversibly inhibit the synthesis of prostaglandins by interfering with the activity of cyclo-oxygenases (COX-1 and COX-2). (Polansky and Weinreb, 1984).

Rationale for Treating Ocular Inflammation

Reducing ocular inflammation is critical because failure to do so may cause patients discomfort, pain, visual loss, and increase the risk for the development of CME.

CME is potentially the most adverse ocular outcome of prostaglandin production. CME is caused by cystic accumulation of intraretinal fluid in the outer plexiform and inner nuclear layers of the retina, as a result of breakdown of the blood-retinal barrier. It is most common following intraocular surgery, and in patients with venous occlusive disease, diabetic retinopathy, and posterior segment inflammatory conditions (Quin). However, CME can develop in surgeries with no obvious compliactions. The condition is often asymptomatic and may only be detected with fluorescein angiography or optical coherence tomography (Quin, Roberts). Although the exact incidence of CME is still unclear, CME is a frequent cause of visual loss following even uncomplicated cataract surgery. Studies suggest that the rate of clinical CME ranges from 1-2% (Ray), while the incidence of angiographic CME may be as high as 9-19% (Ursell, Mentes). In a recent study, patients using ketorolac tromethamine 0.4% preoperatively 1-3 days prior to surgery had no instances of CME, whereas the steroid-only group and the group that got the NSAID just 1 hour prior for anti-miosis had a rate of 12% CME as detected by OCT (Donnenfeld). CME frequently has a late onset, occurring 4-6 weeks postoperatively. CME often presents with blurred or decreased central vision or painless retinal inflammation or swelling. Visual loss is usually temporary but may be irreversible in refractory to conservative treatment. In high risk patients such as diabetics the risk of CME and permanent vision loss is even greater.

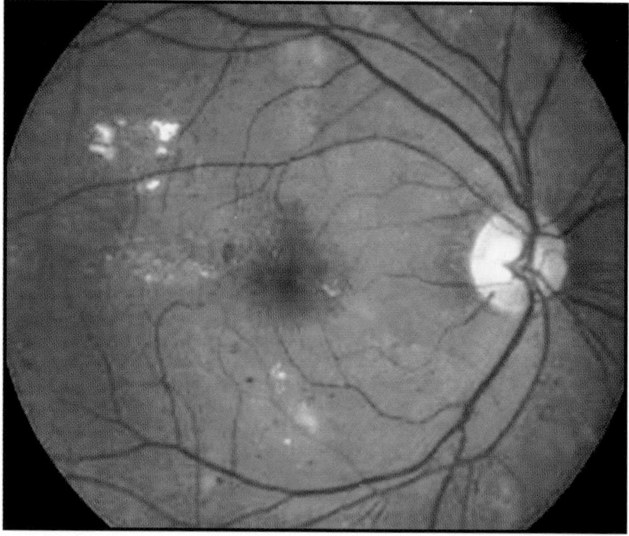

Fig. 28.2: Background diabetic retinopathy increases the risk of CME

NSAIDs are also frequently used to inhibit intraoperative miosis during cataract surgery. Miosis may restrict the surgeon's field of view during cataract surgery, thereby hindering the progression of the procedure, and increasing the risk of complications and posterior capsule rupture (Guzek, Stewart). The NSAIDs prevent miosis by limiting prostaglandin synthesis within the tissues by inhibiting cyclo-oxygenase and reducing inflammation. They also help to maintain increased pupillary size during the surgical procedure thereby helping to reduce complications.

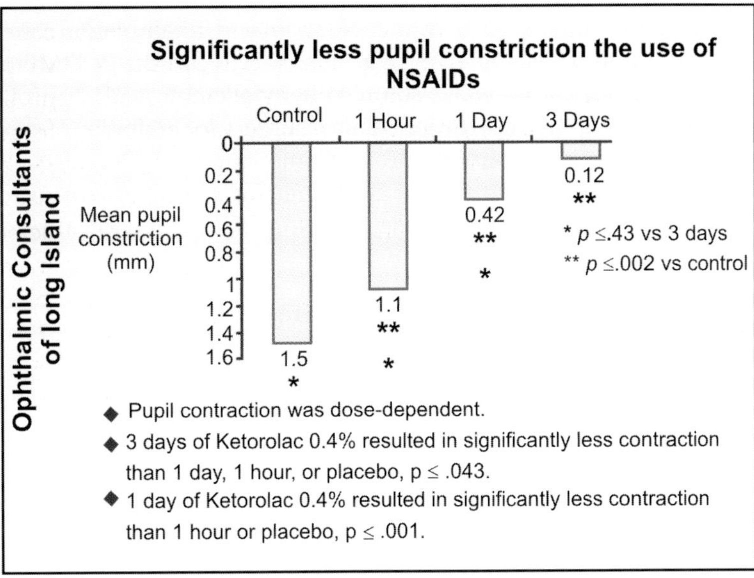

Fig. 28.3: Preoperative NSAIDs reduce pupil constriction during cataract surgery (Donnenfeld)

Pharmacologic Therapy for Ocular Inflammation

Ocular inflammation is currently treated with either topical corticosteroids or NSAIDs. The corticosteroids, considered the gold standard for the treatment of ocular inflammation, are associated with an increased incidence of adverse events that warrant their judicious use. These adverse events include cataract formation, a rise in intraocular pressure, increased susceptibility to microbial infections due to a suppressed host immune-response, retardation in corneal epithelial and stromal wound healing. Steroids are not safe for periods of extended use as prolonged use is associated with development of glaucoma, visual acuity defects and loss of visual field, and posterior subcapsular cataract formation.

A safer alternative to corticosteroids for the treatment of ocular inflammation are the NSAIDs. There are four classes of NSAIDs available for topical ophthalmic use: indoles, phenylacetic acids, an arylacetic acid pro-drug, and phenylalkanoic acids. Indomethacin 1% aqueous suspension is an indole derivative that is available outside of the United States (O'Brien). Diclofenac 1% is a water-soluble phenylacetic derivative approved by the FDA as a treatment to minimize inflammation related to cataract surgery and as a therapeutic option for the reduction of pain and photophobia after cataract surgery. Bromfenac

0.09% is a recently approved twice-daily topical phenylacetic compound indicated for the treatment of postoperative cataract inflammation. Originally available as a systemic medication, the product was removed from the market in the United States because of potentially fatal liver toxicity but has been available as an ophthalmic agent in Japan for several years. Nepafenac 0.1% is approved as a three times a day treatment for pain and inflammation associated with cataract surgery. This agent is an arylacetic acid pro-drug. Flurbiprofen 0.03% and suprofen 1% are water-soluble phenylalkanoic acids approved by the FDA for intraoperative use during cataract surgery for inhibition of excessive miosis during cataract surgery. Ketorolac tromethamine 0.4% is also a water-soluble phenylalkanoic acid and is approved for the treatment of for the reduction of ocular pain and burning/stinging following corneal refractive surgery.

NSAIDs for Control of Pain Following PRK

The recently reported pooled analysis of 2 multicenter, randomized, double-masked, vehicle-controlled, parallel-group studies of 313 patients with unilateral photorefractive keratectomy (PRK) evaluated the safety and analgesic efficacy of ketorolac tromethamine 0.4% ophthalmic solution in postoperative patients (Solomon). After surgery, patients were treated with 1 drop of ketorolac tromethamine 0.4% ophthalmic solution (n = 156) or vehicle (n = 157) four times daily for up to 4 days. Pain intensity, pain relief, use of escape medication, and severity of ocular symptoms were assessed and adverse events, epithelial healing, and visual acuity recorded. Patients in the ketorolac group reported significantly less pain intensity than patients in the vehicle group (P<.001). During the first 12 hours post PRK, 50% fewer patients in the ketorolac group than in the vehicle group had severe to intolerable pain (41.6% [64/154] and 84.5% [131/155], respectively). The median time to no pain was 30 hours in the ketorolac group and 54 hours in the vehicle group (P<.001). Ketorolac patients reported significantly greater pain relief than vehicle patients throughout the study (P<.001) and used significantly less escape medication than vehicle patients for 48 hours post PRK (P<.008). The authors concluded that ketorolac 0.4% ophthalmic solution is safe and effective in reducing ocular pain when used 4 times daily for up to 4 days post PRK.

NSAIDs vs. Steroids

A recent study compared the efficacy, safety and patient comfort of two topical steroids (prednisolone 1% and rimexolone 1%) with ketorolac tromethamine 0.5% after extracapsular cataract extraction in a prospective, randomized, double-masked study of 45 patients. Patients were assigned to receive topical treatment with prednisolone, rimexolone or ketorolac tromethamine ophthalmic solution after phacoemulsification for cataract extraction. Although there were no significant between-group differences in inflammatory cell counts, (P = 0.165), flare readings in the anterior chamber were lowest (P=0.008) in the ketorolac group. One patient in the prednisolone group experienced elevated IOP and had to be excluded. The authors concluded that ketorolac tromethamine provides good control of intraocular inflammation after cataract extraction without the risk of a steroidal IOP increase (Herneiss).

Holzer and associates reported that ketorolac tromethamine ophthalmic solution 0.5% was is effective as loteprednol etabonate ophthalmic suspension 0.5% in reducing inflammation after routine phacoemulsification and IOL implantation, suggesting that ketorolac tromethamine 0.5% is a safe and effective anti-inflammatory alternative to steroids after cataract extraction.

Similarly, Solomon and associates reported ketorolac tromethamine 0.5% is a safe and effective anti-inflammatory alternative to steroids after cataract extraction. In that study, ketorolac tromethamine 0.5% was as effective as rimexolone 1% in reducing inflammation after cataract surgery. There were no between-group differences in signs and symptoms of inflammation, intraocular pressure, or Kowa cell and flare measurements in this double-masked, prospective evaluation of 36 patients (Solomon and Vroman 2001).

NSAIDs for the Inhibition of Miosis

Srinivisin and associates reported that topical ketorolac was a more effective inhibitor of miosis than topical diclofenac during extracapsular cataract extraction and IOL implantation. Ketorolac also provided a more stable mydriatic effect throughout surgery. In a study of 51 patients who were prospectively randomized to receive ketorolac 0.5% or diclofenac 0.1% at 3 intervals preoperatively. In this study, the ketorolac group showed a consistent trend toward larger pupil diameters at subsequent surgical intervals as well as greater inhibition of miosis in the ketorolac group.

Similarly, Snyder and associates reported that the use of ketorolac as a single agent negated the need for use of a combination of preoperative NSAID (flurbiprofen) and postoperative cosrticosteroid for the prevention of intraoperative miosis and postoperative inflammation in cataract surgery. In their study of 26 patients, there were no statistically significant differences in dilation (preoperative versus postoperative) or cell and flare postoperatively. The authors concluded that the use of ketorolac as a single agent could eliminate the expense of using separate anti-inflammatory and antimiotic preparations preoperatively and postoperatively, thereby enhancing surgeon convenience and patient convenience and compliance (Snyder).

Recently, a large study (n=118) compared the effects of topical ketorolac with topical 0.03% flurbiprofen on the inhibition of surgically induced miosis during phacoemulsification cataract surgery. Mean horizontal pupillary diameter measurements for both medications were similar at the start of surgery. However, a consistent trend of larger pupillary diameter was seen in all subsequent surgical intervals in the ketorolac-treated group. Changes from baseline measurements also indicated a more significant inhibition of miosis at all subsequent intervals, and a more stable mydriasis throughout the procedure in the ketorolac-treated group. (Solomon 1997).

NSAIDs and Topical Steroids

It is well accepted that combination topical therapy with a corticosteroid and a NSAID is more effective than either agent dosed individually for treatment of CME following cataract surgery, and a recent study by Rho and associates supports this paradigm. The authors compared combination therapies of diclofenac sodium 0.1% and prednisolone acetate 1%, with ketorolac tromethamine 0.5% and prednisolone acetate 1%, for treatment of CME in 68 patients following uncomplicated cataract surgery. Complete resolution of CME was noted in 28% of diclofenac patients and in 25% of ketorolac patients. Final vision improved three or more lines in 58 and 53% of patients, respectively. None of the patients showed signs of corneal toxicity or significant intraocular pressure rise during the treatment period. The authors concluded that combination therapy with NSAIDs and steroids was effective in reducing the severity of pseudophakic CME and in improving final vision.

The findings of Rho and associates are supported by another recent study by Heier and associates (Heier, 2000). That study evaluated the efficacy of ketorolac, prednisolone acetate 1.0%, and ketorolac and prednisolone combination therapy in the treatment of acute, visually significant, clinical CME following cataract extraction surgery in a randomized, double-masked, prospective trial of 28 patients. Treatment was continued until CME resolved or for 3 months, whichever occurred first and then tapered over 3 weeks. The average improvements in Snellen visual acuity were 1.6 lines with ketorolac monotherapy, 1.1 lines with steroid monotherapy, and 3.8 lines with combination therapy. More patients in the combination group achieved at least a two-line improvement (89% of combination patients versus 67% of ketorolac and 50% of steroid patients). Moreover, these patients improved faster with combination therapy than with monotherapy with either agent (1.33 months for combination therapy compared with 1.43 months for ketorolac patients and 2.75 months for steroid patients). Improvements in contrast sensitivity and leakage on fluorescein angiography tended to mirror improvements in Snellen acuity. The authors concluded that treatment of acute, visually significant pseudophakic CME with ketorolac and prednisolone combination therapy appears to offer benefits over monotherapy with either agent alone.

A study by Arshinoff et al evaluated postoperative pain in 97 PRK patients using different topical NSAID protocols. In their study, treatment with topical homatropine hydrobromide, either diclofenac sodium or ketorolac tromethamine, and a soft contact lens was most effective in achieving post-PRK analgesia. They also found that found that NSAIDs added to topical steroid protocols had a significantly greater effect than steroids alone on reducing myopic regression for one year postoperatively (Arshinoff, 1994).

Prevention of CME

All available evidence demonstrates that ketorolac is an effective treatment for acute and chronic CME. Several studies, however, suggest that ketorolac is also able to prevent CME in postoperative patients. A study by Flach and associates (1990) suggested that ketorolac prevents CME without the risks associated with concomitant topical steroid treatment. In that study, 50 patients with bilateral cataracts were enrolled in a placebo-controlled, paired-comparison, double-masked study. Eleven patients had evidence of angiographic (angiographic aphakic CME) ACME on postoperative day 40. Two of these patients demonstrated bilateral ACME, one patient had ACME in the NSAID-treated eye, and eight patients had ACME in the placebo-treated eye. This was a statistically significant difference favoring drug treatment. In addition, the signs of anterior ocular inflammation were greater in the eyes with ACME.

Roberts presented data from a clinical study at the 2005 meeting of ASCRS that demonstrated that patients using preoperative and postoperative NSAIDs had less postoperative increase in macular thickness than those who did not use NSAIDs. In that study, 200 patients undergoing phacoemulsification were randomized to two pharmaceutical treatment regimens, differing only by the inclusion/exclusion of ketorolac 0.4% into the standard treatment regimen. Outcome measures included macular thickness by OCT at preoperative and 4 weeks post-operative, contrast sensitivity by FACT, and Snellen visual acuity. After 4 weeks, the change in macular thickness was substantially greater without NSAIDs than with NSAIDs (10.4 μm compared with 4.2 μm, respectively). There were no differences in visual acuity. The author concluded that macular edema decreases the quality of postoperative vision and that the use of pre-operative and postoperative NSAIDs decreases the amount of postoperative macular edema.

Many clinicians are hesitant to prescribe topical NSAIDs for long-term use because of prior reports of corneal melting associated with topical NSAIDs (Flach, Gaynes). However, analysis of NSAID-associated corneal events implicates the now defunct generic diclofenac product, diclofenac sodium ophthalmic solution as the agent primarily responsible (Gaynes). The demonstrated safety of ketorolac throughout numerous studies, some as long as 6 weeks duration, suggests that this drug is safe for extended use. In fact ketorolac has actually been recommended for the treatment of post cataract inflammation in a patient with systemic steroid treated rheumatoid arthritis post phacoemulsification. In this patient the fear of "melting" led the physician to avoid topical NSAIDs. However, the severe reaction post-operatively led him to using it successfully in the second eye with excellent results (Caronia).

The available evidence demonstrates that NSAIDs are highly effective analgesics for pain associated with cataract and refractive procedures. The ability to provide relief of patient pain is critical because patients have high expectations and expect almost no pain with ophthalmic surgeries. Patients who experience ocular pain or discomfort may therefore believe that their surgeon may have substandard surgical skills and the resulting patient dissatisfaction and potential for negative word of mouth to the patient's colleagues and friends may have adverse consequences for a surgical practice. Choosing the most effective topical agent for relief of ocular inflammation and pain postoperatively is therefore.

The adjunctive use of NSAIDs with steroids optimizes surgical outcomes as numerous studies have demonstrated that the combination of an NSAID and steroid is more effective for the treatment of postoperative inflammation, CME, and improving visual acuity than either NSAID or steroid monotherapy.

Perhaps the most important effect to surgeons is the increased amount of dilation preoperatively and the tendency for the dilation to remain for the entire procedure. Some surgeons have likened this effect as like having a third hand during surgery. Other studies point out the direct relationship between pupil size and rate of surgical complications (Donnenfeld).

In recent years, there has been a substantially amount of debate in the ophthalmic community regarding the use of NSAIDs prior to surgery to prevent the formation of CME. We understand and accept that increased inflammation postoperatively is associated with an increased risk of developing CME. In fact, a study by Ursell and associates reported that patients who had angiographic CME at day 60 were more likely to have had more postoperative inflammation than patients who did not develop CME (Ursell). It follows, therefore, that preventing inflammation with prophylactic dosing would decrease the risk of developing CME. A recent study by Donnenfeld and associates (Donnenfeld) does provide us with evidence supporting the use of ketorolac 0.4% as surgical prophylaxis against CME. The study was a prospective evaluation of 100 patients randomized in a double-masked fashion prior to phacoemulsification into 4 groups: one group received preoperative ketorolac tromethamine 0.4% four times daily for 3 days and three doses every 15 minutes immediately preceding surgery, another received four doses on the day before surgery ketorolac 0.4% and three doses every 15 minutes immediately preceding surgery, another received ketorolac only 3 times (every 15 minutes) in the hour immediately preceding surgery, and the fourth group was randomized to control. In that study, use of ketorolac for 1 or 3 days reduced the incidence of CME. No patients in these groups had CME at week 2, compared with 12% (3/25) of control patients and 4% (1/25) of patients in the 1 hour group. This study suggests that three day preoperative dosing with ketorolac effectively prevents CME. Other findings of that study demonstrated that ketorolac maintained pupil size, reduced discomfort, limited reductions in epithelial cell counts, and reduced patient need for additional anesthesia. Ketorolac also provided substantial reductions in the amount of time needed to perform surgery, making it a cost-effective pharmaceutical for cataract surgery. Most of these data followed a clear dose-response pattern, suggesting that maximum prophylaxis can be expected with the three day dosing regimen, though even 1 day of ketorolac was consistently superior to 1 hour of ketorolac or to control. This study further confirms the previous work by Flach and Roberts that ketorolac is an effective prophylaxis against CME.

If a 3-day dosing regimen of ketorolac is effective surgical prophylaxis, what is the most appropriate postoperative dosing regimen? In my experience, 4 weeks of QID dosing with ketorolac 0.4% is optimal for most patients, in patients with diabetes mellitus we use at least 6 weeks of therapy and most important in patients with diabetic retinopathy we use ketorolac 0.4% for at least three months to help protect this most susceptible group from developing CME.

BIBLIOGRAPHY

1. Arshinoff S, D'Addario D, Sadler C, Bilotta R, Johnson TM. Use of topical nonsteroidal anti-inflammatory drugs in excimer laser photorefractive keratectomy. J Cataract Refract Surg. 1994;20:216-22.
2. Caronia RM, Perry HD, Donnenfeld ED, J Cataract and Refractive Surg 2002;28 1880-1.
3. Donnenfeld ED, Perry HD, Wittpenn JR, Solomon R, Nattis A, Chou T. Preoperative ketorolac tromethamine 0.4% in phacoemulsification outcomes: pharmacokinetic-response curve. J Cataract Refract Surg. 2006;32(9):1474-82
4. Evans RE, Bucci FA Jr, Amico LM. Efficacy of Ketorolac 0.5% versus Ketorolac 0.4% Following Cataract Surgery. Presented at ARVO, 2005.
5. Flach AJ, Stegman RC, Graham J, Kruger LP. Prophylaxis of aphakic cystoid macular edema without corticosteroids. A paired-comparison, placebo-controlled double-masked study. Ophthalmology. 1990;97:1253-8.
6. Flach AJ. Corneal melts associated with topically applied nonsteroidal anti-inflammatory drugs. Trans Am Ophthalmol Soc. 2001;99:205-10; discussion 210-2.
7. Gaynes BI, Fiscella R. Topical nonsteroidal anti-inflammatory drugs for ophthalmic use: a safety review. Drug Saf. 2002;25:233-50.
8. Goyal R, Shankar J, Fone DL, Hughes DS. Randomized controlled trial of ketorolac in the management of corneal abrasions. Acta Ophthalmol Scand 2001;79(2): 177-9.
9. Guzek JP, Holm M, Cotter JB, et al. Risk factors for intraoperative complications in 1000 extracapsular cataract cases. Ophthalmology 1987;94:461-6.
10. Heier J, Cheetham JK, Degryse R, et al. Ketorolac tromethamine 0.5% ophthalmic solution in the treatment of moderate to severe ocular inflammation after cataract surgery: a randomized, vehicle-controlled clinical trial. Am J Ophthalmol. 1999;127:253-9.
11. Hirneiss C, Neubauer AS, Kampik A, Schonfeld CL. Comparison of prednisolone 1%, rimexolone 1% and ketorolac tromethamine 0.5% after cataract extraction A prospective, randomized, double-masked study. Graefes Arch Clin Exp Ophthalmol. 2005 9; [Epub ahead of print]
12. Kaiser PK, Pineda R 2nd. A study of topical nonsteroidal anti-inflammatory drugs and no pressure patching in the treatment of corneal abrasions. Corneal Abrasion Patching Study Group. Ophthalmology 1997;104:1353-9.

13. McColgin AZ, Heier JS. Control of intraocular inflammation associated with cataract surgery. Curr Opin Ophthalmol. 2000;11(1):3-6.
14. Mentes J, Erakgun T, Afrashi F, Kerci G.Incidence of cystoid macular edema after uncomplicated phacoemulsification. Ophthalmology. 2003;217(6):408-12.
15. O'brien TP. Emerging guidelines for use of NSAID therapy to optimize cataract surgery patient care. Curr Med Res Opin 2005;21(7):1131-8.
16. Polansky JR, Weinreb RN. Steroids as anti-inflammatory agents. In: Sears ML, (Ed). Pharmacology of the Eye. New York, NY: Springer-Verlag; 1984:460-538.
17. Price FW Jr, Price MO, Zeh W, Dobbins K. Pain reduction after laser in situ keratomileusis with ketorolac tromethamine ophthalmic solution 0.5%: a randomized, double-masked, placebo-controlled trial. J Refract Surg. 2002 Mar-Apr;18(2):140-4.
18. Price FW, Tonon E, VanDenburgh AM, Stern K, Cheetham JK, Schiffman RM. Safety and Efficacy of Reformulated Ketorolac Tromethamine 0.4% Ophthalmic Solution in Post-Photorefractive Keratectomy Patients. Presented at ARVO, 2003.
19. Price MO, Price FW. Efficacy of topical ketorolac tromethamine 0.4% for control of pain or discomfort associated with cataract surgery. Curr Med Res Opin. 2004 Dec;20(12):2015-9.
20. Quinn CJ. Cystoid macular edema. Optom Clin. 1996;5(1):111-30.
21. Ray S. D'Amico DJ. Pseudophakic macular edema. Semin Ophthalmol 2002;17: 167-80.
22. Rho DS, Soll SM. Combination Therapy for Pseudophakic Cystoid Macular Edema: Diclofenac Sodium 0.1% and Prednisolone Acetate 1% Versus Ketorolac Tromethamine 0.5% and Prednisolone Acetate 1%. Presented at ARVO, 2004.
23. Rho DS. Treatment of acute pseudophakic cystoid macular edema: Diclofenac versus ketorolac. J Cataract Refract Surg. 2003;29(12):2378-84.
24. Roberts CW. Comparison of the Ocular Comfort of Acular LS with Acular PF in Healthy Volunteers. Presented at ARVO, 2004.
25. Roberts CW. Pretreatment with topical diclofenac sodium to decrease postoperative inflammation. Ophthalmology. 1996;103:636-9.
26. Rossetti L, Autelitano A. Cystoid macular edema following cataract surgery. Curr Opin Ophthalmol 2000;11:65-72.
27. Sandoval HP, Fernandez de Castro LE, Vroman DT, Solomon KD. Comparison of 0.4% Ketorolac Tromethamine Ophthalmic Solution vs 0.5% Ketorolac Tromethamine Ophthalmic Solution to Prevent Inflammation After Phaco-emulsification and Intraocular Lens Implantation: A Prospective, Randomized, Double-Masked, Clinical Trial. Presented at ARVO, 2005.
28. Schechter BA, Wittpenn JR. Evaluation of Ketorolac (Acular LS) During the Induction Phase of Cyclosporine a (Restasis) Therapy to Improve Patient Comfort. Presented at ARVO, 2005.
29. Singal N, Hopkins J. Pseudophakic cystoid macular edema: ketorolac alone vs. ketorolac plus prednisolone. Can J Ophthalmol 2004;39(3):245-50.
30. Snyder RW, Siekert RW, Schwiegerling J, Donnenfeld E, Thompson P. Acular as a single agent for use as an antimiotic and anti-inflammatory in cataract surgery. J Cataract Refract Surg. 2000;26:1225-7.
31. Snyder RW, Siekert RW, Schwiegerling J, Donnenfeld E, Thompson P. Acular as a single agent for use as an antimiotic and anti-inflammatory in cataract surgery. J Cataract Refract Surg. 2000;26:1225-7.

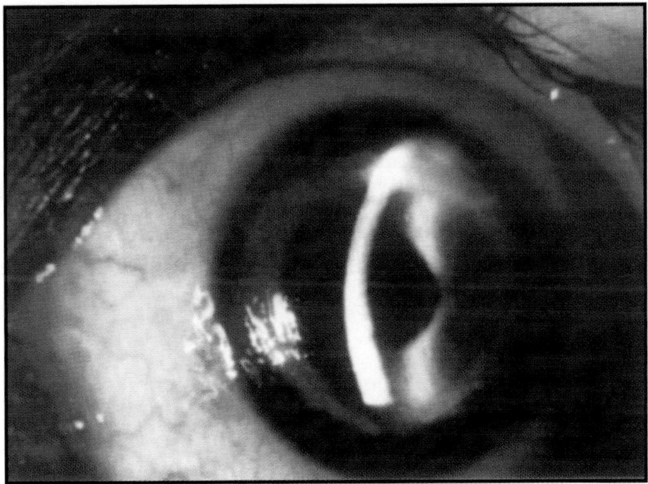

Fig. 29.1: Overlying epithelial defect

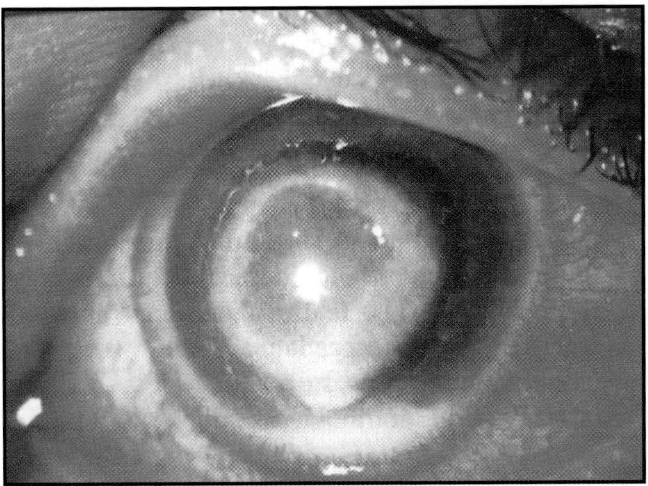

Fig. 29.2: Stromal thinning

infiltration and conjunctival congestion, slow progression and responds to topical steroid therapy. In contrast, the ring infiltration in gram-negative keratitis is fulminant, typically occurs 2-3 days after the onset of symptoms and worsens rapidly if treatment is not started immediately. Another reported feature is the occurrence of multiple scattered subepithelial infiltrates that appear to respond to topical steroid therapy and may be a reaction to the presence of antigen released from killed amoebae. At this stage, this lesion can be confused with the nummular keratitis lesion caused by *Herpes simplex* viruses. Advanced stages of the infection are characterized by central corneal epithelial loss and marked stromal opacity. Vascularization may occur, but it is not usually marked unless secondary bacterial infection has occurred.

2. Scleral changes
   Very often the sclera is not involved with this disease. In advanced cases of Acanthamoebic stromal keratitis, contiguous nodular scleritis may develop. The development of nodular scleritis indicates a poor prognosis for the survival of the eye. Isolated scleral involvement has not been reported.
3. Limbitis
   It has been reported to be a frequent accompaniment, especially in ulcers extending close to the corneal periphery and is characterized by areas of limbal hyperemia and edema.
4. Miscellaneous
   Other anterior segment findings, which can be associated, include hypopyon and glaucoma.[19]

Posterior Segment

Involvement of the posterior segment is extremely rare, although occasional reports exist of optic nerve edema, optic neuropathy and optic atrophy, retinal detachment, choroidal inflammation and macular scar.

PATHOLOGY

Both trophozoites and cysts are seen in histologic sections of infected corneal tissue. Rarely, the parasite has been found in the iris and ciliary body. Evidence of inflammatory response is usually minimal in areas of trophozoite invasion.

DIAGNOSIS

Early diagnosis of Acanthamoeba is important to limit the relentless progression of the disease. The clinical characteristic that helps distinguish Acanthamoeba keratitis from other causes of keratitis is:

a. Ring infiltrate
b. Radial keratoneuritis
c. Pain out of proportion of the clinical findings
d. Elevated epithelial lines
e. Unhealthy, sick looking epithelium with micro-erosions
f. Relative lack of vascularization in light of the chronicity and severity of the disease.
g. History of contact lens use.

DIFFERENTIAL DIAGNOSIS

Acanthamoeba keratitis is often confused with viral keratitis since they share a lot of clinical features. In the initial stages, it may mimic dendritic keratitis and in later stages it may typically mimic viral stromal keratitis and immune ring formation. Like viral stromal keratitis, it may respond to topical steroid therapy initially.

LABORATORY DIAGNOSIS

Once the clinical suspicion of Acanthamoeba keratitis has been raised, laboratory confirmation of the disease should take place prior to starting treatment. The clinically involved epithelium and stroma are scraped vigorously with a sharpened Kimura spatula or a No. 15 Bard Parker blade. Too superficial scrapings may be a reason for non-identification of the organism in smears. If there is deep stromal infiltrate, then a corneal biopsy may be preferred in some cases.

Commonly the cysts and rarely the trophozoites can be identified in corneal scrapings or smears by staining with Gram and Giemsa and potassium hydroxide stain. It has been our experience that Gram staining and potassium hydroxide wet mount preparation are very specific and sensitive for the rapid identification of the organism and may be the only stains required for smear examination. These two smears also show a high correlation with positive cultures. In the potassium hydroxide mount, the cysts stand out as having a double cell wall with cytoplasmic granularity (Fig. 29.3) and the Gram stain reveals the double cell walled nature of these cysts. Trophozoites and cysts stain purple with Giemsa-Wright staining. The trophozoite is characterized

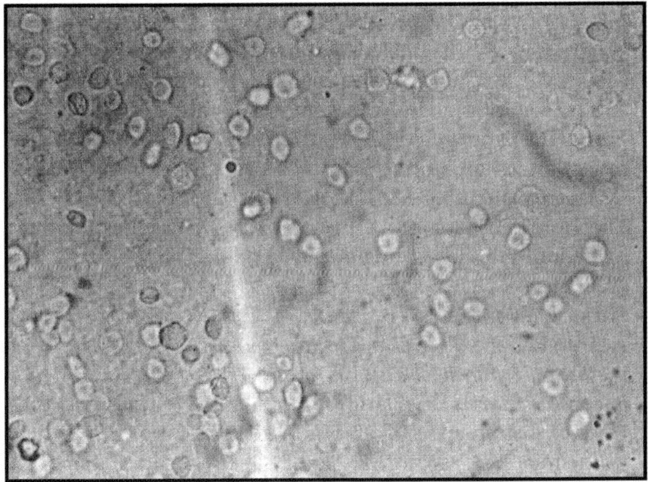

Fig. 29.3: Cytoplasmic granularity

by a large single nucleus and spindle like pseudopodia. It is much easier to recognize the cysts, which are double walled, with the inner wall having a variety of polygonal shapes.

Smears can also be examined using the chemofluorescent dyes such as calcofluor white, and Concanayalin A viewed with a fluorescent microscope.[20] Cysts measuring 10 to 25 mm in diameter appear bright green, and trophozoite measuring 15-20 mm in diameter appears bright orange. Viewed with an ultraviolet light, the chemofluorescent dye appears white. Enzymatic digestion of the background stroma enhances visualization. The method requires a fluorescent microscope and an individual skilled in the identification of Acanthamoeba species, because calcofluor also stains the cell wall of fungi.

The ideal method to be used for growing Acanthamoeba organism is to culture the specimen on a confluent lawn of *Escherichia coli* (monoaxonic culture) plated on nutrient agar.[21] The enteric gram-negative bacteria such as *E.coli* are a food source for Acanthamoeba. In this technique, Acanthamoeba trophozoites now tracks through the lawn of the bacteria. The bacteria will not fill in these paths, because the bacteria are plated in non-nutrient agar. The trailing should be demonstrated on at least one serial plating transfer to be suggestive of Acanthamoeba. Macrophages and polymorphonuclear cells can also produce trails after initial plating (pseudotrails), but leukocytes will not replicate these trails on serial transfer. Two plates are prepared for incubation at 25°C and 37°C, since some species do not grow at higher temperatures. Trophozoites can be identified under the microscope for the presence of contractile vacuoles.

Species identification is based on cyst morphology, immunofluorescent identification, isoenzyme profile, lectin reaction and DNA analysis.

Tandem scanning confocal microscopy has been used in the diagnosis and managing Acanthamoeba keratitis because of the ability to detect the organism on cornea *in vivo*.[22] More recently a study demonstrated that polymerase chain reaction (PCR) analysis of epithelial biopsy specimens could provide definitive verification of the confocal microscopic and histologic identification of Acanthamode organisms associated with keratitis.[25]

TREATMENT

Medical

The initial treatment of choice is using a variety of medical therapies. The various agents described as being helpful in this condition include:

1. Aromatic diamidines [0.1% propamidine isethionate drops and 0.15% dibromopropamidine ointment (Brolene), pentamidine (0.05%)].[23] The diamidines are: frequently used in the treatment regimen. These drops may be started at every half-hour intervals during the day and tapered. Lack of adequate amoebic activity, poor bioavailability, acquired resistance and induced encystment from subcysticidal drug levels are possible reasons for treatment failure.

2. Aminoglycosides (Neomycin): Aminoglycosides with antiamoebic activity include neomycin and paromomycin. Neomycin is commercially available and can be prepared as 8 mg/ml or fortified up to 20 mg/ml.
3. Imidazoles and triazole antifungals (Clotrimazole 1%, Miconazole, Ketoconazole, Itraconazole): Imidazole compounds such as miconazole and clotrimazole can be used topically as a 1-2 percent suspension. Oral therapy with ketoconazole, fluconazole or itraconazole may play an important adjunctive role.
4. Polymyxins.
5. Cationic antiseptics (Polyhexamethylbiguanide and chlorhexidine):[24] Polymeric biguanides are available as a contact lens disinfectant at a low (0.00005%) concentration and as a swimming pool supplement at a high concentration (20%). These biocides interfere with cytoplasmic membrane integrity and inhibit essential respiratory enzymes of multiple microbes. A diluted concentration of PHMB (0.02%) appears clinically useful in the anterior chamber.

At our institute, we commence treatment using 0.02 percent PHMB drops as monotherapy, hourly for the first 15 days and titrate following host response. The treatment is continued at reduced intervals for at least three months after the ulcer has clinically healed. Often the treatment schedules take place for a minimum period of 6 months. The chronic use of PHMB induces severe stromal vascularization, which disappears over a period of time after discontinuation of the drug. Supplementary therapy includes cycloplegics for the treatment of associated uveal inflammation and antiglaucoma medication in cases of increased intraocular pressure. Pain management is an important aspect in the later part of the disease. Sulindac has been found to be of some benefit in the treatment of pain by some investigators.

Topical Corticosteroids

Are used in the early cases of undiagnosed Acanthamoeba keratitis, however their use is controversial. Although steroids may partially suppress the inflammation associated with Acanthamoeba species infection, inhibiting the host response may ultimately prolong the course of the disease.

Penetrating Keratoplasty

The timing and indications for penetrating keratoplasty are not established. Some authors advocate debulking the cornea while the infection is limited. Successful cases with surgery alone have been reported. Others prefer first to treat medically and eradicate the infection.

REFERENCES

1. Kingston D, Warhorst DC. Isolation of amoeba from the air. J Med Microbiol 1969;2:27-36.

2. Culberton CG. The pathogenicity of soil amoeba. Ann Rev Microbiol 1971;25: 231-54.
3. Page FC. Taxonomic and ecological distribution of potentially pathogenic free living amoebas. J Parasitol 1970;56 (Suppl):257.
4. Kyle DE, Noblet GP. Seasonal distributions of thermoloterant free living amoebas. I Willard's Pond. J Protozool 1986;33:422-34.
5. Sawyer TK, Visvesvara GS, Harke BA. Pathogenic amoebas from brackish and ocean sediments. Science 1977;196:1324-25.
6. Mazor T, Hadas E, Jwanika I. The duration of the cyst stage and the viability and violence of Acanthamoeba isolates. Trop Med Parasitol 1995;46:106-08.
7. Sharma S, Srinivasan M, George C. Acanthamoeba keratitis in non-contact lens wearers. Arch Ophthalmol 1990;108:676-78.
8. Stetir Green JK, Bailey TM, Visvesvara GS. The epidemiology of Acanthamoeba keratitis in the Unites States. Am J Ophthalmol 1989;107:331-36.
9. Radford CF, Bacon AS, Part JKG, et al. Risk factors for Acanthamoeba keratitis in contact lens users—a case control study. BMJ 1995;310:1567-70.
10. Stetir-Green JK, Bailey TM, Brandt FH, et al. Acanthamoeba keratitis in soft contact lens wearers—a case control study. JAMA 258: 57-60, 1987.
11. Kilvington S, Larkin DFP, White DG, et al. Laboratory investigation of Acanthamoeba keratitis. J Clin Microbiol 1990;28:2722-25.
12. Seal D, Staphleton F, Dart J. Possible environmental sources of Acanthamoeba sp in contact lens wearers. Br J Ophthalmol 1992;76:424-27.
13. Berger ST, Mondino BJ, Hoft RH et al. Successful medical management of Acanthamoeba keratitis. Am J Ophthalmol 1990;110:395-403.
14. Johns KJ, O'Day DM, Head WS, et al. Herpes simplex masquerade syndrome: Acanthamoeba keratitis. Curr Eye Res 1987;6:207-12.
15. Moore MB, McCulley JP, Kaufman HE, et al. Radial keratoneuritis as a presenting sign in Acanthamoeba keratitis.
16. Perry HD, Donnenfeld ED, Foulks GN, et al. Decreased corneal sensation as an initial feature of Acanthamoeba keratitis. Ophthalmol 1995;102:1565-68.
17. Theodore FH, Jakobiec FA, Juechter KB, et al. Diagnostic value of a ring infiltrates in Acanthamoeba keratitis. Ophthalmol 1995;92:1471-79.
18. Hirst LW, Green WR, Merz W, et al. Management of Acanthamoeba keratitis—a case report and review of the literature. Ophthalmol 1984;91:1105-11.
19. Bacon AS, Frazen DG, Dart JKG, et al. A review of 72 consecutive cases of Acanthamoeba keratitis 1984-1992. Eye 1993;7:719-25.
20. Wilhelmus KR, Osato MS, Font, et al. Rapid diagnosis of Acanthamode keratitis using calcofluor white. Arch Ophthalmol 1986;104:1309.
21. Ma P, Visvesvara GS, Martine AJ, et al. Naegleria and Acanthamoeba infections: Review. Rev Infect Dis 1990;12:490.
22. Cavanagh HD, Patroll WM, Alizadeh H, et al. Clinical and diagnostic use of *in vivo* confocal microscopy in patients with corneal disease. Ophthalmol 1993;100(10):1444.
23. Mathers WD, Nelson SE, Lane JL, et al. Confirmation of confocal microscopy diagnosis of Acanthamoeba keratitis using polymerase chain reaction analysis. Arch Ophthalmol 2000;118:178-83.
24. Wright P, Warhorst D, Jones BR. Acanthamoeba keratitis successfully treated medically. Br J Ophthalmol 1985;69:778.
25. Mandell GL, Bennett JE, Dolin R. In Mandell, Douglas and Bennett's (Eds): Principles and Practice of Infectious Diseases (4th ed). Churchill Livingstone: New York 1997;1118.

Chapter 30

Immunosuppressive Drugs in Ophthalmology

Ashok Garg (India)

INTRODUCTION

Immunosuppressive drugs should be prescribed by ophthalmologist preferably with greater caution and in concert with an oncologist.

Till date there appears to have been very low incidence of severe complications from the combined regimen of corticosteroids and immunosuppressive agents probably because of lower dosage use and better general health of ophthalmic patients receiving them. Patients should be fully informed as to potential risks and benefits.

SELECTION OF PATIENTS

- Selection involves those patients who have progressive, usually bilateral vision threatening disease.
- Failed to respond to conventional Corticosteroid therapy or have unacceptable side effects from them
- Have wegener's granulomatosis, Polyarteritis nodosa or Behcet's disease (Drugs of first choice).
- Have adequate follow-up
- Good compliance about following instructions.
- Are ready to undergo therapy voluntarily with knowledge of potential side effects.
- May benefit certainly from the use of the drugs.
- Have no primary contraindication like active tuberculosis, toxoplasmosis or other infectious process.

Immunosuppressive agents used in ocular inflammatory diseases are classified into three groups:

a. Alkylating agents
b. Antimetabolites
c. Antibiotics

ALKYLATING AGENTS

Common alkylating agents used in ophthalmic conditions are cyclophosphamide and chlorambucil. They work by suppression of lymphocyte T cell (cell mediated immunity) and to lesser extent B cell (antibodies) function.

Clinical Indications

Behcet's disease, sympathetic ophthalmia, rheumatoid arthiritis, Polyarteritis nodosa, Wegner's granulomatosis, Relapsing Poly chondritis, Bullous pemphigoid and Malignancy.

Dosage

Cyclophosphamide

In adult patients start at 150-200 mg/day (1-2 mg/Kg/day) taken empty stomach. A white Blood Count (WBC) is taken at day 1 and after every 2-3 days until at about 7 days. At this point dosage is reduced by 25-50 mg to stabilise the WBC at about 3000 cells/ul. WBC and CBC with differential are than followed weekly and fortnightly once stabilised.

Chlorambucil Dosage

In adult patients start at 0.1-0.2 mg/kg/day and increased every 3-4 days to total dosage of 10-12 mg/day if there is no idiosyncratic reaction. The WBC and CBC with DLC are followed as for cyclophosphamide.

Adverse Reactions

Adverse side effects of alkylating agents include:
- Thrombocytopenia
- Anemia and oppurtunistic infections
- GIT disturbances
- Alopecia, Jaundice
- Pulmonary interstitial fibrosis
- Renal toxicity and testicular atrophy
- Hemorrhagic cystitis is an indication for discontinuing the medication. There is report of increased incidence of myeloproliferative and Lymphoproliferative malignancy in patients on these drugs.

THE ANTIMETABOLITES

The antimetabolites used in ophthalmology are:
1. Azathioprine which interfers with purine metabolism.
2. Methotrexate which interfers with folate action.

   Both functions are essential for nucleic acid synthesis.

Clinical Indications

- In rheumatoid arthiritis, pemphigoid and regional ileitis.
- Sympathetic ophthalmia and VKH syndrome
- Pars planitis and Behcet's disease.
- Recalcitrant cases of Intermediate uveitis.

Dosage

Azathioprine

Azathioprine dosage starts at 1-2 mg/kg/day gradually increasing to 2.5 mg/kg/day. The usual dose range is 100-200 mg/day in one or divided doses. Patient WBC, CBC with differential are taken at regular intervals.

Adverse reaction
- Uncontrolled Leukopenia
- Thrombocytopenia
- Hyper uricemia
- GIT disturbances.

Methotrexate Dosage

Methotrexate dosage is variable due to high drug toxicity. Generally for 1-4 weeks oral, IM or IV dose of 2.5-15 mg is given over 36-48 hours until a therapeutic response is noted and then maintained as per haematologic (weekly) and renal and hepatic (monthly) monitoring.

Adverse effects of methotrexate
- Leukopenia and thrombocytopenia
- Hepatic and renal toxicity
- GIT disturbances
- Interstitial pneumonitis
- CNS toxicity and sterility.

Hematological monitoring (WBC, CBC with differential) is similar to that of cyclophosphamide.

THE ANTIBIOTIC CYCLOSPORIN A

It probably interfers with T cell Lymphocyte activation and interleukin activity and Dapsone may work by lysosomal stabilization.

Indications

Clinical Indications for Cyclosporin A

- Behcets disease (for which corticosteroids are contraindicated).
- Birdshot chorioretinopathy
- Sarcoid, VKH and sympathetic ophthalmia

Relative Indications are

All non infectious cases of uveitis unresponsive to maximum tolerated steroid therapy.

- Eale's disease
- Retinal vasculitis (non-infectious)
- Serpiginous choroiditis.
- Anterior segment diseases include Pemphigoid, Mooren's ulcer, High risk corneal transplant rejection and cataract surgery in uveitis patients.

Dosage

2.5-5 mg/kg/day given orally in an olive oil – ethanol solution with milk or juice. Maximum dose is 10 mg/kg/day.

Adverse Effects

- Systemic hypertension
- Partially reversible renal toxicity
- Opportunistic infections
- Hyperuricemia
- Hepatotoxicity

Monthly and if required weekly blood tests (CBC with differential and WBC) should monitor these effects.

I. A combination of steroid and cyclosporin A therapy augment each other such that addition of Prednisone (10-20 mg/day) or short-term 1 mg/kg/day may allow a lowering of the cyclosporin A dosage. (4-6 mg/kg/day) with no loss of therapeutic efficacy).

II. Chlorambucil or cyclophosphamide and steroid management Module
It involves initial treatment with prednisone 1 mg/kg/day along with cytotoxic drug at an appropriate dose. This treatment should be continued for 4 weeks until the disease is suppressed than steroids are tapered and stopped over 2 months. The cytotoxic drug dose is adjusted to keep the WBC at 3000-4000/ul and continued for one year to induce remission before being stopped. Monitor the CBC and urine analysis weekly until stable than at every 2 weeks.

OCULAR DRUG TOXICITY OF IMMUNOSUPPRESSIVE AGENTS USED IN OPHTHALMIC CONDITIONS

- Decrease in vision
- Visual Hallucinations
- Lids or conjunctiva – redness, conjunctivitis, subconjunctival haemorrhage and hypertrichosis
- Eyelashes or brow losses

- Retinal hemorrhages
- Retinal pigment epithelium disturbances
- Cortical blindness (cyclosporin).

RECENT ADVANCES IN IMMUNOSUPPRESSIVE THERAPY

a. Active research is going on competitive inhibition of IgE binding to effector cells using Fc fragments from human IgE. Isolation of the specific binding site and fragment production with recombinant DNA technology may allow selective inhibition of mast cells or eosinophils in ocular allergic disorders.

b. Adhesion molecules are proteins that allow cells to interact with one another. In patients of SAC and VKC there is a marked increase in conjunctival expression of ICAM-1, ICAM-3 and other adhesion molecules when compared to normal.

   Intensive efforts are going on in developing specific therapeutic agents that can modulate these adhesion molecule (proteins) and diminish the allergic response.

c. Clinical trials are going on in development of suitable therapeutic agents that could modulate the actions of cytokines such as IL-3, IL-5 and GM-CSF suppressing aspects of the immune response that are not strongly affected by current available medications. A better clinical understanding of the role of specific cytokines in the different ocular allergic disorders shall stimulate the development of tailoring therapeutic agents to each of these entities.

Liposomes

New drug delivery systems may offer advantages in future therapy for ocular allergic disorders. Liposomes are vesicles consisting of lipid bilayers alternating with aqueous compartments. They may provide several advantages over current therapeutic modalities in ocular diseases.

- These allow prolonged contact between the medication and ocular tissue by preventing excessive rapid drug removal via tears.
- Changes in lipid composition and liposome struc-ture can alter the amount of intraocular drug absorption.
- Incorporation of monoclonal antibodies into outer lipid bilayer of the liposome would transport the liposome to the target tissue or cell type where the drug is required.

A safe liposome system is now available for ocular use. Cationic lipids such as BDSA can be added to the outer surface of liposomes thereby increasing the contact time of medication with ocular tissues. This liposome system cause minimal eye irritation and may prove valuable in clinical treatment of ocular allergy.

BIBLIOGRAPHY

1. Agarwal Amar. Textbook of Ophthalmology, ed.1, New Delhi: Jaypee Brothers Medical Publishers, 2002.
2. Bartlett JD. Clinical Ocular Pharmacology, ed.4, Boston: Butterworth-Heinemann, 2001.
3. Bartlett JD. Ophthalmic Drug Facts, Lippincott – William and Wilkins, 2001.
4. Bartlett JD, Ross RN. Primary Care of Ocular Allergy, J. Am. Optom Assoc, 1990;61:S3-46.
5. Ciprandi G, et al. Drug Treatment Allergic Conjunctivitis: Drugs 1992;43:154.
6. Crick RP, Trimble RB. Textbook of Clinical Ophthalmology, Hodder and Stoughton, 1986.
7. Duane TD. Clinical Ophthalmology, ed. 4: Butterworth – Heinemann, 1999.
8. Duvall. Ophthalmic Medications and Pharmacology, Slack Inc, 1998.
9. Ellis PP. Ocular Therapeutics and Pharmacology, ed. 7: CV Mosby, 1985.
10. Fechner. Ocular Therapeutics, Slack Inc., 1998.
11. Fraunfelder. Current Ocular Therapy, ed. 5: WB Saunders, 2000.
12. Garg Ashok. Current Trends in Ophthalmology, ed. 1, New Delhi: Jaypee Brothers Medical Publishers, 1997.
13. Garg Ashok. Manual of Ocular Therapeutics, ed. 1, New Delhi: Jaypee Brothers Medical Publishers, 1996.
14. Garg Ashok. Ready Reckoner of Ocular Therapeutics, ed.1, New Delhi, 2002.
15. Goodman LS. Gilman A, Pharmacological Basis of Therapeutics, ed 7, New York: Macmillan, 1985.
16. Havener's. Ocular Pharmacology, ed. 6: CV Mosby, 1994.
17. Kanski. Clinical Ophthalmology, ed 4: Butterworth – Heinemann, 1999.
18. Kershner. Ophthalmic Medications and Pharmacology, Slack. Inc., 1994.
19. Olin BR, et al. Drugs Facts and Comparisons: Facts and Comparisons, St. Louis, 1997.
20. Onofrey. The Ocular Therapeutics; Lippincott-William and Wilkins, 1997.
21. Rhee. The Wills Eye Drug Guide, Lippincott–William and Wilkins, 1998.
22. Steven Podos. Textbook of Ophthalmology, New Delhi: Jaypee Brothers Medical Publishers, 2001.
23. Zimmerman. Textbook of Ocular Pharmacology, Lippincott and William and Wilkins, 1997.

Chapter 31

Management of Cystoid Macular Edema

Arturo Pérez-Arteaga, René Cano-Hidalgo (Mexico)

INTRODUCTION

Cystoid macular edema (CME) is an inflammatory condition of the central retina that can be produced for many causes, since drugs for other ophthalmic diseases until surgical intervention of the eye. If well the initial descriptions of the disease can be found as a surgical complication, now we know much more conditions that can produce these clinical and para-clinical findings, so that we can talk about a multi-factorial disease.

Many drugs are involved in the treatment of this condition. The choose of each one is according the etiology of the inflammatory process, preference of the physician, response of the patient, underlying disease, severity of visual loss and anatomic findings. Even surgical treatment has been described, and so the use of specifical drugs during and after the procedure; so it is a very good way to review the drugs involved in the treatment of this pathologic condition according to the philosophy of this book, the use of anti-inflammatory drugs in ophthalmology. In fact several proven treatment modalities are available and so on new therapies are continuing to expand our horizons.

First the reader will find in this chapter a brief description of CME definition, etiology, clinical findings and diagnostic strategies. Then the drugs that are involved in the treatment of this condition, including those used in the surgical treatment will be described.

Definitions

CME is a pathologic condition of the macula with swelling where multiple cyst-like (cystoid) areas of fluid appear in the central retina, mostly in the outler plexiform layer. It is a painless disorder that according to the cause and severity can be fully reversed or can cause permanent visual loss. Sometimes this condition has clinical manifestations from low to severe, but also can occur in the sub-clinic plane.

Etiology

Post-Surgical, Primary or Secondary (Capsulotomy)

It was first described as the Irving-Gass syndrome; a pathologic condition where Irving in 1953 mentioned a decrease in the visual acuity with vitreoretinal alterations after the intracapsular surgery of the lens, and Gass and Norton described the typical fluoroangiographic changes of this condition. At that time 77% of the eyes operated with intracapsular cataract surgery developed some degree of CME, even sometimes sub-clinical.

During the days of the extracapsular cataract extraction the incidence decreased because the preservation of the posterior capsule and the decrease of vitreous loss. Even so, this incidence increase when there is posterior capsule rupture in an extracapsular technique. With the entrance of phaco-emulsification techniques for cataract surgery the incidence was even less, but again, it was demostrated that the main goal to decrease this condition is the conservation of the posterior capsule and to avoid the vitreous loss. It is still to be proved that the newest technologies of minimally invasive cataract surgery can produce a statistical significance reduction of post-cataract surgery CME.

The posterior capsulotomy is also a very well known procedure that can lead to CME, and it is also related to the rupture of the retinal and aqueous barriers; so in this field new technologies and evolution of intraocular lenses that can reduce the incidence of posterior capsule opacification are very important.

Any kind of intraocular surgery can produce sometime some degree of CME. At the end the cascade of events become from the rupture of the intraocular barriers. The initial trauma (damage, surgery, etc.) produce the liberation of the chemical mediators of the inflammation to the aqueous and vitreous; mainly prostaglandins are produced by the damaged tissue and the traumatized epithelial cells, but many other factors like the complement, the platelet activation factor, lisozymal enzymes, cytokines, nitric oxide, endotheline and interleukine. We can conclude that any factor that contributes to the rupture of the barriers blood-aqueous and blood-retinal is going to increase the possibility to develope CME.

Microvascular Damage

This is commonly found in diabetic retinopathy, occlusive diseases like retinal vein occlusions, and other less commonly diseases like idiopathic juxtafoveal capillary telangiectasia. The main factor is again the rupture of the intraocular barriers that this vascular alterations produce and the liberation of the mentioned mediators during the acute vascular event. Some other factors like the VEGF and IGF-1 liberated by the ischemic tissues, have been involved in the rupture of the intraocular barriers and so in the production of CME. Any syndrome associated with sub-retinal neovascularization can have the same effect.

Inflammatory Diseases

The most well known form of uveitis that can produce CME is pars planitis; in fact CME is the main cause of visual loss in this inflammatory process, but many other forms of uveitis like Behcet´s disease, Crohn´s disease, rheumatoid arthritis, sarcoidosis and some other forms of non-specifical uveitis can produce some degree of CME. The cause is as mentioned before, the liberation of the inflammatory mediators.

Post-medication (Antiglaucoma Drugs and Preservatives)

The first reference about the relation between an anti-glaucoma medication and the development of CME was described by Becker in 1967 and was with the use of epinephrine; was noted years after, that this incidence was more in the aphakic patient. It is well known at this time, that the topical epinephrine increase the prostaglandins in the eye, in particular in the aphakic one, and so the rupture of the intraocular barriers.

Some other medications were described to produce this effect like dipivalilepinephrine, timolol and benzalconium chloride. Recently with the arise of new pharmacologic groups of anti-glaucomatous medication, in particular prostaglandins, the incidence of post-medication CME has increase. A lot of studies have been conducted in this field and what we know currently is that latanoprost, travoprost, bimatoprost and unoprostone can produce some degree of CME and that this incidence can increase with the association of risk factors like cataract surgery, uveitis, posterior capsulotomy and diabetic retinopathy.

This concepts must be taken in count by the physician at the time to prescribe this medications in particular if some risk factors are present in some patient. If the therapy can be done with another medication it will be better, but if it must be continued for some reason, the utilization of non-steroidal anti-inflammatory drugs can avoid the development of CME without loss of the hypotensor effect of the anti-glaucoma drugs. Also a constant follow-up with the explanation to the patient of specific symptoms of macular disease and Amsler test in each visit for glaucoma control, are mandatory.

Peripheral Retinal Lesions

A peripheral lesion, can lead by it self, to the rupture of the intraocular barriers and so the development of CME. It is a good behavior to explorate the periphery of the retina in a case when we find CME and we are trying to know the cause.

Tumoral Diseases

Because of accumulation of leakage and rupture of the barriers, many ocular tumors, like malignant melanomas, peripheral capillary hemangiomas and Coat´s disease can be also cause of CME.

Eye Hypotony

It can be post-traumatic, with or without rupture of the globe, it can be followed cataract surgery, glaucoma procedures or choroidal effusions of any cause. At the end, the low intraocular pressure is the cause for the rupture of the intraocular barriers and so the liberation of mediators.

Optic Nerve Diseases

Optic nerve inflammations like true papilledema, neuropathy or some ischemic diseases can produce CME.

Retinal Traction

Peripheral traction, macular traction, epiretinal membranes, and traction produced by diabetic retinopathy (even without direct macular traction) are common entities that can produce CME.

Final Common Pathway of Underlying Diseases

Ischemic, tractional, inflammatory, toxic and genetic.

Histopathology

The breakdown of the inner blood retinal barrier due to vasogenic and/or cytotoxic causes is the initial event in CME. There is a leaking of the perifoveal capillaries leading the formation of edema. The fluid collects in the loosely arranged outer plexiform layer of Henle; in this layer the fibers are arranged in an horizontal pattern. This is the cause of the petalloid flower appearance that is seen as characteristic of this disease in the angiogram (cystic pattern) (Fig. 31.1). Electronic microscopy has shown accumulation of intracellular fluid within expanded Müller cell processes.

Clinical Findings

There is always a history of previous ocular disease, surgery, medication, vitreous pathology or another condition in the patient that developes CME. Sometimes it can be very easy to obtain, like previous cataract surgey or posterior capsulotomy, but in some others, the physician must be very accurate like in glaucoma medications, posterior vitreous detachment or peripheral tears that may lead to the break of the inner blood retinal barrier.

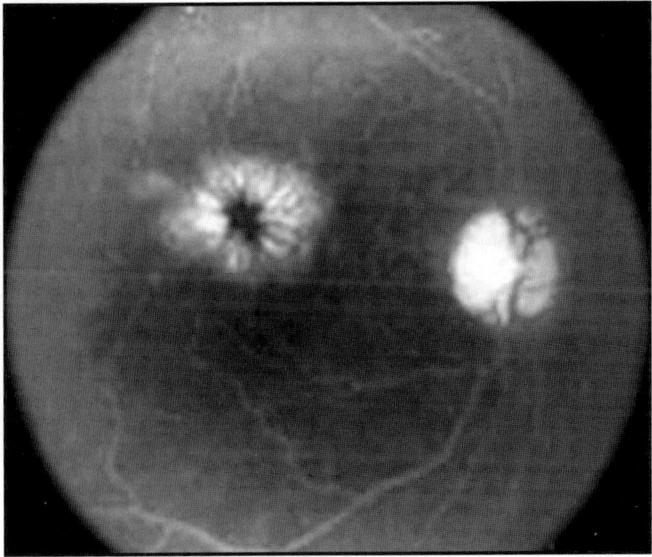

Fig. 31.1: Cystic pattern

The main symptom of CME is the reduction of visual acuity, even so, here are many forms of CME that goes free of visual symptoms. Many patients that undergo a cataract surgery can develope some degree of sub-clinical CME, and the only one evidence can be found in a retinal fluorogram. The degree of the disease and so the severity of symptoms frequently correlates with the degree of complications during the cataract surgery, if this is the case. So the reduction of visual acuity may undergo from a minimal degree, like 20/25 and be not notice by the patient, until very poor visuality like 20/400 or less in severe cases. Like some others macular diseases the patients can experience some degree of metamorphopsia.

At the clinical examination the evidence of surgery, trauma, vascular retinal diseases and others like glaucoma diseases must be achieved. Of course the main study is the fundoscopy where the macular thickening and/or swelling can be found. It also can be found in many degrees depending upon the severity of the disease, and can go since a loss of foveolar reflex without clinical evidence of edema, to a characteristic cystic appearance. This is the typical clinical finding in the ophthalmoscopy, radiating cystic spaces emanating from the macula. Of course, in these cases, there is a complete loss of the red reflex. The red free light examination is mandatory, where a "honeycombed" appearance is seen, and it corresponds to the fluid filled cyst (Fig. 31.2). In severe cases these cyst may coalesce into a macular cyst and then form a hole.

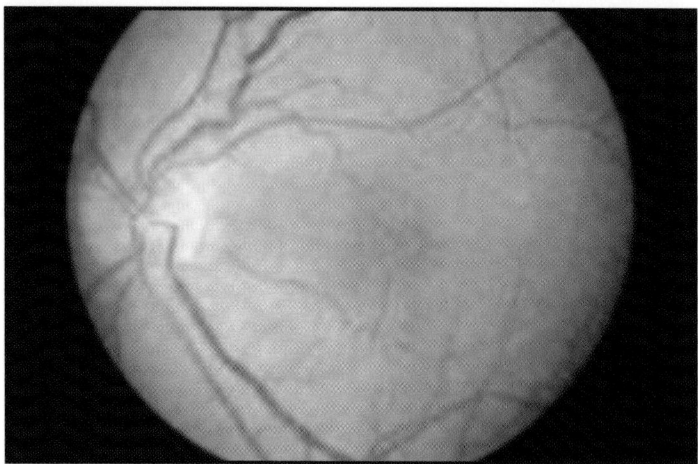

Fig. 31.2: Loss of red reflex

Paraclinical Approach

No laboratory studies are necessary to establish the diagnosis of CME. The main study in the establishment of this diagnosis is the fluorescein angiogram (FA).

In the FA parafoveal retinal capillary leakage is seen in the early and mid phases. These phases are not characteristic of CME because the accumulation of fluid in certain conditions is delayed, so the late phase has a particular importance, and it is about 20 minutes and sometimes can be more, to find the characteristic petaloid pattern of lekage in the macula.

Another related conditions can be seen in the FA according the underlying disease: if lekage microaneurysms are present, diabetic retinopathy can be the cause; vascular collaterals can be due to retinal occlusion; optic nerve findings are also useful in the final etiologic diagnosis establishment.

Optical Coherence Tomography (OCT) is a non-invasive method also very useful in the final diagnosis of CME because the fluid-filled spaces in the retina are easily seen. This cross-sectional image of the retina can also be helpful in the monitoring over time of the disease by quantifying the amount of fluid inside the retina in serial studies. A non-invasive study can be the ideal modality in monitoring the response to treatment.

In particular cases an electroretinogram can also be helpful but not mandatory.

Treatment

The treatment of CME can be divided in two approaches that finally in the practice are combined but in the theory we are going to describe separately.

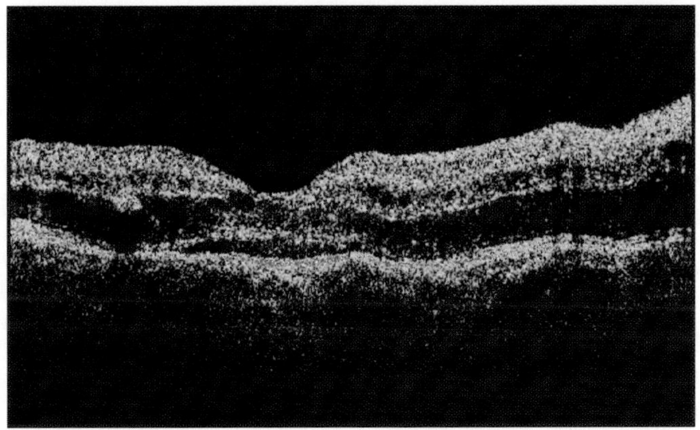

Fig. 31.3: Macular quistic edema

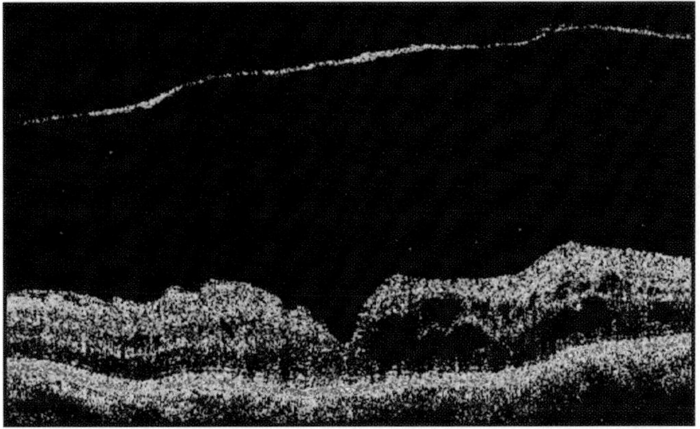

Fig. 31.4: CME plus epiretinal membrane

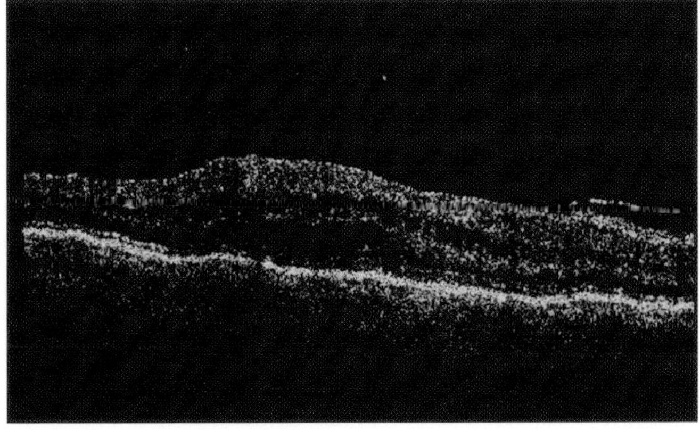

Fig. 31.5: Epiretinal membrane plus macular cystic edema

Non-surgical Approach

Many drugs have been involved for the treatment of CME during the time. Some of them are used as a traditional fashion and some others are emerging as new therapeutic resources.

a. *Non-steroidal anti-inflammatory drugs (NSAIDs)*
   The main effect of this group of drugs is to stabilize the blood-retinal barrier. This effect is because they inhibit the enzyme cyclo-oxygenase. They can be used by systemic way and also in the form of eyedrops. The main examples of this group of medications are:

1. Indomethacine.
2. Ketorolac.
3. Diclofenac.

They inhibit the prostaglandin synthesis by decreasing the activity of the enzyme cyclo-oxygenase. These drugs in the topical form must be used as a medication in the pre-operative and post-operative period of some intraocular procedures like cataract surgery, posterior capsulotomy and peripheral iridectomy for example, to reduce the incidence of CME. This prophylactic form also helps to reduce the postoperative inflammatory process. As has been said before, the development of CME in some way correlates with the degree of manipulation during the ocular surgery and some factors have been demonstrated in the development of CME like the time of light microscope exposure, posterior capsule rupture and vitreous manipulation. Of course, a real "clean" surgery can decrease the incidence of CME, but anyway, the use of NSAIDs is mandatory. New operative devices that avoid the use of direct light exposure during the ocular surgery are promising in the near future to decrease the incidence of CME in uncomplicated surgery cases.

The use of systemic NSAIDs is only reserve for the cases of complete diagnosis of CME; even so some surgeons are using them as a prophylactic medication. There is not a recommended time for the use of systemic NSAIDs for the treatment of CME; the time of use will depend upon the response of each patient in particular according the follow-up.

Because sometimes it is a long term medication, secondary effects of NSAIDs must be always taken in count. In the systemic medication, gastric effects should be monitoring during the visits of the patient. A history of gastric diseases including ulcerative disease and bleeding is mandatory when oral indomethacine is in use. If some of these effects are present the therapeutic must be suspended and replaced by other medication.

Local NSAIDs have also some secondary effects; long-term use may delay wound healing and has been reported cases of corneal stromal thinning or melting in some particular patients receiving diclofenac eyedrops for extended period of time. If symptoms like blurred or diminished vision and signs of corneal deposits, retinal changes and scotoma are present, the medication must be suspended.

b. *Corticosteroids*

Steroidal medication is very useful in the treatment of CME and also in the prevention of it. The routine use of steroids in the eyedrops form before and after surgical procedures, has decrease the incidence of postsurgical CME, even in complicated cases.

The most frequent form of steroid medication for CME is topical, in the form of prednisolone acetate; it is indicated in several conditions of steroid-responsive intraocular inflammation. The presentation is at 1% solution and can be used several times in a day according the severity of the inflammation. The amount and time of administration must be measured according the response of the disease to the treatment. Monitoring of the side effects of topical steroids like, raise in the intraocular pressure and an increased risk of secondary ocular infections, must be evaluating during the time of therapy and this should be discontinued if some of these effects are found. Not all patients have the same response to steroids according the rise in the intraocular pressure; some patients can not tolerate large periods of time without changes in the pressure, but some others can not tolerate too much medication. If the topical steroid therapy is really needed in these cases, the physician can add some glaucoma therapy; medications that can increase the CME should be avoided (e.g. latanoprost, travoprost, epinephrine); the best adjunctive anti-glaucoma medication is dorsolamide that also can have some benefit effect in the macula. Other side effects of long-term topical steroids like subcapsular cataract formation must be addressed.

The use of injections of long acting depot-steroids (eg. triamcinolone) into the sub-tenon space has also a role in the treatment of CME. This external way of administration that can have more penetration to the retina; the drug delivery to the retina is superior by this route in comparison to peribulbar. In some cases of uveitic CME refractory to conventional treatment, the triamcinolone has been used in intravitreous injection alone or in combination with some other drugs. Triamcinolone alone has been effectively in reducing CME and improving vision; some studies are currently underway in the combination of this steroidal drug with other drugs, like bevacizumab (Avastin).

Oral steroids play also an important role in the treatment of CME because the effect in the stabilization of the blood-ocular barrier. They can be useful in some forms of uveitic CME. Nevertheless the secondary effects of systemic corticoid medication must be avoided, and this is why recently the medication of CME is trying to move to the ocular space instead the systemic route.

c. *Carbonic anhydrase inhibitors (CAIs)*

Carbonic anhydrase is an enzyme present in the apical and basal surfaces of the retinal pigment epithelium cell membrane. Its action is to pump and produce a change in the ion flux. CAIs enhance this pumping action of these cells, and helps to improve this ion flux that affects the cellular environment of the retina.

CAIs are commonly used in ophthalmology, in particular in the glaucoma cases, where the topical medication is not enough to control the intraocular pressure, so it is a weel known resource. Also the physician is close to side effects of the CAIs, like the alteration in the ionic composition of blood, increase in urine excretion, and in large doses hepatic and metabolic problems. So it is known that it is not a chronic medication, it has to be used according the severity and response to treatment of CME and the physician has to advice the patient the side effects, the mode to contrarest them and the total communication they both have to mantain in order to manage the dose in good response, but also in good levels of side effects. This medication should be suspended as soon as possible according the evolution of CME.

The presentation of acetazolamide is in tablets of 250 mg and can be given until three to four times a day. Close monitoring of anti-inflammatory and side effects is mandatory.

d. *Intravitreal medication*

Recently new drugs are appearing in the retinal medication field for intravitreal injection, like Bevacizumab (avastin) and Pegaptanib, also called Macugen. These drugs are promising results in many retinal vascular disorders like occlusive diseases and diabetic retinopathy. The side effects are not completely known, and many trials around the world are in progress at this time to achieve consistent results.

The apparently possitive action seen in some vascular disorders lead the possibility to use them in CME. Some of them are including only diabetic patients, some others only postoperative cataract patients and some others are combining the avastin with triamcinolone. During the middle of year 2007 these trials will be finish and we will be able to know the safety, efficacy and probably side effects of these drugs in the treatment of CME.

Surgical Approach and Drugs Related

The surgical treatment is not the first choice in the treatment of CME; nevertheless, some particular situations can lead to the indication of pars plana vitrectomy (PPV):

- Cases of uveitis related CME.
- Remove of vitreous strands that can cave an effect of "pull the retina", from anterior and posterior segment structures.
- Remove inflammatory mediators from the vitreous (eg. memory cells, cytoquines), that can be mantaining an inflammatory response.
- Remove of retained lens fragments.
- Remove of epiretinal membrane.

Because the rupture of the blood-retinal barrier, after the PPV there is an increase in the penetration of topical and oral steroids. Also some surgeons are happy with the use of triamcinolone during the surgical approach, achieving so the beneficial effect of both, vitrectomy and intravitreal medication. We believe at this time, that the PPV by it self is not enough for the treatment of CME; we agree that it must be accompanied by intravitreal medication.

The side effects of steroids in the vitreous cavity must be addressed continuosly because the possibility of changes in IOP; in this particular case sometimes it is very dificult to achieve a good IOP because the deposit effect of the steroid. Even so, sometimes without steroid medication in the vitreous cavity, PPV it self, is able to produce an increase in IOP of dificult control.

The final decision to perform a PPV must be carefuly evaluated and consented between the surgeon and patient, because of the possible side effects.

CONCLUSIONS

At the end of the day a lot of factors are going to influence the prognosis of a patient who develops CME. The main factor of all is the inherent cause of the disease; it will not be the same a patient who develops CME because of a glaucoma treatment (in this case the suspension of the prostaglandin and the medical treatment with NSAIDs can be enough to reverse by complete the disease without any permanent loss of vision), that a CME caused by a chronic pars planitis of difficult treatment (in this case a chronic CME can lead to severe decrease of vision).

Patients who are going to be operated, in particular anterior segment procedures, must be medicated since the preoperative period, through the operation and during the postoperative time, with drugs that can decrease the development of CME, like steroids and NSAIDs according the case. After all we know about this disease, prevention and treatment we believe this should be mandatory. Also in patients with glaucoma control with prostaglandins, this therapy should be avoided and the control must be followed with another anti-glaucoma medication, during the pre, trans and postoperative period. If is not possible to eliminate the prostaglandin and NSAIDs should be started in addition.

Of particular importance is the glaucoma patient, who is receiving medication that can produce CME; the physician must be alert to any kind of sign that can advice the presentation of CME. The adjunctive NSAIDs therapy can be helpful in cases where is impossible to avoid prostaglandins.

New medications are promising good results, even alone or in combination, for the treatment of refractory CME. Like all new products, we are specting some new non-reported adverse effects; the test of time, like always, will lead us to the complete knowledge of their specific indications.

BIBLIOGRAPHY

1. Antcliff RJ, Standorf MR, Chauhan DS et al. Comparison between optical coherence tomography and fundus fluorescein angiography for detection of

cystoid macular edema in patients with uveitis. Ophthalmology 2000;107:593-599.

2. Ayyala RS, Cruz DA, Margo CE, et al. Cystoid macular edema associated with latanoprost in aphakic and pseudophakic eyes. Am J Ophthalmol 1998;126:602-4.
3. Becker B. Topical epinephrine in the treatment of the glaucomas. In New Orleans Glaucoma Symposium: 152-159. The CV Mosby Company. St Louis, 1967.
4. Bhattacherjee PKulkarny PS, Eakins KE. Metabolism of arachidonic acid in rabbit ocular tissues. Invest Ophthalmol Vis Sci 1979;18:172-8.
5. Callanan D, Fellmann RL, Savage JA. Latanoprost associated cystoid macular edema. Am J Ophthalmol 1998;126:134-5.
6. Clinical Trials Gov US National Institutes of Health. The Effect of Macugen in Patients with chronic, post-operative Cystoid Macular Edema. John Hopkins University. July, 2006. Trial ongoing.
7. Clinical Trials Gov. U.S. National Institutes of Healt. To compare Therapeutic effect of Intravitreal Bevacizumab and Triamcinolone in Resistant Uveitic Cystoid Macular Edema. Shaheed Beheshti Medical University. 2006. Trial ongoing.
8. Clinical Trials Gov. U.S. National Institutes of Health. Effect of Prophylactic Ketorolac on CME after Cataract Surgery. Queens University. May, 2006. Trial ongoing.
9. Flach AJ, Jampol LM, Weinberg D et al. Improvement in visual acuity in chronic aphakic and pseudophakic cystoid macular edema after treatment with topical 0.5% ketorolac tromethamine. Am J Ophthtalmol 1991;112:514-19.
10. Furuichi M, Chiba T, Abe K, Kogure S, Iijima H, Tsukahara S, Kashiwagi K. Cistoid macular edema associated with topical Latanoprost in glanulomatous eyes with a normal functioning blood-ocular barrier. J Glaucoma 2001;10:233-236.
11. Gass JDM, Norton EDW. Cystoid macular edema and papilledema following cataract extraction. A fluorescein, funduscopic and angiografic study. Arch Ophthalmol 1966;76:646-61.
12. Handa J, Henry JC, Krupìn T et al. Extracapsular cataract extraction with posterior chamber lens implantation in patients with glaucoma. Arch Ophthalmol 1987;105:765-9.
13. Hanna C, Sharp JD. Ocular absorption of indomethacin by the rabbit. Arc Ophthalmol 1972;88:196-8.
14. Heier JS, Steinert RF, Frederick AR. Cystoid macular edema associated with latanoprost use. Arch Ophthalmol 1998;116:680-682.
15. Irvine SR. A new defined vitreous syndrome following cataract surgery interpreted according to recent concepts of the structure of the vitreous. Am J Ophthalmol 1954;36:599-619.
16. Jaffe NS, Clayman HM, Jaffe MS. Cystoid macular edema after intracapsular and extracapsular cataract extraction with and without an intraocular lens. Ophthalmology 1982;89:25-29.
17. Jampol LM, Sanders DR, Kraff MC. Prophylaxis and therapy of aphakic cystoid macular edema. Suv Ophthalmol 1984;28:535-9.
18. Kass MA, Holmberg NJ. Prostaglandin and throinboxane synthesis by microsomes of rabbit ocular tissues. Invest Ophthalmol Vis Sci 1979;18:166-71.
19. Kent D, Vinores SA, Campochiaro PA. Macular oedema: the role of soluble mediators. Br J Ophthalmol 2000;84:542-5.

20. Kolker AE, Becker B. Epinephrine maculopathy. Ach Ophthal 1968;79:552-62.
21. Liesegang TJ, Bourne WJ, Ilstrup DM. Secondary surgical and neodimium:YAG laser discussions. Am J Ophthalmol 1985;100:164-8.
22. Lima MC, Paranhos A, Salam S, et al. Visually significant cystoid macular edema in pseudophakic and aphakic patients with glaucoma receiving Latanoprost. J of Glaucoma 2000;9:317-24.
23. Malecaze F, Chollet P, Cavrois E, et al. Role of interleukin 6 in the inflammatory response after cataract surgery. An experimental and clinical study. Arch Ophthalmol 1991;109:1681-1683.
24. Mehelas TJ, Kollarits CR, Martin WG. Cystoid macular edema presumably induced by dipivefrin hydrochloride (Propine). Am J Ophthalmol 1982;94:682.
25. Meredith TA, Kenyon KR, Singerman LJ, et al. Perifoveal vascular leakage and macular edema after intracapsular cataract extraction. Br J Ophthalmol 1976;60:765-76.
26. Michels RG, Maumenne AE. Cystoid macular edema associated with topically applied epinephrine in aphakic eyes. Am J Ophthalmol 1975;80:379-88.
27. Miyake K, Ibaraki N, Goto Y, Oogiya S, Ishigaki J, Ota I, Miyake S. ESCRS Binkhorst lecture 2002: Pseudophakic preservative maculopathy. J Cataract Refract Surg 2003;29:1800-10.
28. Miyake K, Ibaraki N. Prostaglandins and cystoid macular edema. Surv Ophthalmol 2002;47(Suppl 1):S203-S218.
29. Miyake K, Kayazawa F, Manabe R, et al. Indomethacin and the epinephrine-induced breakdown of the blood-ocular barrier in rabbits. Invest Ophthalmol Vis Sci 1988;29:332-4.
30. Miyake K, Mibu H, Horiguchi M, et al. Inflammatory mediators in postoperative aphakic and pseudophakic baboon eyes. Arch Ophthalmol 1990;108:1764-7.
31. Miyake K, Miyake Y, Kuratomi R. Long-term effects of topically applied epinephrine on the blood-ocular barrier in humans. Arch Ophthalmol 1987;105:1360-3.
32. Miyake K, Miyake Y, Maekubo K, et al. Incidence of cystoid macular edema after retinal detachment surgery and the use of topical indomethacin. Am J Ophthalmol 1985;100:510-19.
33. Miyake K, Ota I, Ibaraki N et al. Enhanced disruptionof the blood-ocular barrier and the incidente of angiographic cystoid macular edema by topical timolol and its preservative in early posoperative pseudophakia. Arch Ophthalmol 2001;119:387-94.
34. Miyake K, Ota I, Maekubo K, Ichihashi S, Miyake S. Latanoprost accelerates disruption of the blood-aqueous barrier and the incidence of angiographic cystoid macular edema in early postoperative pseudophakias. Arch Ophthalmol 1999;117:34-40.
35. Miyake K, Shirasawa E, Hikita M, et al. Síntesis of prostaglandin E in rabbit eyes with topically applied epinephrine. Invest Ophthalmol Vis Sci 1988;29:332-4.
36. Miyake K, Sugiyama S, Norimatsu I, et al. Prevention of cystoid macular edema after lens extraction by topical indomethacin. Albrecht von Graefes Arch Klin Exp Ophthalmol 1978;209:83-8.
37. Miyake K. Prevention of cystoid macular edema after lens extraction by topical indomethacin. A preliminary report. Albrecht Von Graefes Arch Klin Exp Ophthalmol 1977;203:81-8.

38. Mondino BJ, Nagata S, Glovsky MM. Activation of the alternative complement pathway by intraocular lenses. Invest Ophthalmol Vis Sci 1985;26:905-8.
39. Nishi O, Nishi K, Imanishi M. Synthesis of interleukin-1 and prostaglandin E2 by lens epithelial cells of human cataracts. Br J Ophthalmol 1992;76:338-41.
40. Ohrloff C, Schalnus R, Rothe R, et al. Role of the posterior capsule in the aqueous-vitreous barrier in aphakic and pseudophakic eyes. J Cataract Refract Surg 1990;16:198-201.
41. Ozaki H, Hayasi H, Vinores SA , et al. Intravitreal sustained release of VEGF causes retinal neovascularization in rabbits and breakdown of the blood-retinal barrier in rabbits and primates. Exp Eye Res 1997;64:505-17.
42. Pollack A, Leiba H, Bukelman A, et al. Cystoid macula oedema following cataract extraction in patients with diabetes. Br J Ophthalmol 1992;76:221-4.
43. Rossetti L, Chaudhuri J, Diickersin K. Medical prophylaxis and treatment of cystoid macular edema after cataract sugery. The results of a meta-analysis. Ophthalmology 1998;105:397-405.
44. Schumer RA, Camras CB, Mandahl AG. Putative side effects of prostaglandin analogs. Sur Ophthalmol 2002;47(Suppl 1):S219-S230.
45. Schumer RA, Camras CB, Mandalh AK. Latanoprost and cystoid macular edema: is there a causal relation? Current Opin Ophthalmol 20000;94-10.
46. Sjoquist B, Almegard B, Khalilef V, et al. The bioavailability of Xalatan in the human eye. Invest Ophthalmol Vis Sci 1997;38:S248.
47. Solomon LD. Efficacy of topical flubriprofen and indomethacin in preventing pseudophakic cystoid macular edema. Flubiprofen-CME Study Group I. J Cataract Refract Surg 1995;21:73-81.
48. Thomas JV, Gragoudas ES, Blair NP et al. Correlation of epinephrine use and macular edema in aphakic glaucomatous eyes. Arch Ophthalmol 1978;96:625-8.
49. Ursell PG, Spalton DJ, Withcup SM et al. Cystoid macular edema after phacoemulsification: Relationship to blood-aqueous barrier damage and visual acuity. J Cataract Refract Surg 1999;25:1492-7.
50. Vinores SA, Sen H, Campochiaro PA. An adenosine agonist and prostaglandin E1 cause breakdown of the blood-retinal barrier by opening tigth junctions between vascular endothelial cells. Invest Ophthalmol Vis Sci 1992;33:1870-8.
51. Wand M, Gaudio AR, Shields MB. Latanoprost and cystoid macular edema in high risk aphakic or pseudophakic eyes. J Cat Refract Surgery 2001;27:1397-1401.
52. Wand M, Gaudio AR. Cystoid macular edema associated with ocular hypotensive lipids. Am J Ophthalmol 2002;133:403-5.
53. Wand M, Shields BM. Cystoid macular edema in the era of ocular hypotensive lipids. Am J Ophthalmol 2002;133: 393-7.
54. Warwar RE, Bullock JD, Deepti B. Cystoid macular edema and anterior uveitis associated with latanoprost use. Experience and incidence in a retrospective review of 94 patients. Ophthalmology 1998;105:263-8.
55. Weisz JM, Bressler NM, Bressler SB, et al. Ketorolac treatment of pseudophakic cystoid macular edema identified more than 24 months after cataract extraction. Ophthalmology 1999; 106: 1656-1659. Schumer RA, Camras CB, Mandalh AK. Latanoprost and cystoid macular edema: is there a causal relation? Current Opin Ophthalmol 2000;94-100.
56. Yousufzai SYK, Abdel-Latif AA. Prostaglandin F2a and its analogs induce release of endogenous prostaglandins in iris and ciliary muscles isolated from cat and other mammalian species. Ex Eye Res 19996;63:305-310.

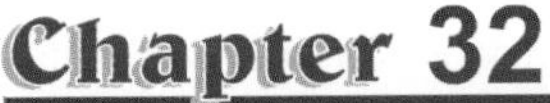

Chapter 32

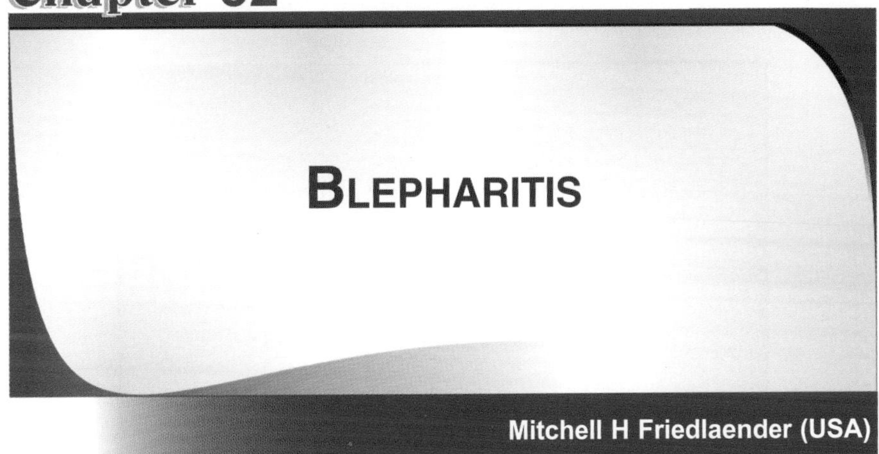

Blepharitis

Mitchell H Friedlaender (USA)

Blepharitis is a classic example of a chronic condition with infectious and inflammatory components. It is one of the most common conditions seen in ophthalmic practice, and probably represents the leading cause of "red eyes". Curiously, blepharitis has received little attention from ophthalmologists and from the pharmaceutical industry.

Classification

Blepharitis may be defined as an inflammation of the eyelids. There are a variety of causes: genetic, infectious, and allergic being the most common. There are three main anatomic patterns of blepharitis: (1) Anterior, affecting the eye lashes and surrounding tissues, (2) Posterior, affecting the meibomian oil glands, and (3) Mixed, a combination of anterior and posterior blepharitis.

Anterior blepharitis (Fig. 32.1) is characterized by seborrheic scales, known as "scurf", adhering to the eye lashes (Fig. 32.2). Fibrin deposits may be lifted from the surface of the lid margins as the lashes grow, forming rings around

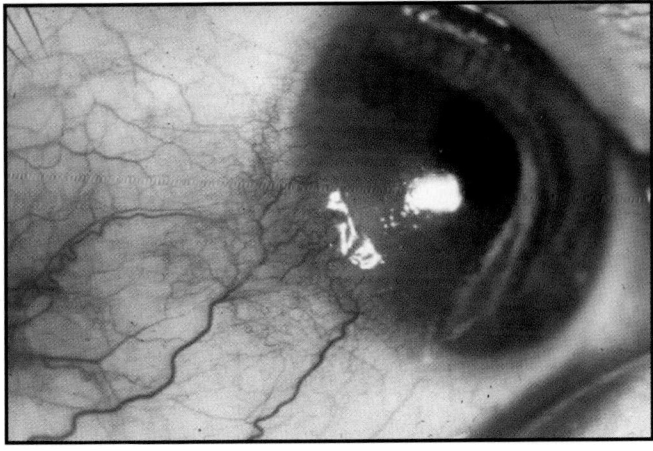

Fig. 32.1: Anterior blepharitis

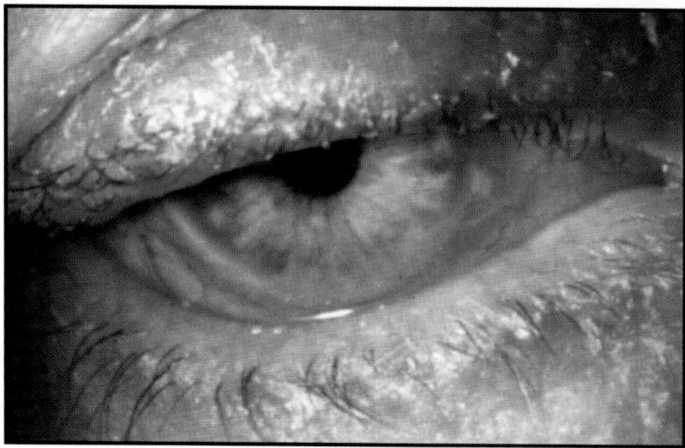

Fig. 32.2: Dandruff, or "scurf" adhering to the eyelashes

the lashes, known as "collarettes". Inflammatory material around the base of the shaft may create the appearance of "sleeves" surrounding the eyelashes.

Genetics

Genetic factors play a role in both anterior and posterior blepharitis. People with a tendency toward seborrhea, and dandruff, will often have scales adhering to the eyelashes. Individuals with rosacea have plugging of the oil glands of the nose, cheeks, and forehead (Fig. 32.3). They also have plugging of the meibomian glands (Fig. 32.4), and sluggish secretions. Complete obstruction may lead to the formation of styes, or chalazia.

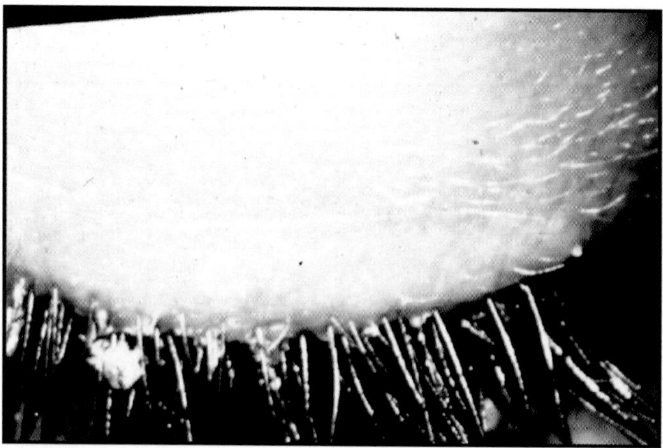

Fig. 32.3: Rosacea

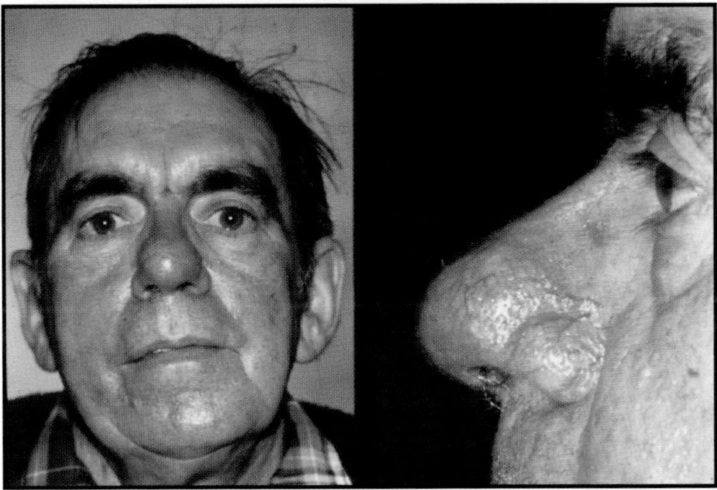

Fig. 32.4: Meibomian gland plugging

Infection

Bacteria, particularly staphylococci, have an affinity for the eyelids. It is common to culture *Staphylococcus aureus* from the lid margins of patients with blepharitis (Fig. 32.5). Other gram-positive and gram-negative organisms have also been recovered. Although swabs from the lid margins often show confluent growth of bacteria, conjunctival cutures from the same patients are often sterile. This may represent antibacterial factors in the tear film, or in the conjunctiva itself, and a resistance of conjunctival tissue to bacterial colonization.

Staphylococcus aureus can frequently be cultured from the eyelids of blepharitis patients.[1] It is widely acknowledged that staphylococcus is capable of colonizing the eyelid margins, creating a chronic, low grade infection. Staphylococcal toxins probably enter the tear film and produce symptoms such as burning, stinging, redness, and discharge. Toxins may cause inflammation and breakdown of the delicate skin of the eyelids (Fig. 32.6). Other organisms have been implicated in blepharits. For example, the parasite *Demodex folliculorum* has been found in about one-third of blepharitis cases.[2] No clear pathologic role has been established for Demodex in blepharitis, and the organism's presence may be an incidental finding. More recently, *Helicobacter pylori*, the bacteria associated with peptic ulcers, gastritis, gastric cancer, and possibly gastric lymphoma, has been found in 76% of blepharitis cases.[3] Again, a causal role for this organism has not been established. We have cultured *Serratia marscesans*, along with *Staphylococcus aureus* from the eyelids of a child with a congenital immunodeficiency syndrome.

Blepharitis is common with viral infections, particularly *Herpes simplex*, and *Herpes zoster*. These conditions are readily identified by the characteristic appearance and distribution of vesicles and pustules on the eyelids.

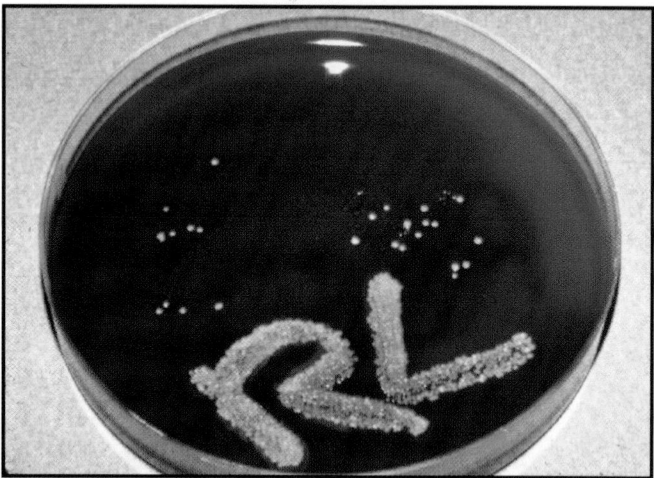

Fig. 32.5: Staphylococcus cultured from the lid margins

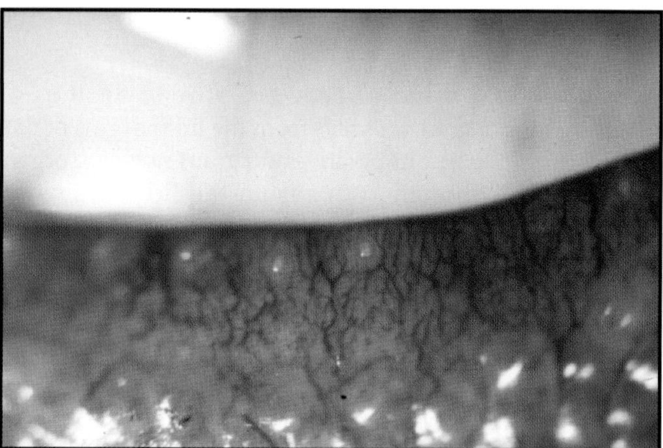

Fig. 32.6: Skin toxicity from staphylococcal blepharitis

Allergy

Allergy, particularly contact allergy, can produce inflammation of the eyelids (Fig. 32.7). Cosmetics, soaps, and shampoos, often contain allergenic substances which can cause a cell-mediated, or delayed, hypersensitivity reaction, of the eyelids. Eyedrops containing neomycin, or sulfa, are frequent causes of contact allergic blepharits Typically, contact blepharitis reactions begin one to three days after exposure to the offending agent. The eyelids become inflamed and itchy. The proper treatment involves the identification of the allergenic substance, and withdrawal of the offending agent. Corticosteroids, usually in cream or ointment form, will help relieve symptoms of itching, swelling, and discomfort.

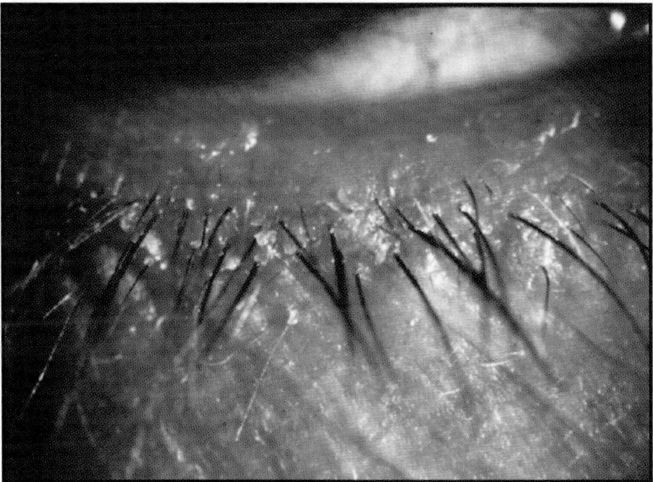

Fig. 32.7: Contact allergy

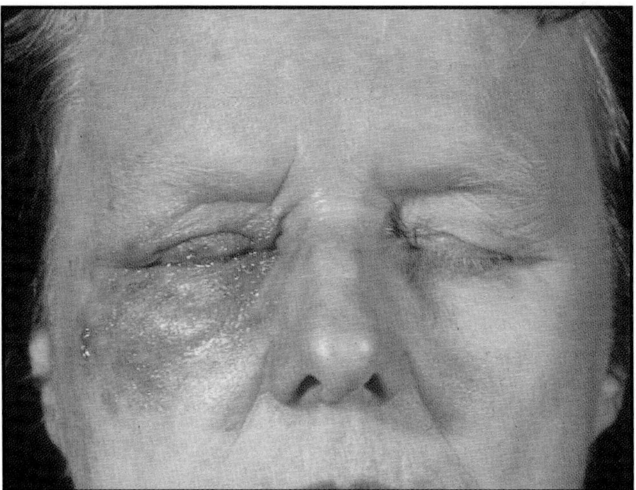

Fig. 32.8: Phlyctenule

Blepharitis can also be seen in IgE-mediated allergy, especially severe types, such as atopic keratoconjunctivitis, and vernal keratoconjunctivitis. It is believed that allergic mediators, produced by mast cells, eosinophils, and other inflammatory cells have a toxic effect on the delicate skin of the eyelids.

Corneal Manifestations

Corneal complications are often associated with chronic blepharitis. Catarrhal infiltrates occur in the peripheral cornea at the 2, 4, 8, and 10 O'clock positions (Fig. 32.8). They usually appear as white, or translucent, infiltrated, but sometimes they are confluent and may form a complete, or incomplete, ring around the cornea, approximately 1 mm central to the limbus. Catarrhal infiltrates may leave spade-shaped scars near the limbus. Sometimes, these contain a leash of blood vessels, extending in from the limbus. The appearance of these characteristic corneal scars is often a clue to the diagnosis of blepharitis. Phylectenules, are much less common than catarrhal infiltrates, but they can be associated with staphylococcal blepharitis, particularly in children.[4]

Chemistry

Considerable work has been done on the chemistry of the lipids and proteins in the meibomian oil gland secretions of patients with blepharitis. McCulley[5] has demonstrated a defect in polar lipids, and suggested this may produce an unstable tear film, and abnormally rapid tear evaporation, and a resultant dry eye. Gilbard[6] has suggested that abnormal meibomian lipids may alter tear film osmolarity, and lead to, or aggravate, a dry eye condition. The profile of tear proteins, analyzed by mass spectroscopy, is different in blepharitis patients, than in normal controls.[7]

Treatment

Treatment of blepharitis usually consists of a combination of lid scrubs and topical or systemic treatment. Lid scrubs, using baby shampoo are highly effective, and should be recommended on a daily basis. When patients include lid hygiene in their daily routine, especially during a bath or shower, they minimize symptoms, as well as periodic flare-ups. An illustrated hand out, or instruction sheet is frequently beneficial (Fig. 32.9).

Topical treatment with a broad spectrum antibiotic ointment, such as erythromycin, bacitracin, or a combination of bacitracin and polymyxin B is often useful. Antibiotic-corticosteroid combination ointments are particularly beneficial. These include tobramycin-dexamethasone combinations (Tobradex®, Alcon, Ft. Worth), and sulfacetamide sodium-prednisolone acetate (Blephamide®, Allergan, Irvine).

More recently, cyclosporine suspension,[8] and tacrolimus ointment[9] have been advocated.

Oral antibiotics may be used in the treatment of blepharitis. Most popular are tetracycline, doxycycline, minocycline, and erythromycin.[10] Often a course of a few weeks to a few months is necessary to achieve the desired effect. Patients should be made aware of the possible side effects of long-term oral antibiotics, such as photosensitivity, and opportunistic infections, such as Candida.

For the treatment of allergic contact dermatitis, the treatment is identification, withdrawal, and avoidance of the offending allergen. For atopic and vernal keratoconjunctivitis, a corticosteroid cream or ointment may be applied to the affected area of the eyelids.

Chapter 33

Toxic Anterior Segment Syndrome

Simon P Holland, Douglas W Morck, Richard Mathias, Tracy L Lee, Gina Chavez, Yumi G Ohashi (Canada)

INTRODUCTION

Toxic anterior segment syndrome (TASS) is increasingly recognized and reported as an early complication of cataract surgery.[1-9] Postoperative inflammation of unknown cause was previously considered as a sterile endophthalmitis although vitritis is uncommon. Multiple outbreaks have recently been reported stimulating extensive research and the creation of a task force. The understanding of TASS is thus rapidly evolving and will likely lead to improved prevention and management of outbreaks.

Diagnosis and Clinical Features

TASS presents as early and severe postoperative inflammation following anterior segment surgery. Symptoms include fibrin formation, corneal edema, minimal or no pain, and the absence of vitreous involvement.[10] Differentiation from conditions such as infectious endophthalmitis (IE) is critical. Table 33.1 summarizes the key differences between TASS and IE. TASS usually presents on the day of surgery or the first day postoperatively, whereas IE presents later, usually day 3 to 7, accompanied by pain and vitreal involvement.[10-13] Figure 33.1 shows a case of TASS with characteristic features presenting on the day of surgery, and Figure 33.2 shows a case of IE. Rarely low grade vitritis may be seen in severe cases of TASS probably from some spillover from the anterior segment. In such cases the vitritis is a result of culture-negative or sterile endophthalmitis rather then infectious endophthalmitis.[10,11] Vitreous taps and more recently PCR can be used to differentiate the two conditions.[14] When the diagnosis is unclear the practitioner should treat as IE due to the severity of its sequelae.[15,16]

Diagnosis
Postoperative
Anterior segment inflammation
Unknown cause

Table 33.1: Differential diagnosis TASS vs. infectious endophthalmitis

Presentation	*TASS*	*Infectious endophthalmitis*
Onset (usual)	6 to 24 hours postoperatively	3 to 7 days postoperatively
Symptoms	Blurred vision	Pain, blurred vision
Cornea	Edema	Edema
Anterior chamber	Cells Fibrin, membranes Hypopyon	Cells Fibrin variable Hypopyon
External findings	None	Variable: Lid swelling Discharge Conjunctival chemosis
Vitreous	Clear, rarely vitritis (culture negative)	Vitritis (primarily culture positive)
Response to topical steroids	Rapid improvement to resolution within days	No improvement

Differential diagnosis
Pain and/or vitritis usually indicates infectious endophthalmitis

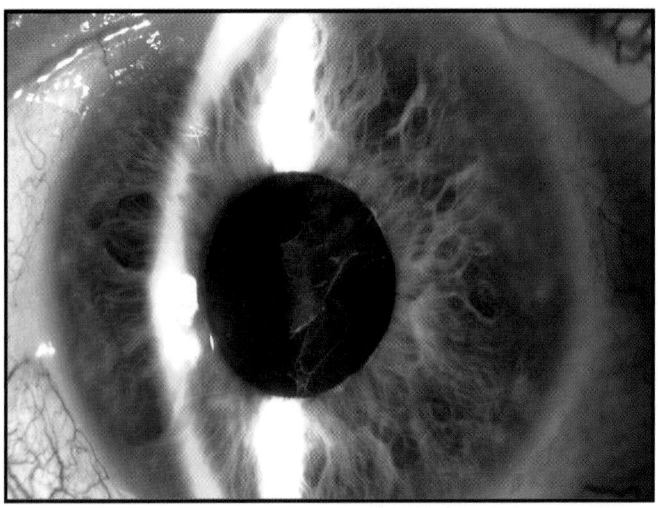

Fig. 33.1: TASS on the first postoperative day (*Courtesy*: SLACK Inc)[10]

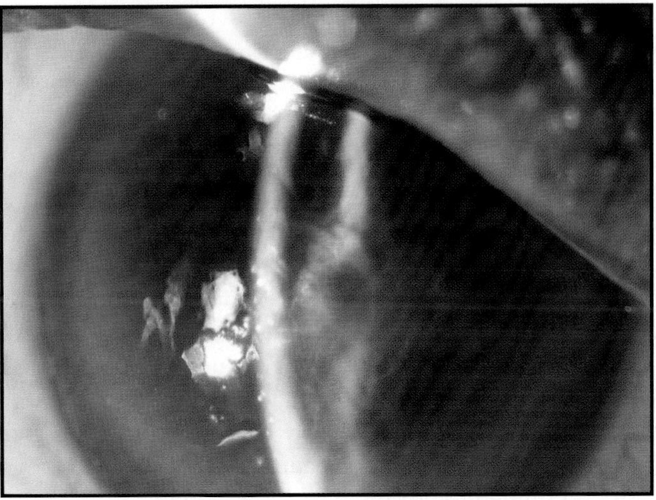

Fig. 33.2: Early endophthalmitis presenting on the day of surgery (*Courtesy*: SLACK Inc)[10]

Toxic endothelial cell destruction syndrome (TECDS) is a related syndrome that specifically indicates localized corneal endothelial damage and is considered to be within the continuum of TASS.[2,5,7,17]

The clinical features of TASS have been well described in previous literature.[1,2,5,7,10,11] Most patients are asymptomatic but may have blurred vision and redness within 24 hours of surgery . Pain is almost never a feature although there may be mild discomfort. Characteristic clinical features include a severe anterior chamber cellular response with fibrin, membrane formation and the occasional hypopyon. Corneal edema, described as limbus to limbus, is frequently present.[10,11,18] When patients present predominantly with corneal edema and less marked anterior chamber inflammation the cause is more likely to be toxic agents (e.g preservatives, ointments).

Features
- Within 48 hours
- Cellular reaction 2-4+
- Fibrin/membranes
- Corneal edema
- No or minimal pain

Pathology

Changes to the pH and osmolality or the inadvertent introduction of an antigen can initiate a cellular response. The histological exams of corneal buttons taken from patients with TASS showed an almost absent endothelial cell layer, with the epithelium thinned and the stroma diffusely thickened.[8] The massive damage to the endothelial layer is a result of its sensitivity to toxic agents.[11]

Epidemiology and Etiology

The epidemic in the United States prompted the American Society of Cataract and Refractive Surgery (ASCRS) to assemble a special task force to deal with the growing problem.[19] The task force reported that over 100 centers experienced an outbreak of TASS prior to May 2006 and this only included clinics that chose to self report.[20] Many outbreaks may be unreported given the potential for poor publicity, and regulatory and liability issues. The increasing incidence of TASS is likely due to an actual rise in numbers rather than simply an increased awareness. Growing interest in TASS is resulting in the rapid expansion of knowledge regarding the cause and therefore the management and prevention of the condition.

The etiology of TASS is speculative, although there is increasing acceptance of its multifactorial causation. The ASCRS task force, and several other researchers have complied a list of possible risk factors and potential causes of TASS.[3,5-8,20-23] These potential etiology factors are listed in Table 33.2.[10] It is likely that individual TASS cases not occurring in an outbreak are due to complications during surgery such as iris stretching, retained cortex and a prolonged surgery.[10] Multiple factors have been associated with TASS outbreaks ranging from inappropriate chemical composition of irrigating solutions to the presence of endotoxins on poorly sterilized instruments.[13]

Intraocular medications, irrigating solutions and balanced salt solution. Many TASS outbreaks have been attributed to contaminants, endotoxins and preservatives gaining access to the anterior chamber during or following surgery.[5,7,12] Outbreaks have been linked to external eye rinses, such as eye

Table 33.2: Potential etiology factors associated with TASS (previously published: SLACK Inc)[10]

Intraocular causes

- Incomplete cortex removal, pupil stretching, and possible immunological differences (as with DLK in atopic patients).

Intraocular medication

- Dosing errors with antibiotics, preservatives, ointments[8], and pH imbalance.

Instrument contamination

- Bacterial endotoxins, dried debris, e.g. inadequate cleaning of cannulas, persistence of detergents, irrigating solutions, endotoxins in irrigating fluids (Endosol),[10,24] incorrect pH or composition of irrigating fluids.

Stream (Alcon, Ft. Worth, Texas) due to the preservative content.[5] Ointments applied postoperatively also have the potential to gain access to the anterior chamber. One study described a TASS outbreak following the application of postoperative ointments and tight eye patching.[8] The use of contaminated balanced salt solution (BSS) has also been associated with TASS outbreaks. Endotoxin was discovered in balanced salt solution (BSS) manufactured by Cytosol Laboratories (Lenoir, NC).[10,24]

Instrument Contamination

Detergent residues left on reusable instruments have the potential to cause corneal toxicity.[2,21] Prolonged cycle sterilization is needed to deactivate enzymes and other active ingredients in detergents.[11] TASS outbreaks have been associated with the dried residue on reusable cannulas.[10]

Impurities can also be present in sterilizer steam.[9,22] An outbreak of TASS was associated with inadequate maintenance of steam sterilizer systems with resulting copper, zinc, nickel, sulfate and silica impurities.[9] Instruments can also become contaminated with endotoxin following short cycle steam sterilization.[25] The sterilization process kills bacteria but does not inactivate endotoxin, which can be a potent initiator of an inflammatory immune response and has been associated with TASS outbreaks.[10,11,22,26]

Ultrasound baths may also be a source of contamination. *Klebsiella pneumonia* and bacterial endotoxin were identified in the ultrasonic cleaning bath during one TASS outbreak.[3]

TASS is often associated with IOL implantation, but more recently has also been observed following placement of phakic IOL.[18] It is important to consider IOL polishing compounds, as well as the chemical structure of the lens as possible causes of TASS.[6,23]

Etiology
- Edema - toxic, e.g.- preservatives
- Inflammation - endotoxin

Causation
- Sterilization issues most common
- Beware of re-usable cannulas

Treatment

Conventional treatment is focused on the suppression of the inflammatory immune response and includes topical steroids given every half-hour to hour for the first three days followed by gradual tapering.[10] During this acute period the patient should be monitored closely for anterior segment inflammation, corneal edema, and intraocular pressure (IOP). In particular monitor for an IOP increase several days following the initial presentation due to damage to the trabecular meshwork.[11] Improvements are generally seen within the first 24 to 48 hours of steroid commencement.

Anterior chamber washout has been reported but outcomes are uncertain and it is not generally recommended.[10,11] When there is corneal and endothelial toxicity a penetrating keratoplasty may be necessary.

Treatment points
Rapid response to frequent steroid drops

Outcomes

Early diagnosis and treatment usually result in an excellent outcome. Most mild cases clear within several days to weeks.[21] Glaucoma is a potential complication due to either initial trabeculitis or fibrin membrane formation.[10] Severe TASS can result in permanent endothelial damage, cystoid macular edema and permanently dilated pupil requiring corrective surgery.[21]

Complications
- Misdiagnosis
- Glaucoma
- Corneal edema
- Cystoid macular edema

Investigation and Reporting

Outbreak investigation is difficult with the multifactorial etiology although sterilization issues usually predominate. Consequences to an affected clinic may be severe with voluntary or mandated closure. Proactive reporting to local regulatory authorities and seeking support from colleagues, as well as academic and public health resources is advisable.[10,27]

Case and Outbreak Definition

Postoperative anterior segment inflammation of unknown cause occurring within 48 hours of surgery with one or more of the following features: anterior chamber response 2+ or greater, fibrin, membranes, corneal edema without significant vitritis.[10] Criteria for a TASS outbreak have not been established as they have for conditions such as DLK.[28] However, any occurrence of more than two affected patients should raise concerns and merit investigation since this may rapidly escalate.

Data Collection

Suggested data include; demographics, VA before and after surgery, symptoms, clinical features, day of surgery, day of onset and diagnosis, any associated conditions, subsequent management and outcome. It is important to record details of the surgical procedure including instrument preparation and specifically any staffing or procedural changes made prior to the onset. Retrospective collection of data is difficult and it is recommended to collect data and note changes as they happen making the creation of an epidemic curve less problematic.

Microbial Investigations

Bacterial culturing, biofilm sampling and analysis of steam distillate and BSS for endotoxin may help determine the cause of the outbreak. The sterilizer reservoir, internal tubing of the sterilizer, ultrasound baths, cannulas and air and water supplies have proved to be useful sampling areas.[10,12,13]

TASS investigations are often difficult and require careful planning. It is usually best to designate one staff member to manage the outbreak, including data collection and media consultation. Another important issue to consider is the disclosure of TASS as a further risk of cataract surgery, particularly during a TASS outbreak.

Once an investigation has been concluded dissemination of the findings will help other practitioners solve their TASS outbreaks or hopefully avoid them. The TASS task force is one example of how this sharing of knowledge has likely reduced the risk of further outbreaks.

Investigation
Suspect everything

CONCLUSION

TASS outbreaks have become of major concern in the ophthalmology community. The assembly of the TASS task force and the numerous recent studies on the subject has assisted in controlling TASS outbreaks. The final task force report concluded that there was no one factor attributable to TASS outbreaks but rather multiple potential etiological factors. It appeared that cleaning and sterilization of instruments for cataract surgery was the most important of the identified factors. It is recommended that all reusable cannulas and instruments be thoroughly flushed with sterile, deionized/distilled water after cleaning at the conclusion of each case.[29]

Although TASS outbreak reports, at least in the United States, now appear to be declining it is important to constantly monitor and improve cleaning and sterilization protocols. Growing awareness resulting in early diagnosis and treatment, with prompt dissemination of new information will hopefully eliminate TASS as a significant complication of modern cataract surgery.

REFERENCES

1. Monson MC, Mamalis N, Olson RJ. Toxic anterior segment inflammation following cataract surgery. J Cataract Refract Surg. 1992;18:184-9.
2. Breebaart AC, Nuyts RMMA, Pels E, et al. Toxic endothelial destruction of the cornea after routine extracapsular cataract surgery. Arch Ophthalmol 1990; 108:1121-25.
3. Kreisler KR, Martin SS, Young CW, et al. Postoperative inflammation following cataract extraction caused by bacterial contamination of the cleaning bath detergent. J Cataract Refract Surg 1992;18:106-10.
4. Nelson DB, Donnenfeld ED, Perry HD. Sterile endophthalmitis after sutureless cataract surgery. Ophthalmolgy 1992;99:1655-7.
5. Liu H, Routley I, Teichmann KD. Toxic endothelial cell destruction from intraocular benzalkonium chloride. J Cataract Refract Surg 2001;27:1746-50.
6. Jehan FS, Mamalis N, Spencer TS, et al. Postoperative sterile endophthalmitis (TASS) with the MemoryLens. J Cataract Refract Surg 2000;26:1773-7.
7. Eleftheriadis H, Cheong M, Saneman S, et al. Corneal toxicity secondary to inadvertent use of benzalkonium chloride preserved viscoelastic material in cataract surgery. Br J Ophthalmol 2002;86:299-305.
8. Werner L, Sher JH, Taylor JR, et al. Toxic anterior segment syndrome and possible association with ointment in the anterior chamber following cataract surgery. J Cataract Refract Surg 2006;32:227-35.
9. Hellinger WC, Hasan SA, Bacalis LP, et al. Outbreak of toxic anterior chamber syndrome following cataract surgery associated with impurities of autoclave steam moisture. Infect Control Hosp Epidemiol 2006;27(13):294-8.
10. Holland SP, Morck DW, Chavez G, Lee, TL. Toxic anterior segment syndrome. In: Agarwal A, (Ed): Refractive Surgery Nightmares: Conquering Refractive Surgery Catastrophes. Thorofare, NJ: SLACK Incorporated. In press.
11. Mamalis N, Edelhauser HF, Dawson DG, et al. Toxic anterior segment syndrome. Review/update. J Cataract Refract Surg 2006;32:324-33.
12. Holland SP, Chavex G, Morck D, Mathias. Toxic Anterior Segment Syndrome After Cataract Surgery Associated with Short-Cycle Sterilization presented at the ASCRS Symposium on Cataract, IOL and Refractive Surgery, San Francisco, USA , March 17-22, 2006. Available at www.ascrs.org. Accessed June 12, 2006.
13. Holland SP, Morck D, Lee T. Update on toxic anterior segment syndrome. Current Opinion in Ophthalmology. In press.
14. Van Gelder RN. Applications of the polymerase chain reaction to diagnosis of ophthalmic disease. Surv Ophthalmol 2001;45(3):248-58.
15. West ES, Behrens A, McDonnell PJ, et al. The incidence of endophthalmitis after cataract surgery among the US medicare population increased between 1994 and 2001. Ophthalmology 2005;112:1388-95.
16. Wallin T, Parker J, Jin Y, et al. Cohort study of 27 cases of endophthalmitis at a single institution. J Cataract Refract Surg 2005;31:735-41.
17. Duffy RE, Brown SE, Caldwell KL, et al. An epidemic of corneal destruction caused by plasma gas sterilization; the Toxic Endothelial Cell Destruction Syndrome Team. Arch Ophthalmology 2000;118:1167-76.

18. Moshirfar M, Whitehead G, Beutler BC, et al. Toxic anterior segment syndrome after Verisyse iris-supported phakic intraocular lens implantation. J Cataract Refract Surg 2006;32(7):1233-37.
19. The American Society of Cataract and Refractive Surgery (ASCRS). (2005). Press release June 22, 2006: TASS task force. Retrieved August 15, 2006, from http://www.ascrs.org/press_releases/Toxic-Anterior-Segment-Syndrome-Outbreak-Preliminary-Report.cfm.
20. The American Society of Cataract and Refractive Surgery (ASCRS). (2005). Press release May 22, 2006: TASS Outbreak Update. Retrieved June 1, 2006, from http://www.ascrs.org/press_releases/upload/UpdateBriefing.doc.
21. Parikh C, Sippy BD, Martin DF, Edelhauser HF. Effects of enzymatic sterilization detergents on the corneal endothelium. Arch Ophthalmol 2002;120:165-72.
22. Whitby JL, Hitchins VM. Endotoxin levels in steam and reservoirs of table-top steam sterilzers. J Cataract Refract Surg 2002;18:51-2.
23. Meltzer, DW. Sterile hypopyon following intraocular lens surgery. Arch Ophthalmol 1980;98:100-4.
24. US Food and Drug Administration. (2006). Patient advisory Feb 13th 2006; FDA-Requested Recall - Cytosol Laboratories, Inc. Product Contains Dangerous Levels of Endotoxin. Retrieved Feb. 14, 2006, from http://www.fda.gov/bbs/topics/news/2006/NEW01315.html.
25. Holland SP, Mathias RG, Morck DW, et al. Diffuse lamellar keratitis related to endotoxins released from sterilizer reservoir biofilms. Ophthalmol 2000; 107(7):1227-1233.
26. Rietschel ET, Brade H. Bacterial endotoxins. Sci Am 1992;267:54-61.
27. Mamalis, N. 2006. TASS outbreaks: What should we do? Cataract and Refractive Surgery Today, July 2006;53-55.
28. Bigham M, Enns CL, Holland SP, et al. Diffuse lamellar keratitis complicating laser in situ keratomileusis; Post-marketing surveillance of an emerging disease in British Columbia, Canada, 2000-2002. J Cataract Refract Surg 2005;31:2340-44.
29. The American Society of Cataract and Refractive Surgery (ASCRS). (2005). Press release September 22, 2006: Toxic Anterior Segment Syndrome (TASS) Outbreak Final Report. Retrieved September 22, 2006, from http://www.ascrs.org/press_releases/Final-TASS-Report.cfm.

Chapter 34

Ocular Pharmacotherapeutics in Corneal Refractive Surgery

Ashok Garg (India)

Ever since Theo Seiler in 1987 and Marguerite McDonald in 1988 did the first corneal ablation in normal sighted eye, excimer laser refractive surgery has produced revolutionary changes in the field of ophthalmology. Refractive Surgery is certainly a high tech advancement in the field of ophthalmic surgery of the last decade of this millenium which has come as a great boon to spectacle weary patients all around the world.

LASIK (Laser assisted *in situ* keratomileusis) and LASEK (Laser assisted subepithelial keratectomy) offer a unique opportunity to provide ametropia to patients with refractive error ranging from –20.00 D of myopia to +8.00 D of hyperopia. The rapid visual recovery and decreased incidence of complications associated with LASIK and LASEK make them far superior to both excimer photoablation (PRK) and automated lamellar keratoplasty (ALK).

LASIK and LASEK provides an extraordinary accurate method of tissue removal (0.20 to 0.25 μm tissue per pulse). The extreme pain, haze, regression and slow visual rehablitation of PRK are absent thus the minimum use of post-precedure medications specially topical steroids and its potential adverse effects.

Although pre-procedure medications are same in Lasik and Lasek as those in PRK surgery while post-procedure medications are drasticaly reduced in Lasik and Lasek surgery leading to quick visual rehabilitation of patient post-operatively.

Development of automated micro-Keratome Hansatome and Laser Microkeatome has make LASIK and LASEK surgery more safe even in the hand of novice refractive surgeon. Indeed the LASIK and LASEK surgery have come of age.

Here, now I shall discuss the ocular therapeutics used in LASIK and LASEK surgery before and after the procedure.

Pre-procedure Therapeutic Medications

Pre-operatively patient is given broad range topical antibiotic eyedrops (Preferably Gatifloxacin (0.3%) or Moxifloxacin (0.5%) at 4 hourly interval starting 24 hours prior to surgery.

A mild oral sedation (diazepam 3 to 10 mg) is given in all cases. Bilateral simultaneous surgery is done in all cases.

TOPICAL ANESTHESIA

For Lasik/Lasek Surgery, refractive Surgeon prefer to give topical anesthesia because of rapid onset of action and lesser irritation to the patient.

Two to five minutes prior to the surgery any of the following topical anesthetic agent can be safely used.

- Proparacaine HCl : 0.5%
- Benoxinate HCl : 0.4%
- Tetracaine HCl : 0.5%

Proparacaine is most commonly used anesthetic agent followed by Benoxinate and tetracaine. Other topical agent like xylocaine (4%) is less commonly used due to problems of irritation, allergy etc.

Proparacaine, benoxinate and tetracaine have rapid onset of action and cause little tingling sensation and irritation to the patient.

Onset of anesthetic action starts with in 15 to 20 seconds with these agents and effects last for 15 to 20 minutes sufficient for the completion of Lasik/ Lasek Surgery. Proparacaine or benoxinate are given topically in the dosage of 2 drops in each eye 2 to 3 times repeated at the interval of one minute.

After topical anesthesia some refractive surgeon prefer to instill pilocarpine 1% in the eye to aid in marking the optical axis.

Pachymetry is performed and patients is carefully centred and eyelids are cleaned with betadine solution (Iodine solution) and operative eye is given a sterile plastic ophthalmic drape to cover the eyelid margins and the cilia.

Post-procedure Therapeutic Medications

The biggest advantage of LASIK and LASEK over PRK is the minimum use of ocular therapeutic in postoperative phase. The visual recovery in LASIK and LASEK is virtually immediate owing to the preservation of the epithelium of the cornea. Typically recovery is painless and post procedure refractions and vision are remarkably stable during the post-operative period. Post-procedure medications are quite significant for early visual rehabilitation and recovery of the patient. During the initial active postoperative phase. Refractive surgeons prefer to give:

a. Oral antibiotic (Gatifloxacin 400 mg OD or Levofloxacin 500 mg OD for 5 days).
b. Topical fluorometholone (FML, 0.1%) eye drops four times a day for two weeks.

c. Topical lubricant like polyvinyl alcohol liquifilm tear drops 4 times a day for two weeks.
d. Topical antibiotic (Moxifloxacin 0.5%). QID for a week. Immediately after LASIK/LASEK procedure some surgeon prefer to give patch for 2 to 3 hours. While other view is to ask the patient to wear a clear eye shield nightly for a week.
e. Oral analgesic (Tab diclofenac 75 mg SR BD for three days if needed but not in routine).

Patient operated for LASIK/Lasek surgery is called for follow up on:

- 2nd day post-procedure
- Ist week
- 2nd weeks
- 3rd weeks

One each follow up following examination are done:

- Vision check up
- IOP with non contact tonometer
- Slit lamp examination for Haze
- Topography to see corneal profile.

Corneal wound healing and its modulations after LASIK/LASEK surgery have multiple components. LASIK/LASEK is a refractive surgical procedure that is performed in several steps and each step involved a different structure of cornea.

Phases of Healing

Following LASIK/LASEK injury healing occurs in several phases. The earliest phase involves the healing of epithelial injury and is characterized by the migration of epithelium which occurs 12 to 24 hr after prcedure 2 to 3 days after the insult, epithelial cell proliferation is evident. Six months after the surgical insult the development of fibrous metaplasia is complete. Throughout these phases of healing the types of cytokine communication are operating to create an integrated repair of injured corneal areas.

Although LASIK/LASEK is safe and reliable procedure yet it is susceptible to all the complications noted in PRK procedure which includes overcorrection, undercorrection, decentration, infection, loss and displacement of flap, central islands and epithelial in growth.

Cornea healing following LASIK/LASEK should be considered as a combination of events involving the response to injury of the epithelium and stroma.

Understanding these events and the molecules that regulate the wound healing response should enable the refractive surgeon to induce fewer complications and aid in developing therapeutic modalities to alter would healing precisely.

Close follow up and attention to postoperative medications and surface lubrication will enable the surgeon to achieve better results.

BIBLIOGRAPHY

1. Agarwal Amar. Textbook of ophthalmology, ed.1, New Delhi: Jaypee Brothers Medical Publishers, 2002.
2. Bartlett JD. Clinical Ocular Pharmacology, ed.4, Boston: Butterworth-Heinemann, 2001
3. Bartlett JD. Ophthalmic Drug facts: Lippincott – William and Wilkins, 2001.
4. Crick RP, Trimble RB. Textbook of clinical ophthalmology: Hodder and Stoughton, 1986.
5. Duane TD. Clinical ophthalmology, ed. 4: Butterworth – Heinemann 1999.
6. Duvall. Ophthalmic Medications and Pharmacology: Slack Inc 1998.
7. Ellis PP. Ocular Therapeutics and Pharmacology, ed. 7: CV Mosby 1985.
8. Fechner. Ocular Therapeutics: Slack Inc 1998.
9. Fraunfelder. Current Ocular Therapy, ed. 5: WB Saunders 2000.
10. Garg Ashok. Current Trends in ophthalmology, ed. 1, New Delhi: Jaypee Brothers Medical Publishers 1997.
11 Garg Ashok. Manual of Ocular Therapeutics, ed. 1, New Delhi: Jaypee Brothers Medical Publishers 1996.
12. Garg Ashok. Ready Reckoner of Ocular Therapeutics, ed.1, New Delhi: 2002.
13. Goodman LS, Gilman A. Pharmacological basis of Therapeutics, ed.7, New York: Macmillan 1985.
14. Havener's, Ocular Pharmacology, ed. 6: CV Mosby 1994.
15. Kanski. Clinical ophthalmology, ed. 4: Butterworth – Heinemann 1999.
16. Kershner. Ophthalmic Medications and Pharmacology: Slack. Inc., 1994.
17. Olin BR et al. Drugs Facts and Comparisons: Facts and Comparisons, St. Louis 1997.
18. Onofrey. The Ocular Therapeutics; Lippincott, William and Wilkins 1997.
19. Rhee. The Wills Eye drug Guide: Lippincott – William and Wilkins 1998.
20. Steven Podos. Textbook of ophthalmology, New Delhi: Jaypee Brothers Medical Publishers 2001.
21. Zimmerman. Textbook of Ocular Pharmacology: Lippincott and William and Wilkins 1997.

Chapter 35

PHARMACOTHERAPEUTICS IN PHACOEMULSIFICATION

Jerome Bovet (Switzerland)

INTRODUCTION

The evolution of cataracte surgery has been to decrease the level of risk; that is to achieve a highly specific, successfull outcome with the least disruption to the patient' physical state. The goal is near immediate visual recovery with minimal correction or better a catarefractive[1] solution which mean no more glasses for far and near. To achieve these goals you need a minimal level of anesthesia, minimal postoperative inflammation and the absence of difficulties during the operation: large pupilla, no pressure inside the eye, no iris inside the wound. As modern cataract surgical techniques have changed,[2] so have the composition of our pharmaceutical treatment. The goal is to use ocular pharmaceutics which are highly effective and very specific in their effects, thus producing minimal side effects. We also want to reduce as far as possible the length and the complexity of the postoperative medication regimen. During the past few years, the main areas of change in the medication routines for cataract surgical patients have been in Table 35.1.

1. Pupil dilatation
2. Anesthesia
3. Postoperative inflammation
4. Prevention of the infection
5. Preservation of the lacrymal film.

Pupil Dilation

The purpose of this chapter is to tell you step by step how to dilate a pupil efficiently for the ambulatory surgery. Most of the patient come one week before surgery in our country.

1. We give a prescription to the patient at the same time we calculate the biometry and we learn the patient the cataract operation procedure and he sign the inform consent formular

Table 35.1: Preoperative, intraoperative, and recovery room medications

Preoperative	
(Exam area and again in preoperative holding area, 30 min prior to transfer to OR)	
Mydriasert	1 tabs
(Chlorhydrate of phenilephrine 5.376 mg	
Tropicamide 0.280 mg	
Novesin (oxybuprocaini hydrochloridum)	1 drop x 1
OT	
Topical anesthesia	Lidocaine (Xylocaïne[R]) 2% 3 drps x 3 (3 min apart with final gtt instilled just prior to beginning)
Around the cornea	
4th quadrant of conjunctival bulbaire	
Desinfection	Gluconate of chlorhexidine 0.5 mg/ml (hibidil[R])
Rincage	BSS solution
Preservation of the lacrymal films and the cornea	Methylcellulose 2%
Intraocular Anesthesia	lidocaine 0.5%:(Xylocaïne[R] 2% 0.5 ml and BSS 2 ml)
Intraocular dilatation if not enough	Homatropine 0.4% Phénylephrine 0.05% 2 ml : Preservative free inside the AC
Irrigation Solution:	
Adrenaline 1 mg/1 ml 0.5 ml	
Preparation:	
To 500 ml bottle BSS add:	
0.5 ml adrenaline	(1:1000)
500 ml bottle BSS	
Vancocin (vancomycin) 500 mg/10 ml	
NaCl 10 ml	
Garamycin (Gentamycin) 60 mg/1.5 ml	
BSS 500 ml	
Zinacef (cephalosporine) 1.5 g/100 ml d'NaCl 0.9%	
Draw up 10 ml NaCl injecting in Vancocin 500 mg/10 ml	
Draw up 3 ml solution Vancocin	
Draw up 3 ml de vancocin and 1.5 ml de Garamycine	
Injecting 0.3 ml de solution in BSS	
Post-op Anterior Chamber Injection fo Indomethacin and Solucortef	
Recovery Room	
Sandwich tea or coffe	

2. He will start NSAID voltaren ophta drops in the operate eye 5 days before the operation 2 times a day.The day of the operation he starts mydriaticum drops every 10 minutes at home 2 hours before he arrives to the clinique.
3. When the patient will arrive at the clinic 30 min before the OT, the nurse will place an insert into the inferior conjunctival fornix of the operate eye Mydriasert[R] contain chlorhydrate of phenilephrine 5.376 mg, tropicamide 0.280 mg and novesine 1 drop
4. If the patient is still not well dilated we use a dilating "cocktail." That we injected before the intracameral anesthesia.[3] We use: Homatropine 0.4%, Phénylephrine 0.05% 2 ml: Preservative free inside the AC.

Anesthesia

Topical anesthesia and intraocular lidocaine

The main indication for topical/intraocular anesthesia is a routine phacoemulsification case. Topical anesthesia was reintroduced by Dr Fichman[4] in October 1991.

The return to topical anesthesia effectively eliminates the risk of complications associated with regional blocks. Topical anesthesia has gained wide acceptance as an effective, efficient, pratical and safe form of ocular anestesia for cataract, refractive and glaucoma surgery.

The ideal agent for topical anesthesia is lidocaine 2% which avoid the corneal epithelium toxicity like we have with tetracaine or marcaine. To protect and lubricate the cornea during the operation we coat the epithelium with hydroxypropylmethylcellulose 2% which give an excellent protection and very sharp vision of the anterior chamber.[5]

Therefore, the surgical assistant will rarely, if ever, need to squirt the cornea.

There are, however, disadvantage associated with topical anesthesia. It can pose probleme when the patient is anxious.

Topical anesthesia does not eliminate all sensation of pressure, cold or discomfort in every patient.

These sensation arise often when we manipulate the iris root.That why many surgeon introduce intraocular anesthesia to avoid this deep pain when the iris is touch.

Topical and intraocular lidocaine are synergistic

The majority of surgeons using topical/intraocular anesthesia use sterile, nonpreserved lidocaine 1%. Because the pH of commercially available lidocaine is in the acidic range (6.4), some patients experience a burning or stinging sensation when it is first injected into the anterior chamber. For this reason,we diluted the lidocaine 2% in BSS to have a lidocaine 0.5% solution. This formulation has a gentler pH and burns a little less when injected.[6]

Step by step[7] topical anesthesia and intraocular anesthesia.

After the patient is place confortable on the operating bed. The nurse instilled lidocaine 2%. 3 drops on the 4 conjunctival quadrant avoiding the cornea to preserve the epithelium.

Then the scrub nurse desinfect with the chlorexidine (Hibidil[R]) rinces the eye with BSS and give some methycellulose drops on the top of cornea.

Immediately after the patient is draped and the speculum inserted.

We make first, a sideport incision. We then inject the lidocaine 1% directly into the anterior chamber through the sideport incision.[8]

After that we exchange the aqueous with a viscoelastic agent, create the clear cornea phaco incision, perform the capsulorrhexis, and then do hydrodissection with the same sterile lidocaine 1%.

SYSTEMIC MEDICATIONS

The main contraindication to topical/intraocular anesthesia is the inability of the patient to cooperate during the surgery. Therefore, significant sedation is not only unnecessary, it also is counterproductive and potentially dangerous.

Now that is not to say that sedation of any kind can never be used.

If a patient cannot tolerate the operating microscope light. If a patient complains about extreme pain and discomfort from either the inflated blood pressure cuff or inserted lid speculum. We will add systemic medications with topical/intraocular anesthesia.

Topical anesthesia patients, like all cataract surgery patients, are about to undergo a new and different experience in unfamiliar surroundings involving their eye and their future vision.[7]

When needed, we have found that 0.5 mg to 1.0 mg of IV midazolam HCl, Roche (Dormicum[R]) is sufficient in the majority of cases. Many surgeons who use topical anesthesia prefer 5 mg of propofol.

In the unusual situation in which more sedation is indicated, the medication should be titrated. Remember, the goal in topical anesthesia is for everyone involved to be relaxed, attentive, and cooperative.

We use for all our patient the hand massage which decrease the psychological anxiety levels, systolic and diastolic blood pressures, and pulse rate.

If the patient is extralarge it maybe transmit some pressure inside the eye just by the way of the Valsalva's maneuver we add in this case mannitol 10 % 5 ml IV, which will decrease temporarily the pressure intraocular.

Postoperative Inflammation the Role of NSAIDs

Over the last decade the use of non-steroidal anti-inflammatory agents has become highly effective in reducing inflammation and the incidence of postoperative cystoid macular edema.

We do not need to rely on a heavy regimen of steroid treatment. We administer diclofenac (Voltaren[R]) 5 days prior to surgery. Diclofenac has been specifically shown to be highly effective in preventing cystoid macular edema and in controlling postoperative inflammation. We had used NSAIDs additionally at the end of surgery to prevent the incidence of cystoid macular edema and because the administered dose will remain in the eye a long time.

The other indication for use of NSAIDs is to prevent miosis during surgery. diclofenac, as well as a number of other NSAIDs have been shown to enhance mydriasis.

At the end of the procedure in the intracameral antibiotic injection, the patient receives diclofenac and solu-Cortef.

Prevention of the Infection (Table 35.2)

When endophthalmitis occurs, the outcome for the patient can be devastating. Therefore, there is much interest in minimizing the occurrence of endophthalmitis.[9] However, because the incidence is so low, there are few well-controlled studies of the risk factors or efficacy of preventive measures. Preoperative disinfection of the surgical site and meticulous attention to sterile technique are essential.

Table 35.2: Check for preventing endophthalmitis
Operating theater air need HEPA filter supply
Identify and treat preoperative blepharitis.
Chlorexidine 5% to cul-de-sac, lids, and skin 2 minutes contact as a preoperative preparation.
Draping techniques, isolate lids and lashes.
Viscoelastics, multiple-use eye drops, avoid prolene haptics.
Surgical insturments, wound leaking, vitreous wick, filtering bleb, irrigating solutions.

The incidence of endophthalmitis was further reduced when both the topical and subconjunctival prophylactic measures were taken together.

Clearly, the use of aIl available routes of prophylactic treatment should be considered.

It has been shown in a randomized experiment that use of antibiotics in the irrigation solution decreased the Iikelihood of a positive postoperative aqueous culture.

ln fact, the benefit of decreasing the rate of endophthalmitis far outweighs the very small risk of developing a resistant strain of bacteria through the use of intraocular antibiotics.[10]

A survey[11] conducted by the American Society for Cataract and Refractive Surgeons has shown that at least 35% of ophthalmic surgeons currently use intracameral antibiotics. Vancomycin was used by 80% and gentamicin by more than 40% of the surgeons surveyed.

Our protocol is to use gentamicin sulfate and vancomicin inside the perfusion bottle like the Gill's protocol[12]: (Garamycin®) solution (0.008 g/cc) filtered through a 0.2 micron millipore and Vancomycin® (0.1 cc at 100 mg/cc in each 500 cc bottle of BSS) to provide protection against gram-positive bacteria which are the most prevalent organisms cultured in endophthalmitis cases.[13]

At the end of the operation we rince the anterior chamber with cefuroxime (Zinacef[R]).

Preservation of the Lacrimal Film

Dry eye syndrome after cataract operation may be du to the desinfection or the topical corticosteroid drops after the operation. To avoid this problem we inject at the end of the operation a cortisone long actin inside the anterior chamber.

Conclusion

Modern phacoemulsification techniques combined with topical anesthesia, intraocular lidocaine and efficient medication regimens provide the patient with a highly comfortable experience. We have reduced the length and complexity of the postoperative medication regimen. Rigorous prophylactic measures protect against endophthalmitis and optimize safety.

REFERENCES

1. J Bovet. Catarefractive Surgery: A next step to phakonit. In mastering the art of bimanual microincision phaco Eds A.Garg Jaypee Brothers Medical Publishers. New Delhi 2005.
2. J Bovet. Management of complications in microphaco in mastering the art of bimanual microincision phaco. Garg A (Eds). Jaypee Brothers Medical Publishers. New Delhi 2005.
3. Dillman DM. Anesthesia for cataract surgery. Chapter 6. In: Wallace RB III (ed). Refractive Cataract Surgery and Multifocal IOLs. Thorofare, NJ: Slack; 2000 Lebuisson DA, Bovet J J. Le concept opératoire pour patients ophthalmologiques ambulants in Laroche L, Lebuisson DA, Montard M Chirurgie de la cataracte chap 6 61-74;ed Masson 1996.
4. Fichman RA. Topical Anesthesia. In: Fine IH, Fichman RA, Grabow HBC Eds. Clear Cornea Cataracte Surgery and topical Anesthesia 1993 Thorofare Slack Inc 97-162.
5. J Bovet, JM Baumgartner, JC Bruckner, V Ilic, O Achard L'anesthésie topique en chirurgie oculaire et sa préparation In: Les Dimensions de la douleur en ophthalmologie AB Safran, T Landis, P Dayer eds Paris Masson, 1998;166-73.
6. Gills JP. Intraocular anesthesia in clear corneal cataract surgery. In: Fine IH, ed. Clear-Corneal Lens Surgery. Thorofare, NJ: SLACK Incorporated 1999;59-69.
7. Lebuisson DA, Chevaleraud E, Bovet JJ. Les anesthésies locales in Laroche L, Lebuisson DA, Montard M Chirurgie de la cataracte Masson 1996;10:109-127.
8. Wirbelauer C, Iven H, Bastian C, Laqua HJ. Systemic levels of lidocaine after intracameral injection during cataract surgery. Cataract Refract Surg 1999; 25: 648-651.
9. Busbee BG. Advances in knowledge and treatment: An update on endophthalmitis. Curr Opin Ophthalmol 2004;15:232-7.

10. Gills JP. Filters and antibiotics in irrigating solution for cataract surgery. J Cataract Refract Surg 1991;17:385.
11. Leaming DV. Practice styles and preferences of ASCRS members-1996 survey. J Cataract Refract Surg 1997;23:527-535.
12. Gills JP. Prevention of endophthalmitis by intraocular solution filtration and antibiotics. J Am Intraoeul Implant Soe 1985;11(2):185-6.
13. Libre PE, Della-Latta P, Chin NX. Intracameral antibiotic agents for endophthalmitis prophylaxis: A pharmacokinetic model. J Cataract Refract Surg 2003;29:1791-4.

Chapter 36

Topical Immune Therapy—A New Hope in Ocular Therapeutics

Ashok Garg (India)

Topical immune therapy is relatively a latest addition in ocular therapeutic armamantorium to treat iatrogenic inflammation following any type of intra-ocular surgery and to make up the decreased levels of ocular immunoglobulins vital for the ocular defence system against external infections during post-operative phase following intraocular surgery.

Before discussing the topical immune therapy monograph let me discuss in nutshell about the ocular defence system and immunity.

As we know that protection from disease results from the detection and subsequent elimination of substances recognized as foreign by the body. This active protection system is called immunity. Immunology is the study of those systems responsible for protection of the individual against external and internal assault.

The eye can manifest virtually any type of immune response as it possesses a number of unique anatomical, physiological and biochemical features, these responses often have a distinct character.

The optical integrity and normal protection function of the eye depends on an adequate supply of fluid covering its surface. The exposed part of the ocular globe – the cornea and the bulbar conjunctiva is covered by a thin fluid film known as pre-ocular tear film. Tears refer to fluid present as pre-corneal tear film and in conjunctival sac.

Tear film is complex trilaminar structure consisting of aqueous layer delimited on both sides by layer of surface active substances. Tear film is directly in contact with the environment and is critically important for protecting the eye from external influences.

The chemical composition of human tears is quite complex as it contain proteins, lipids, metabolites, enzymes, electrolytes and other elements dissolved in fluid scretions of lacrimal gland which play an important role in the defence of the outer eye.

The tear protein fraction forms the first line of ocular defence against external infections.

The antibacterial properties of immunoglobulins, lysozyme, lactoferrin and β-lysin have been well documented by Research scientists.

Immunoglobulins (IgA and IgG) are the major immunoglobulins present in the tears. A small fraction of IgM is also present in the normal tears Normal tears contains an average of 14 mg% of IgA, 17 mg% of IgG and 5-7 mg% of IgM. (Fig. 36.1).

IgA and IgG may act to modulate the normal flora of the ocular adnexa allowing saprophytic growth which prevents less favorable flora from colonizing the ocular surface. They also prevent adherance of bacteria to the mucosal surface, agglutinate bacteria and neutralize viruses and toxins. In the original state any immunoglobulins found in ocular tissues are likely to the mainly derived from the circulating plasma but on the initial exposure to antigen the urea and limbal conjunctiva acquire antibody producing cells, some of which tend to persist.

The conjunctiva has the property of mucous membrane elsewhere in being rich with IgA. IgA present in tears is likely to be derived from both the conjunctiva and the lacrimal gland.

Early diffusion of IgG in the cornea due to its small molecular size in comparison to IgA and IgM is probably responsible for the preponderance of IgG in the cornea. Small quantity of IgM is probably due to blood aqueous and blood retinal barriers. During acute inflammation of the eye, IgG is the most predominant immunoglobulin present in concentration five times more than that of IgA. This significant increase is associated with increased local synthesis and increased vascular permability resulting serum IgG spitting into the tears. Similarly there is increased concentration of IgM in tears following acute inflammation due to transudation of serum proteins into the tears.

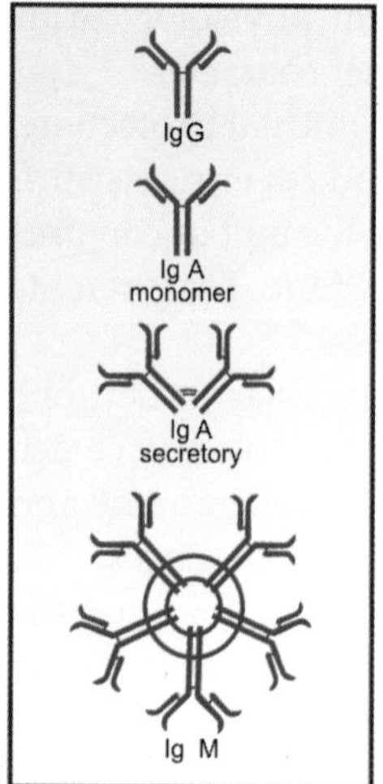

Fig. 36.1: Structural formula of various immunoglobulins present in tears

Extensive Research studies conducted in the last decade by the author and his team had shown the interesting findings which are of paramount importance in relation to ocular defence system during immediate post-operative period following intraocular surgery. These are:

a. In the immediate post-operative period (upto 7 days following intraocular surgery of any type, there is significant decrease in globulin levels of tears predisposing the eye an added risk of infections due to low tissue immunological defence (Figs 36.2 to 36.4).
b. There is tremendous increase in tear secretion rate (confirmed by Schirmer's test) during the immediate postoperative period resulting in a more dilution of immunoglobulins. This increased tear secretion rate is due to mild trauma caused by surgical interference. At this juncture local tissue response to microbial invasion is severely compromised.
c. During the critical period of immediate postoperative phase (1-7 days) the host ocular tissue remains immunocompromised.
d. Meticulous aseptic care and suitable topical anti-inflammatory therapy is needed to protect the eye from external influences and to beef up immuno-compromised ocular defence system due to iatrogenic inflammation of the eye.

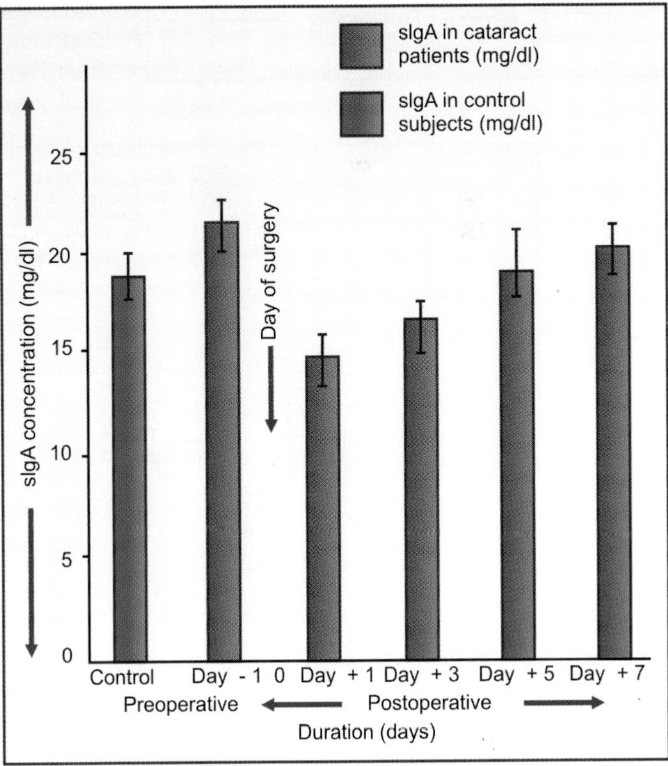

Fig. 36.2: Tear IgA concentration before and after iatrogenic inflammation of the eye

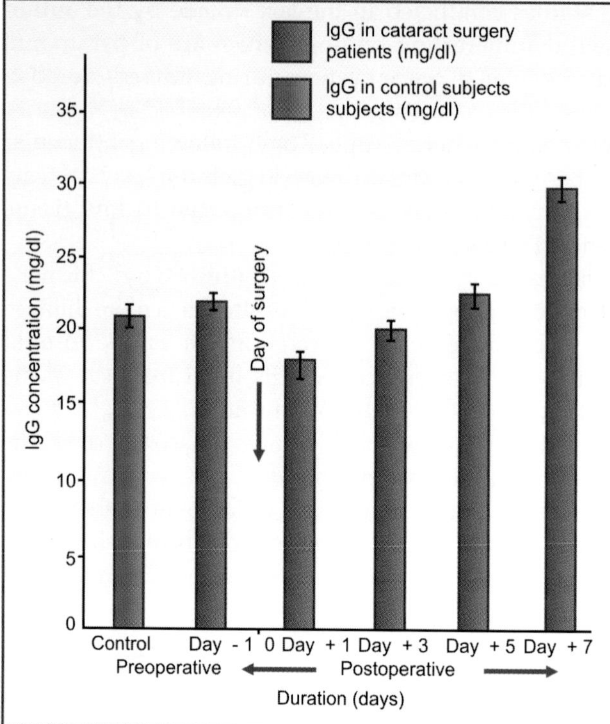

Fig. 36.3: Tear IgG concentration before and after iatrogenic inflammation of the eye

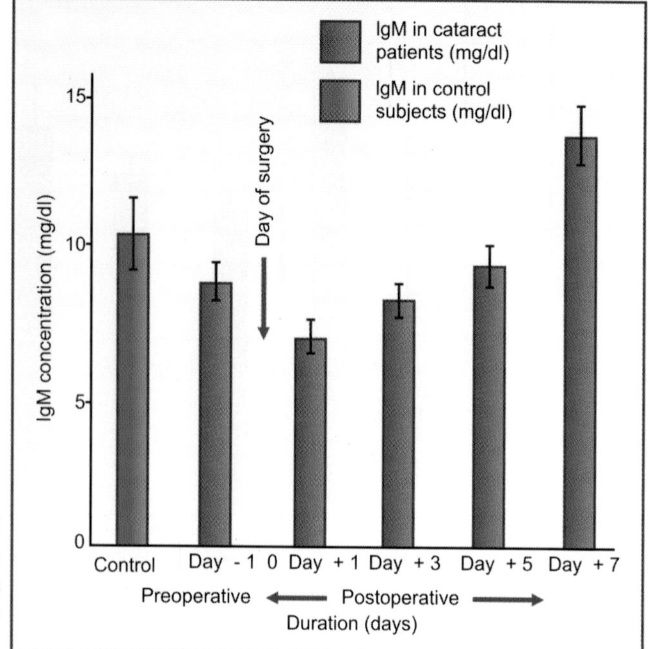

Fig. 36.4: Tear IgM concentration before and after iatrogenic inflammation of the eye

Generally during this critical period topical steroids preparations are advised which have their own ocular and systemic side effects.

Based on above crucial findings. Author prepared a topical non-steroidal immune therapy to be supplemented locally to beef up compromised immune defence system of the eye. Extensive biochemical and clinical trials were conducted of this topical immune therepy before it became commercially available. Trials were conducted in two phases.

1. In Phase I trials were conducted in rabbits eye to ascertain the efficacy of topical globulin eye drops and their possible use in human beings.
2. On getting encouraging response from animal studies (Phase I), extensive biochemical and clinical trials were conducted in human beings.

INDICATIONS FOR TOPICAL IMMUNE THERAPY

- Cataract surgery (ICCE or ECCE)
- Filtering surgery for glaucoma
- IOL implantation and phacoemulsification
- Keratoplasty
- Vitrectomy and posterior segment surgery
- Ocular surgery following trauma
- Lasik surgery
- Squint surgery.

MECHANISM OF ACTION

Topical globulin eye drops (immune therapy) acts by augmenting the severely depleted immunoglobulin levels of tear during immediate postoperative period of (1-7) days following intraocular surgery. It supplements the immunoglobulins present in the tears to fight against external influences.

DOSAGE

It is available as Topical ophthalmic solution (Aspac). It contains 0.1% each of IgG and IgA and 0.05% of IgM in fixed concentrations (available in 5 ml pack). Needs to be refrigerated (2-8ºC) when vial is not opened. Once opened for topical use, the vial can be stored at room temperature.

Usual dosage is to instil 1-2 drops in the affected eye three to four times a day for a week and then gradual tapering over next 7 days.

Topical immune therapy in optimum dose is advocated for a postoperative (1-7 days) because after a week natural globulin levels come back to pre-operative levels. This rise in level of natural globulins may be partially due to fall in tear secretion rate and due to enhanced local globulin production from tear glands. This increase in globulin level is also due to exudation of serum globulins through the blood tear barrier.

A raised clinical score of inflammation during this period is indication of supporting the same view. Topical immune therapy is well tolerated and its intraocular penetration is high.

CONTRAINDICATION

Known hypersensitivity to any of its components.

Adverse Reactions

On topical use it will tolerated and has least side effects.

However, ocular side effects reported are transient burning sensation, irritation, stinging and foreign body sensation, conjunctival injection and hypersensitivity reactions.

Keeping in view of enormous clinical value of topical immune therapy, it will be wonder drug of ophthalmology in near future specially for treating iatrogenic inflammation of the eye.

BIBLIOGRAPHY

1. Agarwal Amar. Text book of ophthalmology, ed.1, New Delhi: Jaypee Medical Publishers, 2002.
2. Bartlett JD. Clinical Ocular Pharmacology, ed.4, Boston: Butterworth-Heinemann, 2001
3. Bartlett JD. Ophthalmic Drug facts: Lippincott – William and Wilkins, 2001.
4. Crick RP, Trimble RB. Text book of clinical ophthalmology : Hodder and Stoughton, 1986.
5. Duane. TD. Clinical ophthalmology, ed. 4: Butterworth – Heinemann, 1999.
6. Duvall. Ophthalmic Medications and Pharmacology: Slack Inc, 1998.
7. Ellis PP. Ocular Therapeutics and Pharmacology, ed. 7: C.V. Mosby, 1985.
8. Fechner. Ocular Therapeutics: Slack Inc., 1998.
9. Fraunfelder. Current Ocular Therapy, ed. 5: W.B. Saunders, 2000.
10. Garg Ashok. Current Trends in ophthalmology, ed. 1, New Delhi : Jaypee Medical Publishers, 1997.
11. Garg Ashok. Manual of Ocular Therapeutics, ed. 1, New Delhi: Jaypee Medical Publishers, 1996.
12. Garg Ashok. Ready Reckoner of Ocular Therapeutics, ed.1, New Delhi: 2002.
13. Garg Ashok. Tear Immunoglobulins status in iatrogenic inflammation of the eye: Internationale Ophthalmologica, 1989; 14: 1-28.
14. Goodman LS, Gilman. A. Pharmacological basis of Therapeutics, ed.7, New York: Macmillan, 1985.
15. Havener's. Ocular Pharmacology, ed. 6: C.V. Mosby, 1994.
16. Kanski. Clinical ophthalmology, ed. 4: Butterworth – Heineman, 1999.
17. Kershner. Ophthalmic Medications and Pharmacology: Slack. Inc., 1994.
18. Koevary. Ocular immunology in diseases: Butterworth – Heinemann, 1999.
19. Olin BR, et al. Drugs Facts and Comparisons: Facts and Comparisons, St. Louis, 1997.
20. Onofrey. The Ocular Therapeutics; Lippincott-William and Wilkins, 1997.
21. Rhee. The Wills Eye drug Guide: Lippincott–William and Wilkins, 1998.
22. Steven Podos. Textbook of ophthalmology, New Delhi: Jaypee Medical Publishers, 2001.
23. Zimmerman. Textbook of Ocular Pharmacology: Lippincott and William and Wilkins, 1997.

Chapter 37

Optimized NSAIDs and Anti-bacterial Regimen is Key to Ocular Surgical Prophylaxis

Ashok Garg (India), Ian Bell (USA)

Cataract surgery is one of the most commonly performed ocular surgery in the world. Given the ability of ocular surface flora to enter the eye during surgery, many of the prophylactic techniques aim is to suppress their number and to limit the growth of those organisms that do enter the eye during intraocular surgery. Antimicrobial prophylaxis is an essential component of both cataract and refractive surgeries. Choosing an antibiotic for surgical prophylaxis in the clinical setting can also be challenging.

The key surgical prophylaxis paradigm shift in recent years for long practicing ophthalmologists is the growing evidence for preoperative use of both topical antibiotics and anti-inflammatory drops. The second shift is the realization that we should discontinue antibiotics more quickly and ensure use of anti-inflammatory for the full course of therapy. These changes are key for limiting post-cataract (iatrogenic) inflammation and infection while they prevent the development of antibiotic resistance in patients. In the pre-operative a fourth-generation fluoroquinolone such as Moxifloxacin 0.5% solution, a non-steroidal anti-inflammatory such as topical Nepafence 0.1%, suspension, and a topical steroid such as prednisolone acetate 1% should all be administered.

Loading the eye with an antibiotic prior to the surgical insult reduces the risk of endophthalmitis. Furthermore studies have shown that the non-steroidal, anti-inflammatory drugs (NSAIDs) and the steroids are synergistic and both work better if the eye is loaded preoperative.

There are two basic ways to approach the preoperative loading. One approach provides the drops within the three-to-four dose delating regimen in the surgical induction area. We can add Neosynephrine 10% Cyclogyl solution (1% Cyclopentolate HCl), an antibiotic, steroid, non-steroidal, so actually they get loaded up with five different drops. Our preoperative routine is three doses of drops starting 30 to 60 minutes before surgery.

Some surgeons prefer to start the drops 24 hours preoperative while others start the drops three days preoperative.

There are select indications where anti-inflammatory drug dosing should begin a week preoperative including high-risk cases for inflammation and secondary macular edema. Such patients includes those with a long-term, history of chronic uveitis and diabetes mellitus and patients with pigmentary retinopathy and macular edema, and those who developed macular edema in the first eye after cataract surgery.

With high-risk patients such as those who are immunocompromised or prone to infection, we can start the antibiotic three days preoperative rather than just on the table.

In our routine cases, I load the entire drop regimen in the eye in the operating room, but the high-risk cases you may start, three to seven days preoperative. There is not yet a consensus, but you may want to go a little longer and by more intense on the high-risk patients.

The research evidence does not clearly identify whether drug delivery shortly preoperative or several days preoperative is better. However, as the patients become higher risk, We tend to have a slightly longer and more intense course of antibiotic and anti-inflammatory drops.

Routine patients that never had a problem generally start to receive the drug in the operating room prior to surgery because it is easiler on the patient.

POSTOPERATIVE SCHEDULE FOR CATARACT PATIENTS

The major changes in recent years from previous antibiotic experience is the perioperative and short postoperative course of the drugs. We now limit antibiotic use because the risk of endophthalmitis drops with in a week when the wound seals. It is the long-term, low-dose use of these drugs that leads to resistant organisms.

Our approach is to administer antibiotics and anti-inflammatory drops (steroid and NSAID) at the end of the case. My staff administer them again in the recovery area before the patient goes home.

We have patients use the antibiotic drops three times a day for one week. Other surgeons have them take the antibiotic for as few as five days.

However, the anti-inflammatory drug is required for longer use. Evidence suggests the blood aqueous barrier breakdown that occurs after cataract surgery persists for four to eight weeks. Because the average breakdown lasts about six weeks, we should treat with anti-inflammatory drops for one to two months in routine cases. This will prevent any rebound of inflammation or other secondary issues.

We need to have patients use the anti-inflammatory drops a big longer than some surgeons think is necessary because often the eyes are quiet and comfortable by two to three weeks after surgery, but there is still some risk for cystoid macular edema up to six weeks postoperative.

For example, for at-risk patients preoperative dosing is recommended for one week and postoperative dosing is recommended for one week and postoperative dosing is recommended for four weeks to several months.

Drug Dosages

The dosing regimen we use instillation of the topical Nevanac, which is a TID drop, a three-times daily drop. We use Moxifloxacin, Nepafenac, and a topical steroid, which seems more than adequate, as these drugs have demonstrated efficacy in contributing to good surgical outcomes.

Ophthalmologists should be aware of adding NSAID drug to their regimen. Most patients recover without complications when surgeons only use an antibiotic and a steroid. However, there are indications that over 10% of patients will develop a very mild macular edema without an NSAID. That's a risk that NSAIDs can eliminate.

We have pretty minimally invasive cataract surgery today, and people work really hard at their surgical technique, but probably the one thing that could have the greatest impact on their outcomes would be to add an NSAID to their regimen.

The incidence of very mild macular edema without an NSAID, even in a good surgeon's hands, is about 12% and adding as NSAID takes it down to less than 1% so you get a hug reduction in one of the most common sight threatening complications of cataract surgery just by adding an NSAID and using it properly.

Proper dosing of antibiotics, NSAIDs, and steroid plays a very important role in preventing complications such as infection or CME.

Minimizing these complications with effective agents and proper therapeutic dosing regimens will improve our surgical outcomes.

Surgeons can greatly improve their chances of a successful surgical outcome if they keep in mind three key criteria in selecting antibiotics: potency, penetration, and safety. A good balance of these aspects – especially potency and penetration – provides the best patient protection.

An antibiotic that is highly potent and effective at killing infections at lower concentrations would lose much of its efficacy if it was unable to penetrate the tissue. Conversely, a medication that penetrates extremely well but lacks potency also would not be very functional.

Clinicians are best served by an effective combination of penetration and potency.

Although researchers are frequently asked whether potency or penetration is more important, the only clear answer is the most effective approach is to combine these factors.

MEASURING POTENCY

Identifying an antibiotics strength in penetration and potency is important, but surgeons should be aware that potency definitions vary. The most common assessment of an antibiotics potency, the minimum inhibitory concentration (MIC), traces whether organisms growth has been stopped. However, the definition still alows viable organisms to remain. This most common term may not be the most important. Another standard, minimum bactericidal concentration (MBC), tracks whether 99.9% of the organism is killed (MBC is approximately 4x the MIC). The final measurement, mutant prevention concentration (MPC), gauges whether the organism was killed with mutations prevented (MPC is approximately 8x the MIC).

Drugs with the lowest potency numbers in MIC, MBC or MPC are among the most potent. With postoperative infections being potentially sight threatening, it is ideal to exceed these levels with the antibiotic concentrations in the target tissues.

PENETRATION TRACKING

Antibiotic tissue penetration plays a key role in protecting against infection.

This issue arises when examining the research on various antibiotics; some may have good potency statistics *in vitro*, but we fail to identify the *in vivo* performance of the antibiotic. The latter will tell ophthalmologists what levels of the drug our patients actually will get in the cornea, the anterior chamber, and the vitreous. Our research administering fluoroquinolones to a cornea transplant model prior to corneal transplant and then examining the antibiotic levels in the cornea showed Moxifloxacin had three times the concentration of Gatifloxacin.

Similar research at various international research centers on aqueous concentrations of antibiotic applied a series of drops preoperative and measured aqueous concentration at the time of cataract surgery. Those researchers identified the same three-fold greater penetration of Moxifloxacin. Protection can be defined by overlaying these concentrations with the MICs for potential pathogens.

In vivo potency after tissue penetration is a better measure of antibiotic efficacy than speed of kill *in vitro*. The latter removes all of the factors that determine how the antibiotic performs in human tissue. These studies disregard the reality of penetration of the antibiotic through human tissue. For these reasons *in vivo* potency and penetration studies will always have more real-world resonance than *in vitro* speed of kill research. The aqueous humor concentrations achieved in the International Research Centers were tested against a *Staph. aureus* ocular isolate using disk-diffusion analysis. The moxifloxacin achieve a 24 mm zone of inhibition, and Gatifloxacin had no zone of inhibition. This surrogate model accounts for tissue penetration and potency at the potential site of infection, thus defining protection.

SAFETY EVALUATION

In addition to potency and penetration, a solid evaluation of antibiotics for surgical prophylaxis should assess whether the drug is nontoxic. Efforts to prevent the use of nontoxic medication should look for epithelial problems or endothelial problems.

As a class of drugs, the Fluoroquinolones have proven to by very safe and nontoxic.

Our experience with all fourth-generation Fluoroquinolones has found that they are very safe. Research comparing corneal epithelial healing post-operative when Moxifloxacin or Gatifloxacin are used have found very similar would healing rates. In fact, an independent well-controlled study evaluating wound healing post-PRK for Moxifloxacin and Gatifloxacin were conducted in USA. The conclusion was that both the drugs are safe. Generally, they found that eyes treated with Moxifloxacin healed faster and had smaller defects than those treated with Gatifloxacin.

Rabbit model studies that created epithelial defects and tracked healing when the two antibiotics are used found similar results. Clinical trials looking at healing after PRK also identified similar healing. Both fluoroquinolones are safe and nontoxic.

Chapter 38

Clinical Applications of Anti-inflammatory and Anti-protease Effects of Tetracyclines in Ocular Surface Disease

Stephen C Pflugfelder, Cintia S De Paiva, De-Quan Li (USA)

The first tetracycline, chlortetracycline, was produced as a fermentation product of *Streptomyces aureofaciens* in 1948. Since then, several tetracycline molecules have been synthesized from chlortetracycline, including tetracycline, doxycycline and minocycline that differ in their absorption, lipophilicity and duration of action (Fig. 38.1). In addition to their antimicrobial effects, tetracyclines have been found to have potent anti-protease and anti-

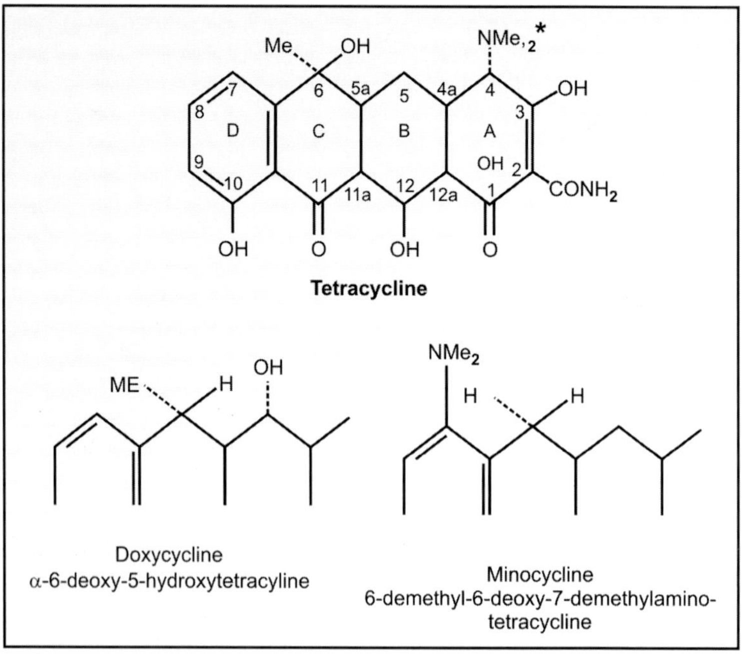

Me OH NMe,2 * OH 7 6 5a 5 4a 4 3 8 D C B A 9 OH 2 10 11 11a 12 12a 1 CONH2 OH O OH O

Tetracycline

ME H OH

Doxycycline
α-6-deoxy-5-hydroxytetracyline

NMe2 H H

Minocycline
6-demethyl-6-deoxy-7-demethylamino-tetracycline

Fig. 38.1: Chemical structures of tetracycline (short-acting, top) and two long-acting derivatives, doxycycline (lower left) and minocycline (lower right). Tetracycline derivatives lacking the dimethylamino group at position 4 on the tetracycline ring structure (asterisk) lose their antibiotic properties

inflammatory effects. Tetracycline derivatives lacking the dimethylamino group at position 4 on the tetracycline ring structure (asterisk in Fig. 38.1) lose their antibiotic properties but retain these non-antimicrobial activities.[1]

Anti-inflammatory and Anti-protease Properties of Tetracyclines

Our group has extensively investigated the effects of doxycycline on stimulated production of inflammatory cytokines and matrix metalloproteinases by the corneal epithelium. Doxycycline was found to inhibit lipopolysaccharide (LPS)-induced production of IL-1β by the corneal epithelium and to stimulate expression of IL-1 receptor antagonist (IL-1 RA), the anti-inflammatory form of this cytokine.[2] Furthermore, doxycycline reduced the steady state level of cellular interleukin 1 converting enzyme (ICE), an enzyme that converts precursor IL-1β to its mature biologically active form. As anticipated, doxycycline significantly decreased IL-1 bioactivity in supernatants from LPS treated corneal epithelial cultures. These anti-inflammatory effects were of comparable magnitude to corticosteroids. Doxycycline also markedly suppressed production of IL-1β, TNF-α and IL-8 by osmotically stressed cultured corneal epithelia (Fig. 38.2).[3] This activity was found to be due in

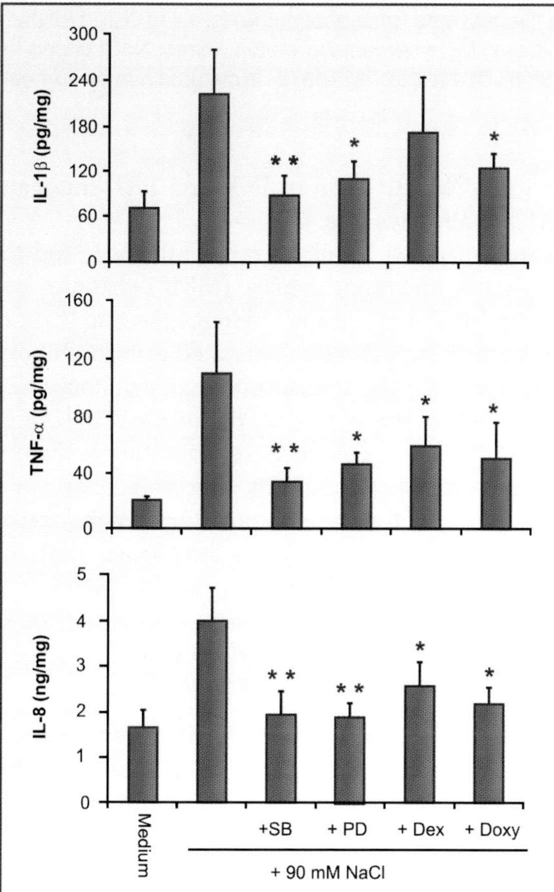

Fig. 38.2: Exposure of cultured human corneal epithelial cells to osmotic stress by adding 90 mm NaCl to their media stimulated production of IL-1β, TNF-α and IL-8. This was blocked by addition of ERK (PD) and JNK (SP) MAPK kinase inhibitors and doxycycline. The corticosteroid dexamethasone inhibited TNF-α and IL-8; *p < 0.05, **p < 0.01 (reprinted from Li DQ et al. Exp Eye Res 2006;82:588-96)

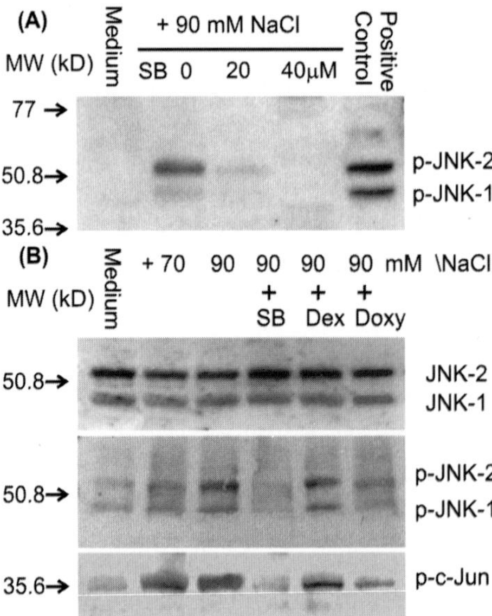

Fig. 38.3: Western blot showing the activated (phosphorylated) forms of JNK-1, JNK 2 and transcription factor c-jun activated by hyperosmolar media (90mM NaCl added to media) and inhibited by SB202190 (A,B) and doxycycline (B) in cultured human corneal epithelial cells

part to doxycycline's ability to block activation of JNK and ERK mitogen activated protein kinase (MAPK) pathways (Fig. 38.3).

Doxycycline in concentrations of 1 and 10 micrograms/ml was found to inhibit production of several matrix metalloproteinase (MMP) enzymes by the corneal epithelium, including MMP-1, -3, -9 and -13 in response to IL-1 or osmotic stress (Fig. 38.4).[4-7] This activity appeared to be related to its inhibition of the stress activated protein kinase JNK.[6] The tetracycline analog minocycline was also found to inhibit stress activated protein kinase pathways in the brain and in cultured microglial cells.[8,9] Taken together these laboratory research studies indicate that tetracyclines have potent inhibitory effects on production of MMPs and inflammatory mediators by the corneal epithelium. With regard to MMPs, the inhibitory activity of tetracyclines surpasses that of corticosteroids.

Clinical Applications of Non-antimicrobial Properties of Tetracyclines for Treatment of Ocular Surface Diseases

Tetracycline antibiotics have been recognized for years as effective therapies for improving signs and symptoms of ocular surface diseases. These salutary effects are most likely due to their non-antimicrobial anti-inflammatory and anti-protease activities. The evidence supporting the clinical efficacy of

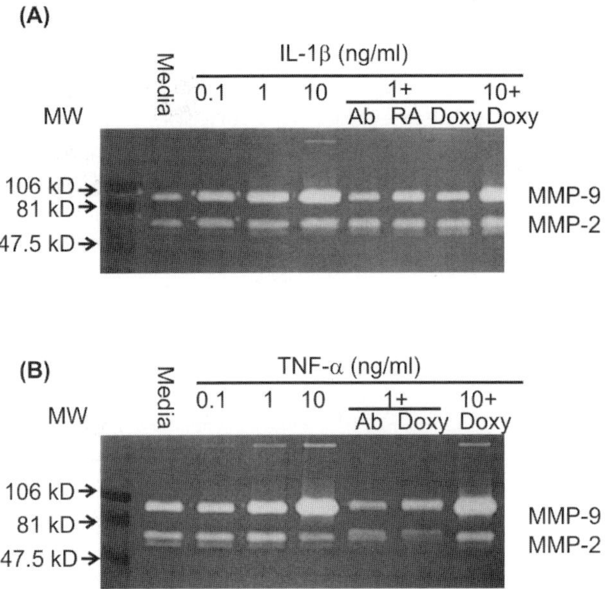

Fig. 38.4: A (top).Gelatin zymogram evaluating regulation of MMP-9 production by IL-1β. Primary human corneal epithelial cultures were grown to sub confluence and switched to serum-free media before treatment with IL-1β at 0.1, 1.0 and 10 ng ml with or without neutralizing antibody (Ab), IL-1 receptor antagonist (IL-1 RA) or doxycycline (Doxy) 1 or 10 mg/ml for 24 hr. The conditioned media were collected for gelatin zymography. B (bottom). Gelatin zymogram evaluating the regulation of MMP-9 production by TNF-α. Primary human corneal epithelial cultures were grown to sub confluence and switched to serum-free media before treatment with TNF-α at 0.1, 1.0 and 10 ng/ml with or without neutralizing antibody (Ab) or doxycycline (Doxy) or 10 mg/ml for 24 hr (reprinted from Li D-Q et al. Exp Eye Res 2001;73:449-59)

tetracyclines, as well as their proposed mechanisms of action for ocular surface diseases including: persistent corneal epithelial defects, recurrent corneal epithelial erosion, corneal stromal ulceration, mucus membrane pemphigoid, phlyctenular keratitis, ocular rosacea and keratitis sicca are provided below.

Treatment of Persistent Corneal Epithelial Defects and Recurrent Corneal Epithelial Erosion

Systemically administered tetracycline (1 gram/day) was found to promote healing of persistent corneal epithelial defects that had been present for 10 days or greater and were unresponsive to conventional treatments, including bandage contact lenses.[10] The most common causes for these epithelial defects were herpetic keratitis, recurrent erosion and dry eye. The corneal epithelial defects healed in 14 of 18 patients, with half of the defects healing within 48 hours.

Doxycycline has been reported to be effective in treating recurrent corneal epithelial erosions in two additional studies. Hope-Ross and associates performed a prospective, randomized, controlled 24 week trial comparing three treatment groups: standard therapies (lubricants, hypertonic saline), oral tetracycline (250mg twice daily) and oral tetracycline and topical prednisolone for recalcitrant recurrent corneal epithelial erosions.[11] The tetracycline and tetracycline plus topical corticosteroid groups both showed significant reductions in the number of recurrent erosions compared to standard therapy during the study period. Furthermore, the tetracycline treated groups had significantly faster healing of epithelial defects than the standard group. Dursun and colleagues reported a series of 7 patients with a history of 1 to 7 prior recurrent erosions that had failed to respond to conventional therapies (artificial tears, hypertonic saline, patching, bandage contact lenses, epithelial debridement) who had resolution of their condition with oral doxycyline (50 mg twice a day) for 3 months and topical corticosteroid (methyprednisolone, prednisolone acetate or fluorometholone) two or three times daily for 3 weeks.[12] Corneal epithelial defects healed in 2 to 10 days when present. No recurrence was observed during a mean follow-up period of 21.9 months.

In a rabbit model of superficial alkali corneal injury, oral doxycycline at a dose of 5 mg/kg/day was noted to significantly speed healing of the corneal epithelial defects.[13]

Prevention of Sterile Corneal Stromal Ulceration and Neovascularization

In 1895, Perry and Golub initially reported the use of oral tetracycline for treatment of sterile corneal ulceration.[14] This was complimented with a study that evaluated the effects of two doses of tetracycline (10mg/kg/day and 50mg/kg/day) in a rabbit model of alkali-induced corneal injury. Both doses of tetracycline were effective in preventing ulceration compared to the untreated control group with the highest dose being the most effective.[15] The tetracycline treated rabbits had a marked reduction in inflammatory cell infiltration of the corneal stroma. Levy and Katz noted that systemic tetracycline decreased corneal performation in a rabbit model of *Pseudomonas* keratitis by approximately 50%.[16] Treatment of two human patients with severe pseudomonas keratitis with oral doxycycline (100 mg BID) arrested stromal ulceration in these patients.[17]

Tetracycline derivatives have also been observed to have potent inhibitory activity for corneal neovascularization in several animal models. A minocycline controlled release polymer implanted into the cornea stroma of rabbits was noted to completely inhibit tumor induced angiogenesis.[18] Doxycycline (2%) administered topically significantly inhibited development of corneal neovascularization after chemical cauterization of the rabbit cornea with silver

desquamation of the superficial corneal epithelia in dry eye, while apical epithelial cells remained intact in eyes that were treated with methylprednisolone or doxycycline (Fig. 38.7C). A concurrent study showed that MMP-9 protein in the corneal epithelium dramatically increased in experimental dry eye and this was prevented by topical treatment with the methylprednisolone or doxycycline 0.025% QID.[37] Gelatinase activity in the corneal epithelium and tears also markedly decreased with these therapies.

SUMMARY

The role of inflammation and increased protease activity in the pathogenesis of ocular surface disease has become evident over the past 2 decades. There is overwhelming evidence indicating that tetracyclines have potent anti-inflammatory and anti-protease effects in treating a variety of ocular surface diseases. They are often effective in low concentrations that minimize systemic side effects and they are synergistic with other commonly utilized immunomodulatory agents. Animal studies and preliminary human experience indicate that tetracyclines, such as doxycycline may be effective when applied topically in sub antimicrobial doses that would eliminate the systemic side effects that commonly accompany oral tetracycline therapy.

REFERENCES

1. Curci JA, Petrinec D, Liao S, Golub LM, Thompson RW. Pharmacological suppression of abdominal aortic aneurysms: a comparison of doxycycline and four chemically modified tetracyclines. J Vasc Surg 1998;28:1082-93.
2. Solomon A, Monroy D, Rosenblatt M, Ji Z, Lokeshwar BL, Pflugfelder SC. Doxycycline inhibition of interleukin-1 in the corneal epithelium. Invest Ophthalmol Vis Sci 2000;41:2544-57.
3. Li DQ, Luo L, Chen Z, Kim HS, Song XJ, Pflugfelder SC. JNK and ERK MAP kinases mediate induction of IL-1α, TNF-α and IL-8 following hyperosmolar stress in human limbal epithelial cells. Exp Eye Res 2006;82:588-96.
4. Li D-Q, Lokeshwar BL, Solomon A, Monroy D, Ji Z, Pflugfelder SC. Regulation of MMP-9 in human corneal epithelial cells. Exp Eye Res 2001;73:449-59.
5. Li de Q, Shang TY, Kim HS, Solomon A, Lokeshwar BL, Pflugfelder SC. Regulated Expression of Collagenases MMP-1, -8, and -13 and Stromelysins MMP-3, -10, and -11 by Human Corneal Epithelial Cells. Invest Ophthalmol Vis Sci 2003;44:2928-36.
6. Li DQ, Chen Z, Song XJ, Luo L, Pflugfelder SC. Stimulation of Matrix Metalloproteinases by Hyperosmolarity via a JNK Pathway in Human Corneal Epithelial Cells. Invest Ophthalmol Vis Sci 2004;45:4302-11.
7. Kim HS, Luo L, Pflugfelder SC, Li DQ. Doxycycline inhibits TGF-beta1-induced MMP-9 via Smad and MAPK pathways in human corneal epithelial cells. Invest Ophthalmol Vis Sci 2005;46:840-8.
8. Zhu S, Stavrovskaya IG, Drozda M, et al. Minocycline inhibits cytochrome C release and delays progression of amyotrophic lateral sclerosis in mice. Nature 2002;417:74-78.

9. Suk K. Minocycline suppresses hypoxic activation of rodent microglia in culture. Neurosci Letters 2004;366:167-171.
10. Perry HD, Kenyon KR, Lamberts DW, Foulks GN, Seedor JA, Golub LM. Systemic tetracycline hydrochloride as adjunctive therapy in the treatment of persistent epithelial defects. Ophthalmology 1986;93:1320-2.
11. Hope-Ross MW, Chell PB, Kervick GN, McDonnell PJ, Jones HS Oral tetracycline in the treatment of recurrent corneal erosions. Eye 1994;8 (Pt 4):384-8.
12. Dursun D, Kim MC, Solomon A, Pflugfelder SC. Treatment of recalcitrant recurrent corneal epithelial erosions with inhibitors of matrix metalloproteinases-9, doxycycline and corticosteroids. Am J Ophthalmol 2001;132:8-13.
13. Perry HD, Hodes LW, Seedor JA, Donnenfeld ED, McNamara TF, Golub LM. Effect of doxycycline hyclate on corneal epithelial wound healing in the rabbit alkali-burn model. Preliminary observations. Cornea 1993;12:379-82.
14. Perry HD, Golub LM. Systemic tetracyclines in the treatment of non-infected corneal ulcers: a case report and proposed new mechanism of action. Ann Ophthalmol 1985;17:742-44.
15. Seedor JA, Perry HD, McNamara TF, Golub LM, Buxton DF, Guthrie DS. Systemic tetracycline treatment of alkali-induces corneal ulceration in rabbits, Arch Ophthalmol 1987;105:268-271.
16. Levy JH, Katz HR. Effect of systemic tetracycline on progression os *Pseudomonas aeruginosa* keratitis in the rabbit. Ann Ophthalmol 1990;22:179-82.
17. McElvanney AM. Doxycycline in the management of pseudomonas corneal melting: Two case reports and a review of the literature. Eye Contact Lens 2003;29:258-61.
18. Riazi-Esfahani M, Peyman GA, Aydin E, Kazi AA, Kivilcim M, Sanders DR. Prevention of corneal neovascularization: Evaluation of various commercially available compounds in an experimental rat model. Cornea 2006;25:801-5.
19. Tamargo RJ, Bok RA, Brem H. Angiogenesis inhibition by minocycline. Cancer Res 1991;51:672-5
20. Peyman GA, Kazi AA, Riazi-Esfahani M, Aydin E, Kivilcim M, Sanders DR. The effect of combinations of flurbiprofen, low molecular weight heparin, and doxycycline on the inhibition of corneal neovascularization. Cornea 2006;25: 582-5.
21. Marks R, Ellis J. Comparative effectiveness of tetracycline and ampicillin in rosacea. A controlled trial. Lancet 1971;2(7733):1049-52.
22. Sneedon IB. A clinical trial of tetracycline in rosacea. Br J Dermatol 1966;78: 649-52.
23. Jenkins MS, Brown SI, Lempert SL, Weinberg RJ. Ocular rosacea. Am J Ophthalmol 1979;88:618-22.
24. Bartholomew RS, Reid BJ, Cheesbrough MJ, Macdonald M, Galloway NR. Oxytetracycline in the treatment of ocular rosacea: a double-blind trial. Br J Ophthalmol 1982;66:386-8
25. Frucht-Pery J, Sagi E, Hemo I,Ever-Hadani P. Efficacy of doxycycline and tetracycline in ocular rosacea. Am J Ophthalmol 1993;116:88-92.
26. Akpek EK, Merchant A,Pinar V, Foster CS. Ocular rosacea: Patient characteristics and follow-up. Ophthalmology 1997;104:1863-7.
27. Zengin N, Tol H, Gunduz K, Okudan S, Balevi S, Endogru H. Meibomian gland dysfunction and tear film abnormalities in rosacea. Cornea 1995;14:144-6.
28. Berman B, Zell D. Subantimicrobial dose doxycycline: A unique treatment for rosacea. Cutis 2005;75(4 Suppl):19-24.

29. Zaidman GW, Brown SI. Orally administered tetracycline for phlyctenular keratoconjunctivitis Am J Ophthalmol 1981;92:178-82
30. Culbertson WW, Huang AJ, Mandelbaum SH, Pflugfelder SC, Boozalis GT, Miller D. Effective treatment of phlyctenular keratoconjunctivitis with oral tetracycline. Ophthalmology 1993;100:1358-66
31. Ahmed M, Zein G, Khawaja F, Foster CS. Ocular cicatricial pemphigoid: pathogenesis, diagnosis and treatment. Prog Retin Eye Res. 2004;23:579-92.
32. Reiche L,Wojnarowska F, Mallon E. Combination therapy with nicotinamide and tetracyclines for cicatricial pemphigoid: Further support for its efficacy. Clin Exp Dermatol 1998;23:254-7.
33. Kreyden OP, Borradori L,Trueb RM,Burg G, Nestle FO [Successful therapy with tetracycline and nicotinamide in cicatricial pemphigoid] Hautarzt 2001;52: 247-50.
34. Dragan L,Eng AM, Lam S, Persson T. Tetracycline and niacinamide: treatment alternatives in ocular cicatricial pemphigoid. Cutis 1999;63:181-3
35. Sacher C, Hunzelmann N. Cicatricial pemphigoid (mucous membrane pemphigoid): Current and emerging therapeutic approaches. Am J Clin Dermatol 2005;6:93-103
36. De Paiva CS, Corrales RM, Villarreal AL, Farley W, Li DQ, Stern ME, Pflugfelder SC. Apical corneal barrier disruption in experimental murine dry eye is abrogated by methylprednisolone and doxycycline Invest Ophthalmol Vis Sci 2006;47: 2847-56
37. De Paiva CS, Corrales RM, Villarreal AL, Farley W, Li DQ, Stern ME, Pflugfelder SC. Corticosteroid and doxycycline suppress MMP-9 and inflammatory cytokine expression, MAPK activation in the corneal epithelium in experimental dry eye. Exp Eye Res 2006;83:526-35.

Chapter 39

Management of Non-Viral Pediatric Keratitis

Anita Panda, Abhiyan Kumar, Shalini Mohan,
Rasheena, V Sujith (India)

Corneal infection is the most common cause of profound ocular morbidity leading to blindness worldwide. Infective keratitis in children (Fig. 39.1) is a cause of great concern to the treating ophthalmologist as it remains an ocular morbidity that is more challenging to diagnose and treat. Scarcity of the literature on the subject adds to the problem of inadequate treatment. Though several large series of adult infective keratitis have been described at great length in various studies[6-14] only few reports are available in pediatric keratitis.[15-22]

The World Health Organization (WHO) has suggested that there are 1.5 million blind children worldwide and 70,000 children have active corneal

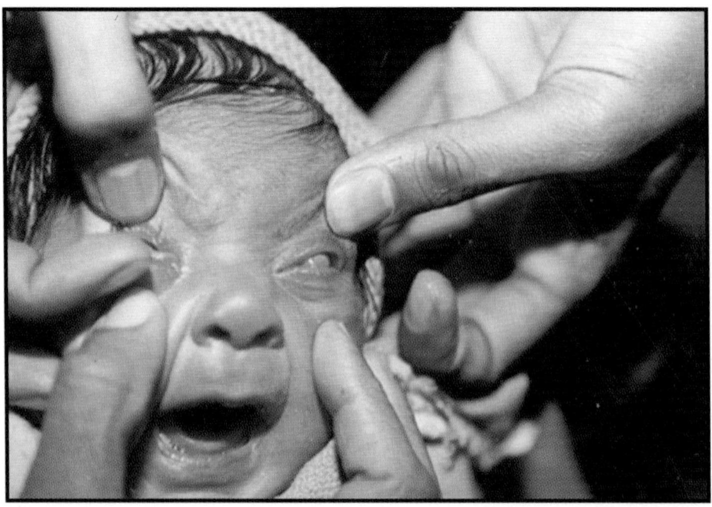

Fig. 39.1: A case of bilateral congenital glaucoma with bilateral corneal ulcer

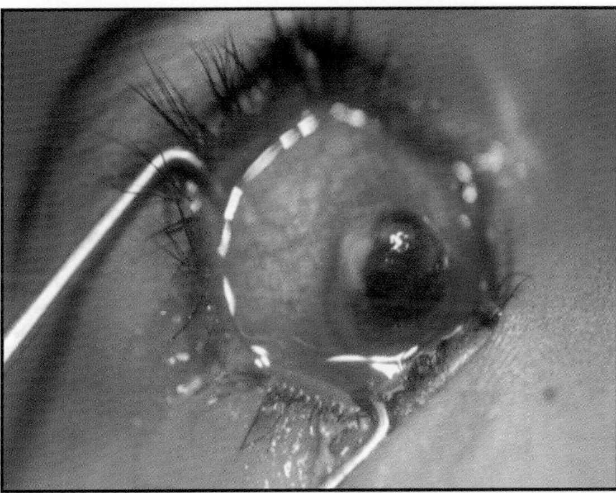

Fig. 39.3: Eye examination using speculum for adequate exposure

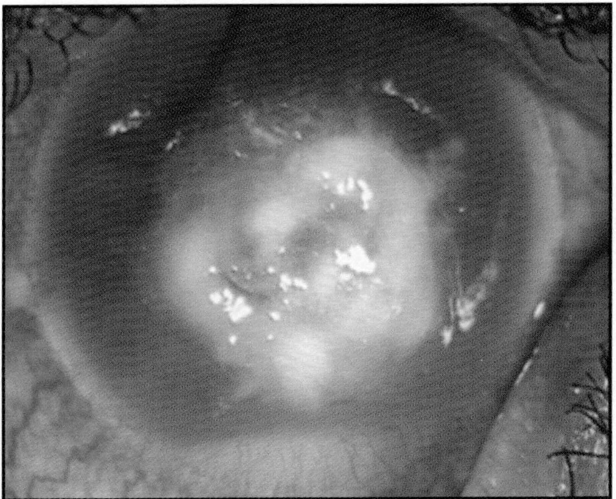

Fig. 39.4: Hypopyon ulcers: Central mixed

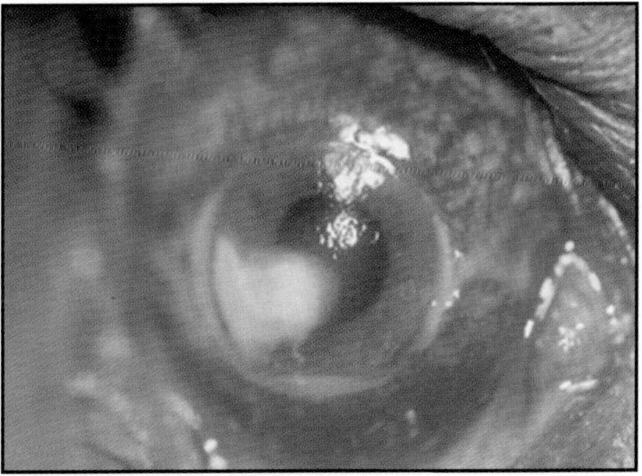

Fig. 39.5: Hypopyon ulcers: Peripheral

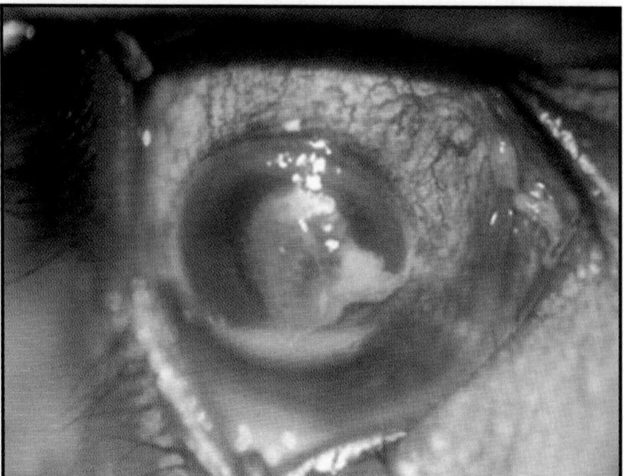

Fig. 39.6: Hypopyon ulcers: Central

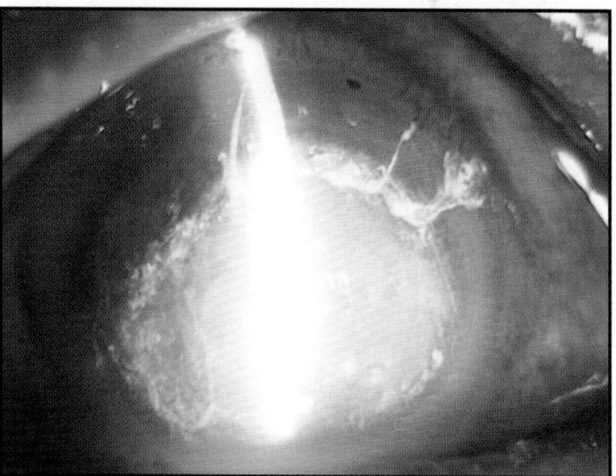

Fig. 39.7: Fungal ulcer (Aspergillus) with hypopyon

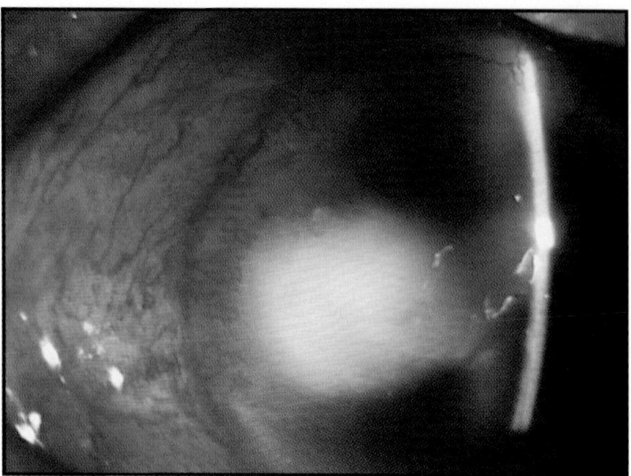

Fig. 39.8: Staphylococcal ulcer resolving with peripheral vascularization

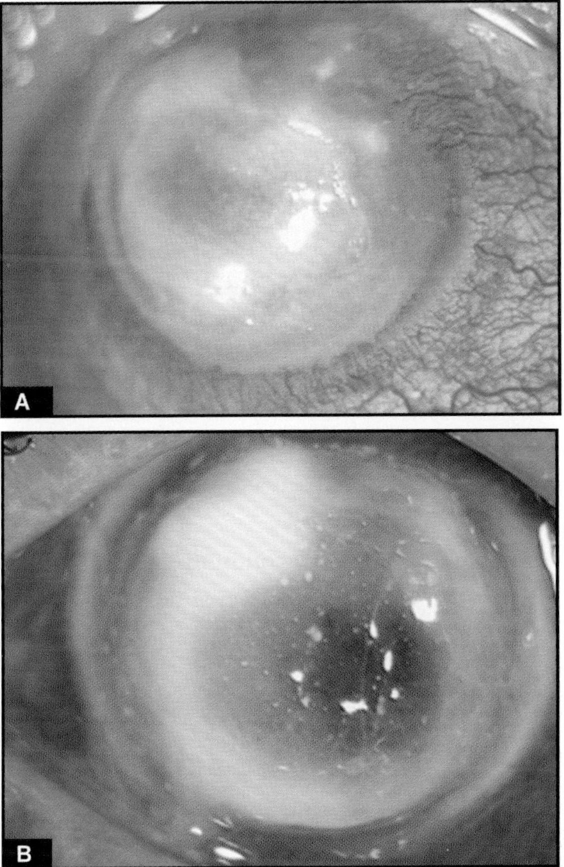

Figs 39.9A and B: Severe ulcer: With impending perforation

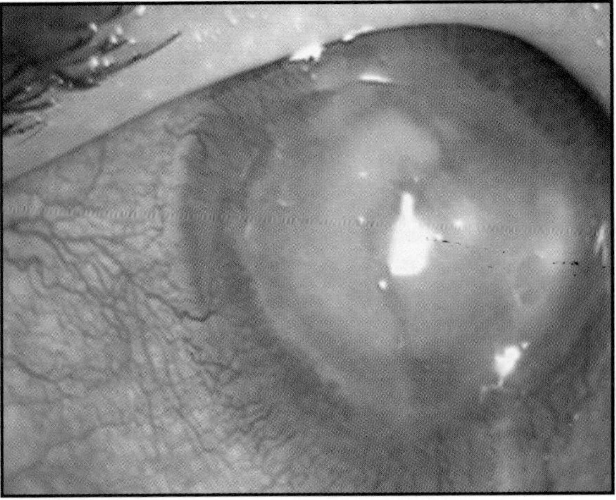

Fig. 39.10: Resolving ulcer: With peripheral vascularization

Clinical signs They can be graded according to Jones criterion[17] (Table 39.2). Bacterial corneal ulcers are non-specific as to the etiology in children with only 30% cases having hypopyon on presentation.[4] Ulcer may be round or oval with centrally or peripherally situated (Figs 39.3 and 39.4). Its sides and floor are gray and ragged in appearance. Conjunctival and cicumciliary congestion is present. Cornea reveals stromal infiltration and edema is present. Iris contour is lost because of iris edema. Increase of vessels permeability in iris leads to anterior chamber cells, flare, fibrinous exudates and hypopyon. If infection is not controlled by appropriate treatment then it spreads both peripherally and deep down. It results in destruction of the stroma as seen in adults and leads to formation of Descemetocele. It can later on perforated by subsequent leukocytic enzymatic degradation, trauma or because of raised intraocular pressure.[11] With appropriate therapy ulcer resolves resulting in cicatrization.

Fungal

Trauma with vegetable matter is most common cause for fungal corneal ulcer. Panda et al reported corneal injury contaminated with vegetable matter was responsible for maximum number of cases.[12] Signs and symptoms do not differ from adults. Signs are more than the symptoms. Ulcer is dry looking ulcer with satellite lesions (Fig. 39.10). It is usually associated with hypopyon.

Acanthamoeba

Acanthamoeba related keratitis is rare among children. These are commonly found in fresh water sources, including bottled water, swimming pools, hot tubs, and bathroom tap water.[20,21] Contact lens solutions are also source of these organisms. It can be seen in children using aphakic contact lens. But non-contact lens related keratitis is also seen commonly.[22] Keratitis occurs in patients with minor corneal trauma and the majority of reported cases have been soft contact lens wearers. Early suspicion is the key to diagnose this condition[22] and prompt medical management results in better treatment outcome.

Table 39.2: Jones criterion for grading of keratitis[14]

Clinical features	*Non-severe*	*Severe*
Area of suppuration	< 6 mm	> 6 mm
Depth of ulcer	Superficial 2/3rd	Deep 1/3rd
Perforation	Unlikely	Present, imminent
Scleral suppuration	Absent	Present

Symptoms

Patients often present with pain, photophobia, and irritation.

Signs

Clinical characteristics[20] include pseudodendrites, stromal ring infiltrate, epithelial haze, endothelial infiltrates and radial keratoneuritis. Later on multifocal stromal infiltrates may lead to disciform keratitis. A ring infiltrate has been described as pathognomonic for Acanthamoeba keratitis.[23] Satellite lesions can be seen causing confusion with fungal infections. The infection is usually unilateral.

Contact Lens-induced Keratitis

The reported incidence of contact lens keratitis is 0.5% in daily wear and 3% in extended wear hydrogel contact lens.[16] It can be of following types:

1. Infective—It is due to stromal invasion of microbes.
2. Non-infective—Keratitis does not imply only infectious etiology. Corneal infiltrates are also sign of keratitis. Corneal infiltrates would be later discussed in details.

Corneal Scraping and Microbiological Evaluations

Corneal scraping/biopsy should be carried out for smear and culture examinations. Scraping should be done with Kimura spatula or No 15. B P knife. It should be immediately inoculated in blood, chocolate, non-nutrient agar with *E.coli*, (in suspected acanthamoeba keratitis) Sabaroud's dextrose agar media supplemented with yeast extract and 50 µg/ml of gentamicin sulfate (without cyclohexamide) to enhance the growth of fungi, potato dextrose agar, thioglycollate broth and brain heart infusion and sent for culture and sensitivity.[21] Slides should be made routinely for gram staining, giemsa staining and KOH wet mount preparation. Other stains include lactophenol cotton blue for fungus, methenamine silver, periodic acid shiff, calcoflour white stain and immunoperoxide stains for Acanthamoeba.[22] Children with Shigella infections must have cultures for their stool done, as it is commomly seen due to fecal contamination.[4]

Corneal biopsy specimens are to be centrifuged and then subjected to all the above tests. If there is availability of sufficient biopsy materials, the same should be also subjected to histopathological study (Fig. 39.11).

Blood agar, chocolate agar and brain heart infusion broth are to be incubated at 37°C while Sabourad's dextrose and Potato dextrose broths are at 25°C.

A culture should be considered positive if there is growth of the same organism on two or more media, confluent growth at site of inoculation on one solid medium, growth in one medium with consistent direct microscopy findings or growth of the same organism on repeated corneal specimens.

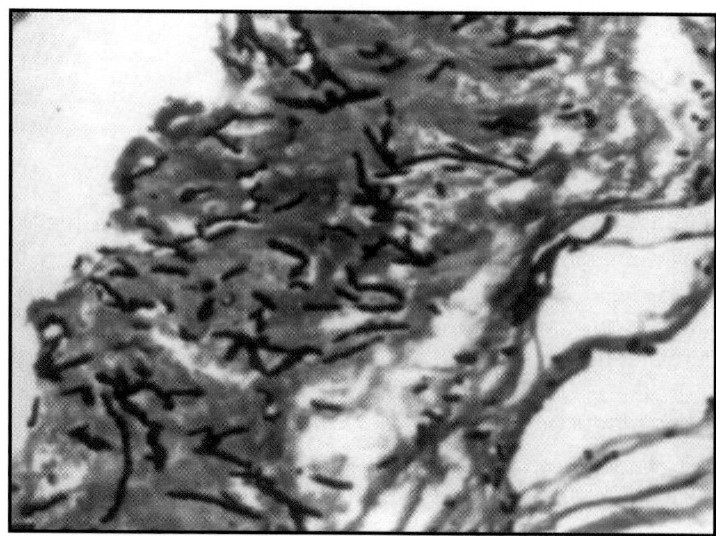

Fig. 39.11: Microscopic picture of fungal hyphae—silver methenamine stain

Management

It is usually the same as in adults except that it is a challenge due to uncooperative nature of the children. They will always need hospitalization to ensure proper examination and treatment. The objective of the therapy is to:

- Rapidly eliminate the infective organisms
- Reduce the inflammatory response
- Prevent structural damage to the cornea and promote epithelial healing.

Medical

i. *Antibacterials*: The recent regimen is fortified cefazolin (5%) and gentamicin (1.4%) in the same manner and the recent initial drug schedules include fortified cefazolin (5%) and tobramycin (1.4%) at same frequency as before in all and vancomycin + tobramycin in fulminating ulcers.

   Antifungals: If the fungal keratitis is clinically suspected, Natamycin suspension (5%) every 5 minutes for 30 minutes and then every 30 minutes till disappearance of infiltration and epithelial defect to be added to the antibacterial regimens. Amphotericin B drop 0.5 mg-10 mg/ml (0.05-0.15%) 5 times a day can be added in deep/non-responsive to Natamycin despite strong suspicion/confirmed fungal ulcer. However, Amphotericin B is irritant to the child's eye. Repeated epithelial debridement is required for better drug penetration.

Anti acanthamoebal: Topical polyhexamethylene biguanide (0.02%) eyedrop with propamidine isethionate eyedrop every 15 minutes to an hour while the patient is awake and Neosporin ophthalmic ointment during night are instilled for confirmed Acanthamoeba keratitis.

Others: Supportive therapy included 1% atropine ointment drop tds, 0.5% Timolol maleate drop BD to all the eyes.

ii. Systemic antibiotic 50 mg/kg body weight and carbonic anhydrase inhibitor at a dose of 1.5 mg/kg body weight are given to all the patients with ulcer size 4 mm or more for 5-7 days. The route of administration is age dependant. Vitamin A (at a dose of 1 lakh IU orally for < 1 year of age and 2 lakh IU for > 1year) should be given to the children with clinical malnutrition. Aprotinin, a plasmin inhibitor, 40 IU/ml 5 times a day can be added in few bacterial ulcers as adjunctive therapy. Topical corticosteroid drop is indicated only in eyes of chronic bacterial ulcer to reduce inflammation after confirming the sterility. If the ulcer is poorly responsive /non-responsive to specific antimicrobial drugs, povidone iodine, having a widest microbial spectrum, can be added to the therapy regimen. It is also effective against bacterial conjunctivitis in children and even prevents conjunctivitis in new born. The advantages include: it is inexpensive, readily available and of all effective in all types of microbial keratitis. Tear substitutes, autologous serum and substance P though do not have much role in active keratitis, have promising role in chronic and non healing ulcers. Autologous Serum – 50% and 100% autulogous serum is used in non healing corneal ulcers, persistent epithelial defects and cases associated with dry eyes. The proposed benefit for the serum is due to.[24]

- Epidermal growth factor (EGF) is present in both tears and serum and has been found to be helpful in healing of traumatic epithelial abrasions. EGF may also facilitate epithelialization because of its anti-apoptotic properties.[25]
- Acidic and basic fibroblast growth factors (aFGF, bFGF) were found to speed up healing of epithelial defects in rabbits.[26]
- Fibronectin another component of serum, has also been found to have some effect in helping epithelialization.[27]
- Vitamin A is found in much higher concentrations in serum compared to tears and may decrease the progression to squamous metaplasia in KCS.[28]
- Mucin expression by cultured conjunctival epithelial cells is upregulated by human serum[28] and this may contribute to the beneficial effects of serum in KCS.
- Serum antiproteases such as α_2 macroglobulin have been thought to inhibit corneal collagenases and be beneficial in conditions such as alkali burns.[29]

Neural factors such as substance P are important for corneal epithelial migration.[27] In neurotrophic ulcers, these substances are decreased and may be supplemented by topical serum.

Healing Criteria

The complete healing of the corneal ulcers is indicated by:

1. Absence of symptoms such as pain and photophobia. (if could be communicated), redness and discharge
2. Absence of epithelial defect as evidenced by the fluorescein staining
3. Absence of infiltration and anterior chamber reaction

Surgical: Ulcers showing signs of impending perforation/perforation underwent surgery

- Glue: For small perforations
  - Fibrin glue
  - Cyanoacrylate glue
- Tarsorrhaphy:
- Patch graft:
  - Corneal?Corneo scleral
  - Amniotic membrane (Fig. 39.12)
- Therapeutic Penetrating Keratoplasty

It is hence imperative to diagnose them at an early stage and formulate an uncompromising management protocol, so as to prevent profound visual morbidity.

Prevention It can be done by decreasing incidence of trauma and malnutrition in children. Ensuring proper Immunization also greatly helps in prevention of infective keratitis in children.

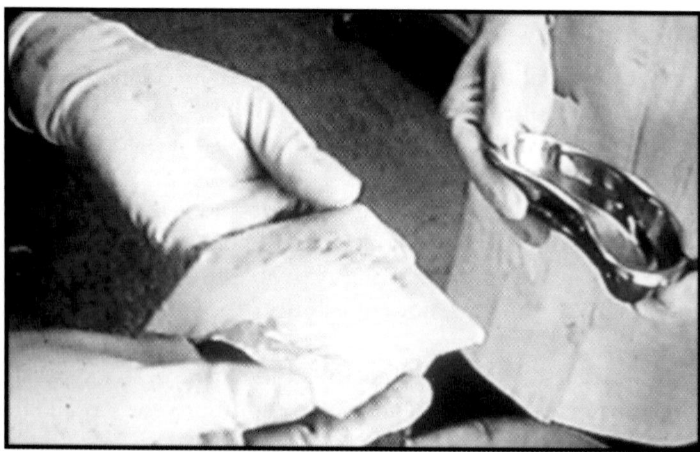

Fig. 39.12: Amniotic membrane for AMT

Early Diagnosis

It is the key to proper treatment and early rehabilitation of the child.

Treatment

Vitamin A Deficiency Disorders

The major cause of blindness in children worldwide is xerophthalmia caused by vitamin A deficiency.[30-32] Vitamin A deficiency is the single most frequent cause of blindness among preschool children in developing countries.[31] The term vitamin A deficiency disorders (VADD) has been introduced to cover the whole clinical spectrum of disease.[30]

Vitamin A deficiency affects growth, the differentiation of epithelial tissues, and immune competence. Vitamin A deficiency occurs when body stores are exhausted and supply fails to meet the body's requirements, either because there is a dietary insufficiency, requirements are increased, or intestinal absorption, transport and metabolism are impaired as a result of conditions such as diarrhea. The younger the child, the more severe is the disease and the higher the risk that corneal destruction will be followed by death.[30]

Clinical Features

It includes:

- Night blindness.
- Bitot's spot—triangular keratotic, foamy areas of interpalpebral bulbar conjunctiva.[23]
- Xerosis of the conjunctiva and cornea—xerophthalmia – dry lusterless poorly wettable surface.[23]
- Corneal ulceration and necrosis of the cornea.

Prevention

- Short-Administration to vulnerable groups of single, large doses of vitamin A on a periodic basis (2 L IU every 3 to 6 months).[30,31]
- Medium-fortification of a dietary vehicle (e.g., sugar or monosodium glutamate) with vitamin A can be initiated.[31]
- Longterm-increased dietary intake of vitamin A through home gardening and nutrition education programs solution to this problem.[31,32]

Treatment

Oral administration of 200,000 IU vitamin A on two successive days[32] and third dose to be given on 15th day.

Non-infective Corneal Infiltrates[33]

These are single or multiple transient discrete collection of grey or white material observed in normally transparent corneal tissue, usually present beneath epithelium.

These can be sterile or non-sterile. These are either inflammatory cells in response to chemotactic factors from damaged local tissues that have migrated cornea through limbal vasculature or from the tears. Or in some cases these may be partially formed of infectious agent as seen in infectious crystalline keratopathy. Catarrhal are sterile, benign and self-limited corneal lesions representing hypersensitivity to ribitol teichoic acid present in bacterial cell wall. This is seen with contact lens wear and is thought to be because of preservative thiomersol in the cleansing solution. Sometimes, these are also seen in contact lens infected with *Streptococcus pneumoniae*. They also occur in cases of staphylococcal blepharokeratoconjunctivitis and phylectenular keratoconjunctivitis.[34-37]

Clinical Feature

In contrast to infective keratitis these have minimal pain, discharge, punctate staining or anterior chamber reaction. These are usually less than 1 mm.

Treatment

Discontinuing contact lens leads to resolution of keratitis.

Miscellaneous Types of Keratitis

Blepharokeratitis/Blepharokeratoconjunctivitis

Whereas blepharitis is common in children, blepharokeratoconjunctivitis is rare.[34] It is a chronic external ocular and adnexal inflammatory condition marked by erythematous and edematous lid margins, crusting and scaling of lid margins, meibomian gland inflammation and inspissation, and conjunctival hyperemia.

The keratitis[35] involves the inferior cornea. The characteristic features are:

- Punctate epithelial keratopathy
- Marginal stromal infiltrates.
- Phlyctenules, marginal keratitis[34]
- Ulceration[34]
- Corneal thinning, scarring, and vascularization.

Treatment: Unlike adult, patients, any children suffered from blepharoconjunctivitis or viral conjunctivitis must be treated with topical antibiotics.

- Lid hygiene - removing debris and crusts along the lid margin, using cotton wool tipped swab sticks with diluted bicarbonate solution, diluted baby shampoo, or warm water

- Topical corticosteroid preparations,
- Topical antibiotics.
- Oral erythromycin (30–40 mg/kg body weight)[34,35] is used in children in place of oral tetracycline and its analogues, doxycycline and minocycline, which are used in adults. But these are contraindicated in children as they can lead to dental anomalies.

Fascicular Keratitis

This is associated with phlyctenular conjunctivitis.[38]

Corneal phlyctenules usually develop near limbus and spread centrally. There is no clear zone between limbus and phlycten. Superficial pannus is associated and ulcer perforates. Peripheral part heals but central ulcer spreads.[36]

Treatment: phlycten can be treated with topical steroid eyedrops. Long-term topical cyclosporin 2% therapy is safe and effective in children with phlyctenular keratoconjunctivitis associated with severe steroid-dependent corneal inflammation.[34]

Shield's Ulcer

Shield ulcer following vernal keratoconjunctivitis, though not frequent is a challenging situation to manage. They tend to occur in young patients in the palpaberal form, with large cobblestone papillae. It has a characteristic appearance—situated in the central part of superior third of the cornea,transversely oval in appearance. It is shallow and has white, shaggy epithelial edges the underlying bowman's layer may appear slightly opacified, with superficial stroma showing cellular infiltration without vascularization. A shield ulcer usually has an indolent course and may persist for weeks or months without enlarging. It may result in corneal scarring, which appears as a gray plaque like opacity of the Bowman's layer and superficial stroma.

Management

The management is similar to that of other forms of kerattis with the addition of topical diluted corticosterids. Use of bandage contact lens provides comfort to the patient and both should be used judiciously.

Acne Rosacea Keratitis[39]

Sterile corneal ulcers are reported to be associated with acne rosacea. Other manifestations include posterior eyelid inflammation including meibomian gland inspissation and lid margin telangiectasis, in conjunction with conjunctival injection or episcleritis.

Eye Exposure and Corneal Infection

The advert effects of eye exposure and corneal infections[40-45] though infrequent in children is another serious problem. Microbial keratitis is a severe complication of corneal exposure in unconscious patients. It holds good for the patient while under general anesthesia and when the patient is ventilated. Therefore, simple method of eye closure must be followed in these situations to prevent the disaster.

Comments

Infective keratitis in pediatric age group is a potentially blinding disorder and gets aggravated due to varied factors. It is difficult to diagnose because not only the children but the parents too are frequently unable to provide a complete history with regards to risk factors such as exact mode of previous trauma, duration of symptoms and others. It is also difficult to obtain the exact history even from the older children as they try to hide the factual evidence due to the fear or possible parental reprisals. Poor patient co-operation is another factor for delay in microbial diagnosis. Management of these eyes is a challenge due to the aggressiveness of the ulcer, poor drug compliance and difficulty in follow up examination.

Demographies (General Epidemiology)

Like male preponderance in adult and geriatric patients.[4,9,47,48] It is also concurrent with pediatric group. This could be due to male children are more prone to the trauma because of their playing habits,[49] more incidence of spring catarrh requiring more use of long term topical corticosteroids and possibly the male children are given more preference over female in some part of the world thus brought more frequently to the hospital to seek medical advice. Children from low socioeconomic group[8,50] and associated low body mass index are more prone for development of ulcer.

Trauma is a common predisposing factor in pediatric keratitis.[8-10] Although anterior segment surgery or previous corneal pathology is among the leading risk factors in developed countries,[10,51] the incidence is receding. Further, as size of the ulcer has a direct correlation in healing, there is a great need to diagnose and treat these eyes at earliest.

Microbiological Evaluation

When to do and when not to culture corneal ulcers is still evolving. Adequate sample collection under patients full cooperation is mandatory to identify the exact nature of the organism is essential to decide appropriate antimicrobial therapy. Considering the sample collection in children is difficult due to poor cooperation the question is more demanding. On the basis of this fact,though microbiological evaluations in all ulcers are ideal, in peripheral ulcer < 4 mm could be treated effectively on clinical basis. However, all the ulcers 4 mm or more in size irrespective of site should be subjected to microbiological evaluation under appropriate anesthesia. Corneal biopsy though a better method of sample collection for microbiological evaluation,[52] should be kept reserved for recalcitrant ulcers only.

Microbes Isolation

There is a decreasing trend in isolation of bacteriae and rising trend for fungal isolation in pediatric keratitis patients. Indigenous bacteria, such as coagulase negative *Staphylococcus* are being isolated with increasing frequency in corneal ulcer, more so in polymicrobial infections.[53] Though clinical characteristics are helpful in postulating the causative organisms such as the staphylococcal ulcers are mainly marginal, *Pseudomonas, Pneumococcal* and *Moraxella* for central ulcers and the complicated ulcers (with hypopyon and perforation) are more commonly associated with gram-negative bacteriae it is not always true. Since, many of the children sustained injuries during playing with sticks, bow and arrow, or exposure to vegetable debris, unusual virulent organisms like Bacillus species can be expected to invade the cornea Though a significant association with *Streptococcus pneumoniae* in the 0-19 year age group is well known[10,54] this is decreased in recent times due to advent of modern lacrimal surgery,[54] Similarly, reduction in *Neisseria gonorrhoeae* isolation could be attributed to improved antenatal, natal and postnatal care, as well as to better prophylaxis available against these organisms.[55]

Fungal infections are particularly common in hot and humid tropical countries and in corneal injury contaminated with soil or vegetable matter[56] besides indiscriminate use of topical steroids and antibiotics.[57] However, the possibility of a referral bias cannot be ruled out in institutional reports as only ulcers not responsive to antibiotics are referred to our tertiary centers.

Medical Therapy

As the child's eye is more prone for infection even after certain type of conjunctivitis, neonatal conjunctivitis and other forms of keratoconjunctivitis known to initiate and enhance corneal ulcer should be treated adequately.

Though initial therapy is determined by the smear report[56,58] It is not always confirmatory as sometime the smear findings may be inconclusive[59] and further there may be lack of facility for specimen collection and microbiological evaluation to all ophthalmologists . Thus a broad spectrum antibiotic/ "shotgun" approach is preferred depending upon the microorganism prevalence data for different geographic location as advocated for all types of corneal ulcers.[58] Considering the increasing resistant effect of gentamicin, the present combination is cefazolin 5% and tobramycin 1.4%. However, care should be taken to use tobramycin on short term basis, as long term topical use is known to cause toxicity. Moreover, as over use of fluoroquinolones might led to bacterial resistance and also induces perforation[25] these drugs are reserved for vision threatening situation only.

Vancomycin is the drug of choice for methicillin – resistant strains of both coagulase negative and coagulase positive staphylococcal infection. In combination with aminoglycoside it provides a synergistic bactericidal effect for the majority of *Staphylococcal aureus* strains. It is also bactericidal against a variety of other Gm + ve aerobic and anaerobic organisms including *Corynebacterium, Bacillus* spp., *Pneumococci, Streptococcus viridans, Clostridium* most *Lactobacillus* spp, *Actinomyces* spp and anerobic streptococci.[59] Despite the potency and other additive properties, use of vancomycin raises a lots of controversy as a promoter of antibiotic resistance. Further, it cannot be administered via intramuscular route as it causes severe pain at the injection site. Orally administered vancomicin is absorbed poorly from GI tract. It is also stated that certain predisposing factors such as immunocomprised status, seriously ill patients may promote vancomycin resistance. Considering the fact that most of the children with keratitis are systemically ill patients with compromised cornea, the drug should be kept reserved for extensive corneal ulcer and its use should be only for 48-72 hr to avoid resistance effect.

As amphotericin is more irritant to child's eye and limited antifungals are available in most parts of the world topical 5% natamycin drop can be used as a first line of therapy and amphotericin B and fluconazole can be added only in specific ulcers. Chlorhexidine, an antiseptic, is a good drug for fungal keratitis.[55]

Surgical Therapy

Various surgical procedures advocated for corneal ulcers in adult may not be helpful for pediatric age group due to technical difficulty and lack of adequate follow up.[60] However, paramedian tarsorrhaphy along with medical therapy for non healing ulcer provides beneficial effects. Vasculoplasty, though considered as an effective procedure for quick healing in adult fungal keratitis is also not suitable for pediatric keratitis. It could be due to dislodgment of the vascular graft following repeated exertion created by the children during drug instillation.

Therapeutic keratoplasty in a child does not behave well due to intense postoperative reaction and other inherent technical difficulties.[61] Sclerokeratoplasty,[62] the procedure of choice for total corneal ulcer in adult is not suitable for children due to thin sclera and low scleral rigidity. However, multilayered amniotic membrane transplant in chronic and non healing ulcers could be an effective procedure.

CONCLUSIONS

Corneal infection in pediatric age group is a disaster because of delayed diagnosis and poor compliance. Non-availability of desirable anesthesia facility and magnifying aids to all the ophthalmologists adds to the problem. The need for repetitive examinations under anesthesia further compounds the situation. A delay in management leads not only to poor visual outcome and delayed visual rehabilitation resulting in amblyopia, especially when severe unilateral corneal infection occurs in the early years of life. On the basis of data available in literature and our own experience, three key settings for implementing childhood keratitis management have been identified:

i. Prevention by proper family and community education about the risk factors,
ii. Prompt clinical and microbiological recognition,and
iii. Effective rational therapy and energetic procedure.

The preventive aspect through primary eye care has not yet received its initial goal. The potential role of both clinical and microbiological recognition seems to be under evaluated and underused. However, the therapeutic aspect is over assessed, as a result of which the unfortunate child is floated with various irrational medicine and sometimes subjected to drastic surgery which could have been very well managed by non destructive surgery. Therefore, it is mandatory for early referral of the child to a referral center for adequate management.

REFERENCES

1. Singh G, Palanisamy M, Madhavan B, Rajaraman R, Narendran K, Kour A, Venkatapathy N. Multivariate Analysis of Childhood Microbial Keratitis in South India. Ann Acad Med Singapore 2006;35:185-9.
2. Whitcher JP, Srinivasan M, Upadhyay MP. Corneal blindness: a global perspective. Bull World Health Organ. 2001;79(3):214-21.
3. Foster A, Sommer A. Childhood blindness from corneal ulceration in Africa: causes, prevention, and treatment. Bull WHO 1986;64:619-623.
4. Cruz OA, Sabir SM, Capo H, Alfonso EC. Microbial keratitis in childhood. Ophthalmology 1993;100:192-6.
5. Krohn MA, Hillier SL, Bell TA, et al. The bacterial etiology of conjunctivitis in early infancy. Am J Epidemiol 1993;138:326-332.
6. Parmar P, Salman A, Kalavathy CM, et al. Microbial keratitis in extreme of ages. Cornea. 2006:25(2);153-8.
7. Kunimoto DY, Sharma S, Reddy MK, Gopinathan U, Jyothi J, Miller D, et al. Microbial keratitis in children. Ophthalmology 1998;105:252-7.
8. Vajpayee RB, Ray M, Panda A, Sharma N, Taylor HR, Murthy GV, Satpathy G, Pandey RM. Risk factors for pediatric presumed microbial keratitis: a case-control study. Cornea 1999;18(5):565-9.
9. Panda A, Sharma N, Das G, Kumar N, Satpathy G. Mycotic keratitis in children: epidemiologic and microbiologic evaluation. Cornea. 1997;16(3):295-9.

10. Ormerod LD, Murphree AL, Gomez DS, Schanzlin DJ, Smith RE. Microbial keratitis in children. Ophthalmology 1986;93:449-55.
11. Lebowitz HM, Frangis JP. Bacterial Keratitis, In: corneal disorders clinical diagnosis and management II Ed WB Saunders. 1998;613-43.
12. Coster DJ. Corneal ulceration In: Fundamentals of clinical ophthalmology—Cornea BMJ books 2002:
13. Basak SK, Basak S, Mohanta A, Bhowmick A. Epidemiological and Microbiological Diagnosis of Suppurative Keratitis in Gangetic West Bengal, Eastern India. Ind J Ophthalmol 2005;53(1):17-22.
14. Parentin F, Liberali T, Perissutti P. Polymicrobial keratomycosis in a three-year-old child. Ocul Immunol Inflamm. 2006;14(2):129-31.
15. Glynn RJ, Schein OD, Seddon JM, Poggio EC, Goodfellow JR, et al. The incidence of ulcerative keratitis among aphakic contact lens wearers in New England. Arch Ophthalmol 1991;109:104.
16. Weissmann BA, Remba MJ, Fugedy E. results of extended wear contact lens—Survey of the contact section of the American Optometric Association. Am Optom Assoc 1987;58:16-171.
17. Jones DB. Decision making in microbial keratitis. Ophthalmology 1981;88: 814-20.
18. Taketazu SH, et al. Outbreak of severe infection due to adenovirus type 7 in a paediatric ward in Japan. J Hosp Infect 1998;39:207-11.
19. Beigi B, Algawi K, Foley-Nolan A, Keefe MO. Herpes simplex keratitis in children. Br J Ophthalmol1994;78:458-60.
20. Hassanlou M, Bhargava A, Hodge WG. Bilateral acanthamoeba keratitis and treatment strategy based on lesion depth. Can J Ophthalmol 2006;41:71-3.
21. O'Brien. Bacterial Keratitis. In: The Cornea by Smolin and Thoft IV Ed; Foster CS, Azar DT, Dohlman CH (Ed). Lippincott Williams and Wilkins 2005;1:236-88.
22. Sharma S, Garg P, Rao GN. Patient characteristics, diagnosis, and treatment of non-contact lens related Acanthamoeba keratitis Br J Ophthalmol 2000;84:1103-8
23. Tauber J, Jehan F. Parasitic Keratitis and conjunctivitis. In: The Cornea by Smolin and Thoft IV Ed; Foster CS, Azar DT, Dohlman CH (Ed). Lippincott Williams and Wilkins 2005;1: 427-46.
24. Alexander C Poon, Gerd Geerling, John K G Dart, Graham E Fraenkel, Julie T Daniels Autologous serum eyedrops for dry eyes and epithelial defects: clinical and in vitro toxicity studies. Br J Ophthalmol 2001;85:1188–97.
25. Collins MK, Perkins GR, Rodriguez Tarduchy G, et al. Growth factors as survival factors: regulation of apoptosis. Bioessays 1994;16:133–8.
26. Fredj-Reygrobellet D, Plouet J, Delayre T, et al. EVects of aFGF and bFGF on wound healing in rabbit corneas. Curr Eye Res 1987;6:1205–9.
27. Nishida T, Ohasai Y, Awata T, et al. Fibronectin: a new therapy for corneal trophic ulcer. Arch Ophthalmol 1983;101:1046. (reported with the use of serum drops).
28. Tsubota K, Goto E, Fujita H, et al. Treatment of dry eye by autologous serum application in Sjögren's syndrome. Br J Ophthalmol 1999;83:390–5.
29. Berman MB. Collagenase inhibitors: rationale for their use in treating corneal ulceration. Int Ophthalmol Clin 1975;15:49–66.
30. McLaren DS. Vitamin A deficiency disorders. J Indian Med Assoc 1999;97:320-3.
31. DeMaeyer EM. The WHO programme of prevention and control of vitamin A deficiency, xerophthalmia and nutritional blindness. Nutr Health 1986;4(2):105-12.

32. Sommer A. Xerophthalmia, keratomalacia and nutritional blindness. Int Ophthalmol. 1990;14:195-9
33. Weissman BA, Mondino BJ. Mocrobial keratitis, In: the cornea – its examination in contact lens practice, Butterworth Heinmann 2001;50-85.
34. Viswalingam M, Rauz S, Morlet N, Dart JKG. Blepharokeratoconjunctivitis in children: diagnosis and treatment. Br J Ophthalmol 2005;89:400-3.
35. Meisler DM, Raizman MB, Traboulsi EI. Oral erythromycin treatment for childhood blepharokeratitis. J AAPOS 2000;4:379-80.
36. Hamilton DR, Davis EA. Phlyctenular keratoconjunctivitis. In: The Cornea by Smolin and Thoft IV Ed; Foster CS, Azar DT, Dohlman CH (Ed). Lippincott Williams and Wilkins 2005;1:509-13.
37. Doan S, Gabison E, Gatinel D, Duong MH, Abitbol O, Hoang-Xuan T. Topical cyclosporine A in severe steroid-dependent childhood phlyctenular keratoconjunctivitis. Am J Ophthalmol. 2006;141:62-66.
38. Taherian K, Shekarchian M, Taylor RH. Fascicular keratitis in children: can corneal phlycten be mobile? Clin Experiment Ophthalmol 2005;33:531-2.
39. Nazir SA, Murphy S, Siatkowski RM, Chodosh J, Siatkowski RL. Ocular rosacea in childhood Am J Ophthalmol 2004;137:138-44.
40. Hilton E, Uliss A, Samuels S, Adams AA, Lesser ML, Lowy FD. Nosocomial eye infections in intensive-care units. Lancet 1983;1:1318-20.
41. Milliken J, Tait GA, Ford-Jones EL, Mindorff GM, Gold R, Mullins G. Nosocomial infections in a paediatric intensive care unit. Crit Care Med 1987;16:233-7.
42. Ommeslaag D, Colardyn F, De Laey J. Eye infections caused by respiratory pathogens in mechanically ventilated patients. Crit Care Med 1987;15:80-1.
43. Farrell M, Wray F. Eye care for ventilated patients. Intensive Critical Care Nursing 1993;9:137-41.
44. B. Parkin, A. Turner, E. Moore, and S. Cook Bacterial keratitis in the critically ill Br J Ophthalmol 1997;81:1060-63.
45. DGEzra, GLewis, M Healy, A Coombes. Preventing exposure keratopathy in the critically ill: a prospective study comparing eye careregimes Br J Ophthalmol 2005;89(8):1068-9.
46. Srinivasan M, Christine AG, George C, et al. Epidemiological evaluation of corneal ulcer in Madurai. Br. Jour Ophthalmol 1997;81:965-971.
47. Derek Y Kunimoto, Sharma S, Garg P, et al. Corneal ulceration in elderly. Br. Jour ophthalmol 2001;82:54-59
48. Panda A, Sharma N, Satpathy G, et al. Childhood keratitis – Epidemiological and microbiological study. Advance Cornea 1997, Plenum publisher. Editor J Lass, New York 491-99.
49. Panda A, Bhatia IM, Dayal Y, Ocular injury. Afro Asian J Ophthalmol 1985;3:163-67.
50. King FS, Burgess A. Anthropometric Reference Values in Nutrition for Developing Countries. Second Edition. New York, Oxford University Press 1993.
51. Clinch TE FF Palmon FE, Robinson MJ, et al. Microbial keratitis in children. Am Jour Ophthalmol 1994;117:65-71.
52. George A, Robert H, Darlene M, Alfonso EC. Corneal biopsy in the management of progressive microbial keratitis. Am Jour Ophthalmology 2000;129:571-6.
53. Liesegang TJ, Foster RK. Spectrum of microbial keratitis in South Florida. Am Jour Ophthalmol 1980;90:38-47.

54. Okaman M, Smolin G. Pneumoccoccal infections of the eye. Am J Ophthalmol 1975;79:719-23.
55. Rahman MR, Minassion DC, Srinivasan M, et al. Trial of chlorhxidine gluconate for fungal corneal ulcers. Ophthalmic Epidemiol 1997;4:141-9.
56. Jones DB. Initial therapy of suspected microbial ulcers II. Specific antibiotics therapy based on corneal smears. Surv Ophthalmol 1997;24:97-103.
57. Polack FM, Kaufman HE, Newmark E. Keratomycosis. Arch Ophthalmol 1971;85:410-22.
58. Asbel P, Stenson S. Ulcerative Keratitis. Arch Ophthalmol 1982;100:77-80.
59. Washington JA. Initial processing for cultures of specimens. In, Laboratory Procedures in clinical Microbiology, New York: Springer, 2nd Edition. Chap 3.
60. Panda A, Khokhar S, Rao V, Das GK, Sharma N. Therapeutic PK in nonhealing corneal ulcer. Ophthalmic surgery 1995;26:325-29.
61. Panda A, Mohan M, Gupta AK. Keratoplasty in children. Canadian Jour Ophthalmol 1988;20:183-7.
62. Panda A, Sharma N, Angra SK, Singh R. Sclerokeratoplasty for total corneal ulcer. Aust. New Z Jour Ophthalmol 1999;27:15-9.

Chapter 40

Topical and Systemic Antibiotics and Anti-inflammatory Drugs in Ophthalmology

Ashok Garg (India)

ANTIBIOTIC THERAPY

Topical Antibiotics Solutions and Ointments

Usual Dosage

Topical drops: Three to four times a day depending upon severity of the infection.

Ointment: One time preferably at bed time dosage can be increased depending upon severity of the infective condition.

1. Gentamicin solution or ointment 0.3%
2. Tobramycin solution or ointment 0.3%
3. Amikacin solution 0.3%
4. Sisomycin solution or ointment 0.3%
5. Neomycin solution 0.17% and ointment 5 mg/gm
6. Framycetin solution or ointment 0.5% and 1.0%
7. Chloramphenicol solution 0.4-1% and ointment 0.5%
8. Erythromycin ointment 0.5%
9. Polymixin B soln. 0.5-1.0% in combination with neomycin 0.35%. Ointment 1-1.5 mg/gm with neomycin.
10. Polymixin B 10000 units and bacitracin 500 units/g in ointment.
11. Sulphacetamide solution 10%, 20%, 30% and ointment 10%
12. Sulfisoxazole solution or ointment 4%
13. Tetracycline ointment or suspension 1% or Chlortetracycline ointment 1%
14. Trimethoprim 0.1% and Polymixin B 10000 units/ml.
15. Norfloxacin solution or ointment 0.3%
16. Ciprofloxacin solution or ointment 0.3%

17. Ofloxacin solution or ointment 0.3%
18. Pefloxacin solution or ointment 0.3%
19. Lomefloxacin solution or ointment 0.3%
20. Sparfloxacin solution or ointment 0.3%
21. Levofloxacin solution 0.5%
22. Moxifloxacin solution 0.5% or ointment 0.5%
23. Gatifloxacin solution 0.3% or ointment 0.3%
24. Gemifloxacin solution 0.3% (under trials).

SYSTEMIC ANTIBIOTICS IN OPHTHALMOLOGY

Dosage

Standard dosage of systemic antibiotics is mentioned alongwith individual drug. However, dosage may vary depending upon type and severity of ocular infection being treated.

1. Benzyl penicillin (Penicillin G)
   Parenteral IM/IV 4-30 million units/24 hours in divided doses 4-6 hourly.
2. Phenoxymethyl penicillin
   Orally 200-500 mg 6 hourly
3. Methicillin
   Parenteral IM/IV 1-2 G 4 hourly.
4. Cloxacillin
   Orally 250-500 mgm 6 hourly
5. Carboxy penicillin
   Parenteral 400 mg- 500 mg/kg/day 4 hourly
6. Ampicillin
   Orally 250-500 mg 4-6 hourly or by parenteral route
7. Amoxycillin
   Orally 250-500 mgm 4-6 hourly
8. Cefazolin
   Parenteral dose 1-6 gm/day 6-8 hourly.
9. Cephalothin
   Parenteral dose 2-12 gm/day 6-8 hourly.
10. Cephapirin
    Parenteral 1-2 gm every 4 hour
11. Cephaloridine
    Parenteral 2-4 gm/day 6 hourly
12. Cephadrine
    Oral, IM/IV : 0.5-1 gm every 6 hourly
13. Cephalexin
    Oral 0.5 g-1 gm every 6 hourly
14. Cefadroxyl
    Oral 1 gm every 12 hourly

15. Cefaclor
    Oral 0.5-1 gm every 8 hourly
16. Cefamandole
    Parenteral 1 gm every 4 hourly
17. Cefoxitin
    Parenteral 1-2 gm every 4 hourly
18. Cefuroxime
    Parenteral 750 mgm-1.5 gm every 8 hourly
19. Cefonicid
    Parenteral 1-2 gm every 24 hourly
20. Cefaranide
    Parenteral 1 gm every 12 hourly
21. Cefotiam
    Parenteral 1 gm every 12 hourly
22. Cefotetan
    Parenteral 1 gm every 12 hourly
23. Cefotaxime
    Parenteral 1-2 gm every 4-6 hourly
24. Cefoparazone
    Parenteral 1-4 gm every 4-8 hourly
25. Cefixime
    200-400 mg/day
26. Cefsulodin
    a. Cefsulodin
       Parenteral 0.5-1 gm 6-12 hourly
    b. Ceftazidime
       Parenteral 1-2 gm every 8-12 hourly
    c. Ceftizoxime
       Parenteral 1-2 gm every 8-12 hoursly
    d. Netilmycin
       Parenteral 3-6.5 mg/kg/day 8 hourly
    e. Kanamycin
       Parentral 15 mg/kg/day 8 hourly
    f. Doxycycline
       Oral 100-200 mg/dose 2-24 hourly
    g. Chlortetracycline
       Oral 250-500 mg/dose 6 hourly
    h. Methacycline
       Oral 150-300 mg/dose 6-12 hourly
    i. Minocycline
       Parenteral 200 mg/dose
    j. Oxytetracycline
       Oral 500 mg 6 hourly

k. Sulfonamides
   Parenteral 100 mg/kg/day 6-8 hourly
   Oral dose 2-4 gm/day 6 hourly
l. Erythromycin
   Oral 1-2 gm/day 6 hourly
   Parenteral 1-4 gm/day continuous drip
m. Roxithromycin
   Oral 150 mg BD before food intake
n. Clindamycin
   Parenteral 1-3 gm/day 6 hourly
   Oral 600 mg - 1.8 gm/day 6 hourly
o. Vancomycin
   Parenteral 2 gm/day 6-12 hourly
p. Spiramycin
   Oral 6-9 million IU/day in 2-3 divided doses.
q. Azithromycin
   Oral 500 mg-1 gm once daily
r. Clarithromycin
   Oral 200-500 mg BD
s. Norfloxacin
   Oral 400 mg BD
   Parenteral 200-400/day 12 hourly
t. Ciprofloxacin
   Oral 500-1500 mg/day 6 hourly
   Parenteral 5-10 mg/kg/day 12 hourly
u. Ofloxacin
   Oral 200-400 mg 6 hourly
   Parenteral 100-200 mg/day/12 hourly
   IV infusion - 200 mg infusion over 30 minutes BD
v. Pefloxacin
   Oral - 400 mg BD
   IV infusion - 400 mg in 100 ml of 5% dextrose solution infusion over one hour
w. Lomefloxacin
   Oral - 400 mg once daily
x. Sparfloxacin
   Oral - 400 mg in divided doses
y. Gemifloxacin
   Oral 400 mg in divided doses
z. Moxifloxacin
   Oral 400 mg in divided doses
   i. Levofloxacin
      Oral 500 mg in divided doses

ii. Gatifloxacin
Oral 400 mg in divided doses
iii. Metronidazole
Oral 400-800 mgm every 8 hourly
Infusion: 15 mg/kg infusion over 30-60 minutes BD
iv. Cotrimoxazole
Oral 1 tablet (Double strength BD (Trimethoprim 160 mg and sulphamethoxazole 800 mg).
Parenteral - 20 mg TMP/kg/day 8 hourly

TOPICAL ANTI-INFLAMMATORY THERAPY

Corticosteroids

Dosage: Disease specific

1. Hydrocortisone:

Acetate suspension	0.5-2.5%
Acetate solution	0.2%
Acetate ointment	1.5%

2. Prednisolone:

Acetate suspension	0.12%, 0.25% and 1.0%
Sodium phosphate solution	0.12%, 0.5% and 1.0%
Phosphate solution	0.5%
Phsophate ointment	0.25%

3. Dexamethasone:

Sodium phosphate solution	0.1%, 0.05% and 0.01%
Suspension	0.1%
Sodium phosphate ointment	0.05%

4. Betamethasone:

Sodium phosphate solution	0.1%
Sodium phosphate ointment	0.1%

5. Triamcinolone acetonide:

Suspension	0.1%
Ointment	0.1%

6. Progesterone like agents:

Medrysone suspension	0.1%
	Fluorometholone
Suspension	0.1% and 0.25% (FML forte)
Ointment	0.1%
	Fluorometholone acetate suspension 0.1%

7. Rimexolone suspension 1%
8. Loteprednol etabonate

Solution	1% and 0.5%

CORTICOSTEROID ANTIBIOTIC COMBINATIONS

Dosage: Based on Desired Corticosteroid Dose and Disease Specific

1. Dexamethasone (0.1%) with neomycin (0.5%) in ophthalmic solution from.
2. Dexamethasone (0.1%) with neomycin (0.35%) and polymixin B (10000 units/ml) suspension or ointment.
3. Dexamethasone (0.1%) with chloramphenicol (0.5%-1%) solution.
4. Dexamethasone (0.1%) with ciprofloxacin (0.3%) solution.
5. Dexamethasone (0.1%) with lomefloxacin (0.3%).
6. Dexamethasone (0.1%) with sparfloxacin (0.3%).
7. Dexamethasone (0.1%) with ofloxacin (0.3%)
8. Dexamethasone (0.1%) with gatifloxacin (0.3%).
9. Dexamethasone (0.1%) with moxifloxacin (0.5%).
10. Dexamethasone (0.1%) with framycetin (0.3%) suspension.
11. Dexamethasone (0.1%) with tobramycin (0.3%) suspension.
12. Dexamethasone (0.1%) with chloramphenicol (1%) and polymixin B 5000 IU solution and ointment.
13. Dexamethasone (0.1%) with gentamicin (0.3%) solution
14. Betamethasone (0.1%) with neomycin (0.5%) solution.
15. Betamethasone (0.1%) with chloramphenicol (0.5%) in solution and ointment.
16. Betamethasone (0.1%) with gentamicin (0.3%) solution.
17. Hydrocortisone (0.5%) with neomycin (0.5%) oint. and solution.
18. Hydrocortisone (1.5%) and neomycin (0.5%) ointment.
19. Hydrocortisone (10 mg/gm), polymixin B 0.5 mg/gm, bacitracin 400 units/gm and neomycin 5 mg/gm ointment.
20. Hydrocortisone (1%) with gentamicin (0.3%) suspension.
21. Hydrocortisone (0.5%) with chloramphenicol (1%) oint.
22. Hydrocortisone (0.5%) with chloramphenicol (0.5%) solution.
23. Prednisolone (1%) with gentamicin (0.3%) suspension.
24. Prednisolone (0.2%) with sulphacetamide (10%) and phenylephrine (0.12%) solution.
25. Fluorometholone (0.1%) with neomycin (0.35%) in solution.
26. Fluorometholone (0.1%) with gentamicin (0.9%) in solution.
27. Fluorometholone (0.1%) with tobramycin (0.3%) in solution.
28. Fluorometholone (0.1%) with ofloxacin (0.3%) in solution
29. Fluorometholone (0.1%) with gatifloxacin (0.9%) in solution.
30. Fluorometholone (0.1%) with moxifloxacin (0.9%) in solution.
31. Prednisolone (0.5%), neomycin 0.35% and polymixin B 10000 units/ml suspension.
32. Prednisolone (0.5%) with ofloxacin 0.3% in solution.
33. Prednisolone (0.5%) with gatifloxacin 0.3% in solution.
34. Prednisolone (0.5%) with moxifloxacin 0.5% in solution.

TOPICAL NON-STEROIDAL ANTI-INFLAMMATORY DRUGS (NSAIDs)

1. Flurbiprofen—0.03% solution
   Dosage: 1 drop every 30 minutes, 2 hours preoperatively (total dose - 4 drops) to prevent intra operative miosis.
2. Diclofenac — 0.1% - 1% solution
   3-4 times a day for 2 weeks for postoperative inflammation and also useful qid for several weeks in cystoid macular edema.
3. Nepafenac — 0.1% suspension.
   3-4 times a day for 2 weeks for postoperative inflammation and also useful qid for several weeks in cystoid macular edema.
4. Suprofen — 1.0% solution
   2 drops at 1, 2 and 3 hours preoperatively or every 4 hours while awake on the day of surgery.
5. Ketorolac — 0.4% and 0.5% solution
   3-4 times a day till the desired effect is obtained.
6. Indomethacin
   Suspension 0.5 - 1.0%
   Solution 0.1%
   Four times a day.
7. Aspirin — 1% solution, four times a day
8. Acetyl salicyclic acid — 0.03% solution, four times a day.
9. Diflunisol — 0.03% solution, four times a day.
10. Oxyphenbutazone — 10% ointment, 1-2 time
11. Phenyl butazone — 10% ointment, 1-2 times.

IMMUNOSUPPRESSIVE AGENTS IN OPHTHALMOLOGY

Alkylating Agents

1. Cyclophosphamide
   Usual dose is 150-200 mg/day (1-2 mg/kg/day) to be taken orally empty stomach. After 7 days (WBC count) dosage may be reduced by 25-50 mg to stabilize the WBC at about 3000 cells/ul
2. Chlorambucil
   Start at 0.1-0.2 mg/kg/day orally and increased every 3-4 days to total dosage of 10-12 mg/day.

Antimetabolites

1. Azathioprine
   Orally start at 1-2 mg/kg/day and gradually incfreased to 2.5 mg/kg/day.
2. Methotrexate
   Dose is variable due to high drug toxicity for first 1-4 weeks orally then IM/IV dose of 2.5-15 mg is given over 36-48 hours.

3. Cyclosporin A
   Oral 2.5-5 mg/kg/day in an olive oil with milk or juice maximum dose 10 mg/kg/day.
   It is also available as topical solution (2%) to be instilled 4-6 times a day depending upon the severity of the ocular condition.

BIBLIOGRAPHY

1. Agarwal Amar. Text book of Ophthalmology, ed.1, New Delhi: Jaypee Brothers Medical Publishers, 2002.
2. Ashok Garg. Ready Reckoner of Ocular Therapeutics, ed.1, New Delhi: 2002.
3. Bartlett. JD, Clinical Ocular Pharmacology, ed.4, Boston: Butterworth-Heinemann, 2001.
4. Bartlett. JD. Ophthalmic Drug facts: Lippincott - William and Wilkins, 2001.
5. Crick. RP, Trimble RB. Textbook of Clinical Ophthalmology: Hodder and Stoughton, 1986.
6. Duane TD. Clinical Ophthalmology, ed. 4: Butterworth - Heinemann, 1999.
7. Duvall. Ophthalmic Medications and Pharmacology: Slack Inc, 1998.
8. Ellis. PP, Ocular Therapeutics and Pharmacology, ed. 7: C.V. Mosby, 1985.
9. Fechner. Ocular Therapeutics: Slack Inc., 1998.
10. Fraunfelder. Current Ocular Therapy, ed. 5: WB Saunders, 2000.
11. Garg Ashok. Current Trends in Ophthalmology, ed. 1, New Delhi: Jaypee Brothers Medical Publishers, 1997.
12. Garg Ashok. Manual of Ocular Therapeutics, ed. 1, New Delhi: Jaypee Brothers Medical Publishers, 1996.
13. Goodman. LS, Gilman. A. Pharmacological Basis of Therapeutics, ed.7, New York: Macmillan, 1985.
14. Havener's, Ocular Pharmacology, ed. 6: CV Mosby, 1994.
15. Kanski. Clinical Ophthalmology, ed. 4: Butterworth - Heineman, 1999.
16. Kershner. Ophthalmic Medications and Pharmacology : Slack. Inc., 1994.
17. Kucers A, Bennett NM. The use of Antibiotics, ed.4, Philadelphia: JB Lippincott Company, 1987.
18. Olin BR, et al. Drugs Facts and Comparisons: Facts and Comparisons, St Louis, 1997.
19. Onofrey. The Ocular Therapeutics; Lippincott-William and Wilkins, 1997.
20. Rhee. The Wills Eye Drug Guide: Lippincott - William and Wilkins, 1998.
21. Seal. Ocular infection Management and Treatment: Martin—Dunitz, 1998.
22. Steven Podos. Textbook of ophthalmology, New Delhi: Jaypee Brothers Medical Publishers, 2001.
23. Zimmerman. Textbook of Ocular Pharmacology: Lippincott and William and Wilkins, 1997.

Chapter 41

OPHTHALMIC MEDICATIONS IN PEDIATRIC AGE GROUP

Rami Pai, Kirit Mody (India)

INTRODUCTION

Many ocular medications are prescribed and used in the pediatric age group. The data regarding their safety in this group of patients are sparse. Considering that the systemic absorption of the ocular drugs in pediatric patients is much greater, it is important that we evaluate the optimum dose with the minimum effective concentration as well as the potential systemic side effects of the various groups of drugs. This will give us a clearer picture of the risk versus benefit of using such drugs in the population.

Most of the commercially available medications have not been well studied in pediatric age group; hence these are prescribed empirically. Great caution is required in using the topical ophthalmic drugs in children especially infants in whom systemic absorption carries a much greater risk. This is because of the following reasons.

1. **Average blood volume:** The average blood volume is smaller in children and to a higher serum concentration of the drug up to 20 folds more.
2. **Absorption:** In children the absorption of drug from the conjunctiva, nasal mucosa and skin contributes significantly. Up to 90% of the drop may be absorbed through the nasal mucosa. Besides this the thin keratin on the skin, reduced tear production and increased incidence of nasolacrimal duct obstruction are factors, which increase systemic absorption.
3. **Drug clearance:** Immature enzymatic pathways and a reduced renal function in neonates slow down elimination of the drug from the blood.
4. **Free drug:** Reduced plasma protein binding and relatively less adipose tissue results in greater amount of free drug available especially in the neonate.

Precautions

Instructions can be given to guardians regarding technique of instillation so that the systemic absorption can be reduced significantly.

1. Only one drop to be instilled at a time.
2. Punctal occlusion with finger for 3 to 4 min after instillation.
3. Wipe the excess overflow of drops immediately.
4. In uncooperative subjects, one to two drops at the medial canthus to be instilled in the supine position. When the eyes open, some of it enters the conjunctival sac, rest is to be wiped with a tissue.

As a general rule it has been suggested that the estimated required topical dosage is as follows:

Birth to two years: One-half the adult dose.
2 – 3 years: Two-thirds the adult dose.
> 3 years: Adult dose.

MYDRIATIC AGENTS

These are frequently used for retinal examination and refraction besides treatment of inflammatory conditions of the iris. They are either sympathomimetics or parasympatholytics. *One has to remember when using these drugs that lighter irides requires much less concentration of the drug than dark irides.*

Adrenergic Agonist

Phenylephrine Hydrochloride

Indications: It is often used with parasympatholytics to cause maximal rapid dilatation of the pupil, especially to examine peripheral retina or preoperatively.

Its action lasts for only 6 hours.

Dosage: Diagnostic purpose 1 drop twice at an interval of 5 to 10 minutes.

Toxicity: As an alpha-adrenergic agent, it can cause hypertension, tachycardia and arrhythmias, besides dry mouth/skin due to systemic absorption. *It should be used with caution in children especially those with hyperthyroidism or tachy-arrhythmias. In children with pheochromocytoma, it might cause sudden and precipitating rise in blood pressure and hypertensive encephalopathy.*

The preparations available in the market are with a concentration of 10% (Drosyn – trade name) or 5% as a combination with tropicamide 0.8% A case of acute gastric dilatation in a preterm infant after two drops each of cyclopentolate 0.5% and phenylephrine 2.5% has been reported. Using phenylephrine in the concentration of 2.5% or less can significantly reduce such type of severe side effects.

The 10% solution should be avoided in children. As 2.5% soln is not available in the market, we can consider dilution of the phenylephrine 5% - tropicamide 0.8% combination for use especially in preterm infants where retinal examination is frequently carried out to rule out or assess Retinopathy of Prematurity (ROP).

Cycloplegic Agents/Parasympatholytics

Indications in children

1. Retinal examination with cycloplegic refraction.
2. Treatment of amblyopia
3. Postoperative cycloplegia
4. Prevent postoperative synechiae formation and relieve pain due to ciliary spasm in uveitis.

This group of drugs being parasympatholytics result if both mydriasis as well as cycloplegia. The relative cycloplegia caused by these drugs is compared below:

Drugs	% Efficiency of cycloplegia
1% Atropine	100%
1% Cyclopentolate	92%
1% Tropicamide	80%
5% Homatropine	54%

Table 41.1 shows the pharmacokinetics of the various mydriatic eyedrops.

Atropine Sulphate

It is a potent anticholinergic used in children for complete cycloplegia.

Dosage

1. *Cycloplegic refraction* 1% eyedrop twice a day or one centimeter of 1% ointment once daily for 1 to 3 days before examination.
2. *Amblyopia* 1% once daily or twice weekly in the sound eye.
3. *Uveitis* 0.5% eyedrop can be instilled three times a day.

Toxicity: The general signs and symptoms include dryness of mouth, skin, fever, delirium, tachycardia and sometime even death. In children toxicity might occur with as little as one drop of 0.5% soln bilaterally. *Lightly pigmented individuals, patients of Down's syndrome and brain damage are more susceptible.*

Dose related side effects of atropine are given below:

Dose of 1% soln	Side effects
1-4 drops	Tachycardia, dry mouth
10 drops	Restlessness, confusion, speech disturbance, hot/dry skin Decreased GI motility and urinary retention
20 drops	Besides above, hyperexcitability, ataxia, hallucination Coma, convulsion and death

Table 41.1: Comparative pharmacokinetics of various dilating agents (mydriatics)

Generic name	*Trade name*	*Concentration*	*Mydriasis*		*Cycloplegia*	
			Max. effect (Min.)	*Full recovery*	*Max.*	*Full recovery*
1. Phenylephrine	Drosyn	10% e.d.			–	–
	Drosyn T	5% e.d.	20-30	6 hr	–	–
2. Atropine	Belpinoatrin	1% e.d./e.o.	40	10+ days	6 hr	14 days
3. Homatropine	Homide	2% e.d.	60	3 days	60 min	3 days
4. Cyclopentolate	Cyclogil	1% e.d.	60	1 day	60 min	1 day
	Cyclopent	0.5% e.d.				
5. Tropicamide	Tropic acyl	1% e.d.	40	6 hr	30 min	6 hr
Tropicamide +	Drosyn T	0.8%		6 hr	30 min	6 hr
Phenylephrine	Tropicalyl plus	5%	20 – 30			

Heading : Comparative Pharmacokinetics of various Dilating Agents

Antidote: Severe anticholinergic toxicity is treated with physiostigmine 0.05% injected intravenously (0.02 mg/kg.) every 5 minutes up to a maximum of 2 mg.

Homatropine

Similar to atropine except that it acts more quickly. It has a shorter duration of action and recovery is also faster (Table 41.1)

Cyclopentolate

In view of the toxic side effects of Atropine this drug is *ideal for refraction* in children.

Dosage: One drop once/twice at 5 min interval and cycloplegic refraction being done 40 minutes later. About 0.5 to 0.75 D hypermetropia might go undetected.

Toxicity:

i. Gastrointestinal disturbances—paralytic ileus, gastric dilatation and necrotizing enterocolitis in infants.
ii. Siezures and behavioural changes—a case of seizure has been reported in cerebral palsy child after instillation of 1% cyclopentolate.
iii. Increased anterior chamber cellular infiltration has been reported. Hence *to be used cautiously in case of uveitis.*

Tropicamide

This is a short acting anticholinergic agent producing rapid mydriasis and incomplete cycloplegia. In combination with phenylephrine it results in rapid mydriasis with a persistant effect making it an *ideal drug for fundus examination and preoperative dilatation.*

Dosage

Cycloplegic refraction : 1 to 2 drops twice at 5 minute interval.
Preoperative mydriasis : 1 to 2 drops at 15 minutes interval 1 to 2 hours prior to surgery.

Toxicity A relatively safe drug but not ideal where cycloplegic refraction is the primary goal especially in infants and young children.

The combination of cyclopentolate hydrochloride 0.2% with phenylephrine hydrochloride 0.1% delivers optimal concentrations desirable for examining premature infants. It offers the advantage of rapid onset and short duration with minimal side effects.

GLAUCOMA MEDICATIONS

Medical treatment of glaucoma in infants is a temporary measure until surgery can be performed. Medications are often inadequate to control intraocular pressure, side effects are concern and compliance can be a challenge, while in the older age group with glaucoma medications play a greater role than surgery. The fact that these medications can cause serious systemic side effects has to be kept in mind as no controlled human studies have been done in children.

Beta-blockers

Mechanism

They decrease aqueous production in the ciliary body by blocking the beta-adrenergic receptor sites.

Advantage

- They are among the least expensive class of agents
- They reduce IOP with little or no effect on pupil size or accommodation.

Potential Side Effects

The ubiquity of beta adrenergic receptor sites in the body can lead to a variety of systemic side effects.

1. Cardiovascular: Bradycardia, hypotension, arrhythmias and heart block.
2. Respiratory: Bronchospasm and apnoea.
3. Central Nervous System: Behavioral changes, depression, dizziness, and cerebral ischemia.
4. Others: Marked hypoglycemia in diabetes.

Contraindications and Toxicity

Due to the above systemic side effects, it is contraindicated in children with cardiac arrhythmias, bronchospasm, asthma and should be used in the lowest possible dose in healthy children.

One drop of 0.5% timolol can cause cardiac block in infants less than two years of age. One neonate developed Cheyne-Stokes breathing and apneic spells lasting up to 30 seconds, that resolved after timolol 0.25% was discontinued.

Table 41.2 shows relative pharmacokinetics of various beta-blockers for glaucoma treatment.

Carbonic Anhydrase Inhibitors

Mechanism of Action

They are sulfonamide derivatives used topically and systemically to inhibit aqueous humor production by slowing the formation of bicarbonate ions with subsequent reduction in sodium and fluid transport.

Table 41.2: Beta blockers

Generic Name	*Trade Name*	*Concentration*	*Dosage*	*Side Effects*	*Remarks*
1. Timolol Maleate	Iotim, Glucomol Ocupress	0.25% - 0.5% eye drops	12 Hourly	CI – Asthma, Bronchitis Heart disease	Good response in children over 10 yrs. 0.25% eye drop/gel preferred in pediatric age group.
	Timolet GFS	0.5% gel	Once a day		
2. Betaxolol hydrochloride	Iobet Optipress Betoptic	0.5% e.d.	12 Hourly	Decreased corneal sensitivity	Greater safety in asthmatics as it is cardioselective.
	Optipress-S	0.25% (suspension)			
3. Carteolol hydrochloride	Ocupress	1% e.d.	12 Hourly	Cardio-pulmonary	Non-selective Beta-blocker
4. Revobunolol	Betagan	0.25% e.d. 0.5% e.d.	12 Hourly	Cardio-pulmonary Dendritic keratopathy	1. Membrane stabilizing 2. Longer duration

Point to Note: The 0.25% sustained release preparation is the preferred agent in pediatric glaucoma due to the lower concentration, decreased systemic absorption and once daily dosing.

Dosage and preparations

Generic name	Trade name	Concentration	Dose
Acetazolamide	Diamox	250 mg Tab 250 mg/ 5 ml	8-30 mg/kg/day
Dorzolamide	Dorzox	2 % e.d	8 – 12 hrly

Systemic forms are used as adjunctives to topical glaucoma therapy. Acetazolamide is administered orally as a liquid suspension at a pediatric dose of 8 to 30 (generally 10 to 15) mg/kg/day. It is available in strength of 250 mg/5 ml.

Though not as effective as oral acetazolamide, topical dorzalamide can be used for short-term treatment. A study reported significant intraocular pressure reductions in one group of 11 pediatric glaucoma patients and was well tolerated. It is available as a 2% eyedrop prescribed 8 to 12 hourly. (Dorzox). In a fixed combination with timolol 0.5% (Dorzox – T) it is reported to be more effective than when the two drops are used separately.

Potential Side Effects

As they are sulfonamide derivatives they are contraindicated in patients allergic to this group.

Gastrointestinal symptoms of nausea and anorexia are common and can be minimized by administering the dose with meals.

Genitourinary symptoms may present as urinary frequency. They are contraindicated in patients with kidney or liver disease or adrenal failure. Occasionally renal calculi are seen.

Other side effects are paraesthesias blood dyscrasias, Steven Johnson's syndrome and metabolic acidosis.

In view of the multiple side effects of systemic CAI, they are not the preferred drug of choice in pediatric age group.

Alpha Adrenergic Agonists

Mechanism of Action

They decrease aqueous production and may increase uveoscleral outflow.

Dosage and Preparation

Generic name	Trade name	Concentration	Dose	Remarks
1. Apraclonidine	Alpha drops Alpha drops DS	0.5% 1%	8 hrly	Short-term use in adults only
2. Brimonidine	Alphagan Iobrim	0.2%	8-12 hrly	More selective than above

Potential Side Effects

These drugs *cross the blood-brain barrier* and are relatively contraindicated in children due to side effects of somnolence and fatigue secondary to CNS depression.

Local allergic reactions are common after prolonged use. Apraclonidine can cause tachyphylaxis within 3 months. Apnea, lethargy, hypotension, hypothermia, hypotonia have been reported after one drop of brimonidine in each eye of infants less than 2 months old. Two young children were unarousable and five others experienced extreme fatigue in another study. Reports of syncopal episodes in two 10 year olds are also known. These symptoms resolved after brimonidine was discontinued.

Apraclonidine should not be used in children. Brimonidine should not be used in children less than 2 years and with great caution in less than 6 years of age.

Adrenergic Agonist (Sympathomimetic)

Mechanism of Action

They decrease aqueous production by vasoconstriction in the ciliary body with prolonged use they improve aqueous outflow and uveoscleral output.

Dosage and Preparation

Generic name	*Trade name*	*Concentration*	*Dosage*
Epinephrine	Eppy	0.5-2%	8 hourly
Dipivalyl	Propine	0.1 %	12 hourly
Epinephrine	DPE		

Potential Side Effects

Ocular side effects include allergy and cystoid macular edema especially in aphakic and pseudaphakic glaucoma patients. Hence, they are contraindicated in these patients. They can also cause conjunctival deposits.

Systemic side effects include sympathetic overactivity like palpitations, tachycardia, hypertension and sweating.

Dipivefrin causes less adverse reactions than epinephrine.

Contraindication

Narrow angle glaucoma and hypersensitivity.

As these drugs cause significant side effects and lower IOP only after prolonged use, they are not the preferred drugs of choice in children.

Parasympathomimetics

Mechanism of Action

Enhances aqueous outflow by ciliary muscle contraction, pull on the scleral spur and trabecular meshwork by acting on the acetylcholine receptors.

They are of two types:

1. Direct acting cholinergics.
2. Cholinesterase inhibitors.

Both these group of drugs cause miosis and ciliary muscle contraction.

Indications

1. Chronic open angle glaucoma.
2. Acute angle closure glaucoma—only pilocarpine.
3. Preoperatively to glaucoma surgery—only pilocarpine.
4. Chronic synechial angle closure glaucoma—pilocarpine and physiostigmine.
5. Postoperatively to cyclodialysis surgery.
6. Accommodative esotropia treatment—anticholinesterase agents.

Dosage and Preparation

Direct acting cholinergics

Generic name	*Trade name*	*Concentration*	*Dosage*
Pilocarpine HCl	Pilocar	1%,2%,4% e.d	4-6 hrly
		4% gel	15 mm o.d
	Occusert	Pilo - 20	20 mg/hr
		Pilo – 40	40 mg/hr
Carbachol	Miostat	1.5%, 2%, 3% e.d	6 hrly

Cholinesterase inhibitors

Generic name	*Trade name*	*Concentration*	*Dosage*	*Remarks*
Physiostigmine	Eserine	0.25%, 0.5% e.d 0.25% e.o	4-6 hrly	reversible
Ecothiophate iodide	Phospholine Iodide	0.06%, 0.125% e.d	12 hrly	irreversible
Isoflurophate	?	0.025% e.o	0.25" 8-72 hr	irreversible

Accommodative esotropia without amblyopia or anisometropia these drugs have to be instilled in both eyes. Dosage is as follows:

Ecothiophate: 0.125% o.d for 2-3 wk

Isofluorophate: 0.25" e.o at bedtime for 2 wks, then once a wk for 2 months.

Potential Side Effects

Ocular

- Miosis resulting in diminished night vision and constriction of visual fields
- Ciliary muscle contraction resulting in myopia, accommodative spasm, headache, forward lens movement and pupillary block glaucoma (Paradoxical increase in IOP)
- Activation of iritis (especially anticholinesterases), iris cyst formation and lacrimal punctual stenosis.
- Retinal tears and retinal detachment.

Systemic

- GI overactivity
- Cardiac irregularities
- Salivation
- Breathing difficulties

Antidote: Overdosage can be treated with parenteral atropine sulfate. The dose is 0.05 mg/kg i.v. initially followed by maintenance with 0.02 to 0.05 mg/kg tritrated.

Contraindications

These drugs are not to be used in inflammatory glaucoma and malignant glaucoma. Anticholinesterases are not to be used in narrow angle glaucoma.

Because the muscle tendon attachments are not well formed in infants, miotics are not very effective in the pediatric age group.

Prostaglandin Analogs

Mechanism of Action

They are analogs of F2 – alpha prostamides and activate metalloproteinases to remodel the extracellular matrix of the uveoscleral pathway thereby facilitating outflow. The also enhance nocturnal ciliary muscle tone.

Dosage and Preparations

Generic name	*Trade name*	*Concentration*	*Dosage*
1. Latanoprost	Latoprost 9 P M	0.005%	At bedtime
2. Bimatoprost	Lumigan	0.03%	At bedtime
3. Travoprost	Travatan	0.004%	od/bd
4. Unoprostone	Rescula	0.15%	bd

Potential Side Effects

Local side effects include increased eyelash growth, increased iris pigmentation, periorbital skin changes and punctate keratitis. Sleep disturbances and sweating have been reported in some children.

When used in a group of pediatric patients, latanoprost was found effective in only a minority of cases, although the drug appears to be well tolerated for short-term use.

These newer class of medications are mainly used in adults due to its impressive potency in adults, once daily dosing, flat diurnal cycle effects and few side effects.

In *summary,* timolol gel once daily is the recommended first line glaucoma medication in pediatrics age group due to its low cost and once daily dosing.

A combination of timolol with dorzolamide (Dorzox T) is more efficacious than taking the concomitant medications. However, the combination does not have the advantage of sustained release and dorzolamide causes stinging which can deter pediatric compliance.

Brimonidine is contraindicated in young children due to the CNS side effects and sympathomimetics are ineffective. The newer agents, prostaglandin analogs seem promising in juvenile-onset open angle glaucoma but long-term studies have to be carried out.

ANTI-INFLAMMATORY DRUGS

Steroids

Mechanism of Action

Corticosteroids are anti-inflammatory drugs for inflammatory eye disease. The inflammatory action is by altered protein transcription in white blood cells (WBCs) results in reduced due to Table 41.3 depicts corticosteroid anti-inflammatory activity.

Table 41.3: Corticosteroid anti-inflammatory activity

Drug	Activity
Hydrocortisome	1
Prednisolone	4
Triamcinalone	5
Methyl prednisolone	5
Betamethasone	25
Dexamethasone	25

Indications

Inflammatory and allergic conditions of the eye. In children the common inflammatory/allergic condition include:

1. Lids: Blepharitis, chalazion
2. Conjunctiva and cornea : Vernal conjunctivitis, phlyctenular kerato-conjunctivitis

3. Uveitis
4. Postoperative: Cataract, squint

Systemic corticosteroids are used in the treatment of severe inflammatory conditions of the eye. Corticosteroid injections are used in intermediate and posterior uveitis and capillary hemangiomas.

Dosage and Preparations

Steroids can be administered topically as drops (solutions, suspension) and ointments. They can be given as periocular injections through subconjunctival, retrobulbar or intralesional routes. Systemic administration either oral or parenteral is also prescribed in certain conditions.

Table 41.4: Lists the various corticosteriod preparations

Generic name	*Concentration*	*Preparation*	*Trade name*
1. Betamethasone	0.1%	e.d./e.o.	Betnesol
Sodium phosphate	0.5 mg	tab	
	4 mg/ml	injection	
2. Dexamethasone	0.1%	e.d.(soln)	Decadron
Sodium phosphate	0.05%	e.d.	Lodex
	0.5 mg	tab	Wymeson
	4 mg/ml	inj	Decadron
3. Hydrocortisone	1%	e.d. (Soln)	Allocort
acetate	2.5%	e.o	Hydrocortistab
4. Prednisolone	0.12%	e.d.	Pred mild
acetate	0.125%	e.d. (suspension)	Ecopred
	1%	"	Predace
		Predmet	
5. Prednisolone	0.125%	e.d. (soln)	AK-Pred/Inflamase
Sodium Phosphate	1%		Inflamase Forte
6. Prednisolone	5,10,20 mg	tab	Wysolone
7. Methylprednisolone	40 mg/ml	inj	Depomedrol
	1 gm/16 ml		Solu-medrol
8. Medrysone	1%	e.d.(Suspen.)	HMS/Flarex
9. Fluoromethalone	0.1%	e.d.(suspen.)	FML/Flomon
acetate		e.o.	FML S.O.P.
	0.25%	e.d.(suspen)	FML forte.
10. Loteprednol	0.5%	e.d. (soln)	Lotepred/Loteflam
etabonate			
11. Rimexolone	1%	e.d.(suspen.)	Vexol.
12. Triamcenalone	1 mg/4 mg	tab	Kenacort
	10/20 mg/ml	inj	Cyanamid
	40 mg/ml		Ledercort

The topical preparations are dosed as 1 to 2 drops every 1 hour to once daily or less, depending on the severity of the inflammation. Ointments are usually used at night for inflammatory conditions of the eyelid.

Dosage, duration and type of systemic steroids use depend on the severity and type of ocular disease. The dose for periocular injections is 0.5 ml in adults. In children the dose can be adjusted according to the age of the child. Systemic administration of steroids needs to be done in consultation with a pediatrician.

Potential Side Effects

Severe undesirable side effects limit topical corticosteroids use. They are

- Ocular hypertension (within 3 to 6 weeks in steroid responsive individual)
- Steroid induced glaucoma
- Posterior subcapsular cataracts
- Reactivation of herpes infections
- Perforation in presence of corneal or scleral thinning
- Systemic effects like headache and hypotension are rare or not commonly complained by children until they are very severe.

Systemic steroids besides having the same side effects like topical can also cause.

- Gastrointestinal—gastritis, peptic ulcer
- Metabolic worsening diabetes, increased appetite, weight gain, sodium and
- Fluid retention
- Vascular—hypertension, capillary fragility
- Skeletal—osteoporosis, aseptic necrosis of the hip
- Infective—exacerbations of infections
- Psychiatric—sleep disturbance and mood problems.

Corticosteroid infections (e.g. Kenacort) have been known to cause ophthalmic artery occlusion during intralesional infection to treat capillary hemangioma. A case of CRAO in a 4-year-old child has also been reported.

Relative Potential Side Effects of Various Corticosteroids

The safety of most of the steroids has not been established in children. Among the newer steroids safety of FML has not been established in children less than two years. *In view of the serious side effects caused by prolonged corticosteroid use, benefits should outweigh the risks of steroid treatment. These drugs should be used with caution in patients diabetes, hypertension, myopia > 5 D or Krukenberg spindle.*

Betamethasone, dexamethasone, and prednisolone are potent corticosteroids with excellent intraocular penetration but high chances of causing IOP spikes. Medrysone has poor intraocular penetration and therefore used for lid inflammations.

The newer generation steroids like fluoromethalone and loteprednol are powerful corticosteroids with fewer propensities to cause rise in IOP. These are indicated for short term treatment and prophylaxis of severe ocular surface disease (VKC). Rimexolone is a derivative of prednisolone that is metabolized to its inactive form in the anterior chamber thus reducing the risk of increased IOP. The ocular hypertensive effect is dose dependent and is more profound than in adults. Although the newer steroids claim to have less effect on IOP, their anti-inflammatory effect is probably limited.

Precautions

1. IOP checked if steroids are used for more than 10 days.
2. Subjects on long-term steroids monitored closely and frequently for complications.
3. Dosage should be titrated for effect from the smallest possible dose and tapered as soon as possible.
4. To consider use of diluted topical corticosteroids (1:10) to produce sufficient anti-inflammatory activity but least side effect.

Nonsteroidal Anti-inflammatory Drugs (NSAIDs)

Mechanism of Action

They inhibit cyclooxygenase and lipo-oxygenase enzymes, which lead to inhibition of inflammatory products. They are unable to modulate inflammatory cytokines other than those generated by arachidonic acid metabolism.

They have synergistic activity with steroids.

Indications

1. Maintain intraoperative mydriasis.
2. Postoperative inflammation.
3. Allergic and giant papillary conjunctivitis.
4. Episcleritis and scleritis (Chronic inflammation associated with JRA).
5. Certain uveitis along with steroids.
6. Cystoid macular edema.

Dosage and Preparations

Topical

Generic name	*Concentration*	*Trade name*
1. Indomethacin	1% e.d (Sol^{n}/Suspn)	Incicin
2. Flurbiproten	0.03% e.d (Soln)	Flur/ocuflur

contd...

contd...

3. Diclofenac	0.1% e.d	Voveran
4. Ketorolac	0.5% e.d	Vcular/Doloket/ Ketlur

They are instilled every 6 hourly. Systemic NSAIDs have an analgesic, antipyretic and anti-inflammatory effect.

Potential Side Effects

The safety and efficacy of these drugs have not been established in children. *The greatest advantage these have over steroids is anti-inflammatory activity without affecting IOP.* The topical formulations do cause local irritation and sometimes allergic reactions. They may increase risk of bleeding in ocular tissues post-procedures.

Oral NSAIDs are useful when tapering corticosteroids. These have to be used carefully as they cause serious systemic side effects.

Diclofenac 0.1% when used for various condition in 208 pediatric patients along with corticosteroids including neonates was found to be effective and safe. In another study of 90 cases of VKC, flurbiprofen was found to be less effective than betamethasone but a safer alternative.

ANTI-ALLERGY MEDICATIONS

Allergic ocular disease is one of the common problems seen in childhood. It might be mild as in allergic conjunctivitis or more severe as in vernal keratoconjunctivitis (VKC). Most of them are primarily type-I hypersensitivity reactions (IgE mediated) with type IV hypersensitivity playing a varying degree of role. Histamine release is responsible for most of the signs, symptoms and sequelae. Current antiallergy medical therapy is aimed at altering mediator production, release or effect on end organ. Besides the anti-allergy groups of drugs mentioned in this section, topical steroids, NSAIDs and immunosuppressors are also being used.

Mast Cell Inhibitors

Mechanism of action

They prevent calcium influx into the mast cells thus inhibiting degranulation.

Indications

These are used in allergic ocular disorders like vernal keratoconjunctivitis, giant papillary conjunctivitis, vernal keratitis and allergic keratoconjunctivitis.

Dosage and Preparations

Generic name	*Concentration*	*Trade name*	*Dosage*
Sodium cromoglycate	2% ed 4% ed	Cromal Cromal forte	qd
Lodoxamide	0.1% ed	Alomide	qd
Ketotifen	0.025% ed	Ketorid	td/bd
Nedocromil	2% ed	Alocril	qd

Potential Side Effects

As there is minimal systemic absorption of the mast cell stabilizer, the toxicity is negligible. Local irritation is common after instillation but these are relatively safe drugs.

In various studies it was found that Lodoxamide and Nedocromil were more efficacious for the treatment of VKC in children. Lodoxamide can be used in children two years or older up to a maximum of 3 months.

Decongestants (Antihistaminics and Sympathomimetics)

Mechanism of Action

Antihistaminics are H_1 receptor antagonists that prevent vasodilatation caused by histamine release. Sympathomimetics are decongestants that cause vasoconstriction by acting on the alpha advenergic receptors.

Preparation and Dosage

These are available as combinations and occasionally along with astringents. Some of the common are listed below

Generic name	*Concentration*	*Trade name*	*Remarks*
1. Phenylephrine HCl Naphazoline HCl Menthol-camphor	0.12% 0.05%	I-kul	Sympathomimetic
2. Naphazoline HCl Chlorpheniramine Antihistaminic Maleate $ZnSO_4$, Boric acid, NaCl	0.056% 0.01%	Andre	Sympathomimetic
3. Oxymetazoline	0.25 mg/ml	Oxylin	Sympathomimetic
4. Naphazoline HCl Boric acid, glycerol	0.01%	Clearine	Sympathomimetic

contd...

contd...

5. Tetrahydrazoline HCl Zn sulfate	0.05%	Visine AC	Sympathomimetic (NA)
6. Naphazoline HCl Antazoline	0.05% 0.5%	Naphcon-A	Sympathomimetic Antihistaminic
7. Levocabastin HCl	0.05%	Livostin	H_1- antagonist
8. Emedastine difumarate	0.05%	Emadine	H_1-antagonist

Usual dosage is 1 to 2 drops 3 to 4 times daily.

Potential Side Effects

None of these drugs have been proven safe in children. While the adverse effect of somnolescence is less likely with second generation as compared to first, none of them are completely free of CNS effects such as impaired concentration, dizziness, headache and insomnia. *They should be used with caution in older children and avoided in those less than 6 years of age. These can precipitate angle closure glaucoma.*

Dual Agents

Mechanism of Action

These provide mast cell stabilizing effect along with H^1-receptor binding.

Indication

These are used in treatment of allergic conjunctivitis.

Dosage and Preparation

Generic name	*Concentration*	*Trade name*	*Dosage*
1. Olopatadine	0.1%	Patanol	b.d
2. Azelastine	0.05%	Optivar	b.d
3. Ketotifen	0.025%	Ketorid	b.d

Potential Side Effects

Besides causing local irritation, the systemic effects include headache, asthenia, pharyngitis and alteration in taste. *The safety of azelastine has been established down to age 3 years.*

ANTIBIOTICS

Antibiotics are routinely prescribed in ophthalmology for both treatment and prophylaxis. The eye is particularly suitable for local application of antibiotics, which can be administered by various routes. Systemic administration of antibiotics has the disadvantage of poor ocular penetration especially in an inflamed eye as well as toxic side effects of the drug to a larger extent. A number of antibiotics that cannot be safely used systemically due to their toxicity can be used locally for external or intraocular infections.

The lipoidal and the blood eye barrier pose significant obstacles in achieving optimum concentrations of the drug in anterior or posterior segement respectively. Drug penetration may be improved by frequent instillation, increasing viscosity of drug, a suitable vehicle, alteration of pH or increasing concentrations of the drug. Delivery of drug into vitreous cavity in severe infections like endophthalmitis can be achieved by intravitreal injections.

To prevent development of resistant organisms follow the following principles:

1. Avoid chronic use of antibiotics.
2. Completely treat all clinical infections.
3. Use antibiotics only when indicated.
4. Limit antibiotic use to diagnosed infections.
5. Use newer antibiotics when there is resistant to traditional therapy.

The antibiotics are subdivided into various groups as follows:

A. Beta-lactams
B. Sulphonamides
C. Aminoglycosides
D. Macrolides
E. Tetracyclines
F. Chloremphenicol
G. Fluoroquinolone.

Indications

Antibiotics are used in ophthalmology for the following conditions:

Prophylaxis

To prevent bacterial infection from occurring as in:

- Foreign bodies and corneal abrasion
- Pre- and postoperatively.

Treatment

To treat ocular infections. These may be
External infections like

- Blepharitis, lid infections
- Dacryocystitis and orbital infections
- Bacterial conjunctivitis

- The common organisms affecting this age group are gram +ve particularly *Staphylococcus* and *Streptococcus*.
- Keratitis

This is rare in children but can be seen after trauma, surgery or contract lens wear. The common pathogens are *Pseudomonas*, staphylococci, alpha-haemolytic streptococci as well as herpes simplex virus.

intraocular infections like:

1. Deep keratitis and corneal ulcers.
2. Endophthalmitis.
   Bacterial/fungal can be by direct microbial penetration or hematogenous spread.

Dosage

In mild infections one drop is instilled four times daily for 5 to 7 days. Ointments have a longer duration in the eye and preferred when the eye needs to be padded. Severe infections can be treated with increased frequency of instillation. These can be given as fortified drops, subconjunctival injections, intravitreal injections as well through the systemic route depending on the severity and site of infection. They are also combined with steroids to prevent detrimental effects of inflammation, which usually accompany any infective pathology.

Table 41.4 gives an overview of various antibiotics and their dosages via the different routes. These are adult doses and need to be given in lower doses in children according to their age.

Beta-lactams

Mechanism of action

These groups of drugs are bactericidal and act by interfering with bacterial cell wall synthesis. They include

1. Penicillins
   - Natural penicillin
   - Semisynthetic penicillin
2. Cephalosporins

These drugs are not available as eyedrops. They can be used for subconjunctival, intravitreal or systemic use. Some of them can be used as eyedrops when reconstituted from the injection form.

Preparations

Penicillin prep	*Type*	*Effectivity*
Penicillin G	Natural penicillin	streptococcal, pneumococcal Gonococcal infections
Methicillin	Semisynthetic	endophthalmitis of penicillinase resistant org

contd...

contd...

Cloxacillin	Semisynthetic	*Staphylococcus, Pneumococcus Streptococcus*
Ampicillin Amoxycilllin	Semisynthetic	gram +ve, gram –ve organisms Ineffective for staph

Cephalosporins	*Type*	*Effectivity*
Cefazolin Cephaloridine Cephalexin	1st generation	Good activity against gram +ve modest activity against gram -ve Ineffective for enterococci
Cefuroxime	2nd generation	gram+ve org esp staph and strep More effective than 1st gen against gram –ve
Cefatoxime Ceftazidime	3rd generation	gram –ve organism only

Cephalosporins are execellent adjuncts to aminoglycosides in the treatment of severe infectious keratitis and endophthalmitis. Ceftazidime with vancomycin or cefazolin with amikacin provide execellent broad spectrum coverage in cases of infective endophthalmitis.

Dosage and Routes of Administration

Side Effects and Safety

Penicillins The commonest adverse reaction is that of hypersensitivity which might be mild to a very severe anaphylaxis. Hence, contraindicated in known cases of allergy to this group of drugs.

Cepholosporins Hypersensitivity reactions, nephrotoxicity, pseudo-memberanous colitis, vitamin K deficiency and pain after im injections are known.

SULFONAMIDES

Mechanism of Action

These are bacteriostatic agents, which inhibit bacterial folate synthetase.

Indications

Superficial ocular infections as in trachoma used to be treated with sulfonamides both systemic and topical. Newer antibiotics have now superceded them. The systemic preparations are also used in ocular toxoplasmosis in combination with pyrimethamine and trimethoprim.

Effectivity

These are effective against both gram +ve and gram –ve organisms.

Resistance

They are not very effective against *Staphylococcus, Neisseria* and *Pseudomonas* organisms.

Preparation and Dosage

The topical eye drops are available as 10%, 20%, and 30% of Sulfacetamide (trade name Albucid). The systemic sulfonamides are sulphadiazine and sulfamethoxazole. Their doses in adult are as follows:
Oral – 2-4 gm day in 4 divided doses.
Parenteral – 100 mg / kg / day in 4 divided doses

Side Effects and Safety

They are cheap drugs but cause significant stinging after instillation. ***They are contraindicated in patients with allergy to sulpha drugs and are not to be used in infants less than 2 months.*** Severe fatalities like Steven Johnson' Syndrome, hepatic necrosis, and blood dyscrasias although rare can occur.

AMINOGLYCOSIDES

Mechanism of Action

Bactericidal agents, which result in abnormal protein production fatal to microbes.

Effectivity

They are broad spectrum antibiotics effective against gram –negative bacilli and *Staphylococcus aureus*

Resistance

Streptococcus and *Chlamydia* organisms are resistant to them.

Preparation and Dosage

The various aminoglycosides used topically are

1. Gentamicin	0.3% soln / e.o.	Genticin
2. Tobramycin	0.3% soln /e.o.	Tobrex
3. Amikacin	0.3% soln	Amikin
4. Neomycin	0.17% e.d. 5 mg/gm oint.	

Other drugs belonging to this group are netilmycin, kanamycin, framycetin and streptomycin.
For dosage refer to Table 41.4

Side Effects and Safety

Corneal toxicity is seen with long-term use. They are ***epithelial and endothelial toxic drugs*** resulting in dryness of eyes, congestion and corneal ulcer. Subconjunctival injections of gentamicin commonly cause subconjunctival hemorrhage. Intravitreal or accidental injection into the eye results in ischemic infarct of retina. Amikacin has the least toxicity and is more effective against aminoglycoside resistance strains. Best used short-term. Neomycin commonly causes contact allergy.

Systemic administration can cause ototoxity, nephrotoxicity and neurotoxicity.

MACROLIDES

Mechanism of Action

These are bacteriostatic agents inhibiting protein synthesis in the bacterial cell.

Effectivity

These are effective against gram-posititive organisms and atypical microbes like *Mycoplasma, Chlamydia, Legionella* and certain *Mycobacteria*. Intravitreal vancomycin has been recommended as initial therapy for exogenous endophthalmitis. Oral clindamycin is also recommended in treatment of ocular toxoplasmosis.

Preparation and Dosage

The various drugs belonging to this group are:
- Erythromycin
- Clindamycin
- Vancomycin
- Roxithromycin
- Azithromycin
- Clarithromycin.

For details of doses and preparations of commonly used macrolides refer to Table 41.3

Side Effects and Safety

They are relatively safe when given topically but are used only in mild bacterial conjunctivitis. Systemic administration can cause GI disturbances

TETRACYCLINES

Mechanism of Action

These are bacteriostatic agents acting by inhibiting protein synthesis in ribosomes.

Effectivity

Gram-positive organisms, gram-negative bacilli, anaerobes, *Mycoplasma*, *Actinomycetes*, *Rickettsia*, *Chlamydia* and *Spirochaetes*. Surface ocular infections respond well to tetracyclines. Topical tetracyclines along with 1% Silver nitrate is recommended in prophylaxis of ophthalmia neonatorum. Acute trachoma is also treated with both systemic and topical preparations. Systemic tetracyclines are indicated in adult inclusion conjunctivitis acquired from genital contact, phlyctenular conjunctivitis, ocular toxoplasmosis, Lyme's disease and ocular rosacea.

Resistance

These are resistant to Proteus and Pseudomonas.

Preparation

Some of the drugs belonging to this group are:
- Tetracycline
- Doxycycline
- Minocycline

Refer to Table 41.4 for details.

Side Effects and Safety

Surface ocular infections caused by susceptible microorganism respond well to tetracycline although intraocular penetration is poor . Topical preparations are relatively safe. Systemic administration can cause GI disturbances, yellow discoloration of teeth, photosensitization, nephrotoxicity and benign intracranial hypertension. Not recommended for use systemically in children due to the side effects.

CHLORAMPHENICOL

Mechanism of Action

It is a bacteriostatic agent interfering with protein synthesis. Being lipophilic it has good intraocular penetration. It is one of the most commonly used topical antibiotic ointment.

Effectivity

It is a broadspectrum antibiotic against gram-positive, gram-negative organism and anaerobes.

Resistance

It is resistant to *Pseudomonas aeruginosa*

Preparation and Dosage

See Detail in Table 41.4.

Side Effects and Safety

The ointment can cause allergic reactions although it is relatively rare. *Bone marrow hypoplasia including aplastic anemia and death has been reported following local application of chloramphenicol. In infants it can cause gray baby syndrome.* Hence, it should not be used when less potentially dangerous agents would provide effective treatment.

FLUOROQUINOLONES

Mechanism of Action

They are bactericidal agents interfering with enzyme DNA gyrase required for bacterial DNA synthesis. They have good ocular penetration.

Effectivity

Broad spectrum antibiotic effective against gram-positive, gram-negative organism including *Pseudomonas, Haemophilus*

Preparation

Generic name	*Concentration*	*Trade name*	*Remarks*
1. Norfloxacin	0.3% soln/e.o.	Norflox	Corneal epithelial toxicity
2. Ciprofloxacin	0.3% e.d./e.o.	Ciplox	Resistant to *Streptococcus*
3. Ofloxacin	0.3% e.d./e.o.	Oflox	More effective

contd...

contd...

			than ciprofloxacin
4. Pefloxacin	0.3% e.d.	Pflox	Inactive against anaerobes. Effective against *N. gonorrhoea*
5. Lomefloxacin	0.3% e.d.		Deep acting
6. Sparfloxacin	0.3% e.d.	Sparflox	Good penetration
7. Levofloxacin	0.5% e.d		Good penetration Safe in children
8. Gatifloxacin	0.3% e.d.	Gatiflox	Safe in children>1 yr
9. Moxifloxacin	0.5% e.d.	Mosi	Safe in children>1 yr

Dosage of topical eyedrops depends on severity of infections. Refer to Table 41.4 for other doses.

Side Effects and Safety

Fluoroquinolones are relatively safe for topical use in children, ***Safety is not established in infants below 1 year of age. They are expensive but extremely effective with good ocular penetration.*** Fourth generation fluroquinolones are active against quinolone resistant strains of *S. aureus*.

ANTIVIRALS (TABLE 41.6)

Viral disease in pediatric patients is often systemic and frequently accompanied by significant ocular inflammation with risk of amblyopia. Immunocompromised children have complex courses with persistence and recurrence of the disease. Unlike bacteria, viruses use host cell machinery for its metabolism and can lie dormant in the host for a long period. Antivirals act on actively replicating viruses only and are toxic to the host cells to a variable extent. As yet no antiviral in available which inhibit viral entry into host cells. Difficulty in diagnosis during incubation and latent period compound the problem.

The common viral infections causing ocular diseases in childhood are:

DNA viruses Herpes simplex
Herpes zoster
RNA viruses Measles
Mumps
Rubella

Mechanism of Action

In general, antivirals act by inhibiting viral DNA synthesis and thereby its replication. These agents are virustatic and cause various degree of host cell toxicity.

Preparations and Dosage

Refer to Table 41.5.

Side Effects and Safety

Host cell toxicity is present to a variable degree, Acyclovir being least toxic and Idoxuridine/trifluoridine most when administered topically.

Local toxicity in the form of superficial punctate keralitis, punctual occlusion, and conjunctival congestion are seen. Safety of gancyclovir implant in children below 9 years is not established.

Oral acyclovir is highly effective for HSV epithelial keratitis, stromal keratitis, recurrence and HZV infections in immuno-compromised pediatric patients, oral valacyclovir may be the preferred substitute of iv acyclovir due to better bioavailability in children although it has been studied only in adults.

Bone marrow suppression and nephrotoxicity are seen with systemically administered antivirals. Therefore renal function and blood cell counts must be monitored.

ANTIFUNGALS

Fungi do not invade the cornea except when it is compromised by injury, or immunosuppression fungal infections are commoner in tropics due to favorable climate. Infections with yeast fungi usually follow alterations in host defenses.

While filamentous fungi infect normal eyes after injury from vegetable matter.

Various antifungals are:

Polyenes

Mechanism of Action

These bind to ergosterol, after cell membrane permeability and disrupt the fungal cell.

Preparation and Dosage

Generic name	*Concentration*	*Trade name*	*Dose*	*Effectivity*
1. Nystatin	100000 units/g Ointment (Oral/I.V)	Nystatin	2 hourly	Fungistatic Superficial Infections
2. Amphotericin B	0.075 – 3 % 0.8-1 mg 5 mg	Fungizone	1 hourly topical SC 24-48 hr Intravitreal intravenous	Deep mycosis
3. Natamycin	5% (Suspension)	Natacyn	5 times/day	Superficial infections Initial drug of choice

Table 41.5: Concentration and dosages of principal antibiotics

Generic Name	*Trade Name*	*Topical*	*Sub conjunctival*	*Intravitreal*	*Systemic*	*Remark*
Amikacin	Amicin (100 mg, 250 mg and 500 mg per 2 ml)	10-15 mg/ml	25-50 μg	100- 400 μg	10-15 mg/kg/day (Total max.dose 15 gm) 3 times/day	Modify dose in Case of renal failure
Amoxycillin	Mox, novamox, Amoxil, Flemoxin	—	—	—	250-500 mg (thrice a day)	—
Ampicillin	Ampillin, Bacipen Roscillin	50 mg/ml	50-250 μg	500 μg	2.0-4.0 g/4 hr	
Bacitracin	Nebasulf	10,000 units/ml	10,000 units	—	—	
Cefazolin	Alcizon, Reflin Azolin	50 mg/ml	100 mg	2.25 mg	2-4 gm/day (in 3-4 doses)	
Cetotaxime	Claforan	33-66 mg/ml	—	2.00 mg	1-2 g (bid)	—
Ceftazidime	Ceftidin	50 mg/ml	100 mg	2.25 mg	2-6 gm/day(in 2 doses)	
Cephalexin	Cephaxin, Nufex	30-60 mg/ml	—	—	1-4 g/day(in 4 days)	On empty stomach
Cephaloridine		—	100 mg	250 μg	0.5-1.0 gm/6 hr	
Cephoxitin		30-60 mg/ml	—	—	—	—
Chloramphenicol	Chloromycetin,	5 mg/ml	50-100 mg	1.0-2.0 mg	50 mg/kg/day	
Ciprofloxacin	Ciftan, Ciplox, Ciprobid, Supraflox Milflox (Milmet)	3 mg/ml	20 mg	100-200 μg	0.5-1.5 g/day(Oral)	
Clindamycin	Dalacin Calcap	5-10 mg/ml	15-50 mg	1.00 mg	900-1800 mg/day (2-3 divided doses)	
Cloxacillin	Klox	—	—	—	250-500 mg(thrice a day)	—
Doxycyclin	Doxy	—	—	—	100-200 mg(times/day)	
Erythromycin	Althrocin, E-mycin Eltocin, Erythrocin	50 mg/ml	100 mg	500 μg	250-500 mg (3-4 times/day)	Max 4 gm daily
Gentamicin	Garamycin,	8-15 mg/ml	20-40 mg	100-400 μg	5.0-7.5 mg/kg/day	
Methicillin		—	150-200 mg	2.0 mg	2.0 mg-4 hr	
Norfloxacin	Norbactin, Norbid Norflox, Normax	3 mg/ml	—	—	200-400 mg(bid) orally	

contd...

Table 41.5 Contd....

Generic Name	*Trade Name*	*Topical*	*Sub conjunctival*	*Intravitreal*	*Systemic*	*Remark*
Ofloxacin	Tarivid, Zanocin	3 mg/ml	—	—	200-800 mg/day	Not recommended for children
Penicillin G	Penivoral, Pentids Crystapen	100,000 units/ml	0.5-1.0 million	200 units	2.0-6.0 mega units/ 4 hr	
Sulfacetamide	Albucid	100-300 mg/ml	—	0.5 mg	4-8 gm/day	—
Tetracycline	Resteclin	0.5%-1.0% (5-10 mg/ml)	2.5-5.0 mg	—	1-4 gm/day (in 4 doses)	Antifungal action Also
Tobramycin	Tobacin	3 mg/ml (8-16 mg/ml) 0.3%	20 mg	100 μg	3-5 mg/kg/day (2-3 doses)	—
Vancomycin	Vancocin CP	5-50 mg/ml	25 mg	1.0 mg (upto 2.00 mg)	2 gm/day (in 2 doses)	Solution remain Stable for 21 days At 4^0 C or 25^0 C

Table 41.6 : Antivirals

	Generic name	*Concentration*	*Trade name*	*Dose*	*Duration*	*Indication*	*Remarks*
1	Indoxuridine (IDU)	0.1% ed 0.5 eo	Ridinox	1 hrly 2 hrly night 6 times	2 weeks	*Superficial HSV Injn.	Corneal toxicity
2	Vidarbine	3% eo 200 mg/ml	Ara-A	5 times 5-15 mg/kg 8 hrly	2- 3 weeks	* HSV keratitis *HSV encephalitis	Decreased host cell toxicity
3	Trifluridine(TFT)	1% ed	Viroptic	6-9 times	2 weeks	* HSV keratitis * Recurrent HSV * Resistant HSV * Deep infection	Less toxic than IDU or Ara - A
4	Acyclovir	3% e.o. 5% dermal cream 200 mg) 400 mg) Tablet 800 mg) 250 mg powder (IV)	Zovirax	5 times 200-800 mg 5 times 5 mg/kg 8 hrly (IV)	2 weeks 10 days 7-10 days	* HSV * Herpes zoster * Acute retinal necrosis * Immunocompromised *Recurrent and deep infections	Potent at antiherpetic and selective to virus cells
5.	Zidovudine	100 mg cap	Retrovir	200 mg 8 hourly Oral		*HIV	Expensive Bone marrow Suppression
6	Foscarnet	24 m/ml viral diluted to 12 mg/ml with dextrose	Foscavir	60 mg/kg 8 hrly IV	2-3 weeks	*CMV in AIDS *Acyclovir resist HSV and VZV	*Nephrotoxic *Administer diluted
7	Famcyclovir			500-700 mg 8 hourly	1 week	HZV	Effective in 1000 doses

contd...

Table 41.6 contd....

	Generic name	*Concentration*	*Trade name*	*Dose*	*Duration*	*Indication*	*Remarks*
8	Gancyclovir	250 mg cap 500 mg powder	Cytovene	5 mg/kg 12 hourly	2-3 weeks	CMV	Bone marrow toxicity
9	Valacyclovir	500 mg/IG (Oral)	Valtrex			HZV	Better *Pani relief *Oral availability Less dosing
10	Fomivirsen sodium		Vitravene	330 mcg intravitreal alternate week X 2 every 4 weeks		CMV in AIDS	
11	Cidofovir	75 mg/ml		5 mg/kg once weekly/ 2 weeks		CMV in AIDS	Nephrotoxic
12	Bromovinyl Deoxyuridine	0.1% ed		8 times	8-10 days	HSV Keratitis	Least toxicity

Side Effects and Safety

These drugs in general are insoluble, cause irritation and are unstable. Natamycin is well tolerated but can cause local irritation and punctate ketatitis. Amphoterin B has poor ocular penetration and can cause anaphylaxis, nausea vomiting and nephrotoxicity when given systemically.

IMIDAZOLE DERIVATIVES

Mechanism of Action

They inhibit ergosterol synthesis, and cause fungal cell inhibition

Preparations and Dosage

Generic name	*Concentration*	*Trade name*	*Dose*	*Remarks*
1. Clotrimazole	1% e.d. 5-10 mg 60 mg/kg 1 day	Mycocid	1 hourly Subconj oral	Fungistatic Effective for *Aspergillus*
2. Miconazole	1% e.d. 5-10 mg 10-40 mg	Micogel	2 hourly Subconj. Intravitreal	Highly effective for *Candida* (Broad Spectrum)
3. Econazole	1% ointment	Ecanol	4-6 times	Poor penetration Sup. infections
4. Ketaconazole	2% Ointment 200 mg Tab.	Fungicide	200 mg- 800 mg o.d.	Highly effective Deep infections
5. Fluconozole	0.3% eye drop 50-200 mg.cap 100 mg	Forcan	4 hourly 200-600 mg/day Intravit	Excellent Ocular penetration Broad-spectrum
6. Intraconazole	100 mg cap 0.01 mg	Sporanox	50-400 mg/day Intravit	Not effective against *Fusarium*

Side Effects and Safety

Topical Imidazoles cause local irritation to a variable degree. Fluconazole, Ketoconazole and miconazole cause the least and are well tolerated when systemically administered they can cause G1 disturbances and hepatotoxicity.

FLUORINATED PYRIMIDINES—FLUCYTOSINE

Mechanism of Action

It blocks fungal thymidine synthesis.

Dosage and Preparation

Generic name	*Concentration*	*Dose*	*Remarks*
Flucytosine	1-1.5% e.d. 250/500 mg cap	1 hrly 50-150 mg/kg/d	Used as an adjunct to other antifungals

Side Effects and Safety

Topical preparations can cause local irritation and systemic use can cause GI disturbances.

CONCLUSION

Many of the medications commonly used in children do not have pediatric dosing labeling presenting a dilemma while treating these patients. Studies on this age group are difficult due to inadequate sample size and objective measurements of signs and symptoms being problematic. It is advisable that physicians analyse risk benefit profile while prescribing in children, establish an appropriate dosage while monitoring the patient closely for local and systemic side effects.

BIBLIOGRAPHY

1. Alm A, Stjernschantz J. Effects on intraocular pressure and side effects of 0.005% latanoprost applied once daily, evening or morning. A comparison with timolol. Scandinavian Latanoprost Study Group. Ophthalmology 1995;102:1743-52.
2. Bielory L. Ocular allergy guidelines: A practical treatment algorithm. Drugs 2002;62:1611-34.
3. Bill A. Uveoscleral drainage of aqueous humor: physiology amd pharmacology. Prog Chin Biol Res 1989;312:417-27.
4. Bito LZ, Racz P, Ruzsony MR, et al. The Prostaglandin analogue, PhXA41, significantly reduces daytime and nighttime intraocular pressure (IOP) by itself, and in timolol-treated glaucomatous eyes [ARVO abstract]. Invest Ophthalmol Vis Sci 1994;35(Suppl):2178.
5. Bowman RJ, Cope J, Nischal KK. Ocular and systemic side effects of bromonidine 0.2% eye drops (Alphagan) in children. Eye 2004;18: 24-6.
6. Camras CB. Comparison of latanoprost and timolol in patients with ocular hypertension and glaucoma: A six month masked, multicenter trial in the United States. The United States Latanoprost Study Group. Ophthalmology 1996;103: 138-47.
7. Carlsen JO, Zabriskie NA, Kwon YH, et al: Apparent central nervous system. Depression in infants after the use of topical brimonidine. Am J Ophthalmol 1999;128:255-6.
8. Controlled evaluation of loteprednol etabonate and prednisolone acetate in the Treatment of acute anterior uveitis. Loteprednol Etabonate US Uveitis. Loteprednol Etabonate US Uveitis Study Group. Am J Ophthalmol 1999;127: 537-44.

9. Egbert JE, Schwartz GS, Walsh AW. Diagnosis and treatment of an ophthalmic artery occlusion during an intralesional injection of cortico-steroid into an eyelid capillary hemangioma. Am J Ophthalmol 1996;121: 638-42.
10. Enyedi LB, Freedman SF, Uckley EG. The effectiveness of latanoprost for the treatment of pediatric glaucoma. J AAPOS 1999;3(1):33-9.
11. Enyedi LB, Freedman SF. Latanoprost for the treatment of pediatric glaucoma. Surv Ophthalmol 2002;47:1:S129-32.
12. Enyedi LB, Freedman SF. Safety and efficacy of brimonidine in children with glaucoma. J AAPOS 2001;5(5): 281-4.
13. Fan DS, NgJS, Lam DS. A prospective study on ocular hypertensive and anti-inflammatory response to different dosages of fluorometholone in children. Ophthalmology 2001;108: 1973-7.
14. Fitzgerald DA, Hanson RM, West C, Martin F, Brown J, Kilham HA. Seizures associated with 1% cyclopentolate eyedrops. J Paediatr Child Health 1990;26(2): 106-7.
15. Foster CS, Alter G, DeBarge LR, et al. Efficacy and safety of rimexolone 1% ophthalmic suspension vs 1% prednisolone acetate in the treatment of uveitis. Am J Ophthalmol 1996;122: 171-82.
16. Gerinec A, Kostolna B. Diclof 0.1% eyedrops in pediatric ophthalmology. Cesk Slov Oftalmol 2001;57(3): 200-3.
17. Katzung, B, et al. Basic and Clinical Pharmacology. ed 8 San Francisco, Lange Medical Books/McGraw-Hill 2001;134-5.
18. Pucci N, Novembre E, Cianferoni A, Lombardi E, Bernardini R, Caputo R, et al. Efficacy and safety of cyclosporine eyedrops in vernal keratoconjunctivitis. Ann Allergy Asthma Immunol 2002;89:298-303.
19. Ruttum MS, Abrams GW, Harris GJ, Ellis MK. Bilateral retinal embolization associated with intralesional corticosteroid injection for capillary hemangioma of infancy. J Pediatr Ophthalmol Strabismus 1993;30: 4-7.
20. Shorr N, Seiff SR. Central retinal artery occlusion associated with periocular corticosteroid injection for juvenile hemangioma. Ophthalmic Surg 1986;17:229-31.
21. Sud RN, Greval RS, Bajwa RS. Topical flurbiprofen therapy in vernal keratoconjunctivitis. Indian J Med Sci 1995;49(9): 205-9.
22. Terasa MM, David Wallace, Sandra Johnson. Ophthalmic medications in pediatric patients. Comprehensive update 2005; 6(2):85-1001.
23. Textbook of Ocular Therapeutics Ashok Garg, 2001.
24. Verin PH, Dicker ID, Mortemousque B. Nedocromil sodium eye drops are more effective than sodium cromoglycate eye drops for the long-term management of vernal keratoconjunctivitis. Clin Exp Allergy 1999;29(4): 529-36.

Chapter 42

Management of Uveitis in Children

Gagandeep Singh Brar, SPS Grewal (India)

Inflammation of the uveal tract when presenting in children and adolescents younger than 16 years of age is termed as pediatric uveitis although some studies advocate using 18 years as the cut-off age.[1] The incidence of uveitis in children has been reported to be less than that of adults and 2.2 to 10.6% of the total number of uveitis patients belong to the pediatric age group.[2-6] Wide variation in the incidence as well as varying prevalence within the same population over time has been reported.

There are some basic differences between childhood uveitis and adult uveal inflammation. Systemic associations of the uveitis are not as common in children as in adults and ANA positive oligoarticular juvenile idiopathic arthritis (JIA) presents as the most common systemic disorder.[7,8] Also, the uveitis is mostly asymptomatic in the early stages in children and they may be presenting to the ophthalmologist at a very late stage. Thirdly, the mainstay of management of uveitis in adults, namely corticosteroids, may not be safe in growing children with permanent adverse effects so steroid sparing agents may have to be employed more frequently for controlling the inflammation. Complications of uveitis are also more common in children because of the chronic and relentless course of the disease in many cases coupled with delayed presentation. Results of surgical intervention in this age group have also been poorer when compared to adults and visual outcomes are less encouraging. Lastly, many children may be at a stage of visual immaturity and attendant amblyopia may further compromise visual rehabilitation.

As with adult uveitis, marked variability has been observed in the patterns of uveitis in children when studied over time and has been attributed to geographical variations, racial and genetic differences, recognition of newer clinical entities, better diagnostic capabilities and better control of infections. In children, in almost one-fourth of all cases, no cause can be ascertained and these are termed as idiopathic uveitis. As already stated, JIA associated uveitis is the most common form of anterior uveitis and toxoplasmosis the most common posterior uveitic entity. Other common entities in children include pars planitis, Behçet's disease and Fuchs' heterochromic uveitis. In one study, anterior uveitis accounted for 30-40%, posterior uveitis for 40-50%, intermediate uveitis for 10-20%, and diffuse uveitis for 5-10% of childhood uveitis.[9]

Juvenile Idiopathic Arthritis Associated Uveitis

In children, juvenile idiopathic arthritis (JIA) has been reported as the accompanying systemic manifestation in 81% of children with uveitis[7] and in 95% of children with anterior uveitis.[10] More recently, JIA was found to be the associated systemic manifestation in 41.5% of 130 children with uveitis.[8] This change has in part been brought about by better recognition of other diseases associated with uveitis in childhood which may strongly resemble JIA. Chronic anterior uveitis may also occur associated with other systemic diseases, such as inflammatory bowel disease and sarcoidosis, and as an isolated phenomenon. Sarcoidosis of childhood frequently manifests in the joints, skin, and eyes and rarely in the lungs.[11] Posterior segment manifestations in the form of retinal vasculitis, peripheral multifocal choroiditis, or choroidal granuloma may help to differentiate this entity from JIA associated uveitis.

Screening guidelines for JIA associated uveitis vary and are mainly based on the perceived risk of developing uveitis: risk factors include the pattern of initial joint disease, the patients' sex, ANA status, and age at onset.

Diagnosis

The uveitis is chronic, non-granulomatous and bilateral in about three-fourth of all cases. Children with pauciarticular involvement are at more risk for developing uveitis than those with polyarticular or 'systemic' JIA. Hypoyon is rare although the intraocular inflammation may be severe. JIA associated uveitis is a 'white uveitis'; the eye is rarely congested even when the inflammation is severe. Girls seem to have a more indolent course than boys and need more careful follow-up. Antinuclear antibody (ANA) positivity may precede uveitis. Seronegativity for rheumatoid factor is the rule. Some cases may be HLA B27 positive and the uveitis may be similar to ankylosing spondylitis associated anterior uveitis. Filiform synechiae with a 'festooned pupil' are common in long standing cases (Fig. 42.1) In chronic cases, complicated cataract develops in more than 50% cases, band shaped keratopathy in almost 40% and secondary glaucoma in 15-20%.

Management

Topical corticosteroids are the mainstay of therapy. They are titrated according to anterior chamber cellular reaction although chronic flare may persist despite

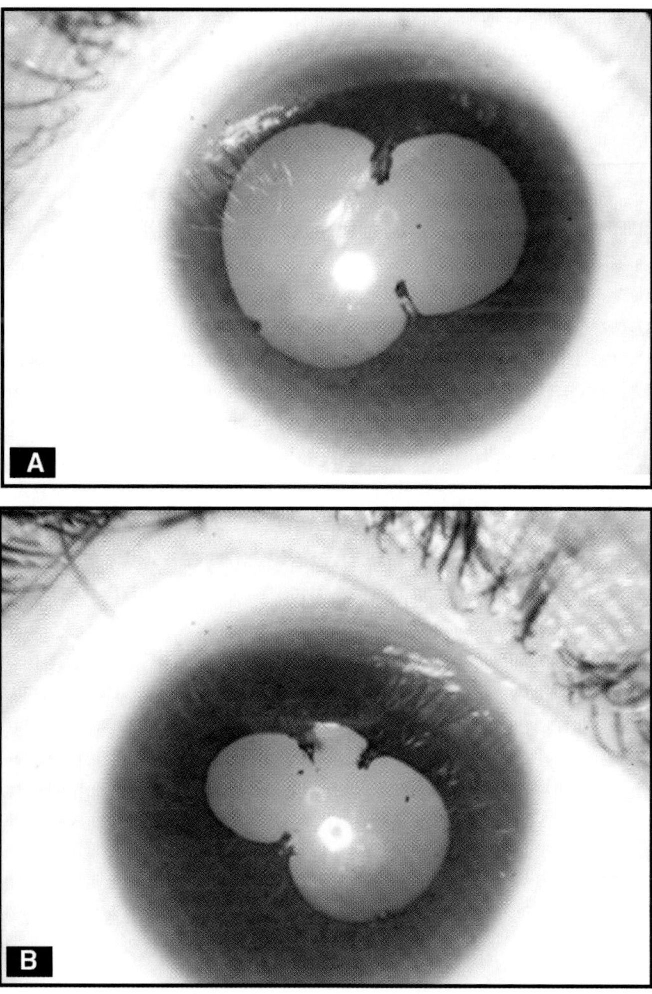

Figs 42.1A and B: Filiform synechiae OU in a 16-year-old child with Juvenile rheumatoid associated uveitis

therapy and should not be aggressively treated. Some children may require depot steroid injections for control of inflammation. A short course of systemic steroids may be necessary in older children but they should be used with caution as they retard normal growth of the child. Systemic immunosuppression has also been found to be useful in severe cases but an internist and pediatrician co-management is mandatory when using systemic therapies in these children. Surgical intervention is warranted for management of cataract, glaucoma and severe band shaped keratopathy. Ideally, inflammation should be controlled prior to surgery. The control of inflammation implies a lack of anterior chamber cellular reaction. At times, in younger children, surgery may be planned despite some inflammatory reaction persisting in order to take care of risk of amblyopia. In some cases with cyclitic membranes, hypotony and low grade inflammation, surgery and removal of these membranes may actually help to control the inflammation and it's sequelae. The two surgical techniques of use today for managing complicated cataracts in JIA associated uveitis are phacoaspiration with or without intraocular lens implantation and lensectomy with anterior vitrectomy. The largest series of cataract surgery in JRA patients reports surgical results in 162 eyes, 61 of which underwent needling and aspiration and the rest underwent lensectomy with anterior vitrectomy.[7] Phthisis bulbi was seen in 25% of eyes undergoing needling and aspiration versus only 3% eyes after lensectomy. Visual acuity of 20/60 or better was achieved in 56% of cases undergoing lensectomy versus 21% with needling and aspiration. However, improvement in microsurgical techniques have also improved the results of extracapsular surgical techniques and Foster et al reported 6 eyes undergoing extracapsular cataract extraction and 4 eyes achieved 20/40 or better and no eye went into phthisis over a follow up period of upto 7 years.[12]

Glaucoma in JIA associated uveitis may be related to inflammation or may be caused by papillary block due to posterior synechiae. Pupillary block may be relieved by an iridectomy which may have to be surgical as laser iridotomies frequently close. Medical management is difficult and many cases require surgical management in the form of trabeculectomy with antimitotic agents or implantation of glaucoma drainage devices. Cyclocryotherapy or cyclophotocoagulation should be reserved as a last resort in eyes with poor visual prognosis.

For band shaped keratopathy, chemical chelation with 0.37M EDTA is done after debridement of epithelium. This improves corneal clarity in majority of cases with severe involvement.

Fuch's Heterochromic Uveitis

Although described by Lawrence in 1843, the syndrome is named after Ernst Fuchs who first analyzed 38 patients and reported features of a 'new' condition in 1906.[13] Although the typical patient is a young adult who presents with visual symptoms and heterochromia, rarely children under 16 years of age may be affected. The uveitis is nonprogressive, mild, and in general nonresponsive to corticosteroid therapy. The diagnosis is usually made on the basis of small, white, diffusely scattered keratic precipitates; minimal cells and flare; lack of posterior synechias; and atrophic changes in the iris. In the full blown case, cataract is invariably present and is most often posterior subcapsular in location (Fig. 42.2). Glaucoma remains perhaps the main sight

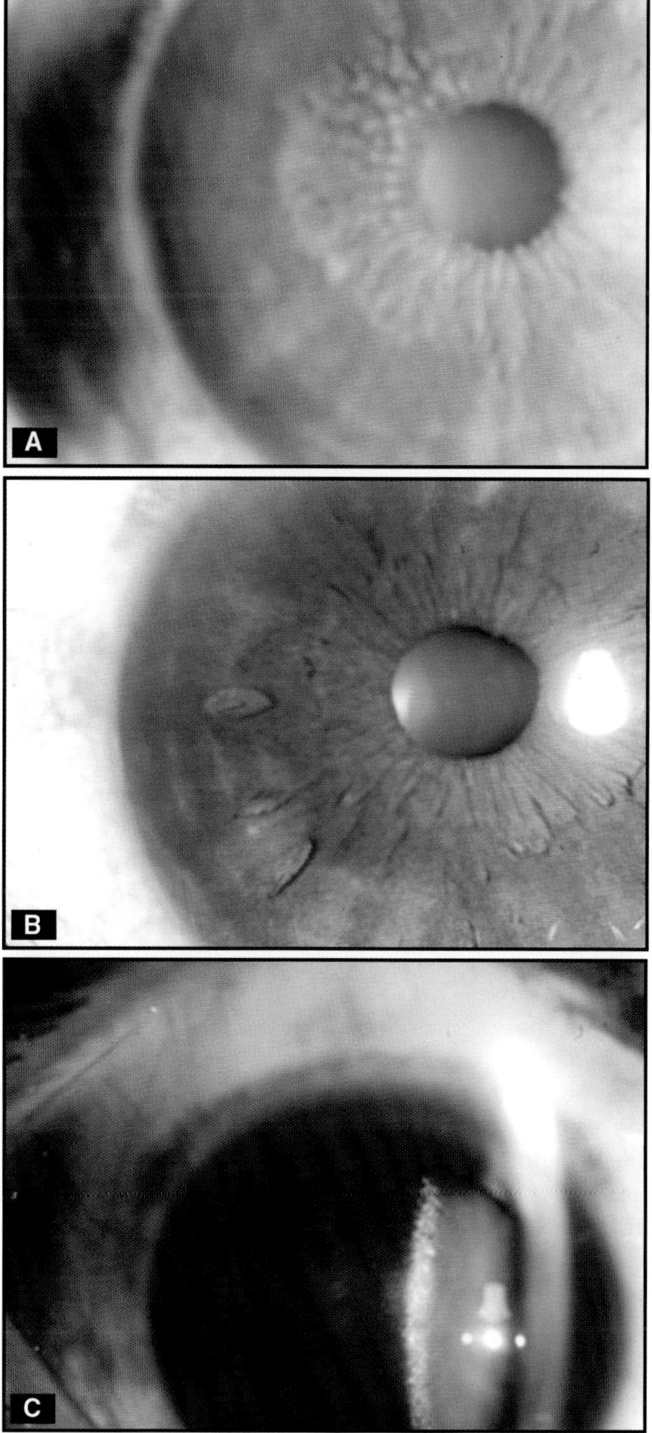

Fig. 42.2A to C

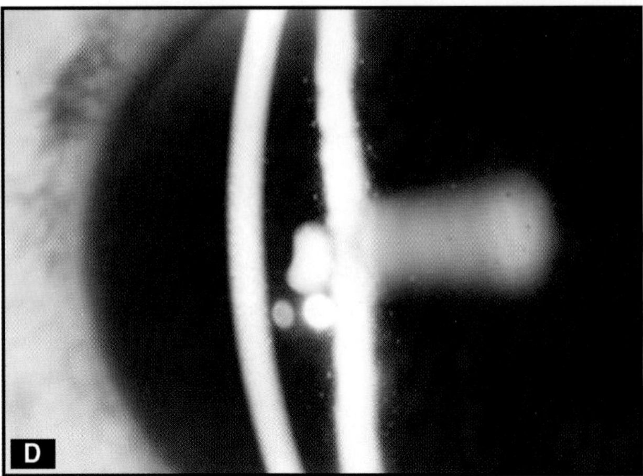

Figs 42.2A to D: A 15-year-old female patient was diagnosed as a case of Fuchs' heterochromic cyclitis on the basis of iris heterochromia, koeppe nodules, stellate keratic precipitates and posterior subcapsular cataract

threatening component of this syndrome and may be seen in 6.3 to 59% of cases.[14]

Management

The inflammatory component usually does not need any treatment as it is mild and does not respond very well to steroids. Complicated cataract is frequently seen, typically posterior subcapsular in morphology, and usually occurs in patients after 40 years of age. It has been managed using different techniques including lens aspiration and intracapsular (ICCE) and extracapsular (ECCE) cataract extraction. The 1990s brought the increasing use of intraocular lenses (IOLs) in patients with FHU. A general consensus has evolved on the good prognosis of posterior chamber IOL (PC IOL) implantation in these patients. However, most studies used manual ECCE and reported postoperative complications such as hyphema, glaucoma, and intractable uveitis. Recently, good results have been reported after phacoemulsification and foldable intraocular lens implantation in FHU.[15]

Management of glaucoma poses the same challenges as in any other form of uveitic glaucoma. Control of inflammation may be required in cases with glaucoma. Surgery for management of glaucoma may be required in a majority of patients with equivocal results.

Intermediate Uveitis

Intermediate uveitis (IU) is a chronic intraocular inflammation, mainly affecting the anterior vitreous and the pars plana. The disease predominantly affects patients under the age of 40 years and forms approximately 8% to 22%[16] of all uveitis in the general uveitic population. The percentage of IU increases in the uveitis population aged less than 16 years.[7,8,17] The visual prognosis in adults is usually favorable.[16] The visual outcome of IU in children is not known. The ocular inflammation in children is frequently discovered late in the disease process, and the child might already be presenting with advanced signs and complications.[18-21] The etiology of IU in adults is considered to be an idiopathic autoimmune disease, and was occasionally associated with sarcoidosis, multiple sclerosis (MS), or infectious diseases.[22] In the pediatric population, the causes and prognosis of IU have not yet been systemically studied. Remission of the disease has been reported, but the incidence of remissions reported was low.[19]

The International Uveitis Study Group has used the term 'Intermediate uveitis' to classify cases with intraocular inflammation restricted to the peripheral retina and adjoining vitreous. Pars planitis refers to a specific form of intermediate uveitis in which white fluffy collection termed as 'snowbanking' is present over the ora serrata and pars plana. Intermediate uveitis is most often idiopathic.

Diagnosis

Patients usually present with a symptom of floaters and occasionally blurring of vision. On examination, anterior chamber reaction is mild to moderate with fine keratic precipitates and usually an absence of posterior synechiae. The main site of inflammation is the pars plana area and peripheral retina and hence anterior vitreous cells are seen. More than half of all cases develop cystoid macular edema resulting in visual impairment. A specific problem noted in the pediatric age group is development of optic disc edema (Fig. 42.3).

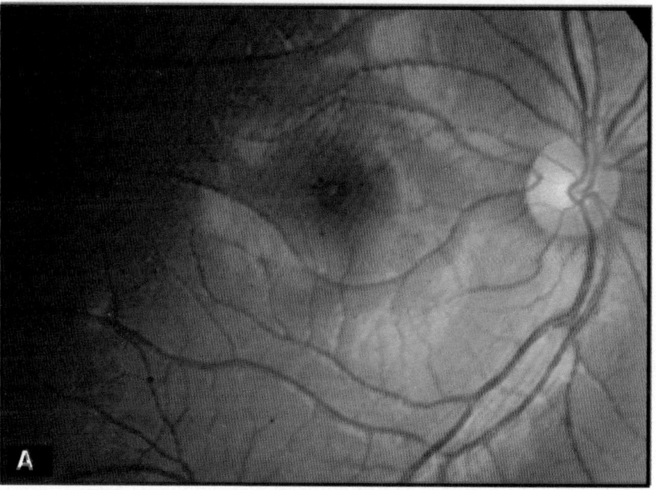

Fig. 42.3A:

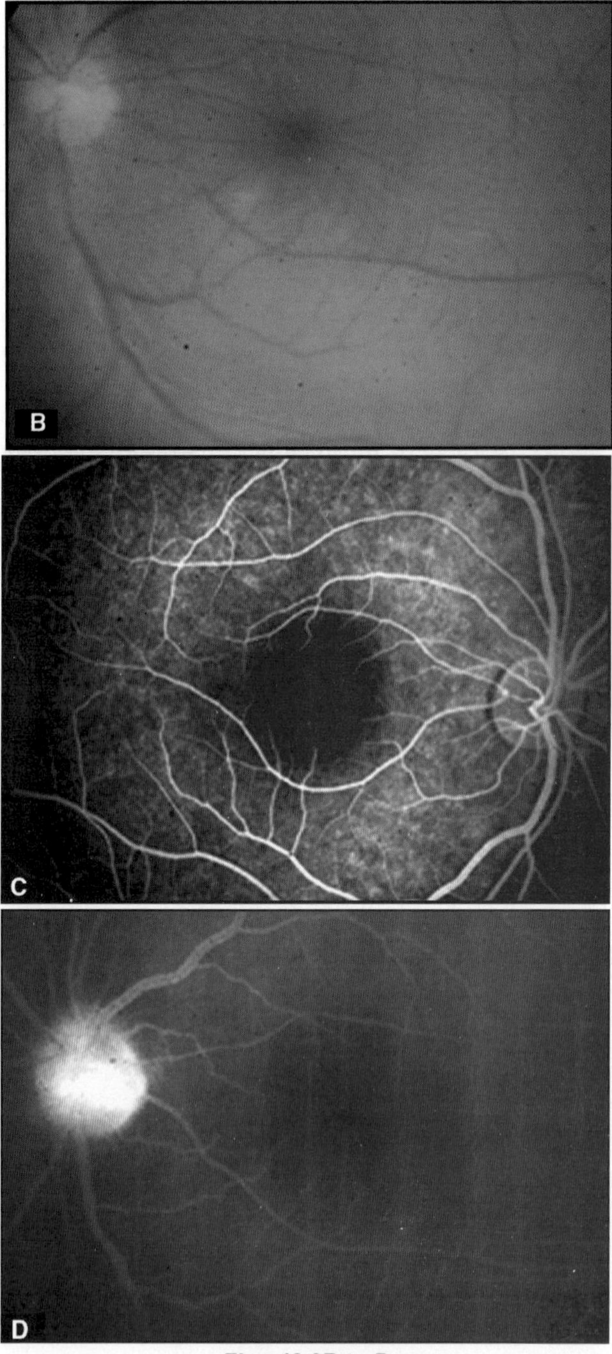

Figs 42.3B to D

Figs 42.3A to D: A 13-year-old girl presented with 6/24 vision in the left eye. Examination showed evidence of pars planitis in the left eye with vitritis, pars plana snowbanking and disc hyperemia. FFA showed left disc leakage

Management

Many cases with mild involvement and without macular edema do not require any treatment. Since the etiology of IU is not very well defined, treatment is mainly symptomatic. In some previous studies, the young patients were less frequently systemically treated than adults.[23] One should consider the presence of CME as an indication for treatment and periocular corticosteroid injections are the mainstay of management of CME. A short course of oral steroids may be necessary in cases with severe anterior vitreous inflammation. Since CME is the major cause of visual loss or impairment of IU in children, early detection and treatment of CME are crucial for the prevention of visual loss.

Behcet's Disease

Behçet's disease is a multi-system inflammatory disorder dominated clinically by recurrent oral and genital ulceration, uveitis, and erythema nodosum. It is characterized by a chronic course, with exacerbations and remissions. Behçet's disease is most frequently seen in adults, although a childhood-onset has been reported. About 2-3% of all affected individuals have childhood-onset.[24] Onset of this disease in children as young as 2 years of age has been reported, but most children develop clinical features after 6-7 years of age.[25] The cause remains unknown, although an autoimmune reaction triggered by an infectious agent in a genetically predisposed individual has been suggested.

Behçet's disease is a vasculitis, affecting vessels of different types, sizes, and localizations. Since the etiology of Behçet's disease is unknown, treatment tends to be empirical and is usually comprised of systemic corticosteroids and immunosuppressants.

The international uveitis study group criteria for diagnosis of Behcet's disease are:[26]

Recurrent oral ulceration	Minor aphthous, major aphthous or herpetiform ulceration observed by physician or patient, which recurred at least 3 times in one 12-month period
Plus 2 of:	
Recurrent genital ulceration	Aphthous ulceration or scarring, observed by physician or patient.
Eye lesions	Anterior uveitis, posterior uveitis, or cells in vitreous on slit lamp examination; or retinal vasculitis observed by ophthalmologist.
Skin lesions	Erythema nodosum observed by physician or patient, pseudofolliculitis or papulo-pustular lesions; or acneiform nodules observed by physician in post-adolescent patients not on corticosteroid treatment.

Positive pathergy test	Read by physician at 24-48 hrs, performed with oblique insertion of a 20-gauge or smaller needle under sterile conditions.

Ocular manifestations include panuveitis, anterior uveitis, posterior uveitis, bilateral disc edema, and retinal vasculitis (Fig. 42.4). Ocular involvement is usually bilateral, although severity of disease may differ between eyes. Ocular disease is the most common cause of significant morbidity in Behcet's disease, since it may lead to visual loss in about five years if not treated.

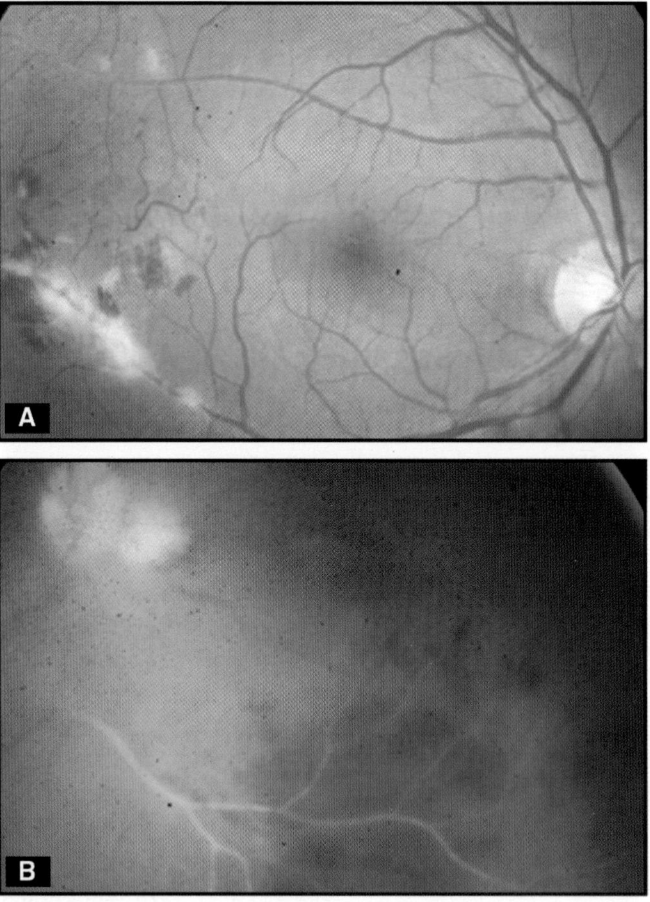

Figs 42.4A and B: A 14-Year-old child presented with poor vision in both eyes. His BCVA was 6/9 in right eye and 6/60 in the left. He had dense witritis in the left eye and evidence of vasculitis in both eyes. He gave history of recurrent oro-genital ulcerations. He was diagnosed as a case of Behcets disease and was treated with oral corticosteroids and immunosuppressive agents

Management

The treatment of BD is symptomatic and empirical, but generally specific to the clinical features of each patient. The acute anterior inflammation may respond well to topical steroids initially. However, posterior segment involvement requires systemic therapy and steroids are usually not effective. Many patients will require immunosuppressive agents in the form of azathioprine, methotrexate or cyclophosphamide which must be prescribed in conjunction with internist or pediatrician.

Toxoplasmosis

Toxoplasmosis is caused by infestation in humans by a protozoan parasite *Toxoplasma gondii* for whom cat is the definitive host and other animals including human beings are the intermediate hosts. While undercooked meat and food contaminated with oocysts from cat feces remain the major sources of infection, contaminated water may be an important additional source in some settings. In most cases, infection is acquired transplacentally when a pregnant mother gets infested.

Clinical Features

If the mother acquires infection in the first or second trimester, the child is either still born or there may be spontaneous abortion or the child may be born with brain damage. In children with inactive disease at birth, most cases are subclinical with chorioretinal scars (Fig. 42.5). Reactivation of disease from these scars occurs between the ages of 10-35 years and manifests as a focal necrotizing retinitis with severe overlying vitritis giving a 'headlight-in-fog' appearance. The active lesion is usually adjacent to an old chorioretinal scar in the posterior pole area.[27,28] Spillover mild anterior segment inflammation may also be present. The choroid and retinal vessels may be indirectly involved. The course may be complicated by development of cystoid macular edema, macular pucker, tractional retinal detachment, rhegmatogenous retinal detachment and choroidal and retinal neovascularization.

Management

Not all lesions require treatment; only vision threatening lesions in the form of those close to fovea, papillomacular bundle and rarely the optic nerve head require to be treated. Treatment is in the form of steroids to control the inflammation and antimicrobials. Steroids may be used orally and topically. Antimicrobials in the form of Clindamycin 300 mg QID, Sulphadiazine 2 gm loading followed by 1gm QID, or Pyrimethamine 75-150 mg loading followed by 25 mg daily, are given for a period of 3-4 weeks. Clindamycin use can

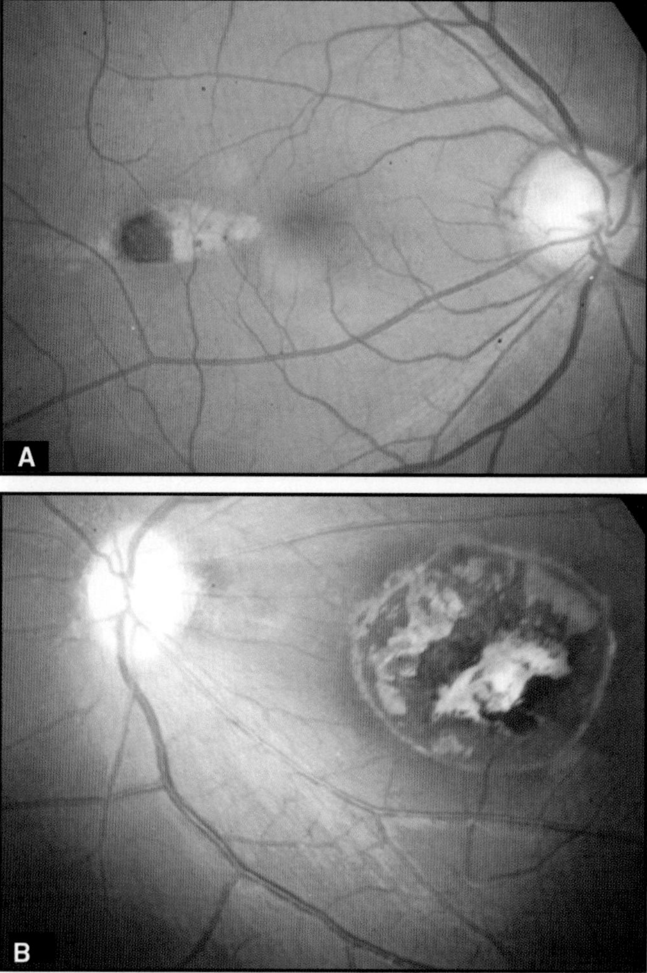

Figs 42.5A and B: A 15-Year-old child presented with poor vision in both eyes. His BCVA was 6/6 in right eye and CF 1meter in the left. Fundus examination showed bilateral toxoplasmosis scars

cause pseudomembranous colitis and one should be careful when using the drug. Patients on Pyrimethamine need follow up for thrombocytopenia and leucopenia.

Toxocariasis

This disease is an infestation with a roundworm found in dogs and cats (*Toxocara canis* and *Toxocara cati*). Young children in close contact with pets or ingesting contaminated food or soil are at risk. The eggs of the worm are ingested which develop into larva which in turn migrate to the lungs, liver,

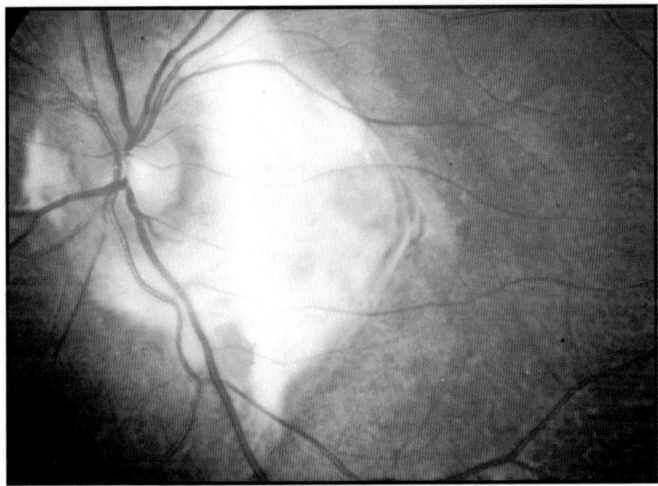

Fig. 42.6: A 6-year-old child presented with esotropia in the left eye. Fundus showed a white dense toxocara granuloma scar in the left eye

brain or eyes. Ocular toxocariasis is characterized by a chronic endophthalmitis-like picture or a granuloma formation in the posterior pole or retinal periphery (Fig. 42.6). The complications could be in the form of cyclitic membranes, macular drag or retinal detachment. Management is restricted to surgical intervention in the form of pars plana vitrectomy for the complications.[29,30]

SUMMARY

Uveitis in children, although less common than in adults, is fairly frequently seen and assumes great importance because of the higher number of complications observed and a poorer visual outcome. The major proportion of cases are either idiopathic or associated with juvenile idiopathic arthritis. Other entities commonly seen are pars planitis, toxoplasmosis and Fuch's Heterochromic Uveitis. In some regions, Behcet's disease may also assume significant proportions. The management of uveitis in children is particularly challenging as the use of aggressive systemic medications may interfere with the growth of the child. The fact that some of these children are in the amblyopic age group further complicates the issue. However, useful vision may be salvaged in a majority of these cases with judicious management.

REFERENCES

1. BenEzra D, Cohen E, Maftzir G. Uveitis in children and adolescents. Br J Ophthalmol 2005;89:444-8
2. David M. Endogenous uveitis in children; associated band shaped keratopathy and rheumatoid arthritis. Arch Ophthalmol 1953;50:443-54.

3. Perkins ES. Patterns of uveitis in children. Br J Ophthalmol 1966;50:169-85.
4. Kimura SJ, Hogan MJ, Thygeson P. Uveitis in children. Arch Ophthalmol 1954;51:80-8.
5. Blegvad O. Iridocyclitis and diseases of the joints in children. Acta Ophthalmol 1941;19:219-36.
6. Kimura SJ, Hogan MJ. Uveitis in children: Analysis of 274 cases. Trans Am Ophthalmol Soc 1964;62:173-92.
7. Kanski JJ, Shun-Shin A. Systematic uveitis syndromes in childhood; An analysis of 340 cases. Ophthalmology 1984;91:1247-52.
8. Tugal-Tutkun I, Harvlikova K, Power WJ, et al. Changing patterns in uveitis of childhood. Ophthalmology 1996;103:375-83.
9. Cunningham ET Jr. Uveitis in children. Ocul Immunol Inflamm 2000;8:251-61.
10. O'Brien JM, Albert DM. Therapeutic approaches for ophthalmic problems in juvenile arthritis. Rheumatol Dis Clin N Amer 1989;15:413-22.
11. Fink CW, Cimaz R. Early onset sarcoidosis: not a benign disease. J Rheumatol 1977;24:174-7.
12. Foster CS, Fong LP, Singh G. Cataract surgery and intraocular lens implantation in patients with uveitis. Ophthalmology 1989;96:281-7
13. Fuchs E. Über Komplicationen der Heterochromie. Z Augenheilkd 1906;15:191-212
14. Jones NP. Fuchs' Heterochromic Uveitis. An Update. Surv Ophthalmol 1993;37:253-72
15. Ram J, Kaushik S, Brar GS, Gupta A, Gupta A. Phacoemulsification in patients with Fuchs' heterochromic uveitis. J Cataract Refract Surg 2002;28:1372-8.
16. AT Vitale, M Zierhut, CS Foster. Intermediate uveitis. In: CS Foster, AT Vitale, (Eds), Diagnosis and treatment of uveitis, WB Saunders Company, Philadelphia 2001; 844-57.
17. Boer de JH, Wulffraat N, Rothova A. Causes of blindness in uveitis of childhood. Br J Ophthalmol 2003; 87:879-84.
18. Smith RE, Godfrey WA, Kimura SJ. Complications of chronic cyclitis. Am J Ophthalmol 1976;82:277-82.
19. Hogan MJ, Kimura SJ, O' Connor GR. Peripheral retinitis and chronic cyclitis in children. Trans Ophthalmol Soc UK 1965;85:39-52.
20. Aaberg TM. The enigma of pars planitis. Am J Ophthalmol 1987;103:828-30.
21. Giles CL. Pediatric intermediate uveitis. J Pediatr Ophthalmol Strabismus 1989;26:136-39.
22. Nussenblatt RB, Whitcup SM, Palestine AG. Intermediate uveitis. In: L Craven, (Ed). Uveitis, fundamentals, and clinical practice, Mosby, St Louis 1996; 279-288.
23. Guest S, Funkhouser E, Lightman S. Pars planitis a comparison of childhood onset and adult onset disease. Clin experiment Ophthalmol 2001;29:81-4.
24. Saylan T, Mat C, Fresko I, Melikoglu M. Behçet's disease in the Middle East. Clin Dermatol 1999;17:209-23.
25. Kari JA, Shah V, Dillon MJ. Behçet's disease in UK children: Clinical features and treatment including thalidomide. Rheumatology 2001;40:933-8.
26. International Study Group for Behçet's Disease. Criteria for diagnosis of Behçet's disease. Lancet 1990;335:1078-80.

27. Holland GN, O'Connor GR, Belfort Jr R, Remington JS. Toxoplasmosis. In: JS. Pepose, GN Holland, KR Wilhelmus, (Eds). Ocular infection and immunity, Mosby-Year Book, Inc., St. Louis, Missouri 1996;1183-1223.
28. Hogan MJ, Kimura SJ, O'Connor GR. Ocular toxoplasmosis. Arch Ophthalmol 1964;72:592-600.
29. Werner JC, Ross RD, Green WR, Watts JC. Pars plana vitrectomy and subretinal surgery for ocular toxocariasis. Arch Ophthalmol 1999;117:532-4
30. Belmont JB, Irvine A, Benson W, O'Connor GR. Vitrectomy in ocular toxocariasis. Arch Ophthalmol 1982;100:1912-5.

Chapter 43

NANOTECHNOLOGY IN OPHTHALMOLOGY

NR Biswas, Alok K Ravi, Madhurjya Gogai (India)

INTRODUCTION

Nanotechnology is a field of science comprising the body of theories and techniques that allow the production and manipulation of minute objects that measure a little as one billionth of a meter (the nanometer). Although research in this field dates back to Richard P. Feynman's work 1959, the term nanotechnology was first coined by K. Eric Drexler in 1986 in the book *Engines of Creation.*

Nanotechnology involves research and technology development at the atomic, molecular, or macromolecular levels in the critical dimension range of approximately 1-100 nanometers. Nanotechnology research and development includes control at the nanoscale and integration of nanoscale structures into larger material components and systems. Within these larger scale assemblies, the control and construction of their structures and components remains at the nanometer scale.

Nanobiotechnology is an emerging area that applies the tools and processes of nano / microfabrication to build devices for studying biosystems. Vice-versa, researchers also learn from biology how to create better micro-nanoscale devices. The field is highly interdisciplinary and features a close collaboration between life scientists, physical scientists, and engineers.

Of relevance to medicine is *Nanomedicine,* which may be defined as the monitoring, repair, construction and control of human biological systems at the molecular level, using engineered nanodevices and nanostructures. The goal is to deliver the potential benefit of discoveries in the laboratory to society.

The power of nanotechnology can be encapsulated in an apparently simple and minute device. Packed with miniature chemical processors, computing, and robotics, it will produce a wide-range of items quickly, cleanly, and inexpensively, building products directly from blueprints. The enabling technologies include optics, nanolithography, mechanochemistry and 3D prototyping.

Although nanotechnology is in the research stage as of now, it is likely to arrive in 20 to 30 years from now. It is being extensively pursued for research on ageing, cancer, and drug development and delivery.

Medicine and Nanotechnology

Medicine attempts to make the best use of the body's natural healing powers and homeostatic mechanisms. The underlying principle is that, all else being equal, those interventions are best that intervene least. The promise of nanotechnology in medicine lies in the potential to achieve this by target specific and controlled delivery of intervention measures at the cellular level. Nanosystems have significantly different biological properties from large-sized systems (e.g. implants or microparticles) that could be used effectively to overcome problems in drug and gene therapy using programmable and controllable microscale robots. This will hopefully unlock the indefinite extension of human health and the expansion of human abilities. The possibility of applying nanotechnology in even traditional Chinese medicine has been explored.[1]

The Medical Nanodevice

Composition

The typical medical nanodevice will probably be a micron-scale robot assembled from nanoscale parts ranging from 1-100 nm (1 nm = 10^{-9} meter), and might be fitted together to make a working machine measuring perhaps 0.5-3 microns (1 micron = 10^{-6} meter) in diameter. Three microns is about the maximum size for blood borne medical nanorobots, the limiting factor being capillary passage.

Carbon will likely be the principal element comprising the bulk of a medical nanorobot, probably in the form of diamond or diamondoid/fullerene nanocomposites—largely because of the tremendous strength and chemical inertness of diamond. Other elements such as hydrogen, sulfur, oxygen, nitrogen, fluorine, silicon, etc. will be used for special purposes.

Properties

The medical nanodevice should be visualized as two spaces : its interior and its exterior. The exterior will be exposed to the diverse chemical brew that makes up our human biochemistry. But the interior of the nanorobot may be a highly controlled environment into which external liquids would not normally intrude, except in specific instance.

The ideal model of the medical nanodevice will consist of an injection of a few cubic centimeters of micron-sized nanorobots. The circulating nanorobots will be designed to accomplish a specific task, and would remain absolutely inactive outside of the target volume. Even once inside the target treatment volume, nanorobots would still remain inactive until the physician tells them to begin the active treatment, or the precise antigenic signature of the target tissue is detected. Knowledge of these antigens will become extensive, soon after the completion of the *Human Genome Project* early in the 21st century.

Nanorobots will communicate their positions, operational status, and the outcome of treatment using encoded acoustic messaging for internal communications as well as for communication with the physician, who will retain complete control. It may not be necessary to image the nanodevices directly, and procedures such as biopsy should be rarely needed. They will have a high level of redundancy to ensure effectiveness and safety. I*n vivo* medical nanodevices could metabolize local glucose and oxygen for energy, or use externally supplied acoustic power. Their exfusion from the body will occur via the usual excretory channels or other scavenger systems. The only physical change to be seen in the patient will hopefully be his recovery.

The Question of Immune Response

Many medical nanorobots will have only temporary residence in the body, and the issue of nanodevice biocompatibility is in principle similar to the biocompatibility of medical implants generally. It is not expected to be a major problem. The design of the exteriors will be critical to minimize bioactivity and opsonization. Passive diamond is one such design.

Replication

Replication is a crucial basic capability for molecular manufacturing, but medical nanorobots need not ever replicate *in vivo* except in the most unusual of circumstances. Replicators will almost certainly be very tightly regulated by governments everywhere.Many medical nanorobots will have very simple computers on board each device. The risk of human like artificial intelligence is unfounded.

Genetics

Of great importance is the use of nanotechnology in genetics. DNA is a unique material for nanotechnology since it is possible to use base sequences to encode instructions for assembly in a predetermined fashion at the nanometer scale. This emerging field of DNA-nanotechnology is now exploring DNA-programmed processes for the assembly of organic compounds, biomolecules, and inorganic materials.[2] Bioconjugated nanoparticles are being evaluated for biosensing and bioimaging, such as cell staining, DNA detection and separation, rapid single bacterium detection, and biotechnological application in DNA protection.[3]

Drug Development

Nanosystems comprising nanoparticles and nanodevices such as nano-biosensors and nanobiochips, are being developed for targeted drug therapy. Among these nanomaterials, carbon nanotubes (CNT) have emerged as an efficient and safe tool for transporting and translocating therapeutic molecules such as bioactive peptides, proteins, nucleic acids and drugs.[4-6]

Many polymerizable surfactants have been synthesized with all possible combination of the various types (anionic, cationic, zwitterionic or non-ionic group) and of classical polymerizable groups (acrylate, methacrylate, acrylamide, vinyl, allyle, diallyle, etc.). The polymerizable group can be located at different parts of the surfactant molecule most often near the polar head or at the end of hydrophobic tail, or even in the counterion (Fig. 43.1).

Another importan parameter, which synergies the release kinetics in different pH, solutions, is the swelling behavior of the polymer. One of the most important characteristics of the present copoly(NIPAAM-VP-AA) micelles is their ability to ionize/deionize at different pH-sensitive polymer.

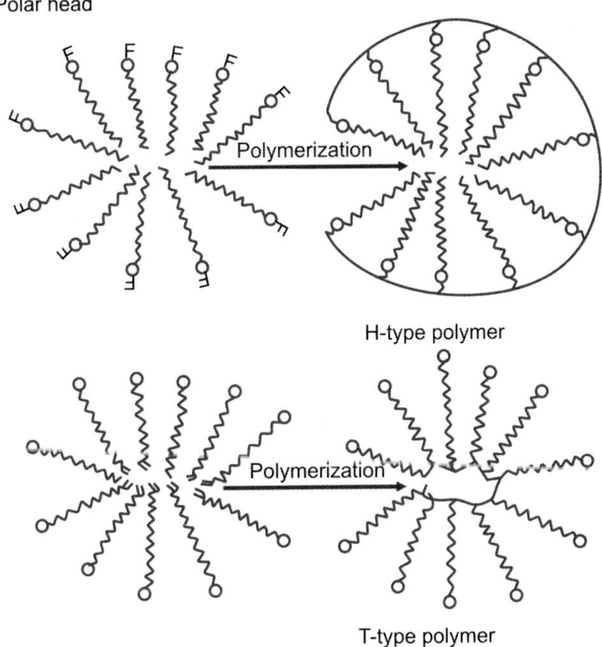

Fig. 43.1: Schematic ideal representation of head and tail monomeric and polymeric

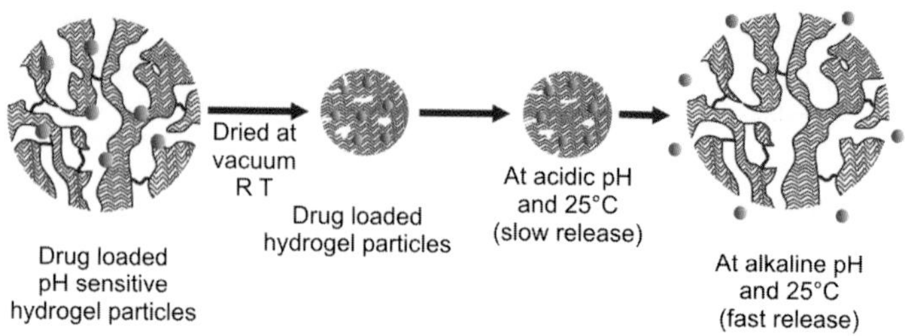

Fig. 43.2

The key to the controlling of the pores of the particles include both overall -COOH content and the ionization of –COOH groups. At acidic pH, the carboxylic groups exhibit inter-chain hydrogen bonding creating a tighter overall network and hence the pore size becomes smaller. Consequently due to small pore size, the release of drug from the micelles is quite slow. At alkaline pH, -COOH groups become ionized and due to repulsion among the ionized –COO groups swelling take place. As a result of swelling, pore size of the polymer increases and the drug release becomes faster (Fig. 43.2).

Nanotechnology in Ophthalmology

The application of nanotechnology in ophthalmology has so far mainly been on the development of drug delivery systems. A few such examples are:

1. Experimental studies have been reported on ocular hypotensive formulation containing biodegradable calcium phosphate nanoparticles (CAP) and 7-hydroxy-2-dipropyl-aminotetralin (7-OH-DPAT) for achieving controlled and targeted drug delivery for treatment of ocular diseases.[7]
2. Gelatin nanoparticles encapsulating pilocarpine HCl or hydrocortisone as model drugs have been produced using a desolvation method.[8]
3. The successful topical application of non-steroidal anti-inflammatory drugs sodium ibuprofen as well as flurbiprofen loaded polymeric nanoparticle suspensions made from inert polymer resins on the eye to counteract the miosis induced by surgical traumas, such as cataract extraction.[9-10]
4. The use of albumin nanoparticles to enhance the antiviral activity of ganciclovir while decreasing its intrinsic toxicity have been evaluated in human fibroblasts.[11]
5. Intravitreal injection of ganciclovir-loaded bovine serum albumin nanoparticles in rats has been studied for treatment of cytomegalovirus infection.[12]

NANOPARTICLES FOR OCULAR DRUG DELIVERY

Studies that have investigated the potential of nanoparticles for ocular drug delivery have been limited and have yet to demonstrate conclusively if they are superior to the conventional eye drop; however, there have been some promising results. Using a radiotracer technique, the ocular disposition of nanoparticles following topical instillation to the rabbit eye was investigated by Wood et al.[14] It was found that although nanoparticles composed of poly-hexyl-2-cyanoacrylate were rapidly cleared from the precorneal site, approximately 1% of the instilled dose was able to adhere to corneal and conjunctival surfaces.

The elimination of ^{III}In-labeled nanoparticles from tear fluid was compared to liposomes and control solutions by gamma-ray scintigraphy.[15] All three preparations were cleared from the cornea much faster than from the inner canthus. Clearance half-life of the solution from the cornea and inner canthus were 1.3 and 5 min, respectively. Positively charged liposomes displayed the longest corneal half-life at 3.7 min, while nanoparticles had the longest inner canthal half-life at 17.3 min and an intermediate value of 2.2 min in the cornea. In comparison, radiotracer technique indicated that polyalkylcyanoacrylate nanoparticles had a half-life in tears of about 20 min.[14] The residence time of these same nanoparticles in inflamed eye tissues was about 4 times higher than that observed in healthy tissues.[16]

The main objective of employing nanoparticles as a carrier for ophthalmic drug delivery is to provide sustained drug release and prolonged therapeutic activity. Using pilocarpine as a model drug, Harmia et al[17] were able to demonstrate prolonged miosis in rabbits following topical administration of drug adsorbed to polybutylcyanoacrylate nanoparticles. A commercial pilocarpine solution was used as a control. Interestingly, when pilocarpine was incorporated into nanoparticle matrix, no significant prolongation of the miotic was observed. It was suggested that an insufficient amount of drug was released from the nanoparticles prior to their removal from the precorneal site; thus, there was also a limited quantity of drug available for absorption. Conversely, when drug was adsorbed to the surface of the nanoparticles, drug release did not restrict the amount of drug available for absorption and may have facilitated a direct interaction with epithelial surfaces of tissues in the precorneal site. In another study, the use of polyalkylcyanoacrylate nanoparticles prolonged the intraocular pressure-reducing effect of pilocarpine for more than 9 h in a rabbit model.[18]

OCULAR DISTRIBUTION OF NANOPARTICLES

The fate of nanoparticles in the body depends on the physicochemical properties of the nanoparticles.[19] Properties such as pH, surfactant, and stabilizers influence the mucoadhesion properties to the ocular membrane and thereby modify the precorneal retention of the nanoparticles. It has been shown that the molecular weight of the polymer influences the residence time of nanoparticles in the precorneal area.[20] As the molecular weight increases, the polymer becomes poorly retained, whereas low molecular weight polymers are retained for a longer time. Experimental data on the disposition of polyhexylcyanoacrylate nanoparticles in tears, the aqueous humor, cornea, and conjunctiva of albino rabbits clearly showed adhesion of nanoparticles to absorbing tissue.[21]

DRUG USED IN PARTICULATE OCULAR DELIVERY

A polybutylcyanoacrylate nanoparticle delivery system for pilocarpine nitrate has been evaluated in comparison to the solution of the drug for pharmacokinetic and pharmacodynamic aspects.[22] Emulsion polymerization technique was employed in preparing nanoparticles, and in vivo experiments were performed by application of the formulations to the eyes of New Zealand white rabbits pretreated with betamethasone to create an elevated intraocular pressure mimicking glaucoma conditions. The results indicated an increase of 23% in pilocarpine levels in aqueous humor and prolonged t½ for the polybutylcyanoacrylate nanoparticle preparation compared to the aqueous control solution. It was possible to prolong the miosis with nanoparticles with lower drug content compared to the control solution. Betaxolol[23] and amikacin sulfate[24] loaded polyalkylcyanoacrylate nanoparticles have shown similar effects. The superficial charge and binding type of the drug onto the nanoparticles are important factors playing a role in the improvement of the therapeutic response. In another study, adsorption of pilocarpine onto polybutylcyanoacrylate nanoparticles enhanced the miotic response by about 22% compared to the control aqueous drug solution.[25]

In a clinical study with Piloplex® (latex emulsion of pilocarpine hydrochloride) a lower level of the drug with less fluctuation compared to the corresponding control solution was observed on the third day of treatment. This study involving nine subjects showed a reduction by 5.25 mmHg of the average diurnal intraocular pressure value compared to the control. Only one out of 30 patients complained of a local sensitivity reaction with Piloplex in the yearlong.[26] Similar results were obtained in yet another study involving 50 patients, where 67.6% of the eyes treated with the formulation were under control, while only 45.2% were under control with the pilocrpine solution.[27]

Nanoparticles appear to offer several advantages in the area of ophthalmic drug delivery. Particularly attractive are their bioadhesive properties which, if optimized, may overcome a major shortcoming of most ophthalmic products, i.e., inadequate retention time in the prcorneal site. Another important feature is the versatility of nanoparticles as a drug carrier. Many different types of compounds can be incorporated or adsorbed to nanoparticles, and depending on the composition, nanoparticles with different release characteristic can be designed. Furthermore, nanoparticles are easy to manufacture and form a stable, yet biodegradable product. Biodegradability suggests that nanoparticles will have low toxicity.

Although most of the investigations provided results that promised an advantage of the nanoparticle ophthalmic drug delivery, there is a need for further studies to elucidate the pharmacodynamic and pharmacokinetic fate of nanoparticle ophthalmic products, the safety of long-term use of this new type of ophthalmic dosage form, and also the aspects of the industrial product development.

Ethics

The ethical debate has seen extreme and opposite positions being adopted. Optimists visualize the best case scenarios, possibly utopian, whereas others present all manner of apocalyptic visions. Many of these are based on incomplete, simplified and outdated visions of a nanotechnology. Therefore, updated information must be made available for an informed debate on ethics. A framework for such a debate has been suggested.[28]

Potential Problems

Problems could relate to biocompatibility, design constraints, and onboard computers malfunctions, and the human factor, a bit small. However, the most serious problems may devolve from the inherent complexity of a multitude of nanodevices independently trying to cooperatively work on a very complex biological task in a short timeframe. Moreover, there is always the possibility of the unexpected.

The Challenge Ahead

No actual working nanorobot has yet been built. Development in these disciplines has proved to be more difficult than expected. The field of nanomedicine is rapidly evolving, and it is necessary to verify realistically how such high technologies may support medicine. The biggest benefit to be gained for human society from nanomedicine is the elimination of all common diseases, medical pain and suffering, and allow for the extension of human capabilities, most especially our mental faculties. Issues of ownership, regulation, ethics, and others will have to be continually addressed as new information becomes available.

REFERENCES

1. Gao YT, Shi SQ, Pan HW. [Possibility of applying nanotechnology to research on the basic theory of traditional Chinese medicine.] Zhong Xi Yi Jie He Xue Bao. 2005;3(6):426-8. [Article in Chinese]
2. Gothelf KV, Labean TH.DNA-programmed assembly of nanostructures. Org Biomol Chem. 2005;21;3(22):4023-37.

3. Tan W, Wang K, He X, Zhao XJ, Drake T, Wang L, Bagwe RP.Bionanotechnology based on silica nanoparticles. Med Res Rev 2004;24(5):621-38.
4. Bianco A, Kostarelos K, Prato M. Applications of carbon nanotubes in drug delivery. Curr Opin Chem Biol 2005;15.
5. Jain KK.The role of nanobiotechnology in drug discovery. Drug Discov Today. 2005;10(21):1435-42.
6. Labhasetwar V. Nanotechnology for drug and gene therapy: the importance of understanding molecular mechanisms of delivery. Curr Opin Biotechnol. 2005;28
7. Chu TC, He Q, Potter DE.Biodegradable calcium phosphate nanoparticles as a new vehicle for delivery of a potential ocular hypotensive agent. J Ocul Pharmacol Ther. 2002;18(6):507-14.
8. Vandervoort J, Ludwig A. Preparation and evaluation of drug-loaded gelatin nanoparticles for topical ophthalmic use. Eur J Pharm Biopharm. 2004 ;57(2):251-61.
9. Pignatello R, Bucolo C, Ferrara P, Maltese A, Puleo A, Puglisi G.Eudragit RS100 nanosuspensions for the ophthalmic controlled delivery of ibuprofen. Eur J Pharm Sci. 2002;16(1-2):53-61.
11. Pignatello R, Bucolo C, Spedalieri G, Maltese A, Puglisi G.Flurbiprofen-loaded acrylate polymer nanosuspensions for ophthalmic application. Biomaterials. 2002;23(15):3247-55.
12. Merodio M, Espuelas MS, Mirshahi M, Arnedo A, Irache JM.Efficacy of ganciclovir-loaded nanoparticles in human cytomegalovirus (HCMV)-infected cells. J Drug Target. 2002;10(3):231-38.
13. Merodio M, Irache JM, Valamanesh F, Mirshahi M.Ocular disposition and tolerance of ganciclovir-loaded albumin nanoparticles after intravitreal injection in rats. Biomaterials. 2002;23(7):1587-94.
14. Wood RW, Li VHK, Kreuter J, Robinson JR. Ocular disposition of polyhexyl-2-cyano[3-^{14}C] acrylate nanoparticles in the albino rabbit. Int J Pharm 1985;23: 175.
15. Kreuter J. Nanoparticles and liposomes in ophthalmic drug delivery, in Ophthalmic Drug Delivery. Biopharmaceutical, Technological and Clinical Aspects, Saettone MS, Bucci G, Speiser P, Eds., Liviana Press, Padua, Italy, 1987;101.
16. Diepold R, Kreuter J, Guggenbuhl P, Robinson JR. Distribution of polyhexyl-2-cyano-[3-^{14}C] acrylate nanoparticles in healthy and chronically inflamed rabbits eyes, Int J Pharm. 1989;54:149.
17. Harmia T, Kreuter J, Speiser P, Boye T, Gurny R, Kubis A. Enhancement of myotic response of rabbits with pilocarpine-loaded polybutylcyanoacrylate nanoparticles. Int J Pharm. 1986;33:187.
18. Diepold R, Kreuter J, Himber J, Gurny R, Lee VHL, Robinson JR, Saettone MF, Schnaudigel OE. Comparison of different models for the testing of pilocarpine eyedrops using conventional eye drops and a novel depot formulation (nanoparticles), Albercht von Graefes Arch Klin Exp Ophthalmol. 1989;227:188.
19. Davis SS, Illum L. The targeting of drugs using polymeric microspheres. Br Polym J. 1983;15:160.
20. Das SK, Tucker IG, Davies NM. A gamma scintigraphic evaluation of the effect of molecular weight of poly(isobutyl cyanoacrylate) Nanoparticles on the precorneal residence in rabbit. Proc Int Symp Control Rel Matter Controlled Release Society, Inc. 1992;19:395.

21. Vezin W, Florence A. In vitro degradation rates of biodegradable poly-N-alkylcyanoacrylates. J Pharm Pharmacol. 1978;30:5P.
22. Zimmer A, Mutschler E, Lambrecht G, Mayer D, Kreuter J. Pharmacokinetic and Pharmacodynamic aspects of an ophthalmic pilocarpine nanoparticle-delivery system. Pharm Res. 1994;11:1435.
23. Marchal-Heussler L, Maincent P, Hoffman H, Spittler J, Couvreur P. Antiglaucomatous activity of betaxolol chlorhydrate sorbed onto different isobutyl cyanoacrylate nanoparticles preparations. Int J Pharm 1990;58:115.
24. Losa C, Valvo P, Castro E, Vila-Jato JL, Alonso MJ. Improvement of ocular penetration of amikacin sulphate by association to poly(butyl cyanoacrylate) nanoparticles. J Pharm Pharmacol. 1991;43:548.
25. Harima T, Kreuter J, Speiser P, Boye T, Gurny R, Kubis A. Enhancement of miotic response of rabbits with pilocarpine-loaded polybutylcyanoacrylate nanoparticles. Int J Pharm. 1986;33:187.
26. Ticho U, Blumenthal M, Zonis S, Gal A, Blank I, Mazor ZW. Piloplex, a new long-acting pilocarpine polymer salt. A long-term study. Br J Ophthalmol. 1979;63:48.
27. Ticho U, Blumenthal M, Zonis S, Gal A, Blank I, Mazor ZW. A clinical trial with Piloplex-a new long-acting pilocarpine compound: preliminary report. Ann Ophthalmol. 1979;11:555.
28. Gordijn B. Nanoethics: From Utopian Dreams and Apocalyptic Nightmares towards a more Balanced View. Sci Eng Ethics. 2005;11(4):521-33.

Chapter 44

Quick Look Tabulated Antibiotics and Anti-inflammatory Drugs in Ophthalmology

Ashok Garg (India)

ANTIBACTERIALS

Drug Name (Generic)	*Dosage form/strength*	*Commercial packing*
a. Aminoglycosides		
Gentamicin Sulfate	Solution 0.3% (3 mg/ml)	In 5 and 10 ml dropper vials
	Ointment 3 mg/g	3.5 g and 5 g tubes
Tobramycin	Solution 0.3% (3mg/ml)	In 3 and 5 ml dropper vials
	Ointment 3 mg/g	3 g and 5 g tubes
Sisomicin	Solution 0.3%	In 3 and 5 ml dropper vials
	Ointment 3 mg/g	3 g and 5g tubes
Neomycin	Solution 0.17% Ointment 5mg/gm	In 5 and 10 ml dropper vials 3 g and 5 g tubes
Framycetin	Solution 0.5 % Ointment 0.5% and 1%	In 5 and 10 ml dropper vials 3 and 5 gm tubes
b. Tetracyclines	Solution 1%	In 5 ml dropper vial
	Ointment 1%	3 and 5 gm tubes
Oxytetracycline	Ointment 1%	3 and 5 gm tubes
c. Sulphacetamide	Solution 10%,20%, 30%	In 5 and 10 ml dropper vial
	Ointment 10% and 30%	3 and 5 gm tubes

contd...

contd...

Sulfasoxazole diolamine	Solution 4%	In 10 and 15 ml dropper vial
d. Chloramphenicol	Solution 0.4-1%	3,5 and 10 ml dropper vial
	Ointment 5 mg/g and 10 mg/g	3 and 5 gm tubes
	Powder for solution/ Injection 25 mg/vial	Preservative free 15 ml pack with diluent
e. Microlides		
Erythromycin	Ointment 0.5% (5 mg/g)	In 3 and 5 gm tubes
Roxithromycin	Ointment 0.5%	In 3 and 5 gm tubes
f. Polypeptides		
Polymixin B	Solution 0.5-1%	5 and 10 ml dropper vial
	Ointment 1-1.5 mg/gm	3 and 5 gm tubes
	Powder for solution 500,000 units	In 20 ml vial
Bacitracin	Ointment 500 units/g and 10000 units/gm	Preservative free in 3 and 5 gm tubes
g. Fluoroquinolones		
Norfloxacin	Solution 0.3%	In 5 and 10 ml dropper vials
	Ointment 3 mg/g (0.3%)	3 and 5 gm tubes
Ciprofloxacin	Solution 0.3%	In 5 and 10 ml dropper vials
	Ointment 3 mg/g	3 and 5 gm tubes
Ofloxacin	Solution 0.3%	In 5 and 10 ml dropper Vials
	Ointment 3 mg/g	3 and 5 gm tubes
Pefloxacin	Solution 0.3%	In 5 ml dropper vials
Lomefloxacin	Solution 0.3%	In 5 ml dropper vials
	Ointment 3 mg/g	3 and 5 gm tubes
Sparfloxacilin	Solution 0.3%	In 5 ml dropper vials
	Ointment 3 mg/g	3 gm tubes
Levofloxacin	Solution 0.5%	In 5 ml dropper vials

Gatifloxacin	Solution 0.3%	In 5 ml dropper vials
Moxifloxacilin	Solution 0.5%	In 5 ml dropper vials
Gemifloxacilin	Solution 0.3%	In 5 ml dropper vials
Clinafloxacilin	Solution 0.3%	In 5 ml dropper vials

COMBINATION ANTIBIOTICS

Bacitracin, neomycin and polymixin B	Combination solution/ Ointment containing polymixin B sulfate 10000 units/g Neomycin sulfate 3.5 mg/g Bacitracin 400 Units/g	In 5 and 10 dropper vials In 5 mg tube
Neomycin sulfate, polymixin B sulfate gramicidin	Combi solution/oint. containing polymixin B Sulfate 10000 units/g, Neomycin sulfate 1.75 mg/g Gramicidin 0.025 mg/ml	In 5 and 10ml dropper vials In 3 and 5 gm tubes
Bacitracin zinc and polymixin B sulfate	Combi solution/ointment polymixin B sulfate 10000 units/g Bacitracin zinc 500 units/g	In 5 and 10 ml dropper vials In 5 gm tube
Polymixin B sulfate and oxytetracycline	Ointment containing polymixin B sulfate 10000 units/g and oxytetracycline HCl 5 mg/g	In 3 and 5 gm tubes
Trimethoprim Sulfate and Polymixin B	Combi solution containing Polymixing B sulfate 10000 units/g Trimethoprim : 1mg/ml	In 5 and 10 ml dropper vials
Sodium sulphacetamide and phenylephirine	Combination solution containing Sulphacetamide 15% phenylephrine HCl 0.125%	In 5 and 15 ml dropper vials

Gentamicin and Vancomycin	Combination solution containing gentamicin 8 ug/ml vancomycin 20 ug/ml	In 5 ml dropper vials

ANTI-INFLAMMATORY DRUGS

Topical Steroidal Agents

	as	
Hydrocortisone	Acetate solution 2%	3 and 5 ml dropper vials
	Acetate suspension 0.5-2.5%	3 and 5 ml dropper vials
	Acetate ointment 1.5%	3 and 5 gm tubes
Prednisolone	as	
	Acetate suspension 0.12%, 0.25% and 1%	5 ml dropper vials
	Sodium phosphate soln 0.12%, 0.5% and 1.0%	5 ml dropper vials
	Phosphate Oint.-0.25%	3 and 5 gm tubes
Dexamethasone	as	
	Sodium phosphate Solution-0.1%, 0.05% and 0.01%	5 ml dropper vial
	Suspension 0.1%, Sodium phosphate	5 ml dropper vial
	Ointment 0.05%	3 and 5 g tubes
Betamethasone	Sodium phosphate Solution 0.1%	In 5 and 10ml dropper vial
	Sodium phosphate Ointment 0.1%	3 and 5 g tubes
Triamcinolone acetonide	Suspension 0.1%	5 ml Dropper vials
	Ointment 0.1%	3 and 5 g tubes
Medrysone	Suspension 1%	In 5 and 10 ml dropper vials
Fluorometholone	Suspension 0.1%, 0.25%	In 5, 10 and 15 ml dropper vials
	Ointment 0.1%	3 and 5 gm tubes
Rimexolone	Suspension 0.1%	5 and 10 ml dropper vials
Loteprednol etabonate	Solution 0.2% and 0.5%	In 2.5,5 and 10 ml dropper vials

Non Steroidal Anti-inflammatory Drugs (NSAIDs)

Flurbiprofen	Solution 0.03%	in 2.5,5 and 10 ml dropper vials
Ketorolac tromethamine	Solution 0.5%	In 5 ml dropper Vial and Single Use 0.4 ml unims
Suprofen	Solution 1%	In 2.5 and 5 ml dropper vials
Diclofenac sodium	Solution 0.1%	In 2.5 and 5 ml dropper vials
Nepafenac	Suspension 0.1%	In 5 ml dropper vials
Indomethacin	Suspension 1%	In 3 and 5 ml dropper vials
	Solution 0.1%	
Aspirin	Solution 1%	In 5 ml dropper vial
Fenoprofen	Solution 0.3%	In 5 ml dropper vial
Ibuprofen	Solution 0.5%	In 5 ml dropper vial
Ketoprofen	Solution 1.0%	In 5 ml dropper vial
Naproxen	Solution 0.5%	In 5 ml dropper vial
Piroxicam	Solution 1%	In 5 ml dropper vial
Diflunisol	Solution 0.03%	In 5 ml dropper vial
Phenyl butazone	Ointment 10%	3 and 5 gm tubes
Oxyphenbutazone	Ointment 10%	3 and 5 gm tubes

TOPICAL STEROID-ANTIBIOTIC COMBINATIONS

	Steroid Per g/ml	*Antibiotic per g/ml*	
Dexamethasone sodium phosphate	Soln.0.1%	0.5%	In 5 ml dropper vial
and neomycin sulfate	Oint.0.1%	0.5%	3 and 5 gm tubes
Dexamethasone Sodium phosphate neomycin sulfate and polymixin B	Susp.0.1%	0.35 (Neomycin) 10000 units/ml Polymixin B	In 5 ml dropper vial
	Oint. 0.1%	0.35 (Neomycin) 10000 units/ml Polymixin B	3 and 5 gm tubes

Dexamethasone Sodium phosphate and chloramphenicol	Soln. 0.1%	0.5-1%	In 5 ml dropper vial
Dexamethasone sodium phosphate and framycetin	Susp.0.1%	0.3%	In 5 ml dropper vial
Dexamethasone sodium phosphate and tobramycin	Susp.0.1% Oint. 0.1%	0.3% 0.3%	In 5 ml dropper vial 3 and 5 gm tubes
Dexamethasone sodium phosphate, Chloramphenicol and polymixin B sulfate	Soln 0.1% 5000 IU	1% Chloram-phenicol Polymixin-B	In 5 ml dropper vial
	Ointment 0.1 5000 IU	1% Chloram-phenicol Polymixin-B	In 3 and 5 gm tubes
Dexamethasone sodium phosphate and gentamicin	Soln. 0.1%	0.3%	In 5 ml dropper vial
Dexamethasone sodium phosphate and ciprofloxacin	Soln..0.1% Oint. 0.1%	0.3% 0.3%	In 5 ml dropper vial In 3 and 5 gm tubes
Dexamethasone, sodium phosphate and ofloxacin	Soln..0.1%	0.3%	In 5 ml dropper vial
Dexamethasone, sodium phosphate and lomefloxacin	Soln..0.1%	0.3%	In 5 ml dropper vial
Dexamethasone, sodium phosphate and sparfloxacin	Soln.0.1%	0.3%	In 5 ml dropper vial
Dexamethasone, sodium phosphate and gatifloxacin	Soln.0.1%	0.3%	In 5 ml dropper vial and 5 gm tubes
Dexamethasone, sodium phosphate and Moxifloxacin	Soln.0.1%	0.5%	In 5 ml dropper vial and 5 gm tubes.
Betamethasone with neomycin	Soln.0.1%	0.5%	In 5 ml dropper vial
Betamethasone with chloramphenicol	Soln. 0.1% Oint. 0.1%	0.5% 0.5%	In 5 ml dropper vial In 3 and 5 gm tubes

Betamethasone and gentamicin	Soln. 0.1%	0.3%	In 5 ml droper vial
Hydrocortisone and neomycin	Soln. 0.5% 1.5% Oint. 0.5-1.5%	0.5% 0.5% 0.5%	In 5 ml dropper vial 3 and 5 gm tubes
Hydrocortisone, polymixin B, bacitracin and neomycin	Soln. 10mg/g	0.5 mg/g Polymixin 400 units/g Bacitracin 5 mg/g Neomycin	In 5 ml dropper vial
	Oint. 10 mg/g	0.5mg/g Polymixin 400 units/g Bacitracin 5 mg/g Neomycin	In 5 gm tube
Hydrocortisone and gentamicin	Susp. 1%	0.3%	In 5 ml dropper vial
Hydrocortisone and chloramphenicol	Soln. 0.5% Oint. 0.5%	1% 1%	In 5 ml dropper vial In 5 g tube
Hydrocortisone and oxytetracycline	Susp. 1.5% Oint. 1.5%	0.5% 0.5%	In 5 ml dropper vial In 3 and 5 gm tube
Prednisolone and gentamicin	Susp.1%	0.3%	In 5ml dropper vial
Prednisolone and sulphacetamide	Soln.0.2% to 0.5% Oint. 0.5%	10%(Sulpha) 10% (Sulpha)	In 5 ml dropper vial In 3 and 5 g tubes
Prednisolone, neomycin and polymixin B	Susp. 0.5%	0.35% (Neomycin) 10000 units (Polymixin)	In 5 and 10 ml dropper vials
Prednisolone and ofloxacin	Susp.1%	0.3%	In 5 ml dropper vial
Prednisolone and Gatifloxacin	Susp.1%	0.3%	In 5 ml dropper vial
prednisolone and moxifloxacin	Susp.1%	0.5%	In 5 ml dropper vial
Fluorometholone and neomycin	Soln.0.1%	0.35%	In 5 ml dropper vial
Fluorometholone and gentamicin	Soln.0.1%	0.9%	In 5 ml dropper vial
Flurometholone and tobramycin	Soln.0.1%	0.3%	In 5ml dropper vial
Fluorometholone and sodium sulphacetamide	Susp. 0.1%	1%	In 5 and 10 ml dropper vials

Flurometholone and ofloxacin	Soln.0.1%	0.3%	In 5 ml dropper vial
Flurometholone and gatioxacin	Soln.0.1%	0.3%	In 5 ml dropper vial
Flurometholone and moxifloxacin	Soln.0.1%	0.5%	In 5 ml dropper vial

Chapter 45

Future Drugs in Ophthalmology

Ashok Garg (India)

Here I shall describe investigational new drugs (INDs), future drugs which are of great interest to ophthalmologists worldwide. These INDs are in the final stages of various clinical trials and shall shortly be approved by Food and Drug Administration FDA (USA) for the commercial use in the ophthalmology.

The investigational new drug (IND) has to pass the following phases of trials before FDA approve it for commercial use.

These stages are:

a. Preclinical Trials:
   In this stage initial drug research and development and animal testing takes place.
b. IND filing:
   Human testing and interstate transport of IND is allowed in this phase.
c. Clinical trials:
   It has three phases.

Phase I

In this phase drug safety and tolerance is evaluated. Pharmaco kinetics are tested in 20-100 normal adults males.

Phase II

In this crucial phase IND is evaluated in 100-200 concerned disease patients to determine effectiveness and dose response.

Phase III

In this final phase IND efficacy and safety is determined in 800-1000 concerned disease patients. Drugs interactions are also recorded in this phase.

d. NDA review
   New drugs analysis (NDA) is submitted to FDA for approval of IND marketing.
e. Post-market surveillance
   This is a ongoing process and in this phase adverse reactions reporting, survey, sampling and inspections are carried out.
   Various investigational new drugs (INDs) which are under various phases of clinical trials and shall be of great use in ophthalmology in near future are tabulated as below Table 45.1.

Table 45.1: Investigational drugs (Topical ophthalmic formulations)

S.No.	*Drug name (Generic)*	*Indications for use*	*Category*
I.	ADL2-1294	For treatment of ocular inflammatory pain	Anti-inflammatory
II.	Alpha-I Anti-chymotrypsin	Inflammatory diseases of the eye	NSAID
III.	Piroxicam	Inflammatory diseases of the eye	NSAID
IV.	Nimesulide	Inflammatory disease of the eye	NSAID
V.	Rofecoxib	Inflammatory disease of the eye	NSAID
VI.	Tenoxicam	Inflammatory disease of the eye	NSAID
VII.	Celecoxib	Inflammatory disease of the eye	NSAID
VIII.	Mitomycin C	To treat refractory glaucoma	Anti-glaucoma
IX.	Adaprolol maleate	Site active targeted delivery system for glaucoma	Anti-glaucoma
X.	AGN-192151	Hypotensive lipid (OHL) for glaucoma	Anti-glaucoma
XI.	AGA	Sitespecific formulation for glaucoma	Anti-glaucoma
XII.	Brimonidinex	Alpha-2 agonist (neuroprotective for optic nerve in glaucoma)	Anti-glaucoma
XIII.	Collagenase	Purified collagease for glaucoma treatment	Anti-glaucoma
XIV.	Dexanabinol (HU-211)	Treatment of glaucoma and optic neuropathies	Anti-glaucoma
XV.	Dronabinol	Treatment of glaucoma	Anti-glaucoma
XVI.	Fibroblast growth factor	Topical glaucoma therapy	Anti-glaucoma

contd...

contd...

S.No.	*Drug name (Generic)*	*Indications for use*	*Category*
XVII.	Glutamate ion channel blockers	Combination blockers for glaucoma	Anti-glaucoma
XVIII.	Memantine	Neuroprotective in glaucoma	Anti-glaucoma
XIX.	Pilocarpine	Treatment of glaucoma using submicron emulsion (SME) delivery system and Durasite sustained release delivery system	Anti-glaucoma
XX.	Verapamil HCl	Treatment of glaucoma	Anti-glaucoma
XXI.	Bromhexine	Mild to moderate kerato conjunctivitis Sicca	Ocular lubricant
XXII.	Cyclosporine Ophthalmic	Treatment of severe Keratoconjunctivitis in Sjögren's syndrome	Ocular lubricant
XXIII.	Dehydrax	Recurrent corneal erosions and dry eye	Ocular lubricant
XXIV.	INS 365	Ocular surface diseases as Dry eye	Ocular lubricant
XXV.	N. Acetyl cysteine (NAC)	Severe Dry eye syndrome	Ocular lubricant
XXVI.	OcuNex	Dry eye syndrome	Ocular lubricant
XXVII.	Acid Implant (Intravitreal)	Cytomegalovirus retinitis	Anti-retroviral drug
XXVIII.	Filgrastim	CMV retinitis	Anti-retroviral drug
XXIX.	Monoclonal antibody to cytomegalovirus	CMV retinitis	Anti-retroviral drug
XXX.	Curdlan sulfate	CMV infections	Anti-retroviral drug
XXXI.	Fomi virsen	CMV retinitis	Anti-retroviral drug
XXXII.	GEM-132	CMV retinitis	Anti-retroviral drug
XXXIII.	Aromatic polycyclic dione (APD-1)	CMV retinitis	Anti-retroviral drug
XXXIV.	ISIS-13312	CMV retinitis	Anti-retroviral drug
XXXV.	Sevirumab	CMV retinitis	Anti-retroviral drug
XXXVI.	Valganciclovir	CMV retinitis	Anti-retroviral drug
XXXVII.	Topical clemastine	Seasonal allergic conjunctivitis	Anti-allergic

contd...

S.No.	*Drug name (Generic)*	*Indications for use*	*Category*
XXXVIII.	Cyproheptadine conjunctivitis	Seasonal allergic	Anti-allergic
XXXIX.	Embramine conjunctivitis	Seasonal allergic	Anti-allergic
XXXX.	Methdilazine conjunctivitis	Seasonal allergic	Anti-allergic
XXXXI.	Lexipafant using durasite delivery	Allergic conjunctivitis	Anti-allergic
XXXXII.	Procaterol	Allergic conjunctivitis	Anti-allergic
XXXXIII.	Tryptase Inhibitor (Second generation)	Allergic conjunctivitis	Anti-allergic
XXXXIV.	Amino caproic acid	Topical treatment of traumatic hyphema of the eye	Anti-hemorrhagic
XXXXV.	Clostridium botulinum toxin type A	Treatment of ocular muscle disorders (Blepharospasm)	Anti-hemorrhagic
XXXXVI.	Clostridium botulinum toxin type F	Treatment of ocular muscle disorders (Blepharospasm)	Anti-hemorrhagic
XXXXVII.	Chlorhexidine 0.02%	Treatment of acanthamoeba Keratitis	Anti-infective
XXXXVIII.	Propamidine isethionate	Treatment of acanthamoeba Keratitis	Anti-infective
XXXXIX.	Chondroitinase	Treating patients undergoing vitrectomy	Surgical adjunct
L.	Fibroblast growth factor	To prevent lens clouding following ECCE/Phaco	Surgical adjunct
LI.	HylanA	Ophthalmic visco surgery	Surgical adjunct
LII.	Vitrase	Treatment of vitreous hemorrhage	Surgical adjunct
LIII.	Epidermal growth factor	Treatment of recurrent corneal erosions	Anti-infective
LIV.	Fibronectin	Treatment of non healing Corneal Ulcers	Anti-infective
LV.	Matrix metalloproteinase	Treatment of non healing Corneal Ulcers	Anti-infective
LVI.	Urogastrone	Acceleration of corneal epithelial regeneration	Anti-infective
LVII.	Permeability increasing Protein	Treatment of corneal ulcers	Anti-infective
LVIII.	Batimastat	Prevention of postsurgical recurrence of pterygium	Anti-infective

contd...

S.No.	*Drug name (Generic)*	*Indications for use*	*Category*
LIX.	Cell Adhesion molecule inhibitors	Treatment of ophthalmic infectious diseases	Anti-infective
LX.	Dehydrex	Treatment of recurrent corneal erosions	Anti-infective
LXI.	Enzyme based Iodine preparation	Treatment of infective eye diseases	Anti-infective
LXII.	GM6001	Treatment of infective eye diseases	Anti-infective
LXIII.	Insulin like growth factor	Treatment of infective eye diseases	Anti-infective
LXIV.	Povidine Iodine (2.5%)	Treatment of infective eye diseases	Anti-infective
LXV.	XMP 200	Bactericidal	Anti-infective
LXVI.	Ciliary neuro-trophic factor	Treatment of macular degeneration and retinitis pigmentosa	Retinal adjunct
LXVII.	CNS-1237	Protection for retinal degeneration	Retinal adjunct
LXVIII.	CNS-5065	Protection for retinal degeneration	Retinal adjunct
LXIX.	Tyrosin kinase antagonist	Treatment of ARMD and diabetic retinopathy	Retinal adjunct
LXX.	FIK-I RTK antagonist	Treatment of ARMD and diabetic retinopathy	Retinal adjunct
LXXI.	Gene therapy	For traction retinal detachment	Retinal adjunct
LXXII.	Hormone growth receptor antagonist	Diabetic retinopathy	Retinal adjunct
LXXIII.	Lisinopril	Diabetic retinopathy	Retinal adjunct
LXXIV.	LGD-1550	Retinal degenerative conditions	Retinal adjunct
LXXV.	Neurotrophic factors	Neuro degenerative conditions of the eye	Retinal adjunct
LXXVI.	NRT technology	Neuro degenerative conditions of the eye	Retinal adjunct
LXXVII.	Oligonucleotide antisense compounds	To treat vascular endothelial growth factor (VEGF) in various retinopathies	Retinal adjunct
LXXVIII.	Retinal pigment cells	Treatment of ARMD	Retinal adjunct
LXXIX.	Tazarotene	Receptor selective retinoid	Retinal adjunct
LXXX.	Tin ethyl etio-purpurin	Photodynamic therapy for ARMD	Retinal adjunct

contd...

S.No.	*Drug name (Generic)*	*Indications for use*	*Category*
LXXXI.	Zopolrestat	Treatment of retinopathies	Retinal adjunct
LXXXII.	Zenarestat	Treatment of diabetic cataract	Anti-cataract
LXXXIII.	Cysteamine hydrochloride	Treatment of corneal cystine crystal accumulation in cystinosis	MIscellaneous
LXXXIV.	SU-101	Treatment of malignant glioma	Anti-cancer in ophthalmology
LXXXV.	Corneaplasty	Refractive correction	Miscellaneous

INDEX

U

V